CLINICS IN DEVELOPMENTAL MEDICINE
Typical and Atypical Motor Development

Typical and Atypical Motor Development

by

DAVID SUGDEN
Professor of Special Needs in Education
University of Leeds
UK

and

MICHAEL WADE
Professor of Kinesiology
University of Minnesota Center for Cognitive Science
USA

2013

Mac Keith Press

© 2013 Mac Keith Press
6 Market Road, London N7 9PW

Editor: Hilary M Hart
Managing Director: Ann-Marie Halligan
Production Manager: Udoka Ohuonu
Project Management: Prepress Projects Ltd

First published in this edition 2013

British Library Cataloguing-in-Publication data
A catalogue record for this book is available from the British Library

ISBN: 978-1-908316-55-4

Typeset by Prepress Projects Ltd, Perth, UK
Printed by Ashford Colour Press Ltd, Gosport, Hants, UK

Mac Keith Press is supported by Scope

Dedication

We dedicate this text to Jack and Barbara Keogh, whose work in the area and the support they have given over the years has been an inspiration to us both.

CONTENTS

FOREWORD

Movement development as an academic topic has often been overshadowed by research into cognitive and social development. Central, however, to the effective implementation of many cognitive intentions or social engagement is the ability to move effectively, and in the manner intended. If that smoothness of interaction is not attained, because of either a developmental issue or an age-related decline, then an individual's quality of life can be markedly affected.

Movement skill development is a core topic for understanding human behaviour. In the past 20 years I have taught in this area to students of psychology, medicine and human movement science, but there has always been a schism between texts that focus on theoretical and empirical accounts of highly skilled adult motor control and the development of those skills from infancy through to adolescence.

In my opinion, the first text to attempt to bridge that gap was Keogh and Sugden's (1985) *Movement Skill Development*. That text cross-referenced current thinking regarding adult movement skills control and the development of those skills from the neonate through to puberty. It also used the innovative approach of introducing the reader to how the empirical data in respective research studies were gleaned by using boxed sections that summarized experimental methods and statistical results. This approach combined the level of description encountered in a conventional textbook with the level of detail provided in a research paper. Following this, Sugden and Keogh (1990) produced a companion text, *Problems in Movement Skill Development*, that used a similar approach to discuss the movement problems that occur across a number of developmental disorders.

This latest book, by Sugden and Wade, combines both previous texts to cover typical development and atypical development in one coherent inter-related format. The authors have retained the use of boxed 'methodological'

sections to enlighten the reader on how experimental work in the different areas was undertaken and how the data that were used to support the conclusions were derived. After consideration and revision of earlier work on typical motor development from birth to puberty, the authors dedicate chapters to cerebral palsy, developmental coordination disorder, visual impairment and the movement skills of children with a range of genetic or developmental disorders, such as Down syndrome, fragile X syndrome, attention-deficit–hyperactivity disorder and autism spectrum disorders.

What is exemplary in this book is the attempt throughout the text to examine whether motor skill problems that are exhibited can be accounted for by current theories of perceptuo-motor control and motor development. It is inevitable that sometimes there is an uneasy fit between models or theories used to explain skilled adult control and the problems exhibited by children with a developmental disorder. But this is a valuable exercise in questioning the appropriateness of some of our current accounts of development across the lifespan. This also introduces a very interesting and topical debate as to why a number of children with very different developmental profiles appear to exhibit difficulties in similar core perceptuo-motor tasks. The book closes with a discussion of assessment methods and how problems in movement skill are defined, identified and managed, which is essential for any student who might be considering an occupation that may bring them into the path of children with atypical development.

Throughout the last decade I have used Keogh and Sugden (1985) and Sugden and Keogh (1990) extensively to introduce undergraduate and postgraduate students to the intriguing area of movement skill development. This new text transcends the two previous books and, I believe, every other text on motor development that is currently available. It provides a coherent treatment of both typical and atypical movement skill development, set within the context of current theory. At the same time it causes the reader to consider such questions as 'How do you identify that a child has a problem?', 'How do you research the nature of that problem?', 'Why do some of the same problems seem to crop up with very different developmental groups?' and 'What can be done to manage those problems?'.

If we can move closer to answering these questions then we will be in a position to give optimum support to the developmental trajectories of children with early movement skill problems. In my opinion, this book takes a major step towards clarifying some of these matters and defining those that still need to be resolved through future research.

Professsor John Wann
Department of Psychology
Royal Holloway, University of London
UK
January 2013

REFERENCES

Keogh JF, Sugden DA (1985) *Movement Skill Development*. New York, NY: MacMillan.

Sugden DA, Keogh JF (1990) *Problems in Movement Skill Development*. Columbia, SC: University of South Carolina Press.

PREFACE

The accomplishment of motor skills is a key part of human development and begins even before birth. The study of this development has been viewed from a number of perspectives incorporating health, medicine, psychology, education and even engineering by both researchers and practitioners from these disciplines. They have in general addressed two questions about motor development: first, what is the course and timing of these developments and how can they best be described? Second, how and why does this change take place and what are the mechanisms involved? Since the beginning of the twentieth century several classic studies have addressed these issues, with the last 20 years or so of research focusing more on trying to answer the second question.

This book addresses both of these questions by describing the process of change in motor development and how and why these changes might occur. It does this by examining development in typical children and contrasting that with an analysis of children who differ in their personal resources, whether those differences are physical, cognitive, social or sensory in nature. This part of the text not only provides insight into how children with a different set of resources develop but also guides us towards a more holistic understanding of development not restricted by typicality. The text also points us in the direction of looking at children in context, emphasizing that the developmental process does not reside solely in the child but is a complex and dynamic result of many interconnecting and often self-organizing constraints arising from both the child and the environment.

David Sugden, Leeds, UK
Mike Wade, Minneapolis, USA
March 2013

ACKNOWLEDGEMENTS

David Sugden thanks Anna Barnett, Carolyn Dunford, Elisabeth Hill, Amanda Kirby and Lorrie Sugden, for their wise comments and reading of various chapters, and Sheila Henderson, for ongoing and continuous debate about motor developmental and impairment issues.

Mike Wade thanks Minnesota colleagues, Tom Stoffregen and Jurgen Konczak, for almost daily opportunities to exchange ideas and elicit input. Thanks are also due to Martha Wade, who patiently helped with the onerous but necessary task of reading and correcting the proofs.

In addition, both authors would like to thank the staff at Mac Keith Press and Prepress Projects, especially Udoka Ohuonu and Evelyn Wilkins, who have been encouraging, patient and helpful in the production of this text.

ABOUT THE AUTHORS

David Sugden is Professor of Special Needs in Education at the University of Leeds, UK, where he heads the Childhood and Inclusive Education Team in the School of Education. His research interests are developmental disorders with specific concentration on motor development and impairment.

Michael Wade is Professor of Kinesiology and a faculty member at the University of Minnesota Center for Cognitive Science. His research interests involve two areas of movement science: developmental change across the lifespan, with an emphasis on individuals with motor difficulties, and the effects of ageing on motor skill performance.

1
AN INTRODUCTION TO MOTOR DEVELOPMENT

Introduction

Movement is the only way we can interact with other human beings, animals, and the environmental context (Wolpert et al 2003). No other human facility allows us to do this in so many ways, whether speaking, walking, writing, climbing, or touching. A child progressing from birth to some level of maturity in movement sheds light not just on this developmental process but also on the evolutionary nature of our being. The two words we use here are 'development' and 'movement', and together they specify the one process of motor development. In this chapter, we take these two terms both together and separately, examining their definitions and characteristics, and paving the way for future chapters that examine the course of motor development in children who have both typical and atypical resources.

Development

From a general perspective child development is a difficult idea to comprehend because changes in human abilities are both broad and complex. Development begins at conception, and at birth the newborn infant is small, essentially immobile, and without verbal communication. In the ensuing 20 years, numerous changes occur that signal larger, more mobile, and more skilful individuals who typically can reason about, and communicate, abstract notions, and who have a personal sense of self and are part of a social system. The examples in this text highlight the many changes in the human abilities concerning movement that attract our attention; some are quite visible, and others are inferred from the more visible ones.

We typically use theory to try to explain how development or a particular part of development takes place. With respect to human development there are theories of cognition, social development, language, and motor development. They seek to explain the observable phenomena from a particular point of view. For example, Newman

and Newman (2007), in their text on human development, group their theories into three categories: those that emphasize biological aspects; those that emphasize environmental factors; and those that place emphasis on the person–environment interaction. As we navigate through this chapter and the rest of the book, it will become evident that, although the bulk of our effort is focused on examining the child's resources, we place much of our emphasis on the interactions among the child, the task, and the environment, which collectively specify the unit of analysis when examining functional motor skills.

Descriptions of change

Physical growth changes are easily recognized, beginning with the observation that children get larger. Humans are microscopic in size at conception and grow to a length of about 20 inches at birth (after only 9 months of life), and a height of 60 inches or more 20 years after birth. Head size at birth represents approximately 25% of the total body length; by the age of 20 a person's head size accounts for approximately 15% of total body length. Changes in body proportions during puberty distinguish male and female physiques, including changes in secondary sex characteristics. Internal systemic changes during puberty provide the capability for reproduction. Also, changes in body-tissue composition and physiological functioning give males relatively more muscle mass than females and a greater capacity for taking in and transporting oxygen to fuel the muscular system.

Pubescence and adolescence are commonly recognized as major periods of change. Pubescence is a time of biological change; adolescence is a time of social change in which an individual becomes more personally and socially independent. These two periods not only influence but also change one another. Changes in secondary sex characteristics, which vary in age at onset and extent of change, often imply greater personal–social development and so change others' expectations and behaviours when interacting socially with these more mature-looking adolescents. The reverse may be true when the social importance of pubertal body changes leads to an increase or decrease in the amount of physical activity undertaken, which can also change body appearance. Our descriptions of change and examples of periods of change should impress us with the scope of human development and should indicate how we can characterize its various aspects.

A complete list of all developmental changes would quickly highlight the enormity and complexity of human development, as well as the realization that development is continuous and ongoing throughout the life cycle. We begin by looking at how periods of change lead to new capabilities that allow individuals to perform new actions they were unable to do earlier. If we think of what we do as requiring some type of internal organization in relation to our surrounding environments, then major periods of change are those times when we reorganize the manner in which we perform tasks – the individual really does change into a different human being – and we recognize the change as another period of development.

Motor development

For all mammals, whether they walk on four (quadrupedal) or two (bipedal) legs, the capacity to walk immediately at birth or relatively soon after is critical to survival. For quadrupeds born in the wild, survival requires nutrition and protection from predators, and walking immediately at birth supports both of these needs, although not always successfully. The newborn human, and our wild genetic relatives (great apes and chimpanzees), enters the world with less urgency for immediate locomotion survival; a set of reflexes enable contact with the mother and necessary nutrition. For the human infant in the ensuing 5 or 6 months, these reflexes support access to resources and nutrition while the infant is undergoing rapid growth of bone, muscle and nervous system; a developing muscular skeletal system that first supports crawling, then upright posture, and finally locomotion, all within the first 40 to 50 weeks post partum. The processes whereby the newborn infant attains first the ability to crawl, then upright posture, and finally walking are central to our understanding of motor development. Beyond an understanding of how coordination and control are achieved, of equal importance is a consideration of the role that movement plays in the overall social and cognitive development of the child's journey to maturity.

From the outset it is important to make a distinction between the forms and variety of natural biological motion and the often artificial motor skills that we need for living in our own particular environment. A constant feature of all living systems is that they move. This movement is both internal and external. Cell death and regeneration, circulation and glandular secretions are internal, and the coordination and control of action through the use of our musculoskeletal apparatus is external. Shortly after conception the closure of the 'neural notch' in the embryo is the precursor to the formation of the motor cortex. Thus, from the beginning of embryonic development, the primacy of movement is established. The interest of both scientists and clinicians has been focused on the change that occurs early in the infant life course (birth to early childhood), and later in life, as we transition from mature adulthood into ageing.

The general sense of development is viewed in this text in relation to movement, which is such a common and ongoing part of our daily lives that to list all movements (motor activities) for a single day would be a continuous and laborious task. We would need to begin with the movements of our fingers and the related body parts in the arm and hand in order to describe using a pen to write this list. Our list would then include movements to dress and feed ourselves, change locations, and participate in work and play activities. Specific tasks might include buttoning a shirt, tying shoelaces, shaving or applying makeup, buttering toast, using a spoon to eat soup, navigating a crowded pavement, riding a bicycle, driving a car, using a keyboard, texting, lifting a box, turning a page, playing a piano, throwing a ball and dealing cards, and many more. The corollary to this is to try and list those activities during a typical day that do not involve movement.

Our capacity to control our movements changes so that we become more accurate and faster in our responses. We also develop more precise force control to increase the range of movements that can be stronger, as well as slower and more subtle. Movements become more coordinated with fewer extraneous movements and appear to be smooth, effortless, and unhurried. A richer repertoire of movements is established to produce variable and elegant solutions to movement problems. Multiple demands can be handled in a shorter time, including the ability to relate our movements to the movements of others. We can plan ahead by knowing what others are likely to do (anticipation). Thus, movement is more than just performing the skill itself; it also involves different contexts and individuals.

What is motor development?

A short definition would be as follows: *Motor development is adaptive change towards competence*. We include the term *adaptive change* because it draws our attention to the transactional relationship between the individual

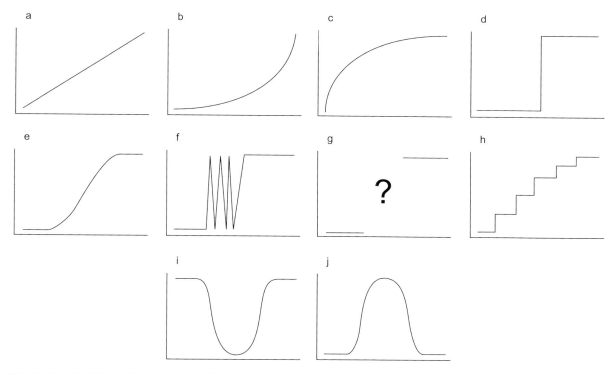

Fig. 1.1 Idealized shape of developmental change: (A) linear, (B) accelerating, (C) asymptotic, (D) step-like, (E) S-shaped, (F) variable, (G) unsystematic, (H) step climbing, (I) U-shaped, and (J) inverted U-shape.

and environment and, as we have noted, change occurs in many different ways. Including the term *competence* directs us to think of the developing child in the process of becoming something other than what he or she is at the moment. Competence conveys the meaning of a larger concern for being effective in our environment, rather than focusing on the achievement of specific skills (Connolly and Bruner 1974). These ideas are not dissimilar to the ecological psychology proposed by James Gibson (1966, 1979), which we discuss later in this chapter. Individuals and environments are seen in a transactional relationship, in which each partner changes in relation to the other. Development is different to, and yet includes, growth, with development being altogether a larger concept that encompasses multiple interacting parts both intrinsic and extrinsic to the child. In addition, learning is in part a consequence of these multiple experiences and, as such, can also be a function of and a contributor to development.

What does change look like?

The obvious manifestations of change indicating development are the behavioural markers ('milestones') that historically denote the trajectory of the developing infant. For example, parents and others often note the

first independent steps of their child. These recognized benchmarks often hide some of the complexities involved in the process of developmental change. Adolph et al (2008) have raised an important methodological issue: namely that, by using a broad generalized longitudinal approach or cross-sectional designs, we have missed critical points of developmental change, which have remained hidden or masked in the broad trajectories of much of the extant data. Adolph et al (2008, p. 527) comment that what we have is 'a gallery of before and after snapshots, studio portraits of newborns, and fossilized milestones but little understanding of the process of development itself. What we need are fine-grained depictions of developmental trajectories'.

They present a graphic illustration of a hypothesized family of the developmental progressions made by a child, varying from smooth, steady-paced trajectories through abrupt step-like changes to those periods that even involve reversals (Fig. 1.1).

The depiction of change shown in Figure 1.1 suggests a multifaceted creature that displays observable behaviours that include variability, continuity, discontinuity, accelerations, and spurts. One has only to work in a classroom to see change happening (i.e. the child who makes steady and often slow but sure progress, picking up the concepts that are being presented. Contrast this with the child who appears to be somewhat disconnected yet takes a major leap forward when the 'penny drops'). In children with atypical resources, change is often more variable, with progress in a forward direction also being accompanied by relapses and the disappearance of behaviours that were already learned.

Adolph et al (2008) argue that the variability in observed changes is a result of statistical sampling methods, which, they believe, examine only the stable endpoints in development. Only by taking more frequent and smaller sampling intervals/observations can we begin to expose such crucial events as when one stable endpoint finishes and another begins. This is a method that Vygotsky (1978) labelled 'micro genetic'. Adolph et al (2008) proposed five guidelines for defining optimal rates of time sampling to adequately capture a true picture of the process of development:

1 Determine the base rate – look for the typical rate at which the skill is expressed.
2 Find the acquisition period – determine the approximate age range for the acquisition period.
3 Sample as frequently as you can – often on a daily basis.
4 Look before the onset – include ages that are before the observable onset.
5 Look for changes in variability – use of smoothing techniques.

For further elaboration of these points see Adolph et al (2008, pp. 527–543).

Characteristics and descriptions of movement

The above brief listing of guidelines reminds us that there are several considerations when defining movement. One important point is that movement often is described in functional terms, when listing actions such as buttoning and throwing. This is quite different from describing the movements harnessed to achieve the functional outcomes of buttoning a shirt and propelling a ball through the air. Movement can be described and analysed strictly as *body movements* or *intended functions*. Both levels of description are useful, though here the focus is mainly on the broader and functional aspects of movement, while including many descriptions and analyses of changes in body movements.

Another consideration is that body movements are situation specific and are required to be adjusted to the extant circumstances, such as walking carefully on an icy pavement in contrast with running full speed in a footrace. The control of movement becomes more complicated when objects and other people are involved, particularly when they are also moving.

One issue in describing movements is determining what we should use as a unit of movement. The difficulty is that every movement is really a combination of many smaller movements. For example, walking and writing are commonly identified as movements, but each is really a composite of many separate movements. We see this when watching infants walking, as they move one foot forward, followed by a pause and the movement of the other foot forward. Also, a pencil can be held in various ways to make single lines in different directions, as well as writing single letters and complete words. The point is that each movement is a combination of other movements and also may be used as a part of another movement. This means that each movement can be labelled in various ways depending on what one chooses to view as the movement unit.

A second concern is describing and analysing movement changes as either continuous or discrete. An important developmental change is the extent to which new movements are a sequence of discrete movements, such as early walking efforts, rather than the more continuous cycle in later walking. The same pattern of change from discrete to continuous is observed in using a pencil, as children initially make a number of discrete or single lines before they move the pencil more continuously. Although many body movements do need to be made continuously, others can be discrete or serial.

Performance and learning, ability and skill

When we describe movement the terms 'performance' and 'learning' are the typical terminology used. While they are often used alongside each other when talking about movement behaviour, it should be remembered that they represent different processes.

Performance

Performance is usually described as involving motor behaviour at a particular moment in time; very often this is a one-shot occurrence and can be readily observed and measured. Thus, a nine-iron golf shot to the 17th hole on a particular day would be classed as performance. Similarly, a 4-year-old child performing a two-footed jump over a rope lying on the floor would also fit this description. Performance does not imply anything other than what one observes at that particular point in time; it says little if anything about how typical that motor behaviour is, or how permanent it is, or whether it can be repeated. Control is closely connected to the issue of performance and involves mechanisms that ensure a more or less smooth and effortless outcome.

LEARNING

Learning, like development, implies that there is a relatively permanent change in motor behaviour, but the two differ in important ways despite being intertwined in many respects. Learning is also intrinsically involved with performance. Learning involves acquiring a set of processes that are instrumental in changing motor behaviour; these processes are assumed and much effort has been expended in determining exactly what these processes are. These processes do often lead to a change in behaviour and in most cases lead to an increased capacity to perform a particular skill or set of skills. Learning typically occurs as a direct result of practice or experience; it is not the result of maturation and growth, two fundamental characteristics of the dynamic processes involved in development. Learning itself is not directly observable but is inferred by measuring performance as defined above on two or more occasions. Finally, learning is relatively permanent and is not simply a one-off occurrence that is influenced by variables such as trait anxiety, illness, motivation, or having an off day. As is often said, 'form is temporary, class is permanent'. Or to put in our language, performance may be temporary but learning is relatively permanent. Of course there is the debate as to what exactly is relatively permanent, but we can say that, when true learning has taken place, the learner has changed in some rather permanent manner. Once you have truly learned to read, or how to ski, the ability to perform may deteriorate but the internal processes that bring about that change are relatively permanent. That does not mean you can maintain the same high standard without practice, but you rarely return to your prior state. For a more detailed review of these concepts see Schmidt and Lee (2011). These concepts are elaborated with respect to intervention in Chapter 12.

ABILITY AND SKILL

These two terms are often confused and occasionally used interchangeably. However, they are different, yet overlapping, and their respective natures have important implications when we look at development across the ability range. The term ability is usually used when referring to a capability or aptitude and is thought to be a relatively stable trait (Schmidt and Lee 2011). Abilities appear to underpin numerous skills, are possibly genetically determined, are not easily influenced by practice, and are thought to be more fundamental than the concept of skill. If we take the area of cognition as an example, intelligence would be ability, whereas reading is probably a skill. Thus, abilities underpin skills, though not in a linear one-to-one relationship; it is much more complex than that: 'abilities represent the "equipment" that a person has at his or her disposal, determining whether or not a given motor task can be performed either poorly or well' (Schmidt and Lee 2011, p. 275).

Abilities can be applied to numerous tasks; for example, the ability of strength will aid in tasks that range from simply lifting a heavy object to pushing a broken-down car to twisting a knob or pulling a lever. The ability to run fast will be of assistance in many sports, in running for a bus, and in escaping a fire. Abilities are very much involved in the concept of transfer or generalization: how the abilities that are used in the performance of one task have relevance to the performance of another.

The way in which authors such as Schmidt and Lee (2011) differentiate between skills and abilities is by describing skills as modifiable by practice and experience and abilities as relatively stable. Thus, skills become the surface outlet of the abilities that underlie them. In linguistic terms, skills would be the 'surface structure' and abilities the 'deep structure' (Chomsky 1966). It is of course more complex than this, as numerous abilities can underlie one holistic skill and numerous skills can be affected by just one ability. For an example of the former, the skill of tennis requires speed, coordination, strength, endurance, and many other abilities. For an example of the latter we have already noted that the ability of speed can underlie many skills in the sporting arena.

We have described these two concepts of ability and skill as they are of great importance in the development of movement in typical and atypical children. First, it is important to know to what degree abilities are a limiting factor. If a certain ability of a child, say with cerebral palsy, is low, how do we address that and should we be spending time working on that ability or would we look to compensatory activities? Second, and closely connected to the first, when a child has difficulties with movement should we be targeting abilities or skills? In the former there is the obvious benefit of a particular ability underpinning numerous skills, and thus if we get the intervention right, we have built transfer and generalization into our programme. The downside of this is that we are not sure, firstly, what these abilities are and what the unit of analysis might be and, secondly, whether or not they are modifiable. Teaching skills gives the advantage of directly addressing the problems the child experiences in daily life with self-care or recreational activities. The downside is that by teaching individual skills we are in danger of foregoing a chance of generalization and there is clearly insufficient time to teach every skill a child requires for adequate functioning. These issues are more fully explored in Chapter 12, in which the questions of what to measure and provide for intervention are paramount.

Consequences of movement

There are different ways to view the consequences of movement activity. The most obvious consequences are the movement outcomes themselves and we have labelled this '*movement by design*'. Here movement is the dependent variable; as in the old saying, we are learning how to move. It is labelled *movement by design* to illustrate that human beings are uniquely designed and have developed (evolved) over thousands of years as a species that comprises approximately 10^{12} neurones, 10^9 receptors, 10^3 muscles, and 10^2 bones! The physical linkages (ligaments, tendons, muscles, and joints) enable the developing human biomechanical system to walk upright, reach, grasp, and explore with an almost infinite capacity to coordinate and control its motor apparatus. This permits the successful execution of numerous skilled activities that satisfy our intents, wants, and desires.

The second we have labelled '*movement that informs*'; in other words, how does a child's growing capacity to move and explore its environment contribute to a wider understanding of the world around us? The answer to this question is directly related to our ability to communicate with others (language), solve problems, and think in abstract terms; in other words, all of the activities which we call cognition.

Movement by design

Clark and Whitall (1989) described four distinct periods of the history of motor development: the precursor period (1787–1928); the maturational period (1928–1946); the normative/descriptive period (1946–1970); and the process-orientated period (1970 to the present day). The first three periods were all essentially descriptive, but the fourth period (process orientated) is driven more by testable theory rather than mere observation and description. The fourth period has been influenced primarily by two distinct theoretical perspectives: information processing theory and the concepts of ecological psychology and dynamical systems theory.

The descriptive period

The British scientist Francis Galton (1876) noted that the study of twins might well show promise for the study of child development because twins share common genetic components.[a] In spite of this important insight, little substantive work on motor development was forthcoming in science until the classic studies by Arnold Gesell

and Catherine Amatruda (1941) and Myrtle McGraw (1963), who compiled careful descriptive data of what they designated as different 'stages' of motor development. Perhaps the most famous were the studies by Myrtle McGraw in 1935 and 1939, in which she reported and discussed the effects of the training of twin males 'Johnny and Jimmy' (McGraw 1935), one of whom was given specific training in a variety of age-appropriate motor skills, and one who received no specific training. These early 20th-century scientists recorded the observed changes that take place from birth through the first 6 or 7 years of life. They were primarily interested in what seemed to them to be the specific stages in the motor development of the child, and from these early observations the term 'motor milestones' was coined. Together the work of Gesell and McGraw formed the basis of much of the clinical work that specified the benchmarks of regular, typical motor development. Their conceptual view was that these motor milestones were reached at specific points in time as a direct function of the orderly development of the central nervous system (CNS). Early developmental theorists thus concluded that brain development was the key and proposed a *neuromaturational* approach to motor development. This theory was based on the assumption that it was the developing neural

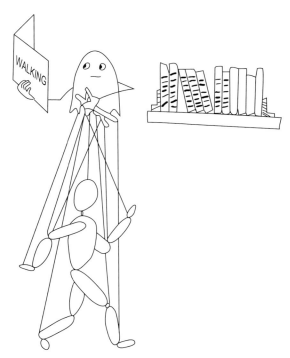

Fig. 1.2 Cartoon of 'motor executive' using scripts based on local terrain in order to control movement. Reproduced with permission from Michaels and Carello (1981).

---

[a] Galton's study is reported in Francis Galton, 'The history of twins, as a criterion of the relative powers of nature and nurture', first published in *Fraser's Magazine* (1875), 12: 566–76 and reprinted with revisions in *Journal of the Anthropological Institute* (1875), 5: 391–406.

apparatus (the brain and associated nervous system) that controlled the timing and emergence of such actions as upright stance and walking. This idea is illustrated in Figure 1.2. Here the CNS is depicted as the 'controller' or 'executive' of the motor apparatus. This viewpoint assumes that, much like a puppet, all motor behaviour is controlled by a 'top down' hierarchical process. This idea was not only part of the *neuromaturational* perspective but, as we shall see later, was central to information processing theory.

During the descriptive period McGraw (1963) developed her ideas of the neuromaturational development of an infant's motor behaviour when she proposed a four-stage description of how the initial reflex abilities of the newborn child gradually fade into the voluntary and more adaptive control capacities of the developing child. McGraw's (1963) four-stage view of development is depicted as follows:

- Stage 1 – the reflexes present in the newborn infant.
- Stage 2 – the CNS develops sufficiently to inhibit these primitive reflexes.
- Stage 3 – the CNS assumes more of the voluntary control of movement.
- Stage 4 – the early reflexes integrate into larger movement patterns.

To illustrate her idea McGraw (1963) used the development of the palmar grasp:

- Stage 1 – pressure on the palm of the newborn infant elicits reflex action of the fingers and thumb to produce the palmar grasp.
- Stage 2 – (after 3–4mo) inhibition by the CNS produces extension of the fingers and thumb, and minimal response when pressure is applied to the infant's palm.
- Stage 3 – the palmar grasp is produced without the need for palmar pressure. This is illustrated when the fingers are extended in anticipation of grasping an object prior to actual contact with the object.
- Stage 4 – a variety of grasping instances emerge, which are employed in a variety of situations and in combination with other movements.

McGraw's (1963) ideas contributed to the adoption of specific periods of child development.

In a similar vein the renowned Swiss biologist Jean Piaget developed the idea of specific developmental periods when he proposed a 'sensorimotor period' in the developing infant, which encompassed one of his proposed developmental stages of the first 2 years of an infant's life. During this sensorimotor or preverbal period, Piaget described in some detail his observations of infant behaviour, as the child developed an understanding of such practical information as object permanence, temporal succession, and sensorimotor causality, which Piaget argued contributed to the formation of 'representational thought'. Here we can see how motor development is seen as a precursor to what Piaget terms representational thought. This has both a 'good news' aspect and a 'bad news' aspect. The good news is that Piaget clearly gives an important role to motor development in his overall theory of development. The bad news is that by distinguishing between motor development and later representational thought, Piaget adheres to the traditional idea of dualism: that movement (regarded as biological) is separate from abstract thinking, which is the central focus of cognitive development. Philosophically this reflects Piaget's adherence to the traditional dualism that has dominated the psychological sciences since the time of Descartes (1596–1650): 'cogito ergo sum'.

The contributions of early developmental theorists such as Myrtle McGraw and Jean Piaget to developmental psychology and the role of motor behaviour went largely ignored by the field of psychology. Other than Piaget's theorizing that cognitive development emerges, in part, from the early sensorimotor stage during the first 24 months of life, only the 19th-century psychologist William James proposed a motor theory of perception (James 1890). As a consequence, the focus of child development was primarily on the abstract processes (cognition), which were regarded as separate and essentially independent from the presumed biologically influenced movement or perceptual motor abilities.

An important theme in this book focuses on the question of whether movement and action are separate, and independent, from what the mainstream psychological sciences regard as cognitive development, or whether the two are linked to reflect two dimensions of the same entity, i.e. *does movement inform?* With respect to motor development, the assumption of the mind–body separation, or dualism, would make it difficult for movement to *inform*. A more contemporary view questions dualism and argues that

The 'mind' is not an abstract 'processor' of information, and sees the 'body' as central to the shaping of mind. This more holistic view regards them as inseparable c.f. 'biological brains are the control systems for biological bodies'.

(Clark 1998, p. 510)

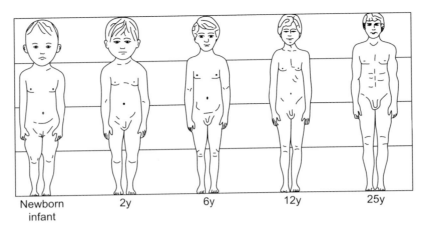

| Newborn infant | 2y | 6y | 12y | 25y |

Fig. 1.3 Changes in body proportions with age. Reproduced with permission from the publisher from Tanner (1981), as replicated from Stratz (1909).

Putting aside the philosophical underpinnings of mind–body dualism, it is important to remember that movement (action) plays an important role in the overall cognitive development of the child. The early theorists (Gesell, McGraw, and Piaget) all recognized this important fact, and were correct in giving movement a critical role in cognitive development, but were probably not fully correct in proposing that it was driven by the development of the CNS, which dictated the timing and emergence of the motor milestones – 'motor readiness'. More contemporary research has clearly demonstrated that a child's ability to master upright posture, walk, and subsequently actively explore his or her environment does not solely rely on a developing CNS and includes other variables such as physical growth trajectory and the accompanying increase in strength and joint development across the skeletal apparatus. For example, it is a consequence of biomechanics (the physics!) that helps to constrain children from walking in the first 7 or 8 months of life. During the first 5 or 6 months of life, the head is larger (and heavier) than the rest of the body, and the overall strength level of the developing infant is insufficient for supporting upright posture until 9 to 15 months. This fact is illustrated in Figure 1.3.

As Figure 1.3 readily depicts, during the first 30 to 36 weeks of life, the size of the infant skull decreases compared with the rest of the body. The change in skull size compared with the rest of the skeletal mass coupled with increased bone and muscle growth permits the child to attain upright posture, begin walking, and begin exploring the world. This redistribution of weight, coupled with increased strength and an optimizing of skeletal size, permits the majority of infants to commence walking between 9 and 15 months. The ability to walk is not 'switched on' by a CNS at some 'critical' point in time; rather, it is a

consequence of ongoing physical development that relies on normal nutrition and the inherent phylogenetic process of the species. Achieving upright postural control and independent locomotion is an emergent phenomenon that is a consequence of the typical physical and neurological development of the infant. This directly challenges the view advanced by the early theorists.

Systems-orientated period

For this introductory chapter, we present a relatively brief overview of three theoretical ideas and orientations that have influenced the psychological sciences generally and much of the motor development and motor learning research since the late 1960s. Each of these theoretical perspectives represents contemporary explanations on how motor behaviour both develops and is formulated. They are: first, information processing; second, the Ecological Psychology of the psychologist James Gibson; and third the dynamical systems theory, the origins of which emanate from the ideas of the Russian physiologist Nicolai Bernstein. All three are further elaborated in Chapter 3 and elsewhere, but a brief outline and their influence on motor development research and thinking are provided below.

INFORMATION PROCESSING

Following on from the descriptive period of early motor development, the post-Second World War period saw the emergence of a new theoretical orientation known as information processing as a way of providing an account of human behaviour. This viewpoint emerged in the behavioural sciences in the 1960s and had its origins in the post-War work of Kenneth Craik (1948), the British scientist, as well as in the development of a theory of communication in the USA (Shannon and Weaver 1949).

(a)
(b)

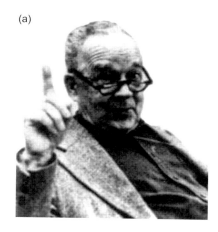
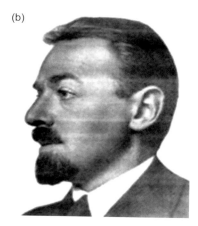

Fig. 1.4 (a) James Gibson (Google images: maquinasdefuego.blogspot.com) and (b) Nicolai Bernstein (Google images: neurotree.org).

Research adhering to the constructs of information processing theory has had, and continues to have, an enormous influence not only in the behavioural sciences psychology but also in engineering, communications and to no less an extent the study of motor learning and control. It has remained the dominant theory in both cognitive psychology and the study of motor behaviour for 50 years and went essentially unchallenged until the mid-1980s. Information processing theory invokes a computer analogy that views the CNS as functioning as a processor of information and a control centre. The focus on motor development and child psychology was to view the developing child as a processor of information, developing an increasingly sophisticated capacity to process incoming environmental information and to interpret that information to develop appropriate responses to whatever task or circumstance were demanded of the child.

Central to information processing theory is the assumption that information from the environment (visual, auditory, etc.) requires interpretation by an internal 'perceptual mechanism' in order to assign meaning, and to ensure the generation of an appropriate response. This in turn triggers the motor system to produce the appropriate action or utterance based on the assigned meaning of the perceptual system. Psychologists have used the information processing model to investigate memory capacity, picture recognition, strategic problem-solving behaviour, reaction time and a wide range of verbal tasks.

The publication of both Adams' (1971) 'A closed loop theory of motor learning' and Schmidt's (1975) 'Schema theory' provided a theoretical basis for a substantial body of research on both children and adults in the context of the information processing paradigm. Both the theories of Adams (1971) and Schmidt (1975) relied on the information processing assumption that skill learning and

performance requires a 'motor programme' to initiate, organize, and execute an appropriate motor response to an environmental task demand. A more detailed treatment of the assumptions and orientation of information processing theory is presented in Chapter 3.

Both motor development and motor learning and control have been influenced by two other theoretical developments. These ideas originated from two scientists: the American psychologist James Gibson of Cornell University and the Russian physiologist Nicolai Bernstein (see Fig. 1.4).

ECOLOGICAL PSYCHOLOGY
James Gibson advanced the idea that information from the surrounding environment is directly perceived. This notion is referred to as 'Gibson's Ecological Psychology' (Gibson 1979). To Gibson (1979) perception and action are not separate systems but are inextricably linked: 'we must perceive in order to move, but we must also move in order to perceive' (Gibson 1979, p. 223).

Both James and Eleanor Gibson went on to contribute a substantial body of knowledge, building on the premise that experience, learning, and knowledge acquisition are a function of changes in perception (Pick 1992), and to producing empirical support for the Gibson (1979) notion of affordances (Adolph et al 1993). The contributions of Eleanor Gibson with respect to motor development are discussed further in Chapter 4.

DYNAMICAL SYSTEMS THEORY
The Russian physiologist Nicolai Bernstein (1967) proposed the idea that coordination and control of movement must to a large degree be essentially self-organizing, and not reliant on the specific motor programme selected from a stored location, presumably in the CNS. This latter

idea formed the theoretical basis for what is now referred to as dynamical systems theory. Bernstein's (1967) idea that skill is self-organizing has its origins in his research produced in the 1930s but was not published in the West until 1967. This idea contributed to the theorizing that supports a dynamical systems approach to motor skill expression. The human body comprises approximately 1000 muscles and 100 bones and associated linkages that require an organizing process to execute a simple motor act. Bernstein (1967) asked how might these many degrees of freedom be controlled or constrained in order for an individual to execute a smooth and efficient action such as reaching for a glass of water? For that matter, how do we perform the many other motor skill activities of daily life? How the many degrees of freedom present in the human skeletal apparatus are constrained is referred to as 'Bernstein's degrees of freedom problem'. Bernstein essentially questions the notion that the CNS alone has the sole responsibility of constraining the available degrees of freedom to execute any specific task. He proposed that skilled activity must rely on 'coordinative structures' (a group of muscles which act synergistically as a functional unit) constrained but not controlled by the CNS. This promotes a more dynamic view of skill production and emphasizes the idea that skilled activity is self-organizing rather than reliant on motor programmes. The concept of coordinative structures is more in keeping with the idea of 'soft assemblies'; that is to say that the CNS has a role to play in all activity, but not in a rigid programme-orientated fashion. The formulation of any motor response will be a function of the constraints of the task performer and the environment (Newell 1986). A typical illustration of this is the hand grasping study reported by Newell et al (1989), whereby infants reach with one or two hands depending on the size of the 'to-be-grasped' cup presented, and the cup's scaled relationship to the hand-width aperture formed by the thumb and index finger. A fuller discussion of this study is presented in Chapter 4.

It is important to remember that the two theoretical orientations of ecological psychology and dynamical systems are not necessarily complementary; that is to say that adherence to the notion that perception is direct (from an ecological perspective) does not require an acceptance of a particular theory of coordination and control of movement. Likewise, those who promote the dynamic systems view that skill production is essentially self-organizing do not need to assume that perception is direct. It is, however, true to say that several researchers referenced in this text support both. This more natural approach to thinking about both perception and action changed both the style of inquiry and the theorizing related to motor development. The late Esther Thelen published extensively on the general idea that developmental motor skills emerge at points along the developmental trajectory, as the developing infant grows in both strength and stature, and the accompanying joint complexes stabilize (shoulder for reaching, lower limbs for both sitting and upright posture). For example, an early dynamical analysis of infant kicking (Thelen and Fisher 1983) provided empirical support that the periodicity (rhythmicity) observed in the kicking of young preambulatory infants (viewed as inconsequential and ignored by earlier theorists) was in fact directly related to the periodicity of the step reflex which young preambulatory infants exhibited when supported over a slow-moving treadmill. Up to this point no relationship was presumed to exist between infant kicking and the development of walking. Thelen and Fisher (1983) demonstrated that the progression to coordinated movement was present in the seemingly random kicking of young infants. Coordinated motor behaviour emerged from changes in the differential growth trajectory of the infant, rather than a consequence of a centrally controlled programme in the CNS. The capacity to walk was present in the design of the coordinative structures but lay dormant until growth changes in limb length and muscular strength were sufficient to support both upright stance (postural stability) and subsequent locomotion.

This more contemporary viewpoint increasingly prevalent in children's motor development focuses on changes in motor development that are synonymous with an increase in *behavioural flexibility*. To better understand the motor development in children the central question to ask is 'How is this flexibility achieved?'. Our earlier discussion about how the maturational approach to this question was addressed by early theorists involved the proposition that the CNS both controlled and timed the appearance of milestones such as upright posture and locomotion. We now know that these milestones are as much a consequence of growth changes in the infant, especially the relative size of the head and increased leg and trunk stability, which enable the child to explore opportunities to attain upright stance and locomotion. The key to motor development from both maturational and empirical evidence is that the developing child must first acquire stability in the key joint complexes required to support a specific skilled action. The research that supports this notion of increasing *behavioural flexibility* is presented and discussed in Chapter 4.

By way of summary, the notion of movement by design represents a musculoskeletal system that has embedded in it the potential for a range of phylogenetic motor skills that emerge as a direct result of the normal growth and development of the infant in the first 2 years of life. These skills emerge as a function of typical growth

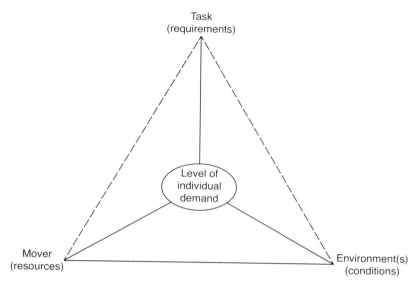

Fig. 1.5 The interrelationships among the mover, the task, and the environment.

and development that assumes adequate nourishment and care, and are honed and improved by interaction with the environment. The major event in this context is the child's ability to master upright posture and locomotion, enabling the child to change location and position and engage in manual exploration of the wider environment. Once achieved the inherent desire to explore quickly opens up immense opportunities to know the world in which the child is born. It is this opportunity to explore that informs, and we now turn to this issue.

Movement that informs
It has long been intuitive to educators in general and especially dance and physical education teachers that movement is important – perhaps critical – to the overall development of the child. Poor coordination observed in young children is often an early warning of more general developmental problems. The ability to move efficiently can be a window on both the trajectory and quality of the child's overall future developmental potential. These observations represent the non-experimental wisdom of experts who spend their lives observing children. As we have already noted, with the exception of the observations of Jean Piaget, much of behavioural science, with some exceptions, essentially ignored investigating the role that movement plays in overall development. By focusing on the abstract aspects of 'mind' the role of movement was seen as more the domain of biology, and the notion that movement might 'inform' cognition was disregarded. The separation of mind and body advanced in the dualism of René Descartes, the 'godfather' of the

psychological sciences, has perpetuated this division. As we have seen, there was recognition by the early theorist that movement was important, even though this view was not widely embraced by psychologists at large; cognition was regarded more as a focus on abstract processes and less connected to movement. An important question to be addressed is whether movement should continue to be regarded as separate from overall cognitive development or whether it is an integral part of cognitive development and a necessary and sufficient condition to optimize development.

Embodied cognition
In the first edition of this text, Keogh and Sugden (1985) illustrated the hypothesized relationships among task, performer, and environment. Figure 1.5 represents the idea that any action or skilled performance must recognize the interrelationship between these three components of the performance extant at any point in time.

These interrelationships among task, performer, and environment were further elaborated by Newell (1986) and presented as a constraints perspective on motor skill acquisition. Any discussion or theorizing about a movement skill or activity must consider this dynamic, tripartite relationship. Gibson (1979) noted that behaviour is regular but not regulated, implying that our motor actions exhibit both stability and flexibility, but these activities are not rigid or stereotypical and have the capacity to be adaptive. This contemporary view of motor development promotes the important coupling relationship between perception and action that contributes to the development of behavioural flexibility in the growing child, which in turn promotes the child's overall cognitive and intellectual development. This embodiment of the relationship between action and cognition has been referred to by Warren (2006) as 'enactive knowledge', that is non-symbolic information grounded in the act of doing. The idea that intelligence emerges from the interaction of the actor and the environment as a consequence of sensory motor activity is now generally referred to as embodied cognition.

To better understand how action or movement is viewed within a larger developmental context, we examine in Chapter 4 how the work of the ecological psychologist Eleanor 'Jackie' Gibson (of visual cliff fame and wife of James Gibson) and the research of the late Esther Thelen and her colleague Beverly Ulrich (Thelen and Ulrich 1991, Thelen 1995), and others, contribute to the notion that argues for a closer relationship between actions and how action enables the development of what we term '*behavioural flexibility*', and how behavioural flexibility is a key contributor to overall cognitive development. Embodied cognition is, in a very real sense, synonymous with the idea of behavioural flexibility:

> The central idea behind the embodiment hypothesis is that intelligence emerges in the interaction of an agent with an environment and as a result of sensorimotor activity. This view stands in opposition to more traditional notions of internal representation and computation and in general has had little to say about symbols, symbolic reasoning, and language... We argue that starting as a baby grounded in a physical, social, and linguistic world is crucial to the development of the flexible and inventive intelligence that characterizes humankind.
>
> (Smith and Gasser 2005, p. 13)

The above quote captures the relationship between embodiment and behavioural flexibility.

Motor development research in the 21st century will promote and investigate how the growing child will acquire the motor skills needed for daily living, play, recreation, and work. We predict that the theoretical orientations of both ecological psychology and dynamical systems theory will produce an upward trajectory of empirical support. This textbook traces not only the history of how scientists have described the observed changes that children exhibit in their movement behaviour but also the conceptual ways in which these changes might be explained. We do not think about movement behaviour as separate from the overall development; we promote the idea that movement behaviour is an integral part of both cognitive and social development. This is perhaps best captured in the following quote by Port and van Gelder (1995):

> Cognitive processes span the brain, the body, and the environment; to understand cognition is to understand the interplay of all three. Inner reasoning processes are no more essentially cognitive than the skillful execution of cognitive movement or the nature of the environment in which cognition takes place. The interaction between 'inner processes' and outer world is not peripheral to cognition, it is the very stuff of which cognition is made
>
> (Port and van Gelder 1995, p. ix)

The trinity proposed by Port and van Gelder (1995) – *brain, body, and environment* – shares an obvious parallel to the *task-mover and environment* proposed earlier by Keogh and Sugden (1985, see Fig. 1.5). Rather than adhering to a rigid separation between motor development and the traditional abstract idea of cognition, contemporary theory embraces the role of movement experiences as a critical feature of overall cognitive development.

Paradigms in cognitive science over much of the last four decades relied primarily on a machine (computer) analogy for studying such things as memory, perception, and verbal learning, and showed little interest in the influence of movement skill. As we have already noted above, this was owing largely to the influence of dualism (mind–body separation), originally proposed by René Descartes. As a consequence, theorizing in cognition has been more concerned with abstract representational phenomena, typically regarded as more difficult to study, whereas motor development and motor skills were regarded as external to this abstract (internal) world of the mind. To many in the psychological sciences, motor skills appeared both mechanistic and somewhat simplistic compared with the abstract process of thinking, seen as the 'true' cognitive science. Any consideration of an interaction between cognition (entirely endogenous phenomena) and sensorimotor coordination was simply ignored. When faced with providing a parsimonious account of addressing something such as Bernstein's 'degrees of freedom problem', serious difficulties occur with a computational approach. Developing computational symbolic logic for the complex movements of sensorimotor output is a challenge that for many in cognitive science is simply ignored. The science of robotics while successful to some degree in building a 'human-like' robot the simulation of adaptable human locomotion is still an as yet unmet goal.

Developing adaptable motor control

Remembering the task–mover–environment triangle depicted in Figure 1.5, growing infants must develop flexibility in their motor activities because the possibilities for action are always changing. Research by Adolph (2005) has demonstrated this dramatically. Earlier we introduced the idea of an affordance as part of Gibson's (1979) theory of direct perception with an affordance being an opportunity for action, which provides information about action possibilities available to the child. Adolph's (2005) research examined affordance thresholds in developing infants to find the go/no-go decision point. When observing young infants walking down a slope, as the angle of the slope increased the infants decided to slide or crawl down rather than walk, again demonstrating movement flexibility and evidence of what Adolph (2005) refers to as an affordance threshold. The threshold thus dictates the motor decision. In the situation above, the affordance is perceived by the infant as a success/failure decision that dictates whether to walk or slide down the incline.

Development generates new perception/action opportunities that improve the infant's behavioural flexibility to respond successfully to an ever-increasing array of motor responses and the context in which they must be performed. Adolph (2005) sees this as not dissimilar to the 'learning to learn' idea first proposed by Harlow (1949). Harlow (1949) promoted the idea of learning sets; that is to say, learners acquire a range of flexible, exploratory behaviours, rather than a specific associative response. Thus, solutions to a particular novel problem could be solved in several ways depending on the conditions extant at any particular moment in time. This in effect is what we refer to as motor equivalence: 'experienced walkers displayed alternative locomotor strategies for coping with risky slopes' (Adolph and Berger 2006, p. 196).

The contemporary approach for explaining the development of motor abilities in children implies a strong link between motor abilities and the general cognitive development of the child. No longer are the two (motor vs cognitive) regarded as separate; there is now substantial empirical evidence to support this perception–action, cognition–action synergy. Now referred to as 'embodied cognition', movement experiences enrich the overall cognitive development of the child by providing 'kinesiological epistemology' (Stoffregen TA, University of Minnesota, personal communication, June 2010). As the developing infant progresses from sitting to crawling, to cruising, and ultimately to walking, each is now regarded as a separate postural state that requires separate motor actions, which do not necessarily transfer to the next developmental state. Infants do, however, build a repertoire of actions in each of the earlier postural states through which they have passed and this provides an ever-increasing range of response flexibility, which can be called upon when novel motor problems are encountered in the environment.

Summary

Treating mind and body as separate entities is losing its appeal as more and more research demonstrates that action (movement) and cognition develop together – they are 'embodied'. The research we have highlighted in this opening chapter demonstrates this important developmental connection. The progression of motor abilities goes hand in hand with the development of the infants' capacity to 'know' about the world at large. Action and thinking are complementary to each other, and the great majority of movement activity is guided by perception, from newborn infants who turn to look at sounds and respond to a turning mobile to the elderly who use body sway to stabilize vision. Being born with the ability to explore and to seek out information about the world produces knowledge that is both flexible and adaptive. When 5 months old, infants know how far they can reach; by 14 months infants know which slopes they can safely walk down. Experience appears to be more important than chronological age; Campos et al (2000), in a lengthy review of the converging research on the impact of self-generated locomotion entitled 'Travel Broadens the Mind', comment as follows:

> So, locomotor experience has effects that can be enduring, even though they are not necessarily predictive of the future; locomotor experience can also explain developmental transitions, even though it cannot determine them; and locomotor experience dramatically changes the relation of the person to that person's environment.
>
> (Campos et al 2000, p. 211)

Our brain develops as a consequence of genetics, but genes do not totally determine its structure or function. Genes make the brain flexible; it is designed to be flexible in order to respond to experience. As we have emphasized in this introductory chapter, physical development, brain development, and experience are all important, but the latter, experience via exploration, is paramount in development. Self-generated movement (exploration) is the critical factor in an infant's ability to acquire knowledge about the wider environment and his or her relationship to the objects and things, living and inanimate, that make up our world.

REFERENCES

Adams JA (1971) A closed loop theory of motor learning. *J Motor Behav* 3: 111–149.

Adolph KE (2005) Learning to learn in the development of action. In: Lockman J, Reiser J, editors. *Action as an Organizer of Learning and Development: The 32nd Minnesota Symposium on Child Development*. Hillsdale, NJ: Erlbaum, pp. 91–122.

Adolph KE, Berger SE (2006) Motor development. In: Kuhn D, Siegler RS, editors. *Handbook of Child Psychology, Volume 2: Cognition, Perception and Language*, 6th edition. New York: Wiley, pp. 161–213.

Adolph KE, Eppler MA, Gibson EJ (1993) Crawling versus walking infants' perception of affordances for locomotion over sloping surfaces. *Child Dev* 64: 1158–1174. http://dx.doi.org/10.2307/1131332

Adolph KE, Robinson SR, Young JW, Gill Alvarez F (2008) What is the shape of developmental change? *Psychol Rev* 115: 527–543. http://dx.doi.org/10.1037/0033-295X.115.3.527

Bernstein N (1967) *The Co-ordination and Regulation of Movements*. New York: Pergamon Press.

Campos JJ, Anderson DI, Barbu-Roth MA, Hubbard EM, Hertenstein MJ, Witherington D (2000) Travel broadens the mind. *Infancy* 1: 149–219. http://dx.doi.org/10.1207/S15327078IN0102_1

Chomsky N (1966) *Topics in the Theory of Generative Grammar*. The Hague: Mouton.

Clark A (1998) Embodied, situated and distributed cognition. In: Bechtel W, Graham G, editors. *A Companion of Cognitive Science*. Malden, MA: Blackwell, pp. 506–517.

Clark JE, Whitall J (1989) What is motor development: the lessons of history. *Quest* 41: 183–202. http://dx.doi.org/10.1080/00336297.1989.10483969

Connolly K, Bruner J (1974) Competence: its nature and nurture. In: Connolly K, Bruner J, editors. *The Growth of Competence*. New York: Academic Press, pp. 3–7.

Craik KJW (1948) Theory of the human operator in control systems. *Br J Psychol* 38: 142–147.

Descartes R (1596–1650) *Descartes, René, The Philosophical Writings of Descartes*, trans. J Cottingham, R Stoothoff, D Murdoch, A Kenny. Cambridge: Cambridge University Press, 3 vols.1984–1991.

Galton F (1876) The history of twins. *Inquiries into Human Faculty and its Development* 5: 391–396.

Gesell A, Amatruda CS (1941) *Developmental Diagnosis: Normal and Abnormal Child Development, Clinical Methods and Practical Applications*. New York: P. B. Hoeber.

Gibson JJ (1966) *The Senses Considered as Perceptual Systems*. Boston, MA: Houghton Mifflin.

Gibson JJ (1979) *The Ecological Approach to Visual Perception*. Boston, MA: Houghton Mifflin.

Harlow H (1949) The nature of learning sets. *Psychol Rev* 56: 51–65. http://dx.doi.org/10.1037/h0062474

James W (1890) *Principles of Psychology, Volumes 1 and 2*. New York: Holt, Rinehart and Winston. http://dx.doi.org/10.1037/11059-000

Keogh JA, Sugden DA (1985) *Movement Skill Development*. New York: Macmillan.

McGraw MB (1935) *Growth: A Study of Johnny and Jimmy*. New York: D Appleton-Century Co.

McGraw MB (1939) *The Neuromuscular Maturation of the Human Infant*. New York: Institute of Child Development.

McGraw MB (1963) *The Neuromuscular Maturation of the Human Infant*, reprint edition. New York: Hafner.

Newell KM (1986) Development of coordination. In: Wade MG, Whiting HTA, editors. *Motor Development in Children: Aspects of Coordination and Control*. Dordrecht: Martinus Nijhoff Publishers, pp. 341–360. http://dx.doi.org/10.1007/978-94-009-4460-2_19

Newell KM, Scully P, Baillargeon R (1989) Task constraints and infant grip configuration. *Developmental Psychobiology* 22: 817–832. http://dx.doi.org/10.1002/dev.420220806

Newman BM, Newman PR (2007) *Theories of Human Development*. Mahwah, NJ: Lawrence Erlbaum Associates.

Pick HL Jr (1992) Eleanor Gibson: learning to perceive and perceiving to learn. *Dev Psychol* 28: 787–794. http://dx.doi.org/10.1037/0012-1649.28.5.787

Port RF, van Gelder T (1995) *Mind as Motion: Explorations in the Dynamics of Cognition*. Cambridge, MA: MIT Press.

Schmidt RA (1975) A schema theory of discrete motor skill learning. *Psychol Rev* 82: 225–260. http://dx.doi.org/10.1037/h0076770

Schmidt RA, Lee TD (2011) *Motor Control and Learning: A Behavioral Emphasis*. Champaign, IL: Human Kinetics.

Shannon CE, Weaver W (1949) *The Mathematical Theory of Communication*. Urbana, IL: University of Illinois Press.

Smith LB, Gasser M (2005) The development of embodied cognition: six lessons from babies. *Artificial Life* 11: 13–30. http://dx.doi.org/10.1162/1064546053278973

Tanner JM (1981) *A History of the Study of Human Growth*. Cambridge: Cambridge Academic Press.

Thelen E (1995) Motor development: a new synthesis. *Am Psychol* 50: 79–95. http://dx.doi.org/10.1037/0003-066X.50.2.79

Thelen E, Fisher DM (1983) The organization of spontaneous leg movements in newborn infants. *J Motor Behav* 15: 353–377.

Thelen E, Ulrich BD (1991) Hidden skills: a dynamic systems analysis of treadmill-elicited stepping during the first year. *Monographs of the Society for Research in Child Development* 56: 1–106.

Vygotsky LS (1978) In: Cole M, John-Teiner V, Schribner S, Souberman E, editors. *Mind in Society: The Development of Higher Psychological Processes*. Cambridge, MA: Harvard University Press.

Warren WH (2006) The dynamics of perception and action. *Psychol Rev* 113: 358–389. http://dx.doi.org/10.1037/0033-295X.113.2.358

Wolpert DM, Doya K, Kawato M (2003) A unifying computational framework for motor control and social interaction. *Phil Trans Royal Soc* 358: 593–602. http://dx.doi.org/10.1098/rstb.2002.1238

2
BIOLOGICAL INFLUENCES ON DEVELOPMENTAL CHANGE

In Chapter 1 children's movement development was described as an adaptive change that occurs as the child progresses towards maturity. This was shown in a dynamic model that portrayed the interplay between the child's resources, the environment in which the activity takes place, and the nature and presentation of the task. The child's resources are a crucial part of this interplay and this chapter examines some of the fundamental biological influences, detailing selected changes in structures and functions as the child progresses to maturity, and a summary of how these biological changes may affect movement development.

Newborn infants change almost as we watch them, becoming bigger in overall size and different in body proportions. Similar changes in internal organs and systems, although not directly visible, can be measured in ways that help us to 'see' internal biological changes. As a starting point for considering biological changes that lead to a mature state, some changes are *structural* and others are *functional*. Physical features may change to create a change in structure, in contrast with a change in how an organ or system functions. It is well established that the regulation of growth is a complex interaction of the child's resources and the environmental context including nutrition. Within the child, genes and hormonal development play a major part, the latter being particularly important for the initiation and regulation of pubertal events (Baxter-Jones 2008). Testosterone, oestrogen, thyroxine, cortisol and adrenal androgens, insulin, and hormones from the pituitary glands are all actively involved in the regulation of growth during the pubertal period, with the central feature of puberty being the maturation of the primary reproductive endocrine axis, often called the hypothalamic–pituitary–gonadal axis (HPG) – see Baxter-Jones (2008) for detail on this topic. Organs such as the brain and heart will change in structure to be larger as well as different in the interconnections of the units within each

organ. Functional changes mean that more can be done or done differently, such as the control of lower neutral units by higher brain centres, lower centres operating independently, a decrease in heart rate, and an increase in the amount of oxygen transported. The distinction between structure and function is not always clear-cut, but it is useful when trying to understand biological change; we have selected certain anthropometric measures to examine structure and neural and sensory measures for function, while recognizing the overlap between structure and function.

Our review of biological change towards maturity covers the period from conception to biological maturity. It is important to note that we are not covering the full age span in biological changes, and thus variables associated with ageing populations are not included. Individuals are expected to change in somewhat similar ways to reach a time when each biological organ or system has and is a complete, fully functioning structure. At that time, an individual is mature in this aspect of biological change. The rate and age of maturity vary among the many biological organs and systems, so aspects of biological change are described separately. However, it is the interplay of each of these aspects in a complex system that produces the end movement product. Maturity can be identified with some certainty for structural changes, whereas maturity of most functional changes is less certain because functional maturity often is difficult to separate from achievements related to the functioning of the organ or system.

Biological influence is used in the title of this chapter to imply a broader sense of change towards maturity because growth too often is limited to *structural change*, particularly size. Our emphasis is also on *functional change* because it has such an impact on the development of movement control. As Baxter-Jones (2008) notes, biological maturation has two components: timing and tempo. Timing refers to when a particular event occurs,

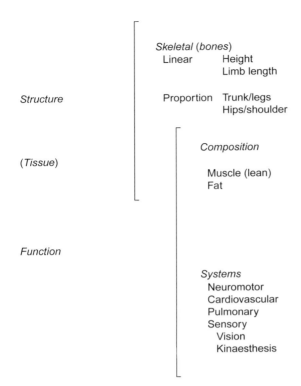

Fig. 2.1 Selected aspects of biological changes towards maturity with important influences upon movement development.

bony structure. Muscles are lean tissue and the means of moving bones and creating movement. The neuromotor system is the coupling of nerves and muscles to control muscle activity; the cardiovascular and pulmonary systems service the neuromotor system's energy needs, primarily oxygen transport and related metabolic needs; and the sensory system involves the use of sensory mechanisms for movement, primarily vision and kinaesthesis.

Selected anthropometric structural changes
Structural changes in body and body part sizes are important as they influence skill development in a number of ways. First, the changes alter the dynamics of child–context interactions in such actions as reaching and grasping and the size of the object to be grasped in relation to the size of the hand, with the action changing spontaneously from a one-handed to a two-handed grasp as the cube increases in size. Another example is shown below in Figure 2.2, in which changes in total body size influence the actions of the individual.

In Figure 2.2a the bench affords sitting on to a fully grown adult, whereas for a toddler in Figure 2.2b it invites cruising around. For a 7- or 8-year-old it may afford jumping off. These three simple examples illustrate the point that the unit of analysis is not simply the child. Change in height has been described and analysed so extensively that we shall present it first and in more detail than the other structural changes. Height continues to be a major topic of interest with recent summaries still taking it as the starting point for descriptions of growth (Baxter-Jones 2008). Analyses of change in height also provoke many of the questions encountered in describing other aspects of structural change, and height is a useful alternative to chronological age as an indicator of general biological maturity.

HEIGHT
Baxter-Jones (2008) alerts us to the difference in growth curves, distinguishing between those that are fitted to a single individual's data over time (longitudinal data) and

such as age of menarche, whereas tempo refers to the rate at which maturation is progressing, such as how quickly an individual progresses from an initial stage through to completion. Timing and tempo vary considerably within individuals of the same age.

A framework is presented in Figure 2.1 that shows three areas of biological change that are important to movement development: bones (skeleton), tissues (body composition), and systems. Bones and tissues provide the basic body structure for size and form and are measured as linear and proportional dimensions. The length of major bones determines linear size and body proportions, with muscle, fat, and other tissues filling out the shape of the

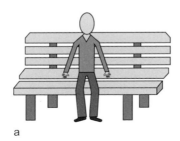

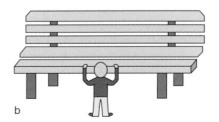

Fig. 2.2 Affordance of action through body–environment scaling.

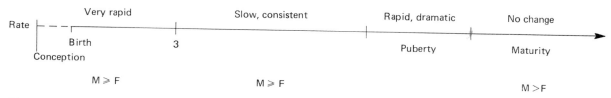

Fig. 2.3 A general representation of four major periods of rate of height change, with general comparisons between male (M) and female (F) average heights (Keogh and Sugden 1985).

curves derived from children of different ages measured once and averaged yearly (cross-sectional data). The latter can be carried out relatively cheaply and quickly and produce group data but cannot show individual growth and the subtle variations that accompany individual analysis. For a review of the pros and cons of longitudinal and cross-sectional data see Baxter-Jones (2008).

Change in height during the growing years is obvious in even casual observations and is the simplest measure of structural growth, although it requires careful measurement procedures to gather useful data. In a classic and comprehensive work, Tanner (1981) compiled a record of the study of human growth in which he found that height was the basic measurement of structural growth from the time of the Ancient Greeks to the present. He lists many reasons why height measurements were recorded, including the identification of people before signatures and pictures were available, selection of military personnel for processional and fighting purposes, and medical–social concerns related to the employment of children. Tanner's historical review is an interesting account of the origins of major issues and related findings, such as daily and seasonal variations in growth measures and growth rates, secular (generation) trends, catch-up growth following interruptions related to trauma and illness, and explanations of growth as body heat (temperature), temperament, and other proposed causal factors. Our review of height growth follows his writings, including an earlier book on growth at adolescence (Tanner 1962).

Patterns of change

Newborn infants are 46 to 56cm in length (height) at birth, which is an amazing amount and rate of change in the 9 months since conception considering that at 3 months the fetus is 8cm long. Children grow to one-half of their mature height by age 3 and two-thirds of their mature height by age 6. The general rate of height change can be divided into four periods, as shown in Figure 2.3. The rate of height change is very rapid from conception through birth to age 3. There is a slow but consistent rate of change from age 3 until the onset of puberty (approximately 5cm per year), when there is another period of

rapid height change accompanied by dramatic changes in body proportions. Small increases in height occur after the end of the pubertal period and full height is usually achieved by age 20 or soon after. Until puberty, males on the average are slightly taller than females. There is a large overlap, though, with some females taller than males of average height at the same age and some males smaller than females of average height at the same age. Females on average enter puberty 2 years earlier than males do, and the age at onset of puberty is quite variable among individuals. This means that height comparisons between males and females during puberty can differ within different samples and at different chronological ages. Adult males are, on average, 10 to 15cm taller than adult females, with much less overlap than during the developing years.

Changes in height can be graphed as height gained or rate of height gain, as in Figures 2.4 and 2.5, which summarize the first longitudinal study on record (Tanner 1981). The two graphs are the work of a French nobleman, Count de Montbeillard, who measured the height of his son at 6-month intervals from birth to age 18 between 1759 and 1777. The general shapes of these two curves approximate findings from many later studies in different parts of the world. The actual measurements may differ, but the curves show the same peaks and accelerations. The distance curve in Figure 2.4 merely indicates the height, or distance, achieved at each age. Montbeillard's son was a little more than 50cm (20 inches) at birth and was approximately 185cm (72–73 inches) at age 18, tall even by modern standards. The rate of height change can be seen by the changes in the slope of the distance curve, but a better view of rate of height change is shown in Figure 2.5.

The rate of height change, which Tanner calls height velocity, is the amount of change per unit of time. The rate in Figure 2.5 is calculated as a rolling, yearly velocity, by calculating the average rate of change over the year for each 6-month interval. This means that the first plotting point at 0.5 years (6 months) is the average rate of increase from birth to 12 months, the second plotting point at 1.0 years (12 months) is the average rate of increase

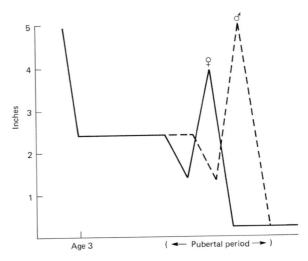

Fig. 2.6 A general representation of height change for females and males (Keogh and Sugden 1985).

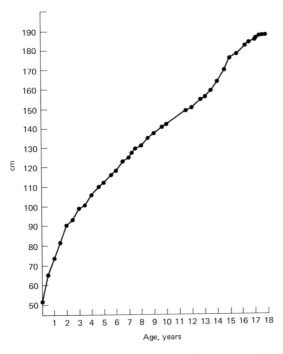

Fig. 2.4 Height of Count de Montbeillard's son, 1759–1777. Reproduced with permission from Tanner, *Growth at Adolescence*, 2nd edition, John Wiley and Sons, 9780632039302, 1981.

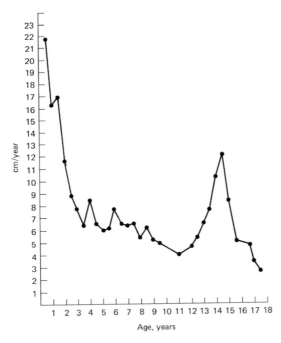

Fig. 2.5 Rate of height change of Count de Montbeillard's son, 1759–1777. Reproduced with permission from Tanner, *Growth at Adolescence*, 2nd edition, John Wiley and Sons, 9780632039302, 1981.

from 6 months to 18 months, and so on. Each plotting point overlaps with adjacent plotting points to remove seasonal effects in which height tends to increase more in the summer and less in the winter. From the general shape of Figure 2.5, we can see the four periods identified in Figure 2.3. The change is very rapid until age 3, followed by a slower and more consistent rate of change until the rapid change at puberty. The fourth period of minimal or no change marks the achievement of mature stature.

It is noticeable that the rate of height change decreased from birth to age 3 but that the absolute rate (amount of increase) is large compared with that at other ages. The rate of height change for Montbeillard's son decreased from 22cm/year in the first year (plotting point at 0.5y) to 9cm/year in the third year (plotting point at 2.5y). The rate of height change beyond age 3, until the decrease in rate preceding puberty, was 6 to 8cm/year. The rate then increased to a peak height velocity of 12cm/year during puberty. The rate of height change for Montbeillard's son varied from nearly 23cm in the first year of life to 5 to 7cm per year during the slower-growing years, followed by an increase of approximately 13cm during one pubertal year. A minimum point in rate, as seen at age 11, marks the onset of puberty, and the peak height velocity (age 14) is a marker that is used to represent the maximal rate of height change during puberty.

A general representation of the rate of height change for males and females is presented in Figure 2.6. Rate and age will vary considerably for individuals and different samples, but the general pattern of change for males and females will approximate the two curves. During the decrease in rate that marks the onset of puberty, the legs continue to grow but the trunk slows its growth for a period of time, as if the body is preparing for the pubertal changes that occur primarily in the upper body. The increase in leg length, with proportionately less change in trunk length, produces a 'leggy' look, which is often quite noticeable, to the embarrassment of the growing adolescent.

The rate of change is similar for males and females up to the onset of puberty for females, with males on the average being slightly taller. Females enter puberty approximately 2 years earlier than males do and tend to go through the pubertal period in less time. Males not only enter puberty later, but also generally have a higher peak height velocity and a somewhat longer pubertal growth period. Males are 10 to 15cm taller than females when they reach mature height, because they grow for several more years and slightly more during their pubertal years.

General influences on mature stature
There are a number of genetic and environmental influences on the height achieved at maturity. Siblings tend to be similar in height because they share some genes and are usually engaged in a similar environment. The correlation of mature heights of identical twins is 0.9, compared with 0.5 for fraternal twins and non-twin siblings (Bloom 1964). Tanner (1989) reports correlations of approximately 0.5 for the heights of parents and the mature stature of their offspring. The larger correlation for identical twins points to genetic influences as the major determinant of mature stature.

Sex is also an important part of genetic influence because males, on the average, are taller at maturity than females. But female–male comparisons must be made within reasonably common gene pools. Height varies considerably in different gene populations, and so women in one gene population may be taller on average than men in another gene population. In addition, people in industrialized societies are increasingly mobile, which makes it difficult to select appropriate samples for female–male comparisons. Tanner (1981) summarizes many earlier studies in which the samples of males and females for each study were from a reasonably common gene pool and the men on average were taller than the women at maturity in all comparisons. The general conclusions are that mature stature is very much determined by the genetic codes transferred by parents and related to sex.

Tanner (1981) also points out those environmental factors that affect mature stature. Nutrition, climate, and socio-economic conditions have been identified as contributing to *secular trends*, which are changes noticed across time. Different generations or cohorts will achieve different mean heights or will have different rates of

height change, which sometimes can be attributed to environmental factors. We generally think of secular trends as increases but there have been decreases, seemingly related to times of war, economic depression, and similar extreme environmental events. Environmental factors need to be quite substantial in 'weight' (e.g. severe malnutrition or superior health services) in order to have an impact. Deprivation also seems to have a larger influence than enrichment.

Individual patterns of change
The rate of height change to this point has been presented as a group of mean changes in relation to chronological age. However, individual children mature at such different rates that chronological age is often a misleading indicator of change. As shown in Figure 2.7, the form and intensity of height change during puberty is underestimated when viewed in relation to chronological age.

Individual rates of height change are plotted in Figure 2.7a in relation to chronological age, with the mean rate of change shown by the dotted line. Individual rates of change in Figure 2.7b are plotted in relation to the peak height velocity. Rather than chronological age, age now is years before and after the time of peak height velocity. Individual curves are strikingly similar, and the mean in the graph to the right is a better representation of their similarity. It is noticeable in Figure 2.7a that earlier-maturing individuals have slightly larger increases at the time of peak height velocity, which is offset to some extent by the longer growing time of later-maturing individuals.

Individual stability
Bloom (1964) examined stability and change in human characteristics with height as a basic model because height data have been reported so extensively and height is probably one of the most stable human characteristics. Bloom defined stability as consistency from one point in time to another. He wanted to know whether individuals maintain a similar position in a group over time, even though everyone is changing. If a child is tall when younger, will he or she be tall when older? Bloom estimated stability by the correlation of height at one age to height at a later age.

One of Bloom's main points was that height is more stable when there is less change. He illustrates this with what he acknowledges is an obvious and absurd question. What is the correlation of height measurements for a sample of people measured at age 20 and again at age 40? The correlation should be close to 1.0 because no change is expected and each person should have the same height measurement at both ages. We also expect a high correlation for height measurements taken at ages 7 and 8 because children change by only a small amount and thus

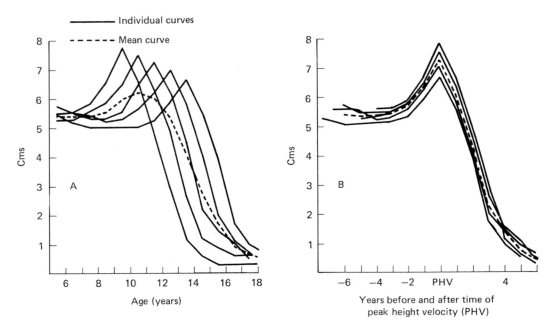

Fig. 2.7 Two views of individual and mean rate of height change during the pubertal growth period, plotted in relation to (a) chronological age and (b) peak height velocity. Reproduced with permission from Tanner, *Growth at Adolescence*, 2nd edition, John Wiley and Sons, 9780632039302, 1981.

cannot be very different after 1 year. The converse is that measures of stability (correlations) will be smaller when individual change is greater; that is, when there is a long time interval with a slow rate of change or a large rate of change in a short time interval. Bloom stresses the amount of change as the most important consideration because the larger the change is the more opportunity there will be for individuals to change positions in the distribution.

Bloom offers much evidence to support his point that stability increases when there is less change. He also demonstrates that stability is erratic during times of great change, particularly when individuals go through a change period at different times and at different rates. This means that stability will be more tenuous when one or both measurements are taken during puberty. His primary concern was to identify the influences on change by studying height and other stable characteristics when individuals encountered extreme environmental conditions. He concludes that environment will have the greatest influence during a period of rapid change and the least influence during a period of slow change. Injury, disease, starvation, and similar extreme conditions will retard height growth more during the early years and puberty when there is more change to be effected.

BODY PROPORTIONS

Individuals grow bigger from birth to the early adult years, as the length of their limbs and trunk and the width of

their hips and shoulders increases. Body dimensions not only increase in size but also at different rates to produce changes in body proportions. These proportional changes are shown in Figure 1.3, in which the body pictures at different ages have been adjusted in order to maintain the same height. Looking first at the newborn infant in the left-hand picture, the head is one-quarter of the total body length and the legs are just a little bit longer than the head. All parts of the body grow, but at mature height (right-hand picture) the head is about one-sixth of the total body length, compared with nearly one-half for the legs. Body proportions change more rapidly in utero, as seen in the changes from the second fetal month through the fifth fetal month to birth.

Baxter-Jones (2008) presents some general summaries about proportions, reporting that from birth to maturity there is a twofold increase in the absolute size of the head, the trunk increases threefold, the arms increase fourfold, and the legs increase fivefold. He observes other gradients of growth with hands and feet increasing before calves, forearms, hips, chest, and shoulders, but after puberty the hands and feet are smaller in proportion to arms, legs, and stature.

Some proportional changes in body breadth are shown in Figure 1.3, but they do not represent changes in girth. The head width approaches the shoulder and hip width at birth, whereas the head width of adults is only one-third of their shoulder width. Shoulder width from birth is greater than hip width, with males' shoulder–hip ratio increasing more than females' during puberty. Some proportional changes in girth can be inferred from these pictures, because a marked change in width is also a change in girth. Thus, the change of the head girth is proportionately smaller than that of the chest girth. The proportion of thigh girth to hip girth changes from quite small before birth to larger at birth, which is followed by a decrease that changes to an increase in the adult years.

Trunk–leg ratio

The length of the legs, trunk, and head can be measured to monitor proportional changes in body segments, which contribute to height changes. The major change occurs in the legs and trunk, with the head contributing only a small amount of absolute increase from birth to the early adult years. The rapid rate of leg growth can be seen by the decrease in the ratio of sitting height to standing height in Figure 1.3. Sitting height is measured as the height from the seat of the chair in which a person is sitting to the top of their head. This measures the change in trunk and head length, and can be compared with a full height measurement, which includes leg length. Sitting height is more than 60% of standing height in the early years but decreases to little more than 50% at mature height.

Differences between the sexes exist at birth and in the early years, with females slightly longer in the leg than in the upper body. Females may be biologically more mature, and thus slightly 'ahead' in the ratio decrease, with the reverse occurring during puberty, when males become slightly longer legged in comparison with their upper-body length.

Hip–shoulder ratio

Hip girth is less than shoulder girth at all ages, although hip girth increases in comparison with shoulder girth. There are no differences between the sexes until age 7, when the hip–shoulder girth ratio increases for females and levels off and later decreases for males. The ratio at age 18 is quite different and is a noticeable difference between the sexes in body proportions. For a detailed description and explanation of anthropometric measures, readers are directed to consult Tanner (1990), whose reports on measurements and calculations are classic and unique.

BODY COMPOSITION AND PHYSIQUE

Bodies are composed of several kinds of tissues, with our primary concerns being muscle, as lean tissue, and fat, both of which can change considerably in a short time, depending on exercise and diet. A number of measures have been used to estimate body composition including body mass index, skinfolds and, in the past, traditional radiography, now becoming rarer because of the associated health risks. Claessens et al (2008) note a number of measures in current use in paediatric populations including densitometry, which involves the ratio of body mass to body volume; dual-energy X-ray absorptiometry; and bioelectrical impedance analysis, which works on the principle that biological tissue can act as a conductor or insulator, with lean tissue having greater conductivity than adipose tissue. However, the most widely used method involves skinfold measures in which the sums of many skinfold measures are entered into a regression equation to predict body density. Although widely used, it has been questioned for its validity within child populations (Claessens et al 2008).

While recognizing the cautionary notes on the various methods of measuring body composition, the general patterns of change in children are somewhat similar. First, infants are fattier than children and there is a loss in fat, rather than a gain, from age 1 to age 5 or 6. Children beyond age 6 have very small gains in fat, with males losing fat during part of their pubertal growth period. The rate of change for bone and muscle resembles that for height, and the rate of change for bone and muscle decreases to a more steady rate from age 4 until the onset of puberty. The female rate of change increases during puberty, as does the male, and the males have a slightly higher peak muscle–bone rate of change. Looking across the full age range, males have a higher rate of change for bone and muscle and a lower rate of gain for subcutaneous fat. The overall effects are that children progressively increase their ratio of muscle to fat and males have a higher ratio of muscle to fat at maturity than females. There is a change in the ratio of fat to lean tissue in males and females.

Bone and fat measurements derived from radiographs of the calf have been plotted in relation to one another, for children at age 7 and adults, and a discriminant function has been calculated to find the line that best separated males and females. A count can be made to determine how many individuals are misclassified, indicating females that appeared on the male side of the line and vice versa. Misclassification was nearly 40% at age 7 and only 5% for adults.

Differences in body build are noted informally when, to describe general tissue composition, we say that a person is lean, muscular, or round. Physique is not body size (being large or small in length and mass), but it is a composite of proportional relationships among sizes of body parts and measures of body composition.

Various ratios of height and weight have provided simple and quick estimates of physique. Bayley and Davis

(1935) used the ratio of weight/(height)^2 to measure the lateral–linear relationship during an infant's first 3 years. Wetzel (1941, 1943) devised a grid based on height and weight for seven different growth channels, which represent different body builds. Children are measured at regular intervals with the expectation that a change in growth channel will indicate a change in health status. Ratios of height and weight are obviously quite limited estimates of physique, but they have the advantage of using readily available measurements and simple calculations, and these early measures are noted because they were used at a time when classic longitudinal data on children were being collected.

More elaborate systems of describing physique have been devised with the concept of somatotype, which was introduced by Sheldon and coworkers (Sheldon and Stevens 1942, Sheldon et al 1954). The Sheldon method is a complex rating of three standardized photographs in combination with a ponderal index score. Three components are rated separately on a seven-point scale from 1, as the least indicative, to 7, as the most indicative. The three components are endomorphy, mesomorphy, and ectomorphy, suggesting the embryonic tissues of endoderm, mesoderm, and ectoderm. Endomorphy implies a softer, rounder body build, in comparison with the better-defined musculature and balanced body proportions of mesomorphy and the leaner, linear dimension of ectomorphy. An important limitation of Sheldon's somatotypes is that the ratings are organized to classify adult males and were not intended for use with women and children. Most women are endomorphic in Sheldon's ratings, and children change markedly depending on the characteristics being rated. Another controversial issue surrounding Sheldon's somatotypes was that he viewed them as being predictive of genotype and this provoked much criticism as we now know to what degree somatotype can be changed by diet and exercise. Modifications of Sheldon's original work that utilize both photographic and anthropometric measures (Carter and Heath 1990) and view somatotype as the phenotype that describes the body at a moment in time have been proposed and largely accepted. Anthropometric measures dominate the rating with 10 body measurements taken, but again complete agreement on its validity is not present, with the lack of trunk measurement being one criticism of the system (Claessens et al 2008).

There is an obvious limitation in the lack of a well-established and acceptable method of physique classification that can be adopted for use with children. Malina and Rarick (1973) summarize evidence that points to a larger similarity between parents and children in linear height than in breadth and girth dimensions. Parnell (1958)

reported that 34 of a sample of 45 children followed their parents' physique pattern in terms of their phenotypic ratings.

All of this suggests an expected genetic link, but still leaves us with the problem of describing physique changes during the growing years. Proportions change for body measurements and tissue composition, which makes it difficult to organize a scheme for physique classifications at one age that is appropriate for a later age. Malina and Rarick (1973) summarize evidence that points to a consistency in physique components for individuals during short intervals of 3 or 4 years, except during adolescence. However, there is little evidence showing consistency in physique from the early years to maturity. This is a particularly difficult problem because the physique during the early years is quite different in its proportions or ratios at later ages.

Males and females probably have similar physiques from birth through the prepubertal years because they are similar on many separate measures of body proportions and body composition. Males have a slightly leaner body mass than females before puberty, but this becomes greater during and after puberty and by young adulthood they have 50% more lean body mass than females (Baxter-Jones 2008). Males also are bigger after puberty, and there are noticeable differences in female–male comparisons after puberty on many structural characteristics. As noted earlier, the overlap or mismatch is often less than 10% when classifying adults as female or male on measures such as hip–shoulder width and lean–fat ratio. This means that female–male differences in physique changes must be recognized when describing patterns of change.

Structural growth provides much of the foundations for movement skill development. For example, the anthropometric changes such as height and body ratios and composition affect the control of movement. A reduction in fat, the growth of long bones, and an increase in muscle mass and lean tissue are all constraints on movement skill, and as these change so will the accompanying skilled performance. This is particularly true in periods of great change such as in the first 2 years of life and during puberty. There is not a discrete dividing line between structure and function, as they act on each other with a bidirectional effect, but it is useful to examine them separately while remembering this connection.

PUBERTAL PERIOD
Males and females are alike in most biological characteristics before puberty, although they are quite different in many respects after puberty. Changes during the pubertal years are quite important in regard to increased potential for fitness and strength, which are needed for

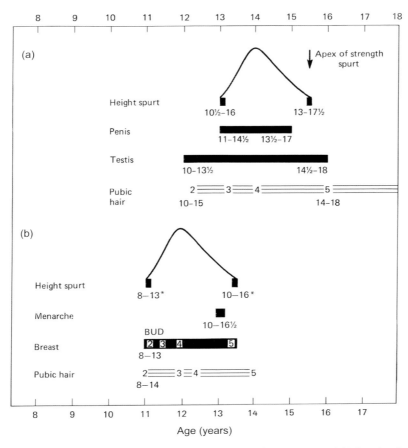

Fig. 2.8 Range of ages for onset and completion of selected pubertal changes for (a) males and (b) females. Range of ages for onset and completion of height spurt for females is from data reported by Faust (1977). Reproduced with permission from the publisher from Tanner (1962).

high-level performance in some movement skills. During puberty, which usually occurs in females from 10 to 13 years and in males from 12 to 15 years, there is an increase in the number of hormones entering the bloodstream in response to signals from the hypothalamus. This results in the pituitary releasing growth hormones to stimulate production of thyroxine and sex hormones, with the end product being an increase in body size accompanied by skeletal, tissue, and metabolic changes. These in turn have a profound effect on movement skill performance. For detail on these constitutional changes, Tanner (1990) is recommended.

As individuals go through puberty at such a wide range of chronological ages, changes are presented in regard to several measures of pubertal age, as a way of adjusting individuals to a common growth time, rather than using chronological age as a baseline measure of age.

Secondary sex changes

The secondary sex changes in Figure 2.8 are listed in relation to chronological age and the pattern of height

change. The onset and completion of some changes are marked with a range of chronological age to illustrate individual variability. For example, age ranges are noted for breast development and first menstrual flow, or menarche, for females and changes in the testes and penis for males. The pattern of height change at puberty, called the height spurt, provides a general means of marking the onset and completion of puberty. Notice that menarche occurs late in puberty and really marks the beginning of the completion of puberty. The apex of strength increase tends to come near the end of puberty, probably because some time is needed to incorporate and use the biological changes, such as the increase in muscle mass, to produce strength (Asmussen 1973). The exact ages of pubertal markers vary over cultures and over time but the phases of progression remain similar.

Females undergo their pubertal changes approximately 2 years earlier than males and also go through the pubertal years in a somewhat shorter time. Add the wide range of ages at which individuals enter puberty and it becomes obvious that individual difference is the rule

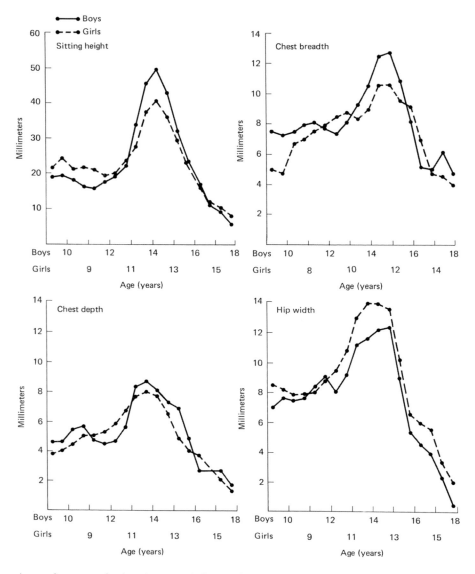

Fig. 2.9 Comparisons of patterns of pubertal structural changes for sitting height, chest breadth, chest depth, and hip width. Peak height velocities for males were at ages 14 or 15 and for females were at ages 12 or 13. Reproduced with permission from the publisher from Tanner (1962), as drawn from data reported by Shuttleworth (1939).

rather than the exception in pubertal changes in relation to chronological age. When children become adolescents at age 13, many females are completing their puberty, whereas most males are just entering it.

Structural and functional changes

Adjustments have been made to represent biological changes during puberty in ways that remove the confounding effect of individual variations in maturity level as related to chronological age. An example is the alignment of individual rates of height change on peak height velocity, as shown earlier in Figure 2.7. Another way is

shown in Figure 2.9 in the four graphs of rate changes of selected structural features. Tanner (1962) used data from Shuttleworth (1939) and made a number of adjustments to compare the patterns of change for males and females. He began by including only males with peak height velocities between the ages of 14 and 15 and females with peak height velocities between the ages of 12 and 13. This provided comparable samples of males and females who were at relatively the same level of maturity within their sex group. In other words, Tanner eliminated earlier- and later-maturing males and females and then aligned the patterns in relation to peak pubertal changes, with the chronological age baselines adjusted accordingly. Notice that the baseline adjustments are similar in each graph, except that the changes in chest breadth occur slightly earlier for females.

Tanner's comparisons demonstrate the similar patterns of change for males and females when adjusted for the level of maturity. There are differences in absolute amount of change, as noted earlier for males gaining more height and wider chests and females gaining more hip width, yet the patterns of change are strikingly similar in the times of rises and falls in the curves and the overall lengths of the pubertal change period for these structural functions.

Faust (1977) made extensive analyses of the pubertal height growth of the females in the California Adolescent Study (Jones 1939) to derive a procedure for marking the onset and end of pubertal height growth. She showed that females increase slightly in rate through the time period, in contrast with males' more steady rate of change, and females have a higher rate of change (increase) at each developmental point. Other findings included changes in the hip–shoulder ratio, which increased in males because of their increase in shoulder width and decreased in females because of their increase in hip width.

The patterns of biological change during puberty are quite similar for individuals when considered in relation to level of maturity, or what might be called pubertal age. Additionally, those biological systems that serve a common function seem to develop uniformly, as demonstrated by the similar timings among patterns of change when adjusted to pubertal age. Although sex differences in patterns of change are quite striking for many aspects of pubertal development, both females and males improve their resources substantially for maximal movement performance.

MATURITY

The principal concern in our review of biological changes has been progress towards maturity, with the general criterion that the structure is complete and fully functioning. It is apparent that maturity is an elusive and changeable state depending on which biological change is being described and what the criteria for maturity are. As noted earlier, it is easier to identify structural maturity than functional maturity, although it is difficult to obtain some structural measures. Here some structural measures of maturity that are used to label individuals as early, average, or late maturers are examined. These measures are useful in studying the relationship of the level of maturity to many movement performance achievements. A first step is to look at the differences in the rate of maturity for different types of biological change.

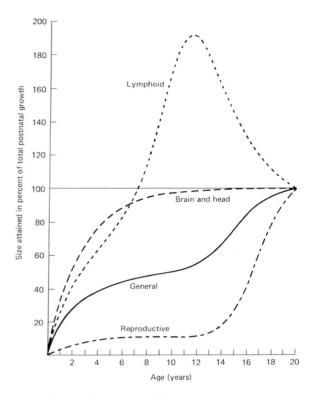

Fig. 2.10 Growth curves of different parts and tissues of the body. Reproduced with permission from the publisher from Tanner (1962), as redrawn from Scammon (1930).

General maturity differences

Differences in the rate of maturity among several aspects of biological change are shown in Figure 2.10. These are structural changes in size, with maturity marked as size at age 20. The curves are different from the distance and rate curves used to this point in that they represent the percentage of postnatal development from birth to maturity (age 20). Each curve begins at zero and ends at 100%. The brain and head grow rapidly in the early years, and achieve 90% of their growth beyond birth by ages 6 or 7. General growth, which includes many of the biological changes we are reviewing, is not yet at 50% by age 6. Remember that these percentages describe the proportion of growth from birth to age 20 and do not consider the amount of growth achieved in utero.

The reproductive system grows very little until the pubertal years, when growth is very rapid. We also know that the reproductive system is not functional until pubertal changes occur and that functionality of the reproductive system matures very rapidly to provide the potential for procreation. Functional maturity cannot often be defined and measured with the clarity and precision we desire, and there is considerable variation in maturity states for men and women.

The pattern of lymphoid change also points out the differences in maturity among biological changes. The lymph system increases in size and function during the pubertal years in order to serve the pubertal change processes, which are primarily biochemical and hormonal in nature, and then decreases in size and function. This means that maturity for the lymph system should really be recognized as occurring at an earlier age, with a decrease occurring more rapidly than for other biological changes.

There is evidence that body systems make an effort to catch up, as seen by accelerated growth rates after interruptions by disease or injury (Tanner 1962). Recalling Bloom's ideas regarding stability and change (1964), he suggests that more is lost and not regained when disruption occurs during times of rapid change. If a proportion, such as one-half, is regained during the catch-up period, the final loss will be greater if the initial loss is greater. There is much to be learned about catch-up growth, beyond knowing that the body does try to accelerate growth during catch-up periods.

Individual level of maturity
It is often desirable to specify the level of maturity for an individual, such as how far an individual has progressed towards maturity and how an individual compares in level of maturity with others. Measures of distance and rate might indicate that an individual is nearing maturity, even though he or she is relatively late in reaching it. Another individual of the same chronological age might be an early maturer who has already reached maturity. Chronological age is often used in the early years as a general estimate of biological maturity, but it measures only the passage of time and not biological change.

Skeletal or bone maturity is widely recognized as the best single indicator of maturity status, with the bones in the hand and wrist usually providing the best estimates of the development of cartilage to the full ossified skeletal structure. Radiographs of the hand are often used to estimate skeletal age or bone age because the hand's many bones offer many growth centres to rate. Standards have been established from radiographs of children at many ages, meaning that on average children are expected to have growth centres of the size and shape seen in the standard radiograph for that age. There are several ways to use these standards, as explained by Tanner (1962), but the general idea is to specify the level of maturity for skeletal development. When an individual is measured as having a particular skeletal age, we compare skeletal age with chronological age to determine whether an individual is early or late in skeletal maturity. Everyone, whether early, average, or late maturers, reaches a point of complete skeletal maturity.

Females are more biologically mature than males until they reach a chronological age when both are mature. Tanner (1962) estimates that a male's mean skeletal age is approximately 80% of that of a female's of the same chronological age from birth until near the time of maturity. The absolute difference at age 1 is about 2 months and at age 10 about 2 years.

The level of maturity can be assessed in other ways by choosing a particular biological characteristic and establishing norms or standards to mark progress towards maturity. Peak height velocity is used in several ways to provide a point around which maturity in stature can be defined and measured. However, an important limitation in using these maturity measures is having to wait until they occur, and also we must make a series of observations or measurements over a period of time if pre- and postmarkers are required. Although skeletal age can be used at a single time to estimate the level of maturity, considerable professional skill is needed to obtain useful measurements, and individuals are not now as willing to have radiographs and other measures taken unless they have a medical problem.

There is often concern with the development of individuals who seem to be late maturers or early maturers. Despite the many problems encountered in measuring level of maturity, extreme levels can be established with more assurance than levels in the middle range of maturity. This is because a specific score or age is not needed; we need only to find those who are beyond a particular score or age. For example, we could identify all of the 10-year-old males within two standard deviations of the mean as being within a normal range (sometimes labelled as within normal limits [WNL]). Late maturers would then be those with a skeletal age of less than 8 years 0 months, and early maturers would have a skeletal age of more than 12 years 0 months. This would mark 2 to 3% as being late maturers and 2 to 3% as being early maturers. Thus, designations of late and early are arbitrary and depend on our judgement of where to place a cut-off. A less extreme cut-off in this example would be to choose a standard deviation of 1.5, which would establish the normal limits as 8 years 6 months and 11 years 6 months. Assuming a normal distribution, the less extreme cut-off would identify 7 to 8% as late maturers and 7 to 8% as early maturers. Another method of identifying late and early maturers is to make a percentage cut-off, for example, of the lowest 10% and the highest 10%. Extreme designations, such as early and late, are in the eye of the beholder, which means that a check is made of the basis for such designations to determine whether they match what is acceptable as appropriate cut-off points.

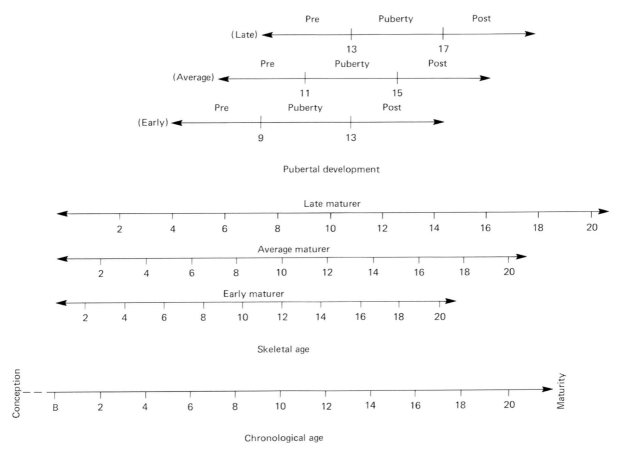

Fig. 2.11 General comparisons of different rates of maturity for skeletal age and pubertal development of males in relation to chronological age (Keogh and Sugden 1985).

A general representation of the rate of maturity in relation to chronological age is shown in Figure 2.11 for male skeletal age and pubertal development. Late and early maturers for skeletal age were chosen as being 20% behind or ahead of the mean skeletal age. According to chronological age 10, the average maturer is skeletal age 10, in comparison with skeletal age 8 for a late maturer and skeletal age 12 for an early maturer. A similar comparison with other chronological ages should find a 20% lag or acceleration for the late or early maturer, respectively, with skeletal age matching chronological age for the average maturer. This demonstrates that early maturers take 4 to 5 years fewer to reach skeletal age 20. Furthermore, early maturers tend to go through the pubertal growth period in a shorter time than late maturers do.

Our representation of pubertal development is based on a 4-year period of pubertal development, which underestimates early–late differences and is conservative. Note that the early maturer finishes puberty at a time when the late maturer is entering it.

Biological change towards maturity is reviewed in relation to the structural and functional aspects of skeletal, tissue, and system changes. The rate and age of maturity vary greatly among the many different biological characteristics, so maturity must be defined and described separately for each. With this limitation in mind, some general patterns of change can be described.

The neurological system matures quite early so as to provide the basis for the early development of movement control. The development of some functions, such as brain lateralization, may not be complete until later years, but the neurological system is mature in most respects by the early school years. The rate of change varies among different parts of the neurological system and seems related more to functional need than to structural order. The rate of change also varies within a particular area of the brain, seemingly to serve one aspect of movement before another. For example, the neural development of arm and trunk movements in motor and sensory areas occurs before the neural development of leg movements in the same areas. Also, sensory and motor areas develop in relation to one another in ways that reflect their roles in specific aspects of movement control.

The pattern of height change provides a general pattern of change for body size and some aspects of muscle functioning. These changes go through four periods, beginning with rapid early development and followed by a consistent period of change until puberty. The third period of change during puberty is rapid and produces important structural and functional changes. The fourth period is a time of little or no change when individuals reach a mature state. Changes across these four periods are quite substantial and lead to an increase in body size, changes in body proportions, an increase in the muscle–fat ratio, and changes in cardiorespiratory functioning to provide more oxygen to fuel muscular activity. These changes are unified and so have a greater potential for producing forceful movements.

Individuals vary greatly in maturity state when measured by skeletal age, peak height velocity, and similar measures. It is possible to label individuals as early or late maturers by using one or more of these measures, but individual patterns of change for height are quite similar when adjusted to an age baseline reflecting maturity level. Individual patterns of change for other biological characteristics have not been described in sufficient detail to make comparisons of this type.

Physiological, neural, and sensory functional changes
Functional and some structural changes are taken together in this section, as both growth of the structures and the effects of growth on movement are considered. Functional aspects of biological changes are limited here to systems that might influence the development of movement control. We consider the development of physiological functioning for oxygen transport and the related metabolic needs, followed by the nervous system and the sensory systems. Physiological functioning is related to endurance more than to movement skill, but the neuromotor system depends on these physiological resources to a certain level in order to function. For greater detail of these functions, see Armstrong and van Mechelen (2008).

PHYSIOLOGICAL SYSTEMS

Oxygen uptake and usage
The physiological changes important to muscular activity are centred on the intake, transportation, and use of oxygen. The cycle consists of taking air into the lungs, extracting oxygen from the air, transporting oxygen through the cardiovascular system to muscles and other functional units, and gathering carbon dioxide for transport back to the lungs, where the cycle continues by expelling carbon dioxide and gathering additional oxygen. This is a simple and superficial description of the route taken by oxygen to supply a necessary commodity in the energy operations of muscular activity. Oxygen uptake and usage are important in a number of ways, including the ability to take in large amounts of air, transport large amounts of oxygen, and exchange large amounts of oxygen at the places where it is needed. These are functions of the pulmonary and cardiovascular systems. It is thought that oxygen uptake and usage improve from birth to maturity and that males and females are similar in this respect until just before the pubertal years, when males improve their oxygen uptake and usage more than females.

The data for aerobic measures are consistent with body size appropriately controlled for; males' peak V_{O_2} increases with age through childhood to young adulthood, whereas females' peak V_{O_2} levels off at around 14 years of age. Similarly, anaerobic measures present age related increases and in addition show a marked more increase than aerobic fitness during adolescence. Armstrong and Fawkner (2008) review exercise metabolism in children and conclude that there is interplay of both anaerobic and aerobic metabolism, with young people exhibiting higher oxidative activity than adults.

Armstrong et al (2008) argue that peak V_{O_2} is the best measure of aerobic fitness, with males and, to a lesser extent, females (the latter peaking at 14) showing almost linear increases from childhood through adolescence into emerging adulthood. Peak V_{O_2} is higher in the prepubertal years for males and this difference increases with age. Measures of peak V_{O_2} are often clouded by body size, and when this is controlled a different picture emerges. Males remain remarkably consistent when this measure is factored out, whereas females show a progressive decline. However, this statistic is obtained by dividing V_{O_2} by body mass, and Armstrong et al (2008) argue that this favours light subjects and penalizes heavy ones. This ratio scaling has led to misinterpretation of physiological variables, and more sophisticated models of controlling for body size are now beginning to show different results. Using multilevel regression models on longitudinal rather than cross-sectional data, there is a conflict with conventional wisdom as outlined above, with both sexes showing progressive increases in peak V_{O_2}, independent of the influence of body size. With body size controlled, males have a higher peak V_{O_2} than females, and this difference increases with growth. Armstrong et al (2008) conclude by saying that, no matter how peak V_{O_2} is measured, it is higher in males than females from 10 years of age onwards.

The interesting variable of locomotor economy is described in detail by Morgan (2008) who defined it as 'the mass-related oxygen consumption (V_{O_2}) for a given sub-maximal speed' (p. 283). These types of data would be particularly useful for designing therapeutic regimes for children with physical difficulties. His general conclusions are that children increase in economy with age into adolescence and adulthood, and from walking and running studies the explanations for this include higher stride frequency, a larger body surface-area-to-mass ratio, and greater muscle coactivation of the legs. As with many of these measures, there is interindividual variability, which can be reduced by treadmill practice. Females tend to be more economical than males in running and walking energy costs, which is thought to be because of a greater reliance on anaerobic metabolism, more stable limb movement coordination patterns and less fat-free mass. In children with cerebral palsy there is an increase in energy expenditure with age that shows less economy than in children without cerebral palsy. From the few studies that are available, Morgan (2008) concludes that this is due to greater motor dysfunction, a lower leg-strength-to-body-mass ratio, excess lower-limb muscle coactivation, and less mobility, and thus restricts options. He does, however, note an important point, which is relevant to our emphasis on dynamical explanations of movement: basic gait parameters such as speed, stride length, and height appear to be geared to the minimization of aerobic demand. In other words, the system is self-organizing to the parameters and constraints that are present.

Thermoregulation plays its part in activities for children of all ages, and children's responses to changes in hot and cold environments differ from those of adults. Children have a larger surface-area-to-mass ratio and a smaller volume of blood, making them rely on dry heat loss more and sweating when warm less, and this lower sweating rate in children is a major difference between children and adults. Hot and cold environments change body temperatures in children more than in adults, and this is accompanied in children by a higher metabolic cost in the cold and a greater intolerance to heat. However, unless there are extremes of high temperature, children manage their core temperatures pretty well through lower sweating rates but relatively high surface area. Falk and Dotan (2008) when summarizing this also note that there is much to be done in this area on such topics as the developmental interaction between all of the variables involved in temperature regulation, what happens during adolescence, sex differences, and the effect of training and acclimatization.

Fawkner (2008) in examining the developmental changes in the pulmonary system notes that its aim is to maintain blood–gas homeostasis under all conditions, requiring the maintenance of the partial pressure of oxygen and carbon dioxide. She concedes that much is not known in this area in children but makes a number of tentative conclusions. First, the lungs increase in length and width in relation to height and weight, with females' velocity peaking at 12 to 13 and males' at 14 to 15 years of age. Similar increases are seen in thorax size, airways, alveoli number, and muscle strength, which all contribute to increases in lung function with age. As females go through puberty earlier than males, there is a short period when their lung volume and functions are superior to those of males, but at all other times males outperform females in these measures.

When any form of activity is undertaken, the supply of blood and its constituent parts is crucial; thus, the developmental adaptations of the cardiovascular system are of particular importance. Rowland (2008) makes the point that this is true for both adults and children, but the difference being that children's systems are in a constant state of evolution. He summarizes a number of variables associated with cardiovascular functions and how they change developmentally. Heart rate progressively falls with age from 85 beats per minute (bpm) at age 4 to about 60bpm at age 18, with mean rates in females about 2 or 3bpm faster at all ages. This decline is linked to size-relative basal metabolic rate because, although calorie expenditure rises in absolute terms with age, when adjusted for body size it actually declines by 23% from 6 to 16 years of age, paralelling the decrease in heart rate (Rowland 2008). There is a dearth of studies on stroke volume in early childhood, but Rowland (2008) reports that it does seem to remain stable between the ages of 10 and adulthood. He also concludes that the responses of the cardiovascular system to exercise are no different in growing children (from age 10) than in mature adults, but that there are a number of gaps in our knowledge such as whether sex differences in cardiac responses are independent of body composition.

Vital capacity
Respiratory ability is measured in a number of ways, with vital capacity as a representative pattern of change. Vital capacity, which is maximal expiration following maximal inspiration, increases at a similar rate in both males and females until about age 12, when males improve at a faster rate to have an approximately 20% greater vital capacity at age 20. As males are larger than females at maturity, their increased vital capacity might be merely a matter of greater size with relatively the same vital capacity. This seems to be the case in the prepubertal years, when males are slightly larger and have a slightly larger vital capacity. Females enter puberty earlier than males, and there is a period when their lung volumes and

dynamic lung capacity are superior to males' (Fawkner 2008). Vital capacity is related to body size, with no sex differences until the older ages, when body sizes are larger for both males and females. Males at maturity are both larger than females and have a larger vital capacity in relation to body size.

Heart rate, blood pressure and red blood cells
The mean resting (basal) heart rate decreases by between 15 to 20bpm from the early years to age 10, with males and females being similar until age 10, when males continue to decrease and provide more pressure per pulse for fewer pulses per minute. Pulse pressures increase during the pubertal years, with females' levelling off at age 13, while males' continue to increase. Males at maturity have more pressure per pulse for fewer pulses per minute than females. Systolic blood pressure rises steadily during childhood, and, during the pubertal years, females' systolic blood pressure increases less than males'. There is very little change in diastolic blood pressure during the pubertal years, and thus the increased changes in pulse pressure during these years are in systolic blood pressure, which is related to greater basal stroke volume. Finally, blood volume increases from birth to maturity, with males and females having similar blood volume until the pubertal years, when males' volume increases more than females'.

A greater blood volume means a larger number of red blood cells to transport more oxygen to the muscles and carry more carbon dioxide away from the muscles. The general pattern of change, as expected from the changes in blood volume, is that males and females have a similar pattern of increase until the pubertal years, with males increasing noticeably beyond age 12, when females level off.

In summary, oxygen uptake and usage improve to provide a greater supply of energy resources for muscular activity. Males and females develop at a similar level and rate until puberty. Mature males tend to have better intake, transport, and use of oxygen.

Sex differences before puberty have minor implications for movement development, except that females are approximately 20% more mature than males in many of the biological characteristics described here. Changes during the pubertal years lead to males being larger and potentially stronger than females. Strength potential is related to males having more muscle mass and increased cardiorespiratory functioning. Individuals vary so much in their chronological age of entering and completing puberty that developmental comparisons of any kind are confounded from chronological ages 10 to 18 by the individual's pubertal state.

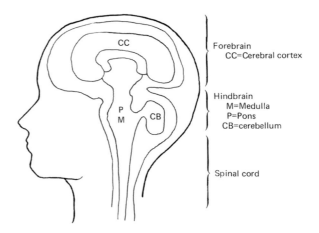

Fig. 2.12 A general representation of selected neural structures (Keogh and Sugden 1985).

NERVOUS SYSTEM
The nervous system extends to all regions of the body and participates in all body functions by gathering, organizing, and transporting information. The cerebral cortex is the structural top of the nervous system, interacting with others on the structural–functional scale through to the individual neurone, which combines with other neurones to transmit neural signals. A general representation of several important neural structures is shown in Figure 2.12. Areas of importance are the spinal cord, hindbrain, and forebrain. The spinal cord contains nerve fibres in the spinal roots and nerves and their branches. The hindbrain contains the medulla, pons, midbrain, and cerebellum, and the forebrain is dominated by the cerebral hemispheres, which contain the cerebral cortex.

Brown et al (1997) point out that the development of the brain and nervous system is not totally genetically led but an interaction of the genetic information and environmental factors. They continue by noting that neural development is not a simply linear increase of new cells, but involves the removal of excess ones and the remodelling of others. A good example of this is that most cells in the nervous system generally start in a different place to where they eventually end up in the mature organ.

Neural growth
The neurone is the basic cellular structure of the nervous system, with nerve impulses travelling along the neurones to transmit information. Information is relayed from one cell to another via a synapse, which is a junction between two cells. Information is transmitted throughout the nervous system by the neurones and their synapses. The axon, which is the part of the neurone along which the nerve impulses travel, is surrounded by a sheath of fatty

material known as myelin. One of the functions of myelin is to insulate each axon from its neighbours, thus avoiding confusion in the messages passing down each one and being a catalyst for increased neural conduction velocity.

Neurones develop over a long time, with different ones forming at different times. In general, large neurones are produced before small ones, with local circuit neurones usually being the last to be formed (Brown et al 1997). Neural conduction velocity changes quite dramatically in the early months to add to the functional complexity of early neural development. The conduction velocity of the nerve is directly proportional to the diameter of the nerve, and in the peripheral nervous system the motor nerve conduction time increases by about 1m/s per week between 20 and 30 weeks' gestation from 20 to 30m/s, with above 60m/s being customary in adults; much of this is due to myelinization (Brown et al 1997).

Tanner (1990) cautions on the use of brain size or weight as a measure of development because different parts of the brain grow at different rates and reach maximum velocities at different times. However, coarse-grained descriptions show that the brain at birth is approximately 25% of the weight of an adult brain. This proportion is 50% at 6 months, 75% at 2 years and 6 months, and 90% at 5 years. Contrast this with the weight of the whole body, which at birth is about 5% of the weight of a young adult's and about 50% at 10 years. The rate of growth in brain size is near its maximum at birth, and by 6 years of age children have achieved almost all of their adult brain size (Kessen et al 1970). The midbrain, pons, and medulla occupy 8% of the total volume at 3 months fetal age, but by birth this has fallen to 1.5%. From 1 to 10 years, the percentage increases again slightly because of fibre tract growth. The cerebrum increases in percentage in utero and then decreases as the cerebellum increases in relative size.

Much of the early growth in brain size and weight can be attributed to myelinization, and Brown et al (1997) note that myelin makes up one-quarter of mature brain weight. In some parts, myelinization in the brain takes place in the first year of life, but myelinization in other parts of the nervous system continues into the pubertal growth years. The process of myelinization has been extensively examined as an index of neural growth. Before myelinization, neurones have slower transmission rates, are prone to fatigue, and are limited in their rate of repetitive firing. Myelination increases conduction velocity by up to ten-fold, and the relative rates of myelinization in different areas of the brain give a rough idea of when these areas reach adult levels of functioning (Bronson 1982, Brown et al 1997). Both sensory and motor pathways begin myelinization 5 to 6 months before birth. In the sensory system, subcortical afferents are in a relatively advanced

stage of myelinization by birth, but the pathways in the neocortex begin the process only at or shortly before birth. A similar sequence is found in the motor system with, for example, the pyramidal tract, which is the major efferent pathway from the motor cortex, beginning myelinization a month before birth and achieving full myelinization by the end of the first year. Brown et al (1997) note that myelinization of the peripheral nerves, spinal cord, brainstem, cerebellum, basal ganglia, thalamus, and cortex occur in a caudal to rostral order. Myelinization is rapid in some areas, being completed between 38 weeks of gestation and 6 weeks after birth in areas such as the pons, cerebellar white matter, and brainstem, with the cerebellum being poorly myelinated at birth but completely myelinated and resembling that of an adult by 3 months of age. The corpus callosum begins myelinization 8 weeks after birth. The relationship between myelinization and function is complex. For example, Brown et al (1997) report that the leg myelinates early, yet function in the form of walking is relatively late, although one could speculate that spontaneous kicking may be a result of early myelinization.

Cortical development

The human cerebral cortex is identifiable at about 8 weeks following conception and by 26 weeks shows a typical structure. All nerve cells present in adults are thought to be formed during the first 20 or 30 weeks in utero, and subsequent development is from cell differentiation, axon and dendrite growth, and myelinization, with only a few new nerve cells appearing. The cortex at birth is functioning but poorly organized. In the first 2 years of life, development occurs in a regular order with the primary motor and sensory areas being among the first to develop, illustrating the primacy of perception and movement early in life. The development spreads to the association areas and the frontal lobe, followed by areas such as the hippocampus and cingulate gyri. In the first year of life, the parietal and frontal lobes develop rapidly, whereas the second year is characterized by growth of the temporal and occipital lobes and the cingulate gyrus, with the latter not complete by 2 years of age. At this time, the primary sensory and motor areas have reached equivalent states of development, but the brain as a whole keeps developing at least until adolescence. Tanner (1990) makes the key point that fibres providing impulses to the cortex myelinate at the same time as those taking impulses away, proposing that maturation occurs in functional units not geographical areas.

There is considerable growth after birth in many structures, including marked changes in both surface areas and fissurization, especially during the first year. There is considerable debate as to the extent to which environmental conditions can influence brain maturation and organization. From comparisons of preterm with typically developing term infants, it seems that most of the changes in cortical activity are related to age rather than environment; that is, early neural development is primarily a matter of biological maturation. However, extreme environmental conditions, such as malnutrition, can influence neural development, and there are times when the neural system is more vulnerable to disease and injury.

Neural plasticity
One of the characteristic features of the nervous system is the ability to reorganize itself as a consequence of experiences. Typically, as the child learns, neural pathways are developed and when there is atypical development, as following some insult to the brain, there is often the capability to compensate for any loss of function or to maximize those parts that remain. Closely connected to neural plasticity is the concept of a sensitive or critical period, referring to times within a child's life when some functions appear to have optimum development with a decreasing development before or after that time. Human abilities such as language have been extensively studied with particular attention on children who, for a variety of reasons, have not developed language at the typical time. Specifically, if there has been damage to the language centres in the brain, the question asked is whether other centres can take over and whether there is a time limit for this to occur. We do know that the brain is amenable to change or is plastic and that experiences are influential in facilitating this plasticity. This capability is of particular value for children who have other forms of disability, such as cerebral palsy, autistic spectrum disorder, or attention deficit disorder, for example, and an exciting area for future research that may change the way we work with them. Currently, the work is in its infancy, with questions surrounding which areas of the brain are most amenable to change, what time periods in an individual's life are most susceptible to change, and what type of experiences directly lead to any structural plasticity.

Growth and function
There is a usefulness in the gross distinction between the subcortical (spinal cord, brainstem) and the neocortical (cortex) systems, especially at the neonatal period. At the time of birth, human infants are in a transition period in which cortical influence is marginally present or about to emerge. Newborn infants are largely influenced by the better-developed subcortical systems, and the emergence of neocortical influence is reflected in early changes in infant behaviour. Thus, in the early postnatal period, reactions such as reflexes, which usually require only subcortical control, should be more readily elicited. In reactions requiring neocortical participation, there should be a wide range of individual differences, and there should be a rapid postnatal advance in motor abilities, as neocortical control starts to provide a more complex level of neural organization.

An example of functional development in the higher centres is the differentiation of functions between the right and left hemispheres. Owing to their physical separation and the results of some early split-brain experiments, it has been customary to view the different hemispheric functions in dichotomous terms. Analytic processing in the left hemisphere versus Gestalt or holistic in the right is an example. These rigid dichotomies have been questioned (Henderson 1982), although it is clear that different processing functions are preferred by each hemisphere. The left hemisphere of adults generally contains mechanisms for speech, and damage here is more likely to show language deficits in patients than damage to the right hemisphere, which tends to specialize in spatial relations (especially visual cues).

There are many questions regarding the two hemispheres' specialization of function, such as when specialization or lateralization of function occurs. Hand dominance is seen quite early in infants, often as young as 3 months old when they will make more 'fists' with one hand than the other (Michel and Harkins 1986), but there is not a complete one-to-one correspondence between the preferred fisting and later-established hand dominance. Brown et al (1997) note that the young infant probably uses both sides of the brain in learning skills and employs a mirroring strategy, which is superseded by a lateralization effect involving suppression of one side to favour the other and usually occurring between the ages of 3 and 6 years. Some have argued for a propensity for lateralization at birth, with lateralization by 5 years of age (Hiscock and Kinsbourne 1978). Others feel that hemispheric lateralization occurs later. What is relatively clear is that it is practically complete by 10 to 12 years of age. Much of the evidence comes from studies of aphasia, in which recovery is much more common below ages 10 to 12 than at older ages. It is as though the brain is relatively plastic in the early years, and so speech function can be taken over by the right hemisphere. After about 12 years of age, however, the prognosis is poor.

Structure and function seem to be interrelated in a complex manner. For example, fibres associated with auditory stimulation myelinate as early as the sixth fetal month and continue to myelinate up to 4 years of age. The visual system starts to myelinate later, just after birth, but myelinization is then completed very quickly. If we relate these comparisons to function, audition is analysed at subcortical levels in utero and becomes cortical after birth through a slow development. Vision is not needed in utero, but its development must proceed rapidly after birth to provide a functional system in a short period of time. Audition can function adequately with the slower rate of myelinization, whereas visual development requires a more rapid rate of myelinization at a particular time. Myelinization is related more to functional units than to neuroanatomical regions.

There are two clear divisions of neural development in the first 2 years of life after birth. First is the order in which the various areas of the brain develop, and second is the order in which the body functions associated with these areas develop. The primary motor area, for example, is the most advanced, followed by the primary sensory area, and gradually development spreads out from these areas. Within the motor and sensory areas, the nerve cells controlling movements of the arms and upper trunk develop ahead of those controlling the legs. Although the motor cortex develops earlier than the other neural areas, the legs remain the last to develop in the motor cortex. By 2 years of age, the primary sensory area has caught up with the primary motor area, and the association areas have developed further, but other areas are still immature. In summary, the human brain undergoes both quantitative and qualitative changes from conception to maturity. The brain grows bigger and increases its number of cells, folds, and fissures; myelinization occurs; and the amount of water decreases. The brain also changes in function, as illustrated by hemispheric lateralization, which is complete by ages 10 to 12.

This section reviewed change towards maturity for body size, proportions and composition and neurological and cardiorespiratory functioning. Although variability is the rule for different biological characteristics and individuals, there is an underlying organization and order that seems to reflect functional development. We noted this in our summary statements about changes in neurological development being related to the early development of movement control, and changes in body make-up and muscle functioning being related to the later development of speeded and forceful movements. Although we cannot capture this complex organization and larger order, there appears to be an overall unity that is lost when looking at smaller pieces of the total picture.

SENSORY SYSTEMS

Vision and kinaesthesis are crucial elements in the control, performance, and learning of skilled movements. We are describing them separately, but in our actions they work together providing us with information about our movements and the contexts in which they occur. Working in unison, they enable us to specify the environmental context, provide ongoing control of our movements, and supply continuous feedback. This section describes the fundamental processes involved in vision and kinaesthesis. The development of these processes in the production of movement are analysed in many of the following chapters.

Vision

The role of vision

First, vision gives an instant and simultaneous picture of the environmental context. There is no other sense that gives us this in so much detail and with so much clarity. Vision shows where objects and people are located in the environment, helping us to negotiate these objects according to our goals. Of great importance is the information vision provides about moving objects and people that are part of our everyday experiences. Crossing a road without vision is hazardous, and even using our acute auditory sense there are still bicycles and other pedestrians who provide little information other than what is gained from vision. In sporting environments we use vision in skiing to pick out a route and keep away from danger. Skiers often talk of the difficulty they have in 'white out' conditions when they cannot see the environment and are often confused in some light when the snowline becomes indistinguishable from the horizon, often with nauseous consequences. More routinely, vision is the primary source for locating objects in our everyday activities, such as in self-care, cooking, work, and recreation. Audition is the only other sensory system that is useful in obtaining spatial information about objects that are out of reach, yet audition can only provide that information if the object or person emits sound, and even then the information is not as rich, accurate, or detailed as that from vision.

Second, vision allows us to predict events within environmental contexts, something no other sense can give us. Thus, we are able to see two moving objects about to collide with one another and take evasive action; we are able to anticipate the outstretched arms of a child or loved one rather than having to wait until there has been contact; and we are able to simply reach out to shake hands. In all of these and other activities, vision is our guiding sense. Whether it is to avoid danger, to express our feelings, or simply to engage in the normal actions of daily life, vision provides us with the rich information to enable this to occur.

Third, vision often acts as a control of movement. When reaching and grasping a cup or another object, vision can act as a guide towards the cup aiding not only the spatial trajectory of the arm–hand action but also in a temporal sense by assisting the hand with the correct timing for the shaping of the hand towards the cup and the ultimate closing of the hand to grasp. This does not imply that vision is constantly altering and guiding the hand, as the movement is often ballistic with little ongoing feedback. It does, however, mean that guidance is often included, and when it is not, it is most likely that vision has provided the information that allows the timing and spatial characteristics of the ballistic movements to be appropriate. In a complex skill such as driving, we constantly use visual cues to determine how much to accelerate and how much to brake as well as in the very obvious act of steering. In these two examples of how vision helps to control movement there are distinct differences. The first example is a rather short movement, both in time and in space, involving one arm. The other involves both arms and legs, being continuous over time, and incorporating the movement of another object, in this case a car, almost as part of the extended body. These two examples serve to illustrate how vision takes on different roles according to the demands of the task.

Fourth, vision allows us to correct any errors we make by providing feedback not just about the end product but also the manner in which the errors have been made. For example, when a ball is thrown to another person, vision provides information about time and space: the ball being thrown too far, too hard, at the wrong time, or all of these. Vision allows us to check the legibility and accuracy of handwriting or keyboard inputs. It also allows us to note when everything is progressing according to plan and when adjustment is required.

Fifth, vision links with other sensory information, particularly kinaesthesia, to provide information that is intersensory in nature and not simply a one plus one of visual and kinaesthetic sensory input but a complete and different whole that is forged from the two modalities.

A final, and often overlooked, feature of vision is that it provides redundancy in terms of allowing many ways of knowing the same thing, from different angles in different lights, from different distances, and by verifying information obtained from other sources. Thus when a sculptor is examining his or her work, he or she can do so from various sides, the top, or the bottom and from a distance or close by. No other sense gives us this detail of information. Through this, vision is not only providing information but also becomes motivational by providing the individual with information that acts as an incentive for the person to engage in the environmental context (Sugden and Keogh 1990, Schmidt and Lee 2005, Magill 2007). This motivational quality of vision is one that is later described with respect to overall development.

The importance of vision in movement is demonstrated by the term perception–action coupling, which is often used to describe the close connection between the eyes and the hands or feet in actions such as writing and drawing, driving a car, or kicking and trapping a ball, emphasizing the link between the eyes and the limbs and body. This link between vision and action has been found across many contexts to involve both temporal and spatial coupling of the limbs and body and eyes.

Aspects of visual development

The roles that vision plays are supported by the development of a number of separate yet interconnected visual processes, all contributing to the resulting richness of information that vision supplies. The processes that develop begin with the fundamental ones of acuity and accommodation, which lead to the utility of vision in more complex and demanding situations as the child develops and starts to move in a changing environmental context. Many of these are detailed in Chapters 4, 5 and 6.

Visual acuity is an attribute that develops early in life and is the ability to detect fine spatial patterns. It is often measured by grating, which involves parallel vertical lines separated by a background of regular spaces which are made narrower to the point where the observer can no longer differentiate the lines from the background. The development of visual acuity enables the infant to see the detail of any object, with the focal distance for acuity at birth being 4 to 10 inches and increasing rapidly to normal adult acuity within the first year of life. How quickly infants develop acuity following visual deprivation was examined by Maurer et al (1990), who studied infants deprived of visual input because of cataracts they had been born with in one or both eyes. After 3 months the cataracts were removed and contact lenses inserted, resulting in newborn-like acuity after 10 minutes across all of the infants and further improvement after 1 hour of focused visual input.

Location in depth of objects and people is an important spatial dimension and there are numerous cues for depth perception, one being binocularity, which is available by virtue of the fact that we have two eyes. At birth the eyes' muscles do not work together smoothly and the infant uses monocular vision which changes to binocular functioning, which consists of the convergence angle of the two eyes and stereopsis, the disparity between the two images received by each eye. Through the use of different behavioural and electrophysiological methods, we find that the onset of binocularity usually occurs between the ages of 10 and 16 weeks, with considerable variation even in typically developing children (Braddick 1996).

Accommodation enables us to see objects close up by bringing them into focus, and in humans this occurs by altering the power of the lens. This is done through the ciliary muscles attached to the lens, which cause it to thicken, increasing its curvature and enabling the eye to focus on nearby objects. Like many visual features this facility improves rapidly in the first 3 to 4 months of life and reaches adult-like responses by the end of the first year.

Objects have a constancy in that they will remain the same shape even when the retinal image has changed, and through constancy we are able to recognize different sensory input as having the same perceptual meaning. As young as 6 weeks, infants will attend to the actual size of objects, not just their retinal image. Objects must also be perceived in relation to other objects in order to recognize perceptually the whole display. Thus figure–ground perception is studied to examine how and why some objects become figures and others background.

Figure–ground relationships are changeable and complex, but young infants do have sufficient perceptual development to identify people and objects as separate from the background.

The perception of depth is another much-studied aspect of visual perception that enables us to judge how far to reach for a glass of water (absolute distance judgement) or whether a man is further away than a boy even though the man looks smaller because he is 200m further away (relative distance judgement). By 4 months of age infants are relatively accurate in reaching and grasping, which suggests that their absolute distance judgement for close objects is reasonable even if their motor control limits them. The ability to judge relative distance involves using a number of visual cues, such as binocular parallax, with each eye giving a slightly different retinal image or visual picture. The visual system integrates the two retinal images into one visual picture, with the two inputs providing depth and distance cues. An interesting developmental consideration in binocular parallax is that adults' eyes are twice as far apart as newborn infants', which means that ongoing calibration is required throughout the growing years. Motion parallax is another visual cue in which objects on the retinal image are displaced when the head is turned and moved. The amount of retinal displacement of objects is a function of their distance and direction from the point of focus. The direction and rate of retinal displacement indicate the objects' relative distance. Motion parallax is not subject to the same growth problems as binocular parallax because changes in retinal image as a function of head movement are independent of physical growth changes. Another visual cue for distance is optical expansion, which occurs whenever the distance between the perceiver and another person or object changes. Optical expansion as well as contraction specify proportional changes from the staring point rather than distance in absolute terms.

Another important feature of the visual system is the ability to detect motion, with this facility being found in every species. This ability is fundamental to perception, cognition, and action, contributing and elaborating, for example, knowledge of action of the individual and the control of actions. Anticipation, coincidence, and tracking of moving people and objects, so important to actions in our daily life, are all reliant on the detection of motion. Braddick et al (2003) acknowledge some sensitivity to dynamic stimuli very early in life, but what they label 'the classic criterion' of directional selection, that is a differential response to a target that moves at the same speed in the opposite direction, they believe comes a little later. There is evidence that some direction of movement is registered early, but Braddick et al (2003) argue that this is a subcortical reflex system and that infants start to use cortical control systems around 2 to 3 months of age. This continues to develop through early childhood and reaches adult levels, depending on the task, by around 10 years of age.

How does vision provide information?
The roles of *central* and *peripheral* vision provide different sets of information in the control of movement. Central vision, sometimes called *foveal* vision, detects information in the environment in the middle 2 to 5 degrees of the visual field. Peripheral vision detects information in the wider environmental field, which can be around 200 degrees horizontally and 160 degrees vertically (Magill 2006). Both of these are used in everyday activities such as walking, with central vision guiding the person on the correct path and peripheral vision monitoring other events in the environment. Peripheral vision is important in the detection of optical flow, which involves patterns of light striking the retina from the environmental context. This enables the detection of moving objects, or the change in the optical array when we move, thus helping us to move effectively through the environment. As the individual moves or if the environment changes, the angles of the rays of light change, thus providing different information. To take a sporting example, on a putting green where the surface of the green is not constant, there will be more optical flows from the balls and the undulation of the green will provide the golfer with many pieces of, often complex, visual information, making the putting action difficult.

One popular theory of how vision provides information proposes two distinct methods of visual processing, known as the ventral and dorsal streams (Goodale and Milner 1992). The two streams take in information from the environment through the retina and subsequently process the information in the primary visual cortex, but they have two different roles. The ventral stream is argued to be responsible for specifying the layout of the environment, providing a rich source of information and the location of objects and people and their movements. The ventral stream has often been called the 'vision for perception system'. The dorsal stream, on the other hand, is proposed to be responsible for the visual control of movements. Thus when walking into a room, the ventral stream would specify the layout of the room and where the door is, whereas the dorsal stream would guide the hand towards the door handle such that it could be turned to open the door. The dorsal stream has often been called the 'vision for action system' (Goodale and Milner 1992, Brown et al 2005). Support for the two streams has come from studies of patients with brain injuries, with some patients being able to recognize objects but not use them effectively and other patients exhibiting the opposite in not being able to recognize the objects but being able to use them in an appropriate manner (Goodale and Milner 1992). Schmidt and Lee (2005) remind us that both streams would work in tandem in a task such as hammering a nail, with the ventral stream specifying the location of the nail and the dorsal stream controlling the action of hammering. The absence of both of these streams, as in blind children, would cause different and serious blockages to movement competence. Much of the evidence for the two streams comes from specific populations of individuals with particular forms of brain damage, and the results may not be generalizable to typical populations. For example, the streams are not necessarily absent in children with dorsal and ventral stream dysfunction. Some of the children with this disorder may have normal acuity and visual fields and thus differ from other children with severe visual impairment.

The visual processing research also notes the concept of 'time to contact', offering an explanation as to how we process fast-moving visual information such as car driving or ball catching. Time to contact or tau was first proposed by Lee (1980, 1990, 1998) and Lee and Young (1985), emanating from earlier work and theorizing by James Gibson (1966). As a moving object (e.g. a ball) approaches, the light rays from the ball increase in a specific manner. The ball casts a retinal image that increases in size as it approaches and increases in size faster the higher the speed of the ball. This is illustrated in a formula that relates the speed and size of the approaching ball to the optical/retinal expansion, and Lee called this 'tau'. This can be specified mathematically with tau being the inverse of the relative rate of change in the visual angle made by a moving object with the speed of the object remaining constant. It allows predictability by affording the start of an action to occur with no real central cognitive processing, simply relying on optical expansion, which drives a time-to-contact. Again this theory has come under scrutiny with some researchers noting that tau is an important variable but not sufficient to totally explain vision's role in activities such as ball catching and becomes much more complex when a person has to move to catch a ball that does not come directly to them (Magill 2006).

A more recent visual property, and discussed in Chapter 9, is the bearing angle, which is the angle between a moving object, the interception point, and the individual who is trying to intercept the object and can be considered as an on-line control strategy. If the bearing angle is kept constant, it provides enough information for interception without the need for continuous computing of input data. Recent work, on tasks such as walking to intercept a moving ball, has found the bearing angle to be kept constant and used more successfully in adults and older children aged 10 to 12 years than in younger children aged 5 to 7 years (Chohan et al 2006, 2008). It remains to be seen how much potential this variable can offer to explain interceptive movements, but it is showing another visual cue with potential use.

The role that vision plays in movement is substantial in the many ways that have been described above. Vision also interacts with other sensory systems such as proprioception, with terms such as visuoproprioception being used to describe this link (Lee and Aaronson 1974). When skills are being learned, depending on the nature of the task, we often rely on vision in the first instance and as we become more proficient we shift more to proprioceptive control. One has only to look at beginners learning to play soccer or basketball who appear to need constant visual monitoring of the hand and foot on the ball compared with skilled players who have their 'head off' the ball, seeking out cues in the constantly moving context. Vision's importance in the performance and learning of motor skills cannot be overemphasized because it provides information in so many different ways. The effect that vision has on the movements of the developing child is described and analysed through many studies presented in Chapters 4 to 6.

Kinaesthesis
A traditional definition of kinaesthesis refers to a person's knowledge, without the use of vision or other perceptual inputs, but kinaesthesis also has a strong relationship with other sensory perceptual modalities, particularly vision in our actions. Kinaesthesis is widely acknowledged to play an important role in motor skill learning and performance, providing information concerning the body and its parts at the beginning, during, and at the end of any movement. Kinaesthetic information is gathered through a number of

quite different sensory receptors that combine to provide knowledge about the body's position and movement; these tend to be internal (within our body). Below, five types of sensory receptors are reviewed and the contributions of each are described. We cannot document their developmental progress and precise involvement in the development of body knowledge, but kinaesthesis is information available across the lifespan, as long as the musculoskeletal system functions in an optimal fashion. Clearly the very young and the very old have less than optimal functioning because of the early development of infants and the process of ageing in the elderly, which can mask optimal information from muscle and joint complexes.

Receptors

Numerous receptors, located in the muscles, tendons, bones, and moveable joints, respond to mechanical distortion. Mechanoreceptors are found in bone and muscle structures, and are stimulated by joint movement and changes in muscle length and tension; these are collectively called proprioceptors. Proprioceptors specify joint position and movement (direction, rate, and duration) and information about muscle length and tension. The information is a form of perceptual information that influences motor output. This sensory information goes to all levels of the nervous system, including the spinal cord, cerebellum, and cerebral cortex.

Sensory receptors convert one form of energy, mechanical distortion, into another, bioelectrical. It is thought that the mechanical distortion of unmyelinated sensory endings leads to an enlargement of the membranes' pores, making them more permeable to small ions such as sodium. The electrical current generated when the sensory ending is mechanically distorted is called the *generator potential*, and it is unique to the sensory ending. Once this generator potential reaches a critical level or threshold, the current triggers a nerve impulse. The rate at which each successive nerve impulse is triggered is related proportionately to the size of the generator potential. The number of impulses per unit of time is the frequency code of the receptor, which can signal the strength and location of a single stimulus.

If a stimulus is applied to a receptor for a long period of time, the frequency code will begin to decline in a process known as adaptation. Some mechanoreceptors adapt slowly, thus providing a stable frequency code for an extended duration (5min to over 2h), and others adapt quickly (1min to less than 1s). Slow- and fast-adapting receptors together provide information about the onset, intensity, and duration of the stimulus. Details about the mechanisms of neuromuscular control and the role it may

play in development are limited. We can however survey some of the receptors and their contributions to kinaesthesis. These include vestibular receptors that are not part of the mechanoreceptors in skeletomuscular structures but are important in providing position data with respect to head position.

VESTIBULAR RECEPTORS

Vestibular receptors are different in form and function to other proprioceptors, with a location in the inner ear, and provide information about the position of the head. They are found in the membranous labyrinth, which is loosely located in the bony labyrinth of the skull's temporal bone at the internal end of the external auditory canal. There are two types of receptor organ in the vestibular labyrinth: *cristae* in the semicircular canals and *maculae* in the utricle. Cristae can detect acceleration, deceleration, and the direction of rotary head movement, but they cannot detect head position or the constant velocity of head movement. These receptors are very important to oculomotor reflexes, in which eye movements are matched to head movements. Maculae detect the position of the head relative to gravity and help in righting reflexes. The vestibular system senses acceleration, but when a steady state of motion is obtained, optic flow is used to indicate that movement is occurring; thus vestibular mechanisms are essential for postural stability and change of motion but less so for continuous steady state egomotion.

JOINT RECEPTORS

Nerve branches are distributed in the joint capsule, fibrous cartilage, hyaline cartilage, and articular fat pads, with the receptors being divided into four main categories based on their morphology, location, and physiological characteristics. Three types function as mechanoreceptors, and the fourth is part of the pain receptor system. The first three provide information about joint movement and position, as they respond to the mechanical stresses applied to the nerve ending (Table 2.1). Responses can be classified by location, and joint receptors fall into the two categories of slow- and rapid-adapting receptors. *Slow adapters* respond to both joint position and joint movement, with each receptor having an activation range from 15 to 25 degrees over which it is excited. Joint positions outside this range have no effect, and the receptor remains silent. Within the excitatory range, the receptor has a characteristic frequency rate for different angles. Movement within the activation range produces a transient discharge that quickly declines to a steady state determined by position. *Rapid adapters* are excited by a rapid joint movement in any direction and adapt rapidly when the movement stops. Speed is generally a critical parameter, and motor units

TABLE 2.1
Proprioceptive information available from joint receptors

Movement parameter	Type of receptor	
	Slowly adapting	Rapidly adapting
Joint position (static)	Differential adaptation rates to joint positions within excitatory range	Cannot differentiate
Direction of movement	Differential transient response to movement in opposite direction	Cannot differentiate
Speed of movement	Frequency of transient response related to movement rate; rate of adaptation differs with movement	Different threshold to movement rate

appear to have different thresholds. Joint receptors specify the following information:

1   static position of joint
2   onset, duration, and range of joint movement
3   velocity and acceleration of joint movement
4   pressure and tension on joint structures and joint torque
5   pain in joint structures.

TENDON RECEPTORS

Golgi tendon organs (GTOs) are located predominantly at musculotendinous junctions and less frequently wholly within the tendon. The GTOs are nerve endings that are compressed when tension is placed on the collagen fascicles. When the muscle is relaxed, there is no tension on the loosely packed collagen fibres and no compression of nerve endings. When the muscle stretches or contracts, the collagen fibres are pulled together to compress the nerve endings. Most GTO endings are extremely sensitive to contractile tension placed on the collagen fascicles, which constantly monitor and provide information to the central nervous system on muscular tension. Each GTO probably samples the tension level of several different motor units, and the combined response from all participating receptors provides detailed information concerning the state of the contraction.

PACINIAN CORPUSCLES

These ellipsoidal structures are located in the various connective tissues, such as subcutaneous tissue, fascia of muscle and tendon, and periosteum. The pacinian corpuscles are responsive to the slightest compression, and because of their location in the connective tissues surrounding bone and muscle, they signal pressure caused by muscular contraction. They are capable of adapting rapidly to a maintained pressure and have no capacity to signal different intensities of contraction. However, each pacinian corpuscle has a distinct threshold, and the

nervous system can use the range of stimulated receptors to determine the magnitude of the pressure.

MUSCLE SPINDLE

The muscle spindle is an unusual structure in that it is both an auxiliary motor unit and a sensory organ, which combine to regulate muscle stiffness.

It is located in somatic muscle between the muscle fascicles and parallel to the extrafusal fibres (see Fig. 2.13). It consists of a variable number of intrafusal fibres surrounded by a connective tissue capsule, which is continuous with the connective tissue of the extrafusal fibre fascicles. These intrafusal fibres are innervated by fusimotor neurones, also known as gamma motoneurones. Contraction of the intrafusal fibres does not appreciably add to the gross muscle tension produced by the extrafusal fibres because the intrafusal fibres are fewer in number and smaller in size than the extrafusal fibres. On the other hand, the fusimotor neurones influence gross muscle contraction via the circuit called the gamma loop. Activation by the gamma motoneurones has a triple effect at the spinal level. First, a proprioceptive code is sent through the ascending pathways to the cerebellum and cerebral sensory cortices; second, alpha motoneurones of the same muscle are facilitated; and, third, alpha motoneurones of the antagonistic muscle are inhibited.

The spindle as a motor and sensory mechanism is part of a theory of neuromuscular control known as alpha–gamma coactivation, which states that all muscular contractions are controlled by independent but cooperative signals to the target muscle's alpha and gamma motoneurones. Owing to these cooperative signals, the spindle can be passive or active during gross muscle stretch, which means that it can respond to the length of the muscle but does not always do so. When the spindle is passive, its output is related in a near linear fashion to the length of the passive muscle; that is, it follows the muscle. When the spindle is active, the spindle discharge is a result of both the true muscle length and the rate of gamma activation.

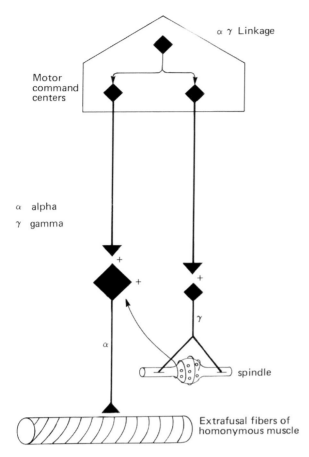

Fig. 2.13 Alpha–gamma coactivation. Reproduced with the permission of J.L. Smith.

In effect, the spindle is set by the gamma motoneurone to expect a certain amount of muscle stretch for an activity, such as walking. Muscle action for walking takes place via the alpha motoneurones, and spindle activity is

a result of muscle stretch plus what has been set by the gamma motoneurones. If the muscle stretch is greater than expected, such as when missing a step while walking downstairs, the spindle will fire its Ia afferents (see Fig. 2.13), which link with the alpha motoneurones and in turn adjust the muscle action. This is the spindle working as a *sensorimotor* organ. Owing to its unique sensorimotor properties, the spindle has become an important part of current theories on motor control.

The functions of sensory receptors described in this section are summarized in Table 2.2. The body is wired in an intricate and interlocking manner to produce position and movement information from many sources. Specific functions can be pinpointed, such as detecting the acceleration of head movements and detecting and regulating muscle stiffness, but we do not know how the more specific functions are combined or used in more complete movements and in adjusting to different movement situations. Also, as noted earlier, we do not know what developmental changes to expect in individual receptors and in the combined use of the information they provide. The sensory receptors described here are the sensory basis of the traditional view of kinaesthesis.

Acuity and recognition
Research on kinaesthesis has typically been investigated as discrimination *acuity* in detecting and being sensitive to differences or matching quantities, such as location, distance, weight, force, time, speed, and acceleration. The stimulus to be detected or matched is usually present, so only acuity is measured. If the stimulus is removed after presentation, kinaesthetic *memory* will also be measured. Kinaesthetic acuity and memory are measured mainly as the extent to which individuals can discriminate stimuli or reproduce a movement. *Discrimination* confirms that a difference exists and judges its extent. Simple examples

TABLE 2.2
Functions of kinaesthetic sensory receptors

Receptor	Type	Function
Type I (Ruffini)	Joint mechanoreceptor	Slow adapting to joint movement and position
Type II (Pacinean)	Joint mechanoreceptor	Fast adapting to rapid movement in any direction
Type III (Golgi)	Joint mechanoreceptor	Slow adapting to joint movement and position
Golgi tendon organ	Tendon mechanoreceptor	Fast adapting to muscle contraction and stretch
Pacinean corpuscle	Connective tissue mechanoreceptor	Fast adapting to muscle contraction pressure
Spindle	Sensorimotor organ	Regulates muscle stiffness through muscle length and gamma bias; provides information about muscle length
Cristae	Vestibular receptor	Detects acceleration, deceleration, and direction of rotary head movements
Maculae	Vestibular receptor	Detects head position in relation to gravity

are comparing the weights of objects and the location, distance, and speed of limb movements. *Reproduction of movements* is used to indicate that a person recognizes certain kinaesthetic information, such as the location, distance, and speed of a previous movement, by accurately repeating it. Kinaesthesis can be measured in terms of space, force, and time, and these variables can be analysed in active, passive, and constrained movements. *Active movements* are measured by requiring individuals to reproduce a movement that they set as a criterion. Typically, blindfolded individuals will actively move a certain distance and then try to reproduce the movement. In *passive movements*, the experimenter moves the participant's limb, and then the subject tries to reproduce the movement. In a passive situation, the participants receive less information during the criterion movement than when they actively set the movement criterion because only sensory and no motor information is available in a passive movement. Between passive and active modes are *constrained movements*, in which the participants actively move but are stopped at a predetermined location. This allows the experimenter to control the distance travelled and the location of the stop. These three types of measurements are often compared to evaluate the efficiency of afferent versus efferent information in a given movement. For example, a task could be performed by using each of the three movement modes. If active movement is superior, the subjects are presumably benefiting from efferent or motor output information. If there is no difference among the movement modes, sensory information is dominant.

As an example of the development of kinaesthesis, Laszlo and Bairstow (1980) and Bairstow and Laszlo (1981) investigated the effects of age on acuity and memory. In the 1980 study, children aged from 5 to 12 years and a group of young adults were tested in an active movement mode on a runway apparatus and a stencil pattern apparatus. In the second study (1981) children had to perform in a passive movement mode. Kinaesthetic acuity in both studies approached adult levels by age 8, although kinaesthetic memory had not reached an adult level at age 12. Other studies have supported this developmental trend, but ages of achievement vary as a result of the demands of different tasks (Smothergill 1973, Sugden 1980).

Kinaesthesis: a contemporary perspective

It is certainly the case that the development of kinaesthesis is important to movement skill production. When absent or in a diminished form regular movement is severely constrained or impossible. Heretofore kinaesthesis has been defined as knowledge about the orientation of the body and its parts in space. It has often been described as the 'feel' of a movement from which the individual gleans preparatory, ongoing, or terminal information about it. At a basic level, infants and young children become able to differentiate their own bodies from the environment, recognize and know their body parts, recognize their orientation in relation to one another, and know their movement functions. The kinaesthetic system also specifies body position and movement through a network of receptors. Kinaesthesis has traditionally been labelled as the 'body-knowledge system' that provides the actor or mover with spatial information with respect to a chosen movement.

A major contemporary development to better understand this so-called 'feel' is to recognize that 'feel' is in fact a dimension of perception globally represented. First by vision (the dominant modality), and second by kinaesthesis, which includes a haptic system, the sense of touch. Haptics, however, provides far more information than mere touch. When we move the muscle–joint system in space, whether we are wielding a hand-held object or moving an arm in space, information is detected via three-dimensional joint motion. This extension of haptic information as a key element of perception provides a more theoretically focused understanding of what we call 'kinaesthesis'. A more contemporary, and empirically supported, description of kinaesthesis is what is referred to as 'dynamic touch' (Turvey 1996). Dynamic touch is the perceptual process that detects (via 'feel') the properties of the moments of inertia generated at the different joint complexes engaged during any particular motion of the body.

> The muscle sense, or dynamic touch (Gibson, 1966; Turvey, 1996), is one of several subsystems making up the haptic perceptual system, which is responsible for perceiving the body (proprioception) and the adjacent environment (exteroception) by means of the body.
> (Carello and Turvey 2004, p. 25)

The importance of muscle sense is dramatically illustrated in individuals with some form of neuropathy. With the loss of muscle sense regular postural control, locomotion, and reaching and grasping are extremely challenging and in some cases impossible. While much has been written about 'kinaesthesis', an empirical understanding of this modality of global perception has gone unnoticed and to a large degree underappreciated (Carello and Turvey 2004). Reliance on vision alone produces a laboured form of coordination and control. Visual control of locomotion demands specific monitoring of each step in terms of both initiating and ending each component of the step cycle.

TABLE 2.3
General achievements in the functional development of body knowledge[a]

Age (y)	Identification of body parts	Laterality	Directionality	Lateral preference: handedness
0–2	Begin to 'show' major body parts (eyes, nose, ears, hands, feet)			Preference changes during first year depending on task
2–5	80% identify eyes 50% identify eyebrows	Left–right discrimination no better than chance Ages 4–5: realization that left and right are opposite sides of the body; unsure of which is which	Very little knowledge of directionality	Ages 3–5: increase in right-handedness
5–7	Ages 5–6: 70% identify all major body parts Age 7: 70% identify minor body parts (elbows, wrists, heels)	Consistent in response whether right or wrong Age 7: mistakes are infrequent	Age 6: mirror and imitate movements Age 7: begin to use body as directional reference of object, but still subjective	Handedness may shift or be inconsistent
7–12	Ages 8–9: mistakes are rare	Beyond ages 7–8: identify all left and right body parts	Age 9: make objective directional references Age 10: identify right and left of person facing them Age 12: begin to use natural reference systems	Ages 9–10: right-handedness stabilizes for approximately 80% Right-eyedness increases Ages 10–11: right hand–eye coordination preference increases

[a] Keogh and Sugden (1985).

This new focus on dynamic touch provides support for the ecological view of direct perception, whereby dynamic touch takes on the mantle of the traditional term 'kinaesthesis', and this view provides a common theme for how visual perception is interpreted.

BODY KNOWLEDGE

In the broadest sense of the word, kinaesthesis would include the development of body knowledge. Body knowledge develops by being sensitive to, and detecting information about, body parts and their functions, recognizing direction of the body, and establishing hand preference.

Movement occurs in a three-dimensional world with the body acting as a central reference point; thus, knowledge about the body is a necessary part of movement. As children grow, they must establish *body knowledge* in many ways and must continuously adjust and calibrate it. A general achievement of infants and young children is becoming able to differentiate between themselves (egocentric) and their environment (allocentric). They come to the realization that there is a separation (boundary) between their body and other objects and persons. Part of this body knowledge is functional, such as a physical knowledge of separateness, and the other part is affective,

such as knowing that one has an existence in thought and emotion. The sum of this physical separateness and identity of self provides a basis for the body to be a reference point in the environment.

Body knowledge can be represented in two ways: first, there is the *functional knowledge* of knowing body parts – their functions and dimensions of external space in relation to body dimensions – and, second, there is *affective knowledge* – how one feels about one's own body. Our discussion here is limited to functional knowledge because it is more directly related to understanding the development of movement control. A summary of achievements in the functional development of body knowledge is presented in Table 2.3, which was compiled from several sources. The achievements are divided into four areas.

Knowledge of body parts

In response to, 'Show me your hands,' infants will look at or raise their hands; from this the infant learns the *verbal identification* of these body parts. In response to a person touching a body part and asking, 'What is this?', children will correctly state, 'This is my arm.' Before they are 18 months old, they can show or touch major parts of their body: eyes, nose, ears, hands, and feet. As they grow older they can recognize other parts, such as elbows and knees, and identify body parts verbally.

Laterality culminates in children using natural frames of reference based on permanent areas and invariant points of reference, such as horizontal–vertical, east–west, and north–south positioning. These progressions appear to be gradual, with sizable changes at ages 7 and 8, and a slower but continued increase to age 12. Closely associated with the knowledge of body parts is children's perception of sides of the body. As they grow older, children realize that their body has two sides, with two hands, two eyes, two legs, and so on. The corresponding parts are similar in size and shape but occupy different positions on the body. Laterality is thought by many to be an important foundation on which the delineation of other spatial dimensions is built.

Laterality in the simplest sense means that infants and children know that two body parts are similar but are on opposite sides of the body, even though they do not recognize and cannot accurately use the words 'right' and 'left' to label the two sides. The simple knowledge of *sidedness* is a perceptual distinction, whereas the attachment of right–left labels is a learned distinction to create general directions that apply, eventually, to spatial dimensions. Infants make the perceptual distinction quite early; that is, they will use one hand to hold a cube while using the other to explore it or to pick up another cube and bang it on the first one. They can interchange the function of their hands, and they can use both hands to do the same movement.

The distinction between right and left to label body parts is assessed initially by observing children's behaviour when asked, 'Show me your right leg,' or 'Touch your left knee with your right hand.' There is considerable variability in the age at which children can accurately identify and use right and left body parts, which can be explained by the informal and formal instructions to which children have been exposed and by differences in testing procedures. Despite the wide range in individual achievement, the distinction between the body's right and left dimensions is generally only a chance response before about age 5, in contrast with an accurate response by ages 7 or 8. Belmont and Birch (1963) used seven measures of right–left discrimination of body parts and reported that 95% of the children over 7 years of age responded correctly to all seven questions, compared with only 69% of those under 7 years.

Directionality

Children must also establish a sense of direction in the space around them, including labels such as right–left, up–down, and forward–backward. We call this knowledge of dimensions of external space *directionality*, which

children often organize in relation to their position. For example, when looking at a house, we see a car parked on the left. If we change our position to view it from the back of the house, the car will now be on the right, as we look at it. When we give directions to someone for finding a place of interest, we often use our body as a reference point, because if we do not the instructions may be ambiguous. We say, 'If you are travelling towards the beach, the camera store will be on your left.' Of course, when leaving the beach, it will be on the right. As there are no invariant spatial references in external space, children begin with their own body as a reference to the dimensions of external space. Eventually, they are able to do this without consciously referring to their own body.

Long and Looft (1972) found that children at age 6 are aware of vertical and horizontal identification of up–down and are able to imitate or mirror many movements made by the experimenter. Children at age 8 begin to relate their body laterality to other objects, in that they start to use their body for the directional reference of another object in one position (e.g. 'The book is on my right'). However, if the children change position, they will not change their reference position. Thus children can make judgements that are not egocentric but that are still subjective. By age 9, children base their answers on objective directional relationships. For example, when they change their position to the opposite side of a table, they then see a book as being on their left. They can also follow directions based on two-directional references (e.g. 'Draw a triangle at the *bottom left-hand* corner of the paper'). By age 10, children can correctly specify the right and left of a person facing them. By age 11, they are able to judge correctly that certain objects are adjacent to other objects, and, by age 12, children begin to use natural reference systems (e.g. 'The sun sets in the west').

Children progress from a subjective and egocentric perspective towards a more objective view of space. Piaget and Inhelder (1956) saw this as a transition from an egocentric to an allocentric laterality, culminating in a knowledge system which supports perceptual–cognitive organization of the visual world. Body knowledge seems to be a significant aspect of the early organization of spatial knowledge because it is an essential point of reference.

Lateral preference

A universally observed behaviour is that humans use one of their eyes, hands, or feet in preference to the other. When we kick a ball, write our name, or cross our legs, we favour one side of our body over the other. Preference sometimes is labelled as dominance to suggest the prevalence of one of the cerebral hemispheres in controlling the preferred eye, hand, or foot. If children develop a preference for an eye, hand, and foot on the same side of the body, they are said to have pure dominance. If any one of the preferred body parts is on the opposite side of the body, the child is said to have mixed dominance. We shall use the word *preference* rather than *dominance*, except when referring directly to control by the right or left cerebral hemisphere.

Limb preference is measured by observing how children perform a variety of movements; eye preference can be observed when looking through a telescope. Variations in task presentations may favour one side or the other, such as handing objects to infants to observe. To determine true preference a number of tasks must be observed at different times. It helps if the requirements for accuracy and speed are minimal such as opening doors or carrying small objects. Most humans regardless of age are somewhat ambidextrous in using the non-preferred hand when convenient or necessary. Preference is just that: it does not imply that the other hand is not used and is less useful.

Hand preference seems to exist and change quite early in life. Seth (1973) observed infants from 5 to 12 months of age and found a marked preference for the left hand from 4 months through 7 months. He filmed the manipulation of objects such as a cube and a bell and found in the early months a tendency for the left hand to predominate over the right. Also, infants had a better success rate with their left hand than with their right hand. There was a shift, however, in the later months when infants used their right hand more and with a higher success rate. Hand preference has not been studied in the second and third year of life after birth, although we do know that most children by age 3 will show a right-hand preference for many everyday activities and that there will be some changes in hand preference until about age 10. Hand preference to this point has been limited to unimanual tasks in which one hand or the other, but not both, will be used. The ages and percentages will vary depending on the task being observed and the preference criteria being used. Foot preference appears to be similar, except in hopping.

Why do humans prefer one side to the other? A well-known answer to this question was proposed by Annett (1985, 1996), called *Annett's right-shift theory*. This theory proposed a genetic 'right-shift' that has evolved into the cerebral symmetry that is present for most individuals. The genetic, learning, and pathological antecedents of human handedness have been examined. Earlier work by Hicks and Kinsbourne (1976) concluded the following. First, they noted that there is little to suggest that handedness is learned, but if learning is a reason, then we should find cultures in which left-handers predominate, which appears not to be the case. They report that indirect evidence, such as paintings, suggest that across cultures people have been predominantly right-handed since prehistoric times. Recent studies have found a general invariance in handedness from childhood through young adulthood. Second, they noted that there are some pathological conditions associated with left-handedness, including an increased frequency of left-handedness in persons diagnosed with intellectual disability, epilepsy, cerebral palsy, stammering, developmental aphasia, articulating apraxia, and specific learning disorders, but that the relationship between handedness and dysfunction is very complex and appears not to be directly connected. Indeed, most left-handers do not have any noticeable pathological disorders, and the majority of individuals with these disorders are right-handed. In addition, a casual observance of top-class sports individuals would not suggest being left-handed is a detriment. Finally, Hicks and Kinsbourne (1976) support a genetic hypothesis for the genesis of handedness, with the warning that, although the evidence for this is strong, the appropriate genetic model is far from clear. Seeking an established explanation for lateral preference is not new; all conclusions seem to converge on a genetic, evolutionary cause. Van Strien (2000) in a more recent review of handedness supports this long-term historical quest for an answer.

Influences on motor development

The biological changes described allow us to think in the broadest terms about how these changes affect our actions and these are described throughout the book. Here we are presenting in the broadest sense some of the consequences of the biological changes, recognizing that most of these are described in more detail in the following three chapters together with the second section of the book, which examines atypical development.

Early Development of Motor Control

The development of motor control is a combination and dynamic interaction of the neuromotor system and the development of perceptual–cognitive abilities together with extrinsic constraints in our child–task–environment model. Although these are separated here for study, no one part of the system operates in isolation and the dynamic should always be kept in mind.

The neuromotor system is an obviously crucial part of early motor control, being responsible for producing movement with interrelationships among essentially all of the body's physiological systems and the external context. Even within the nervous system, it is difficult to separate the neuromotor system from other neural systems or parts, which means that we generally will be speaking of changes in the neural system rather than confining our discussion to the neuromotor system.

An important limitation is that early motor functioning is used often to estimate the adequacy of other aspects of development, including neural development. That is, holding the head upright, reaching and grasping an object, and similar achievements are used to indicate adequate development of the neural, vestibular, visual, and other biological systems, as well as adequate development of perceptual, cognitive, and social functioning.

Reflexes
Reflexes are used to check on certain aspects of neural development and are discussed in Chapter 4, which examines their role in movement and describes changes for selected reflexes. We note that some reflexes disappear (or at least are suppressed) and that others remain active throughout life. Reflexes in the form of more automatic movements also become part of the development of voluntary movement control. Until recently, the dominant theory of reflexive to voluntary control was a neural-based maturational approach inspired by the classic work of early researchers such as Gesell (1928), Shirley (1931), Bayley (1943) and McGraw (1963). For example, McGraw (1963) proposed a four-stage view of reflexes fading into voluntary control and more adaptive control moving from the appearance of the reflex to voluntary control. McGraw had no real empirical support for her statement that a reflex becomes part of later movements, but reflexive to voluntary control in McGraw's terms can be described as progressing from flexion to extension to anticipation.

More contemporary views on reflexes incorporate dynamic systems, as described in Chapters 1 and 4. They are often considered to be precursors of voluntary actions such as crawling and stepping and later the cortically controlled movements of walking, despite there being a gap between the end of the reflex period and the beginning of the voluntary movements (Zelazo 1983). Thelen (1995) notes that the reflex movements of stepping disappear but they do continue in the form of spontaneous kicking when the child is laid on his or her back. Thelen (1995) in summarizing a number of her investigations proposes that stepping behaviour has multiple aetiologies and is not simply dependent upon maturation, as McGraw would favour, which invokes voluntary cortical centres inhibiting reflexes while later facilitating voluntary control by higher centres. Thelen and Fisher (1982, 1983) note that the random kicking movements that infants make when they are laid on their backs have a similar pattern to the 'stepping' reflex, except that they are spontaneous and do not disappear, suggesting that they are the same movements but in different postures and that cortical suppression of one movement and not the other does not really make any sense. Their explanation invokes a dynamical systems perspective whereby other resources of the child interplay and it is not simply a neural maturation progression. For example, Thelen and her colleagues (1981, 1982) have shown that, at the same time as the stepping reflex disappears, infants have a rapid gain in mass and their legs are simply too heavy for them. They provided evidence of this by placing the children in the supine position when the movement was still present or placing the child in water when the stepping reflex was 'restored'. Thelen and Fisher (1983) then added weights to the children, thereby imitating the natural weight gain in the legs, and found the result to be the same: the stepping reflex was inhibited. Goldfield et al (1993) further supported the notion that the child's resources rapidly adapt to any constraints by showing that, when they used a baby bouncer, infants adapted to gain optimum bounce for the minimal expenditure of energy, with the authors noting that 'infants assemble and tune a periodic kicking system akin to a forced mass spring homing in on its resonant frequency' (Goldfield et al 1993, p. 1137).

Spontaneous movements and motor synergies
Spontaneous movements are discussed in Chapter 4 in regard to a type of movement very common in young infants. Thelen et al (1981) note that spontaneous movements may be precursors to later development, in much the same way that reflexes may provide a basis for the later voluntary control of movement. For example, they point out that reflexive stepping has been considered as the developmental precursor to walking, whereas spontaneous kicking shows a spatial and temporal structure like that of mature locomotion in humans and other species, and also may be a developmental precursor to walking.

Well-coordinated kicking begins at around 1 month, increases in frequency up to 7 months of age, and then declines with the onset of crawling and walking. Thelen and colleagues (1981) videotaped eight term infants from 4 to 6 weeks of age and used frame-by-frame analyses. The repetitive cycle of flexion and extension in the hip, knee, and ankle joints was morphologically much like the cycle of a single leg movement in mature locomotion, for both spatial and temporal characteristics. Mature locomotion has two distinct temporal phases: (1) the swing phase when the foot is off the ground and the body is moving forward, and (2) the stance phase when the foot is on the ground and the body is moving forward over the stance foot. As the walking speed increases, the stance phase decreases in duration, but the swing phase remains constant or increases. Thelen and colleagues equated various parts of the spontaneous kicking action to the swing and stance phases and then compared them with locomotion

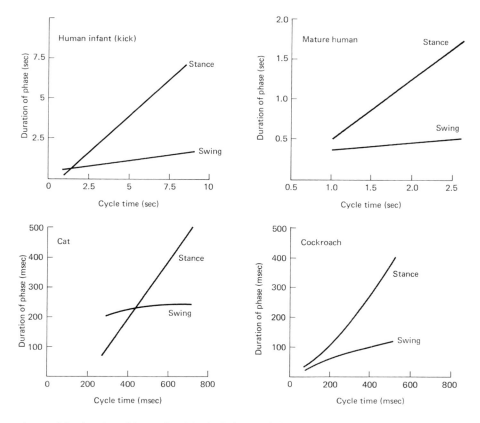

Fig. 2.14 Comparisons of the duration of 'stance' and 'swing' phases of single-leg kicking, as step cycle time increases, in human infants with mature humans, cats, and cockroaches. Reproduced with permission from Thelen et al (1981).

in mature humans, cats, and cockroaches. The results presented in Figure 2.14 show the similarity of the time durations. As the cycle time increases (*slower* walking), stance time increases; swing time is only marginally affected by cycle time.

Spontaneous kicking is different from reflexive walking in that there is no input from either weight-bearing changes or tactile feedback from the feet. Kicking therefore may be controlled by a central motor programme or central pattern generator. Thelen and colleagues conclude that both spontaneous kicking and early reflexive stepping may be forerunners of mature locomotion. They view kicking as manifesting a central patterning of the limbs and reflexive stepping as reflecting a system that modifies or tunes movements to environmental specifications.

DEVELOPMENT OF MAXIMUM PERFORMANCE

A common way of studying biological changes and movement development is through the maximal performance of specific movement skills. The normative summary of play-game skills in Chapter 4 considers these movement skills, which require a high level of force production to create speed or impart force to objects (including one's own body), which means that a functional use of strength is important.

The functional use of strength is so important to producing maximal performance particularly in closed movement skills that it must be recognized as a major consideration. Throwing for distance demonstrates the need for functional strength in an effective summation of force. The analyses of throwing indicate how the ordering and timing of movements among arm and trunk segments lead to a more effective summation of force. Jumping for distance requires the same functional use of strength, but to propel the body rather than an object. Running for speed is somewhat similar, except that the movements are repeated in a series of coordinated movements of body parts to propel the body forward. More force could be generated in these movement skills if children were stronger and if available strength could be effectively utilised. This means that 'skilful' summation is often limited by children's ability to create muscular tension. The converse is that additional strength in creating greater muscular tension is not useful unless the movement parts are coordinated to summate the potential available in the muscles. The desirable combination is 'strong' muscles and 'skilful' coordination to achieve maximal force output appropriate to the task requirements.

The relationships between structural changes and the development of maximal performance involving the functional use of strength tend to be greater at the upper and lower ends of distributions. Performance extremes are examined separately, and some general comments on the development of fitness and strength in relation to more functional biological changes are made.

General relationships

The development of maximal performance has been studied primarily in terms of structural changes, except for the development of muscle in relation to functional strength. The principal finding is that structural differences among children of the same chronological age cannot predict maximal movement performance as defined here. Few of the measures of height, body proportions, body composition, and physique for children at age 6 correlate substantially with their maximal performance scores for running, jumping, throwing, and similar movement tasks. Malina and Rarick (1973), in a critical review of related literature, concluded that 'performance in motor skills during elementary school ages is largely unaffected by body build and constitutional factors, *except at the extremes of the continuum*' (p.150, italics added). They acknowledge that physique and related structural characteristics can limit or enhance performance but are not good predictors of maximal performance scores (also see Malina 1975).

Strength

A measure of muscle strength that is often employed is the muscle cross-sectional area (CSA). There are debates about how to use this and associated measurements, but here we stay with the anatomical CSA, which is recommended by De Ste Croix (2008). The CSAs of muscle fibres are at their adult size by age 14 in males and age 10 in females, with De Ste Croix (2008) reporting that many differences between the sexes in CSA favoured males but the differences were small up to these ages. After these ages differences increased with adult females, for example, showing CSAs of the arm and thigh about 57% and 73% of the adult male. However, although CSA does affect strength development, it is less of an explanatory variable once body size is taken into account. De Ste Croix (2008) concludes by noting that we know little about muscle fibre types in children probably because of ethical issues concerning the collection of data through muscle biopsies.

De Ste Croix (2008) reports that there is some debate on when sex differences become evident, but before puberty there is considerable overlap between the sexes and by 16 or 17 years of age there are few females outperforming males on strength tests with males on average performing 54% higher than females. There have been reports of notable differences being seen as early as 3 years of age. However, in a review of studies De Ste Croix (2008) reports that 14 or 15 seems to be the age when large differences are established but also cautions against firm conclusions especially when measuring upper body strength with sociological explanations coming into play. The reasons for these differences are associated with stature and mass, with peak height velocity being particularly important.

Some of the findings from the classic Medford Growth Study (Clarke 1971) are presented in Table 2.4 to show the relationships among biological measures and movement performance. The Medford Growth Study annually tested males in an Oregon town from 1956 through 1968, and the cable-tension strength test in Table 2.4 is the average of 11 strength measures.

The measures in the table are all correlated to 11 measures of strength. Looking at Table 2.4, body size and muscle size (arm girth) correlated 0.3 to 0.6 with strength. This was probably owing to greater muscle mass in males with larger body structures, as when measuring strength in a more direct outcome (cable tension), muscle mass is more important in force production than in a skilled movement. Physique and maturity correlations with strength were at a lower level and were a more erratic set of values. This is a complicated set of relationships because more mature children presumably have acquired more of their muscle mass, and the three physique ratings are based partly on estimates of muscle mass. It is noticeable that skeletal age correlated higher (0.40 and 0.56) with strength during the pubertal years (ages 12 and 15), when early maturers were probably acquiring muscle mass at a higher rate than late maturers were. Mesomorphy (well-defined musculature) correlations also were positive, in comparison with negative correlations for ectomorphy and low positive correlations (neutral) for endomorphy. In general, the physique and maturity correlations were low (0.3 or less).

The cable-tension strength test correlated 0.3 to 0.5 for jumping and running, which need force production to achieve maximal distance and speed. The importance of strength was emphasized when correlations increased to 0.5 to 0.7 for jumping performance times weight. For example, two males at age 7, weighing 27kg and 32kg, would score 300 points and 350 points, respectively, for jumping the same distance of 127cm. The male weighing 32kg must generate more effective force to jump the same

TABLE 2.4
Relationship[a] of cable-tension strength test to measures of maturity, size, physique, and
movement performance for males in the Medford Growth Study[b]

Measure	Chronological age				
	7	9	12	15	17
Number of participants	113	175	278	343	272
Maturity					
Skeletal age	34	24	40	56	15
Structure (size)					
Height	44	34	43	49	21
Weight	48	35	53	59	46
Leg length	41	25	35	30	11
Arm girth	52	34	50	54	46
Physique					
Endomorphy	01	15	28	03	07
Mesomorphy	37	27	33	42	35
Ectomorphy	−20	−18	−31	−22	−39
Movement performance					
Standing log jump					
Distance	37	38	30	44	25
Distance×weight	59	52	65	70	53
Shuttle run (60 yards)[c]	49	51	29	31	29

[a]Pearson product moment correlations with decimal point omitted. [b]Based on data from Clarke (1971). [c]Sign reversed.

distance, which is a more functional use of strength, but the heavier male generally has more muscle mass.

Correlations with reaction time and movement time show the lack of a relationship between structural characteristics and movement performance when force production is minimal. Reaction time, which is the time taken to initiate a movement, did not correlate significantly with level of maturity, size, and strength. Movement time also did not correlate significantly with these structural characteristics, probably because the arm-hand and body movements were so limited that the generation of force was not critical.

In the introduction to this section we said that the functional use of strength is a major consideration in maximal performance, and therefore muscle mass becomes important in concert with skill in summating force. Various structural characteristics and the level of maturity may be related to maximal performance because they reflect muscle mass and functional strength.

Despite some of the generally neutral findings, structural differences are probably important to maximal performance for the movement skills we are reviewing here. The problem seems to be in matching specific structural

characteristics to specific task requirements. For example, it seems too much to expect that a general measure of physique will predict a specific movement achievement, but the general physique category of mesomorphy does combine the body proportions and composition that should contribute to better performance in many play-game and athletic skills. Task requirements should be analysed more carefully to find specific aspects of physique that contribute to maximal performance. This means that we must find ways to assess the coordination of movement parts, which leads us back to the development of motor control. Some individuals are probably better equipped than others to coordinate movement parts in summating force, although they can make great improvement with good instruction. Our comments here do not change our conclusion that structural differences among children of the same chronological age do not greatly predict maximal performance with the exception of extremes of biological states.

Fitness and strength

Exercise as physical activity will increase work fitness and a lack of exercise will lead to a decrease in fitness and strength. Although training effects confound analyses of developmental changes, our comments are appropriate for children who are physically active within a similar, normal level of activity. The general pattern of change in fitness is that children steadily increase their oxygen uptake and usage, which contribute to the potential for improved fitness. Level of fitness can vary noticeably among children at a particular age because they vary in their activity level, but their potential for fitness improves with chronological age. Physiological changes during puberty also greatly enhance fitness potential.

Strength should be considered in two ways. First, strength can be the direct and primary outcome, such as when exerting pressure on a dynamometer or lifting a certain amount of weight. Second, strength can be part of a movement skill when using it functionally to contribute to maximal performance, such as when going faster or imparting force to objects. We know that children improve their strength in both respects to have larger grip strength scores, greater running speed, and longer jumping distances. An important contributing factor must be the absolute and relative (to weight) increases in muscle mass. Again, muscle mass increases particularly during the pubertal years, with males having greater absolute and relative increases. Strength potential improves with chronological age, and level of strength can change when participating in appropriate physical activities.

General considerations
The rate of change in relation to maturity and the age of achieving maturity vary noticeably among the many aspects of our biological make up. As noted earlier, we can measure level of maturity for selected biological characteristics, but we cannot single out one level of maturity for all aspects of biological change. Chronological age, though a convenient indication of level of maturity, is not useful except to mark the passage of time. Skeletal age, peak height velocity, and similar measures are appropriate for certain purposes, yet often are too general. Microscopic measures of change, such as dendritic growth in a specific neural area, can precisely measure level of maturity, but cannot be easily related to movement changes. There is no easy solution when trying to choose an appropriate measure of maturity, but a first step is to consider the appropriateness of maturity measures when reading research reports and proposed explanations.

The other side of the coin is to measure movement changes in a way that matches maturity and movement, and thus we must use changes in movement components rather than general achievements and general performance scores. Longitudinal measures also are needed to trace maturity and movement relationships, with an emphasis

on the development of movement control rather than maximal performance.

The distinction between level and rate of maturity must also be kept in mind. The level of maturity for a biological characteristic indicates the level of development for a particular resource at a particular time. The rate of maturity makes a comparison across time and in relation to other individuals, and has been the general maturity concern in regard to studying early and late maturers. The level of maturity, if well measured, is a more definitive approach because we can match changes in movement development to the level of the development of resources.

We organized our brief review around, first, the early development of movement control and, second, the maximal performance of forceful movements. The early development and initial refinement of movement control seem to be determined largely by the development of higher-level neural control centres interacting with the environmental context, with movements being organized into larger and more adaptable packages. Reflexes and spontaneous movements are the prominent observable movements in the early months and there are substantial changes that increase the potential for a more complex and adaptable organization of movement.

The development of maximal performance involving the functional use of strength has been studied in relation to many biological characteristics. One conclusion is that the structural differences among children of the same chronological age do not greatly predict maximal performance, with studies limited in that the biological and performance measures have been too general to reveal a relationship and many measures are needed to predict performance, with task requirements matched to the biological characteristics of interest. However, when this matching does occur, there is a strong relationship generally obtained for performance on strength or exercise fitness tasks and measures of muscle mass or oxygen uptake and usage. It is more difficult to find such relationships for motor control, even for maximal performance of forceful movements.

An important qualification is that extremes in level of biological state may be quite predictive of extreme levels of performance. Extremes may serve both to limit and to enhance, as often seen in individuals who achieve a high level of performance. These individuals tend to have common biological characteristics, particularly those that pertain to a high level of performance in the specific movement task. Particular biological characteristics may be helpful and almost necessary to achieve a world-class level of performance, but no set of biological characteristics is likely to be sufficient without the addition of certain personal–social qualities.

Summary

In this chapter we have attempted to choose those biological variables that pertain to the development of motor control and maximal performance – for detail on much of this work see Armstrong and van Mechelen (2008). Throughout this text there is reference to a model that incorporates the child's resources, the task and the environmental context. The biological changes (child resources) are described here in isolation, and although we can get some idea of their development, it is only when they fit into the dynamic constraints model involving the other two parts of task and environmental that we obtain the full picture. Yet, clearly, the biological development of the child's resources are a crucial part of how a child progresses to maturity in the performance and learning of skilled actions.

The chapter has concentrated on the structural and functional development of the biological structures, and at times these are difficult to separate. For example, the structural development of oxygen uptake has a strong relationship with the functional development of endurance; likewise, the structural development of the nervous system influences many skilled actions. However, the overall development of the child involves both structural and functional progressions, and throughout the lifespan of the child these are influenced by the types of tasks and opportunities a child receives.

REFERENCES

Annett M (1985) *Left, Right, Hand and Brain: The Right Shift Theory*. London: Erlbaum.

Annett M (1996) In defence of rightshift theory. *Percept Mot Skills* 82: 115–137. http://dx.doi.org/10.2466/pms.1996.82.1.115

Armstrong N, Fawkner SG (2008) Exercise metabolism. In: Armstrong N, van Mechelen W, editors. *Paediatric Exercise Science and Medicine*, 2nd edition. Oxford: Oxford University Press, pp. 213–226.

Armstrong N, van Mechelen W (2008) Maximal intensity exercise. In: Armstrong N, van Mechelen W, editors. *Paediatric Exercise Science and Medicine*, 2nd edition. Oxford: Oxford University Press.

Armstrong N, McManus AM, Welsman JR (2008) In: Armstrong N, van Mechelen W, editors. *Paediatric Exercise Science and Medicine*, 2nd edition. Oxford: Oxford University Press, pp. 269–282.

Asmussen E (1973) Growth in muscular strength and power. In: Rarick GL, editor. *Physical Activity: Human Growth and Development*. New York: Academic Press, pp. 60–79.

Bairstow PJ, Laszlo JL (1981) Kinaesthetic sensitivity to passive movements and its relationship to motor development and motor control. *Dev Med Child Neurol* 23: 606–616. http://dx.doi.org/10.1111/j.1469-8749.1981.tb02042.x

Baxter-Jones ADG (2008) Growth and maturation. In: Armstrong N, van Mechelen W, editors. *Paediatric Exercise Science and Medicine*, 2nd edition. Oxford: Oxford University Press, pp. 157–168.

Bayley N (1943) Size and body build of adolescents in relation to rate of skeletal maturity. *Child Dev* 14: 47–90. http://dx.doi.org/10.2307/1125513

Bayley N, Davis FC (1935) Growth changes in growth size and proportions during the first three years: a developmental study of sixty-one children by repeated measures. *Biometrika* 27: 26–87.

Belmont L, Birch HG (1963) Lateral dominance and right–left awareness in normal children. *Child Dev* 34: 257–270.

Bloom BS (1964) *Stability and Change in Human Characteristics*. New York: Wiley.

Braddick O (1996) Binocularity in infancy. *Eye* 10: 182–188. http://dx.doi.org/10.1038/eye.1996.45

Braddick O, Atkinson J, Wattam-Bell J (2003) Normal and anomalous development of visual motion processing: motion coherence and dorsal stream vulnerability. *Neuropsychologia* 41: 1769–1784. http://dx.doi.org/10.1016/S0028-3932(03)00178-7

Bronson GW (1982) Structure, status and characteristics of the nervous system at birth. In: Stratton P, editor. *Psychobiology of the Human Newborn*. New York: Wiley, pp. 99–118.

Brown JK, Omar T, O'Reagan M (1997) Brain development and the development of tone and movement. In: Connolly KJ, Forssberg H, editors. *Neurophysiology and Neuropsychology of Motor Development*. London: Mac Keith Press, pp. 1–41.

Brown LE, Halpert BA, Goodale MA (2005) Peripheral vision for perception and action. *Experimental Brain Research* 165: 97–106. http://dx.doi.org/10.1007/s00221-005-2285-y

Carello C, Turvey MT (2004) Physics and psychology of the muscle sense. *Curr Dir Psychol Sci* 13: 25–28. http://dx.doi.org/10.1111/j.0963-7214.2004.01301007.x

Carter JEL, Heath BH (1990) *Somatotyping: Development and Applications*. Cambridge: Cambridge University Press.

Chohan A, Savelsbergh GJP, Van Kampen PM, Wind M, Verheul MCG (2006) Postural adjustments and bearing angle use in interceptive actions. *Exp Brain Res* 171: 47–55. http://dx.doi.org/10.1007/s00221-005-0239-z

Chohan A, Verheul MCG, Van Kampen PM, Wind M, Savelsbergh GJP (2008) Children's use of the bearing angle in interceptive actions. *J Motor Behav* 40: 18–28. http://dx.doi.org/10.3200/JMBR.40.1.18-28

Claessens AL, Beunen G, Malina RM (2008) Anthrometry, physique, body composition and maturity. In: Armstrong N, van Mechelen W, editors. *Paediatric Exercise Science and Medicine*, 2nd edition. Oxford: Oxford University Press, pp. 23–37.

Clarke HH (1971) *Physical and Motor Tests in the Medford Boys' Growth Study*. Englewood Cliffs, NJ: Prentice Hall.

De Ste Croix MBA (2008) Muscle strength. In: Armstrong N, van Mechelen W, editors. *Paediatric Exercise Science and Medicine*, 2nd edition. Oxford: Oxford University Press, pp. 199–212.

Falk B, Dotan R (2008) Temperature regulation. In: Armstrong N, van Mechelen W, editors. *Paediatric Exercise Science and Medicine*, 2nd edition. Oxford: Oxford University Press, pp. 309–324.

Faust MS (1977) Somatic development of adolescent girls. *Monographs of the Society for Research in Child Development* 42, 1, Serial no. 169.

Fawkner SG (2008) Pulmonary function. In: Armstrong N, van Mechelen W, editors. *Paediatric Exercise Science and Medicine*, 2nd edition. Oxford: Oxford University Press, pp. 243–253.

Gesell A (1928) *Infancy and Human Growth*. Oxford: Macmillan.

Gibson JJ (1966) *The Senses Considered as Perceptual Systems*. Boston, MA: Houghton Mifflin.

Goldfield EC, Kay BA, Warren WH Jr (1993) Infant bouncing: the assembly and tuning of action systems. *Child Dev* 64: 1128–1142. http://dx.doi.org/10.2307/1131330

Goodale MA, Milner AD (1992) Separate visual pathways for perception and action. *Trends Neurosci* 15: 20–25. http://dx.doi.org/10.1016/0166-2236(92)90344-8

Henderson L (1982) *Orthography and Word Recognition in Reading*. London: Academic Press.

Hicks RE, Kinsbourne M (1976) On the genesis of human handedness: a review. *J Behav* 18: 257–266.

Hiscock M, Kinsbourne M (1978) Ontogeny of cerebral dominance: evidence from time-sharing asymmetry in children. *Dev Psychol* 14: 321–329. http://dx.doi.org/10.1037/0012-1649.14.4.321

Jones HE (1939) Principles and methods of the adolescent growth spurt. *J Consult Psychol* 3: 157–159. http://dx.doi.org/10.1037/h0050181

Keogh JF, Sugden DA (1985) *Movement Skill Development*. New York: Macmillan.

Kessen W, Haith MM, Salapatek PH (1970) Human infancy: a bibliography and guide. In: Mussen PH, editor. *Carmichael's Manual of Child Psychology*, 3rd edition. New York: Wiley, pp. 287–445.

Laszlo JL, Bairstow PJ (1980) The measurement of kinaesthetic sensitivity in children and adults. *Dev Med Child Neurol* 22: 454–464. http://dx.doi.org/10.1111/j.1469-8749.1980.tb04350.x

Lee DN (1980) The optic flow field: the foundation of vision. *Phil Trans Royal Soc B Biol Sci* 290: 169–179. http://dx.doi.org/10.1098/rstb.1980.0089

Lee DN (1990) Visuo-motor coordination in space–time. In: Warren R, Wertheim AH, editors. *Perception and Control of Self-Motion*. Hillsdale, NJ: Erlbaum, pp. 487–505.

Lee DN (1998) Guiding movements by coupling taus. *Ecol Psychol* 10: 221–250.

Lee DN, Aaronson E (1974) Visual proprioceptive control of standing in human infants. *Percept Psychophys* 15: 529–532. http://dx.doi.org/10.3758/BF03199297

Lee DN, Young DS (1985) Visual timing of interceptive action. In: Ingle D, Jeannerod M, Lee DN, editors. *Brain Mechanisms and Spatial Vision*. Dordrecht: Martinus Nijhoff, pp. 1–30. http://dx.doi.org/10.1007/978-94-009-5071-9_1

Long AB, Looft WR (1972) Development of directionality in children: ages six through twelve. *Dev Psychol* 6: 375–380. http://dx.doi.org/10.1037/h0032577

McGraw MB (1963) *The Neuromuscular Maturation of the Human Infant*, reprint edition. New York: Hafner.

Magill RA (2007) *Motor Learning and Control: Concepts and Applications*, 8th edition. New York: McGraw-Hill.

Malina RM (1975) Anthropometric correlates of strength and motor performance. *Exerc Sport Sci Rev* 3: 249–274. http://dx.doi.org/10.1249/00003677-197500030-00012

Malina RM, Rarick GL (1973) Growth, physique and motor performance. In: Rarick GL, editor. *Physical Activity: Human Growth and Development*. New York: Academic Press, pp. 125–153.

Maurer D, Lewis TL, Brent HP, Levin AV (1990) Rapid improvement in the acuity of infants after visual input. *Science* 286: 108–110. http://dx.doi.org/10.1126/science.286.5437.108

Michel GF, Harkins DA (1986) Postural and lateral asymmetries in the ontogeny of handedness during infancy. *Dev Psychobiol* 19: 247–258. http://dx.doi.org/10.1002/dev.420190310

Morgan DW (2008) Locomotor economy. In: Armstrong N, van Mechelen W, editors. *Paediatric Exercise Science and Medicine*, 2nd edition. Oxford: Oxford University Press, pp. 283–296.

Parnell RW (1958) *Behaviour and Physique: An Introduction to Practical and Applied Somatometry*. London: Arnold.

Piaget J, Inhelder B (1956) *The Child's Conception of Space*. London: Routledge and Kegan Paul.

Rowland TW (2008) Cardiovascular function. In: Armstrong N, van Mechelen W, editors. *Paediatric Exercise Science and Medicine*, 2nd edition. Oxford: Oxford University Press, pp. 255–268.

Scammon RE (1930) The measurement of the body in childhood. In: Harrison JA, Jackson CM, Patterson DG, Scammon RE, editors. *The Measurement of Man*. Minneapolis, MN: University of Minnesota Press, pp. 171–215.

Schmidt RA, Lee TD (2005) *Motor Control and Learning: A Behavioural Emphasis*. Champaign, IL: Human Kinetics.

Seth G (1973) Eye hand coordination and 'handedness': a developmental study of visuomotor behaviour in infancy. *Br J Educ Psychol* 43: 35–49. http://dx.doi.org/10.1111/j.2044-8279.1973.tb00735.x

Sheldon WH, Stevens SS (1942) *The Varieties of Human Physique*. New York: Harper and Row.

Sheldon WH, Dupertuis CW, McDermot E (1954) *Atlas of Men: A Guide for Somatotyping the Adult Male of all Ages*. New York: Harper and Row.

Shirley MM (1931) *The First Two Years: A Study of Twenty-Five Babies, Volume 1: Postural and Locomotor Development*. Minneapolis, MN: University of Minnesota Press.

Shuttleworth FK (1939) The physical and mental growth of girls and boys aged six to nineteen in relation to age at maximum growth. *Monographs of the Society for Research in Child Development* 4,3, Serial no. 22.

Smothergill DW (1973) Accuracy and variability in targets in the localisation of spatial targets at 3 age levels. *Dev Psychol* 8: 62–68. http://dx.doi.org/10.1037/h0033839

Sugden DA (1980) Developmental strategies in motor and visual short term memory. *Percept Mot Skills* 51: 146. http://dx.doi.org/10.2466/pms.1980.51.1.146

Sugden DA, Keogh JF (1990) *Problems in Movement Skill Development*. Columbia: University of South Carolina Press.

Tanner JM (1962) *Growth at Adolescence*, 2nd edition. Oxford: Blackwell.

Tanner JM (1981) *A History of the Study of Human Growth*. Cambridge: Cambridge University Press.

Tanner JM (1989) *Foetus into Man: Physical Growth from Conception to Maturity*. Cambridge, MA: Harvard University Press.

Thelen E (1995) Motor development: a new synthesis. *Am Psychol* 50: 79–95. http://dx.doi.org/10.1037/0003-066X.50.2.79

Thelen E, Fisher DM (1982) New born stepping: an explanation for a 'disappearing' reflex. *Dev Psychol* 18: 560–575.

Thelen E, Fisher DM (1983) The organisation of spontaneous leg movements in new born infants. *J Motor Behav* 15: 153–377.

Thelen E, Bradshaw G, Ward JA (1981) Spontaneous kicking in month old infants: manifestation of a human central locomotor program. *Behav Neural Biol* 32: 45–53. http://dx.doi.org/10.1016/S0163-1047(81)90257-0

Turvey MT (1996) Dynamic touch. *Am Psychol* 51: 1134–1152. http://dx.doi.org/10.1037/0003-066X.51.11.1134

Van Strien JW (2000) Genetic intrauterine and cultural origins of human handedness. In Mandal MK, Bulman-Fleming MB, Tiwari G editors. *Side-Bias: A Neurological Perspective.* Dordrecht: Kluwer Academic, pp. 41–61.

Wetzel NC (1941) Physical fitness in terms of physique, development and basal metabolism. *JAMA* 116: 1187–1195. http://dx.doi.org/10.1001/jama.1941.02820120001001

Wetzel NC (1943) Assessing the physical condition of children. *J Pediatr* 22: 82–110. http://dx.doi.org/10.1016/S0022-3476(43)80144-X.

3
DEVELOPMENTAL MODELS AND THEORIES

Motor control and development theories

The two intertwining topics of motor control and development permeate this text, yet they have different origins and history. In short, the origins of motor control have predominantly concentrated on adult motor behaviour, whereas developmental theories have rarely emphasized motor control as their starting point. There are of course exceptions, and this text concentrates on the literature where the two come together. In order to understand this state of affairs, this chapter analyses prominent, selected, theoretical positions starting from historical aspects of motor control and development leading to our current theoretical stance. In Chapter 1 we examined both motor control and development as separate components, whereas here we analyse how researchers have pulled them together to influence the study of the development of motor control.

What constitutes processing?

We have employed the term 'processing' as it is used widely in both the motor control and developmental literature, often in different ways, yet traditionally agreeing that from the time information enters the system it undergoes a series of transformations through to the production of movement. The components of these transformations differ according to individual models but usually contain mechanisms for how information is brought into the system from the environment; how this information is attended to and selected out as being relevant to the task on hand; and how memory systems organize the information for a response and some kind of programme that contains parameters of force, timing, and space for the movement. Various types of feedback are then employed to evaluate the movement and prepare for a future response. Permeating the whole process is the concept of time, with some components requiring speed of responding as a major feature, and researchers in the developmental field have used this as a measurable variable of development in many studies. Some models have proposed the concept of a limited processing space where an individual can be overloaded to the detriment of the final movement performance, again a concept that has featured in the developmental field. Earlier models of processing were simple, sequential, and linear, with more modern ones embracing complexity and simultaneous channels and components. This type of research has and still does provide us with valuable information about the development of motor skills. However, it is not without its critics, with Ulrich (1997) noting that these approaches still rely on existing structures such as motor programmes and do not tell us how they originate. They could be labelled simply as descriptions at a deeper level.

This traditional view of processing has a rival in dynamical systems and ecological explanations, as introduced in Chapter 1. Here, instead of the solutions to a particular challenging motor problem residing in the above transformations within the individual, it is the matching of the internal resources of the person to the specific environmental context that provides the solution. This involves a move away from internal structures such as genes, programmes, and cognitive processing to those that involve a complexity of these internal constraints as well as the external ones of exploration, adaptation, repeated cycles of perception, and action and the contextual and self-organizational nature of development.

Early research on motor development began primarily with descriptive studies that analysed the changes observed in the developing infant; the use of 'theory', as it related more specifically to motor development, did not appear in the scientific literature until the late 1940s and early 1950s. It was not until 1970, a further 20 years, that a serious attempt was made to exploit the specific theoretical predictions encompassed in information processing and relate it to the development of motor skills in children.

As we noted in Chapter 1, the publication of *Mechanisms of Motor Skill* (Connolly 1970) was the first to present empirical research on motor development in children from a theoretical (primarily information processing) perspective. The Connolly book reported a range of experimental studies, analysed and interpreted from an information processing orientation.

The information processing paradigm for studying the development of motor skill interprets the earlier reference to 'motor milestones' as changes in the child's capacity as a processor of information. The developmental aspects of the coordination and control of skill development were viewed as a motor 'problem' to be solved. The information processing model provided a blueprint to map how motor skills were organized and executed. A central tenet of the information processing model was the processing speed necessary to generate a response, and the amount of information to be processed (bits) to both organize and execute the skill. Studies of children's reaction times and movement times produced developmental research literature that was a welcome addition to the earlier descriptive studies of children's skill development. This style of inquiry viewed the central nervous system (CNS) as a 'communication channel', which processed the input of information, made sense of inputs (perception), and organized an appropriate response. The information processing model was an important catalyst to move beyond description and develop a theory to account for motor skill development. Children were seen as developing what in computer language is referred to as 'subroutines', and as the sophistication and the efficiency of children's movement skills increased, this was interpreted as an increase in the complexity and sophistication of those subroutines.

The information processing theory has held sway in the research literature on the skill development of adults and children for 50 years or so. Much of the motor development research was featured in the first edition of this text (Keogh and Sugden 1985). Since then the focus of research from an information processing theoretical view has not changed from the fundamental assumption that the brain functions as a computational engine, which both interprets and creates the motor responses necessary to execute intentional movement. There have been important developments, especially with respect to brain science technology, which directly records changes in brain activation via functional magnetic resonance imagery, which measures changes in blood flow in different locations of the cortex. However, the latest editions of current textbooks that deal with the control and coordination of motor skills, cf. Schmidt and Lee (2011) and Magill (2009), contain only limited information on newer brain

science research, which features the use of such technology, as it relates to motor learning and control. Perhaps an exception is a series of articles by Wolpert and colleagues (Davidson and Wolpert 2005, Wolpert et al 2001), which continue to promote the notion of 'internal models' and their adherence to the computational perspective. This view is best summed up by the following: 'Generally in motor learning we consider how the brain adapts to control the body' (Wolpert et al 2001, p. 487).

Despite this more recent look at control from a processing viewpoint, which we discuss in more detail later in this chapter, there is little new information or research on the associated issues such as memory, attention, processing capacity, and so forth, which can impact on motor development. From an information processing perspective the majority of research has focused mostly on the structure of practice, contextual interference, and variations in how to provide feedback as well as in what form: knowledge of results or knowledge of performance to the learner.

We review some of the traditional research on information processing with reference to the developmental differences, such as they are (i.e. adult–child and intellectual differences). What is clear is that the more recent dynamic systems perspective on the development of control and coordination has had a profound impact on how motor behaviour (coordination and control of motor skills) progresses across the lifespan; what exactly constitutes 'information'; and how we (adults and children) detect and process that information (perceive) and act (respond) on it. This chapter reviews the developmental literature from both theoretical viewpoints.

The chapter is divided into two major parts.

- First, we present a review of the key elements and topics of the traditional *information processing* perspective, including developmental memory; the role of attention; the nature and limits of processing capacity; and feedback designated as knowledge of results, from a developmental perspective.
- Second, we present a review of alternative theoretical approaches and how definitions of information and processing are addressed by these alternative approaches.

As a backdrop it is important to again bear in mind, first, the distinction between phylogenetic and ontogenetic skills. By phylogenetic we refer to the characteristics that the developing child carries with him or her as part of the evolution of the human species: in motor control and coordination this includes the development of posture, locomotion, reaching and grasping, and the skill set, referred to in the motor development literature as 'fundamental motor skills'.

Ontogenetic motor development relates more to the development of individual skill sets that form part of and are necessary for an individual's activity in their own societal or cultural context. Activities of daily living – skills needed for employment, and skills that enhance opportunities for successful social interaction and participation in recreational and sport-related activities that themselves promote relationships and friendships – would be included here.

As a second backdrop, all expressions of skilled behaviour are constrained by the dynamic and ongoing interaction between the *task performer* and the *environment*. This is a model we refer to consistently throughout the text, and we firmly believe that it is this triad of parameters that form the basis of analysis for motor skill development, and not simply the resources of the child.

Traditional information processing
A central tenet of traditional information processing is the concept of memory, and there is no doubt that we all develop a memory; further, it is axiomatic that we engage in both short- and long-term memorial behaviours, which allow us to recall information for immediate use and for later. Perhaps the best-known memory researcher from the traditional perspective was Endel Tulving. He has described memory as 'the capacity that permits organisms to benefit from their past experiences' (Tulving 1985, p. 385). The distinction between the traditional view (promoted by Tulving) and the contemporary view of memory is whether or not this remembering behaviour actually requires a set of structures or devices in our head. Traditional models, in one form or another, adhere to this structural notion by employing a whole range of terms such as buffers, sensory registers, or rehearsal to infer activity of a functional memory system.

Over time new technologies have produced a shift from essentially inferring different kinds of (internal) structures in the head to explain data to the more recent use of brain imaging techniques that seek to identify where, in the brain, different responses appear to stimulate brain activity. Recording this kind of neural activity represents an increase in blood flow to the specific neural location of interest. The more recent brain imaging techniques continue to adhere to a 'structural' explanation of memory activity, except that, now, rather than inventing names for the inferred 'devices' that are presumed to process information, brain imaging can pinpoint the locus of the neural activity. This certainly is an advance on the earlier inferential approach, but still requires some level of conjecture in regard to describing the presumed function

of memory. Here we note only the models of memory that are essentially developmental.

MEMORY DEVELOPMENT
Most models of memory, whether dealing with cognitive or motor events, draw a distinction between *structural* and *control* features. Structural features are assumed to be independent of age, with young children having the same structural features as adults (presumably 'hard wired' at birth). However, control operations vary and can change according to the child's development level. We discuss two of the best-known models of memory, which reflect much of the research on memory. These two models, one developmental but not motor and the other motor but not developmental, have enabled researchers to adapt them both when looking at developmental motor control.

Brown: memory as knowing
The late developmental psychologist Ann Brown approached the concept of memory as *knowing* rather than as remembering and forgetting, which shifted the general focus to what people know and how they come to know it. In her model (Brown 1975), she specified three kinds of knowing:

Knowing: our knowledge base, which is our semantic memory and provides a dynamic knowledge system underlying all cognitive activity.
Knowing how to know: our repertoire of processing skills.
Knowing about knowing: our metamemory or knowledge about our own memory.

Brown's model had clear developmental implications given her focus on both typical development and those with intellectual disabilities. Her model was organized to demonstrate some of the changes seen in developmental memory.

Knowing. Brown notes that most of what we know and remember about our world comes from a continuous interaction with a meaningful environment to produce a knowledge store, or *knowledge base*. General features of events are retained in what Brown calls *semantic memory*, which provides *more meaningful knowing*. Brown also recognized that we process information related to particular events, or episodes, such as reading the letters on an eye chart or reading a list of nonsense syllables in a laboratory experiment and that such *less meaningful knowing* may be retained as *episodic memory*. The episodic–semantic distinction is a continuum from more a specific to more a general knowledge of events, with the idea that the more semantic memory is, the more useful it will be.

Brown used children's memory for narratives to illustrate the general development of knowing, pointing out that preschool children can reconstruct meaningful narratives to provide the gist of a story but have problems with the sequence of events. They later improve at retelling stories and can use meaning to produce the most probable order of events. Here the children are remembering not so much a copy of events but are employing their semantic knowledge of the world to *reconstruct the course of events*. The meaning in their knowledge base aids in retrieval and, more importantly, in the use of what is known. The development of semantic knowledge is also essential in the use of episodic memory.

To Brown, memory is not separate from intelligence and, not dissimilar from a Piagetian view, which holds that cognitive development is responsible for memory development (Piaget and Inhelder 1973), memory is not a copy of events but a continuously changing *constructive process, with the individual actively organizing the material to be remembered.* For Brown and Piaget, understanding, knowing, and remembering are inseparable parts of intelligence. As children's general operational levels change, so does their ability to remember meaningful events.

Knowing how to know. Brown used the phrase *knowing how to know* to describe the *development of control operations*, particularly strategies, for deliberate memorization. Brown (1978) reviewed the literature on processing strategies and memory development and came to three conclusions. First, children who are chronologically or cognitively young are deficient in using strategies. They do not use rehearsal and similar strategies spontaneously. Second, young children can be trained to use some strategies, and this has been confirmed in studies on both typical children and children with an intellectual disability. Third, these trained processing skills tend to be abandoned unless they are actively used. Two terms are introduced here: first, what is called a 'production deficiency', when poor use of a control operation is evident; second, a 'mediation deficiency', when a participant is trained to use a particular strategy but fails to apply it as a mediator.

Knowing about knowing. Children's knowledge of their own memory develops in that they become better able to evaluate situation requirements and discover more about their own memory operations. Adults know that it is harder to remember 12 rather than four items, and they consciously know how they change their strategies for remembering. They may group the items by common characteristics or in relation to an artificial ordering system, such as assigning numbers to each item. Adults also know other things about how they go about knowing. They know that they have a repertoire of strategies and whether they have a preferred approach such as dividing the information or the problem into two groups before analysing it further. They may also know that they retrieve or remember on the basis of how they code the information for storage, such as being aware that, 'It begins with a "B",' or 'It is very large and soft', when verbally describing their search for something in memory. Children seem to know less about their knowing. Knowing about knowing is often labelled *metamemory*. In their studies of metamemory, Kreutzer et al (1975) found that, as they grew older, children recognized that older children studied differently and remembered better. Younger children seemed to be *aware* that familiarity and similar abstract properties affect the retrieval of information, whereas older children seemed to *know* this. As early as kindergarten, children can verbalize about memory being affected by study time, number of items, and knowing that it is easier to relearn a forgotten activity than to start on a totally new task.

The concept of 'knowing about knowing' improves with age as a result of increases in overall knowledge and increasing use of strategies, as well as a growing awareness of memory (Schneider and Pressley 1997, Flavell et al 2002). There is reason to believe that the same concepts might apply to the development of a child's ability to coordinate and control movement. However, important though memory might be to movement, the study of memory and movement has received little empirical attention, with studies limited primarily to a multistore view of memory, in regard to movement performance and adult learning, and with few studies on children. Research using a short-term motor memory paradigm (STMM) has yielded some limited insights into the memory processes involved in movement. These studies typically involve blindfolded participants making a criterion movement by moving an arm a designated distance on a linear or curvilinear track, such as that illustrated in Figure 3.1.

The criterion movement can be performed in active, passive, or constrained movement modes. After returning to a starting position and waiting a certain length of time, participants attempt to reproduce the criterion movement. Waiting time (intertrial delay) is varied to manipulate the retention interval in which the participants are presumed to retain the criterion movement in memory. Retention intervals may be unfilled (e.g. no activity), which is

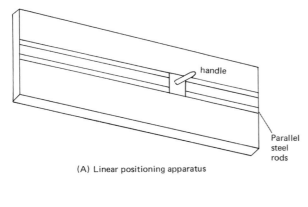

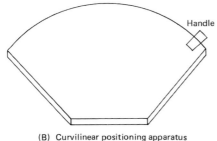

Fig. 3.1 Apparatus for assessing short-term motor memory.

presumed to permit rehearsal, or they may be filled with a secondary task designed to disrupt rehearsal. Participants are blindfolded, allowing only proprioceptive information to be available. Vision is sometimes available but it is limited because environmental cues must be masked when the participants are not blindfolded. The drawback of this research is that the laboratory tasks used are not typical of human movement skills. This calls into question the validity of the results.

Traditional models of memory continue to drive a substantial research enterprise in both adults and children. Diamond (2000) promoted the idea that motor development and cognitive development share a close interrelationship, based on the evidence of cerebellar development, which is important for both motor and cognitive function. The basis and stimulus for current work in memory, with emphasis on children, continues to assume that a memory system has a structural basis, as evidenced by research by Mandler and McDonough (1995) and more recently by Bauer (2004). The focus of this work has been on infants' ability to imitate, via recall, non-verbal activity.

Motor programmes as schemas
A second form of memory comes from the motor control field and involves Schmidt's (1975) schema theory of a generalized motor programme (GMP), organized around

rules called recognition and recall schemas. The general sense of schemas is that a mover has rules defining the relationships among the information involved in the production and evaluation of a movement. For example, more force is needed to produce greater velocity, or a longer distance when throwing an object. Schmidt named four features of information required for an individual to make an intended movement: initial conditions that exist prior to the movement, response specifications for the motor programme, sensory consequences of the movement, and the outcome of the movement. When several similar movements have been attempted, the mover can abstract the relationships among these four sources of information in order to formulate both the recognition schema and recall schema.

A fundamental proposition in schema theory is that the variability of experience (practice) will lead to the establishment of stronger schemas, especially when it relates to a common set of tasks. The logic is that the variability of experience offers richer and more varied information to the mover, who can extract from this information a more complete rule about means–ends relationships. It follows that a more complete schema allows the mover to organize movements better in unfamiliar or novel situations, which involve the class of movements covered by a GMP. The studies of children and schema development suggest that children only have some means of organizing movement around their general knowledge about the relationship between outcome and intent, whether we call this relationship a schema or some other construct. Variability of practice benefits skill learning in children (Yan et al 1998). The whole issue of GMPs, which schema theory addresses, does not provide a complete account of skill production in children or adults. It does, however, point to a less specific need for separate programmes to be stored in the context of a traditional information processing theoretical context.

A recent review of schema theory (Shea and Wulf 2005) noted that, irrespective of any critical evaluation of Schmidt's schema theory, the consistent results of variability of practice studies suggest that any re-evaluation of GMPs must take into account the ideas expressed by the original schema theory. It is perhaps important to note that the way in which we structure practice, and the benefits derived from organizing practice to reflect the variability idea, does not require a specific theoretical account: there is something intuitive about practising a range of skilled activities around a common theme. It is also an empirical fact that structure of practice studies have bolstered the central message in schema theory rather than providing more general support for the GMP aspect it was originally intended to address.

The traditional approach (information processing) assumes that movement production is the neuromotor system's control of the movements and positions of the body parts. A movement's force, speed, accuracy, and related outcomes are external manifestations of neuromotor activity. Motor control is the general designation of a field of study that focuses on the production of movement by the neuromotor system. Motor control is expanding rapidly as a field of study, although it is mainly concerned with mature performance and often with high-level, elite performance. This section is a brief and speculative look at some of the issues and concerns involved in the development of motor control.

Motor control research has been concerned primarily with how the neuromotor system produces movements. Some research has dealt directly with this issue by examining the structural and functional characteristics of certain aspects of the nervous system. Another approach has been to infer motor control functioning from behavioural measurements. Whereas discussion here is limited to a behavioural approach, work in both areas has progressed rapidly in combining the direct study of neuromotor functioning with behavioural inferences.

Internal models redux

Generally in motor learning we consider how the brain adapts to control the body.
(Wolpert et al 2001, p. 487)

Skilled motor behavior requires both inverse and forward internal models…appropriate for different tasks and environments.
(Wolpert et al 2001, p. 488)

The above two quotes by Daniel Wolpert and colleagues remind us that the long-held assumption that motor skills are constructed and controlled by the brain, via computational activity, is alive and well. The continuing challenge for computational neuroscience in general, however, is to solve the problem of redundancy (referred to as 'Bernstein's problem'). With respect to natural biological motion the system makes redundancy a virtue, not a problem. Neuroscience continues to adhere to a strategy of seeking to solve the challenge of how the brain exploits the virtue of redundancy. Wolpert et al (2001), quoted above, specify three principal ways in which the learning system interacts with the environment, and these are represented by three computational paradigms: supervised learning, reinforcement learning, and unsupervised learning. The unifying framework for understanding these principles is Bayesian learning (i.e. Bayesian decision theory). From the research published by Wolpert and his group (Wolpert and Flanagan 2010) and others working on this problem, progress has been mixed. In a far-ranging review of computational motor control, Karniel (2011) continues the 'promissory' message of this approach to understanding human motor control and notes, 'We have a lot of work before us as we strive to formulate a reasonable computational model for motor control for the motor system' (Karniel 2011, p. 403).

The work of Wolpert has provided new impetus to the well-established computational approaches to understanding motor control, but the problem of simulating natural biological motor control remains a challenge. The engineering idea of system 'noise' remains an explanation that to a large degree is conjecture, for a less than perfect simulation. While progress has been made, the successes remain more robotic than human. From a developmental perspective this more recent work on internal models has had no impact on our understanding of emergent motor behaviour in the child. In fact nothing new has been forthcoming since the insights offered by Connolly (1970): the maturing child was depicted as developing more mature subroutines that reflect more efficient and precise motor behaviour and skill.

Information processing and motor development
Traditional information processing has provided us with a plethora of detail concerning the development of motor control. In this section we provide examples of the types of paradigms and studies that have been used over the last 50 years and that have utilized this theoretical approach as the base. These examples are selections that illustrate the fundamental principles of traditional information processing in which the information is transformed through a series of operations from the taking in of information to the final movement product.

SHORT-TERM MOTOR MEMORY
Research by Adams and Dijkstra (1966) initially questioned whether STMM followed the same laws as verbal short-term memory. Using adult participants the results contradicted the verbal studies of Adams and Dijkstra (1966) and Posner and Konick (1966). Verbal memory, but not motor memory, appeared to be differentially affected by the difficulty of the secondary task used in the filled retention interval. However, some of the earlier inconsistencies were explained by the finding that different encoding processes were used for different reproduction cues, particularly location and distance cues. Location cues represent final limb position; distance cues determine how far the limb travels in space. Few studies exist on the development of movement memory in children, and these

have been concerned mainly with mnemonic strategies, such as rehearsal. A series of studies by Sugden (1978, 1980a,b) examined the development of rehearsal in the visual–motor and motor memory in typically developing children (TDC), and males with intellectual disability. Sugden's research confirmed that for visual–motor and motor tasks, as for verbal tasks, a characteristic feature of immature memorizers was the lack of spontaneous use of control operations, such as rehearsal. Immature memorizers include both TDC who are young in age and children young in cognitive functioning. Likewise, Reid (1980a) also found evidence for rehearsal in 10- and 16-year-old TDC on a STMM task, whereas children with intellectual disabilities showed no evidence of rehearsal. In a follow-up study, Reid (1980b) attempted to aid memory in children with intellectual disability by teaching them a mnemonic strategy. The teaching was successful, with the participants with intellectual disability being more accurate in an instructional than a non-instructional condition. Reid suggested that the problem was a production deficiency because training resulted in improved performance.

Kelso and colleagues (1979) allowed children with intellectual disability to select their own movement to reproduce, rather than having the experimenter specify the movement criterion. Their findings suggested that active involvement in producing the criterion movement aided retention and might help overcome a production deficiency. Reid (1980b) noted, however, that the children with intellectual disability in these experiments were instructed to remember the movement's end location, which may have led to unintentional rehearsal and, thus, may not have been spontaneously producing a rehearsal strategy. Memory for location and distance was tested by Thomas et al (1983) in a large-scale environment. Children (ages 4 to 12) jogged (ran) through a course and then were asked to recall the location, or distance, covered in an event. The results from the two experiments in this study were similar to the findings from the arm-positioning movements in laboratory studies.

With minimal research focus on 'memory for movement' the findings that have been reported rely a great deal on 'conjectured' inferences such as 'access to central processing space' or 'processing strategies are age related'. Overall, the study of memory to better understand motor development has been a less than interesting area of study. Only age effects (well known) and intellectual differences (also a well-established fact) show reliable differences from a developmental perspective.

The focus on the motor aspects of the memory system's short-term or working memory and long-term memory abilities is an area that has added little to our

knowledge save the fact that by 6 months of age children can recall information and by 2 years of age this ability is firmly established. Likewise, as children develop, typical activities such as rehearsal and retrieval become evident with respect to memorizing information. What remains an unsolved issue is how memory functions 'in the head'. Brain imaging has moved the exploration beyond conjecture and has now found the location of brain activity. What remains a challenge is the inherent plasticity of the brain, such that it has a known capacity to 'reorganize' activities in different locations. Memory function may well be a 'moving target' from this perspective. The only true motor domain issue is the fact that we all remember well continuous motor skills and are less capable of remembering more discrete motor activities. Why is this? One conjecture (Schmidt and Lee 2011) is that discrete skills may have a higher verbal–cognitive component than the more periodic, continuous skills, such as swimming or riding a bicycle.

ATTENTION

When we think about attention, what immediately comes to mind is our level of 'alertness' with respect to initiating a motor activity. Sport psychologists refer to this as 'focus'. The other common feature, with respect to attention, is our ability to do more than one thing at a time. The recent problem of mobile telephone use while driving is a classic example of what is referred to as 'divided attention'. Finally, there is the concept of 'selective attention', which distinguishes our ability to focus on relevant versus irrelevant aspects of a task or activity. The majority of research on these aspects of attention point to a general age effect (Harnishfeger and Pope 1996). As one might expect, younger children are more easily distracted and cannot stay 'on task' as well as older children (Goldberg et al 2001).

With the information processing system having structures and control operations, attention is a prerequisite. Attention is typically viewed as having a *limited capacity* that can be allocated as needed. It is logical, therefore, that attention allocation will show a developmental trend, as improvement in allocation requires the selection of task-relevant variables. The concept of selective attention is often investigated in dual-task or time-sharing paradigms, in which a central task and a secondary task are performed separately. When both tasks are performed simultaneously, any differences between them indicate how children allocate their limited processing capacity. In a series of studies by Hagen and associates (Hagen 1967, Hagen and Fisch 1968, Druker and Hagen 1969), performance on a primary task improved with age, but performance on a secondary task did not, or sometimes declined. This suggested that younger children allocate their available attention somewhat equally between the two tasks. Older children seemed to recognize the importance of the primary task and allocated more attention to it. Other research (Conroy and Weener 1976, Dusek 1978, Hale and Alderman 1978) supported these findings. Simon (1972) reviewed this literature and concluded that the structural limits of attention are fixed but can be reallocated. As they grow older, children become more adept at distributing the allocation of their attentional resources by adopting deliberate, though not necessarily conscious, strategies.

Wickens and Benel (1982) refer to capacity allocation as *time-sharing efficiency*, which improves with age. They suggested four possible sources of improvement:

1 *Automation*: performance on one task stays the same with less attention, making more resources available for doing a concurrent task.
2 *Expanding resources*: a structural increase in capacity.
3 *Functional differentiation of resource reservoirs*: the existence of more than a single capacity, so that two tasks interfere with each other only to the extent that they draw from the same reservoir.
4 *Attention deployment skills*: the use of strategies (control operations) as a functional means of processing more information.

CAPACITY ALLOCATION

Assuming that attentional capacity can be variably allocated to parts of the processing system as needed, it follows that when young children first acquire a movement pattern, most of their attentional capacity is required to control the movement. This suggests that *time sharing* must exist in some form. Some individuals can perform several tasks at once, such as walking, bouncing a ball, and seeing what is happening around them. The processing demands for a mature adult do not exceed the available attentional capacity for such multitasking. Young children trying to perform several tasks simultaneously may well exceed the amount of available capacity. Investigations of dual-task performance are one way to study time sharing in capacity allocation from a developmental perspective.

Bruner (1970) outlined the action of sucking, which, in young infants, changes on a week-to-week basis. Sucking behaviour is a well-established, reflexive action at birth, which eventually becomes a voluntary behaviour. At first, young infants suck with their eyes shut. If their eyes are open during sucking, object tracking begins and the sucking is disrupted. At 9 weeks, infants suck in bursts and look up during the pauses; at 3 to 4 months, infants

appear to be able to suck and to look up simultaneously, but this may be misleading because looking reduces suction amplitude. Bruner referred to this as 'place holding', which maintains the structure of a more inclusive act while executing the various parts separately. Later, infants can look up without reducing their suction power, thus achieving a functional dual-task behaviour. To examine the infant's growing repertoire of dual-task behaviours, Bruner (1970) placed a toy in a box with a see-through lid, which slid open. An efficient way to obtain the toy would be to slide open the lid with one hand, and then hold it open while reaching for the toy with the other hand. The two hands need to be sequenced with all the constituent parts in order. Bruner observed infants from 6 to 17 months and found overall success for 6% of the younger group, rising to 37% success for the older group. Another illustration of two-handed skill is described in Chapter 5 for the marble game used by Elliott and Connolly (1974) *(see Fig. 5.10)*. The overall results indicate that younger children could execute individual movements but had difficulty in performing simultaneous or sequential movements; as they grew older, they were better able to turn the knobs together and with correct timing.

PROCESSING SPEED

The speed of responding to a stimulus is an important consideration because many movement situations have a time constraint connected to the response. In information processing history, responding as quickly as possible to a stimulus has produced a plethora of research on groups of humans across the lifespan. The research focuses on what is referred to as *response time*, which is the sum of two rapid movements. The first is reaction time and the second is movement time. Research on both reaction time and movement time clearly demonstrates that they share a common relationship. Additional detail is provided on the developmental aspects of these topics in Chapter 6.

Reaction time

Reaction time is the usual way in which speed of processing is measured, on the assumption that reaction time reflects the time needed to process information from the stimulus signal and initiate movement. If the information load is known, the processing speed will be the information load divided by the reaction time. The linear relationship between information load and reaction time was first reported by Hick (1952) in what has become known as Hick's law: reaction time increases linearly with information load, when load is specified as the logarithm of the number of equally occurring alternatives. Connected to this explanation, it is important to know that a 'bit' (shorthand for binary digit) is the amount of information

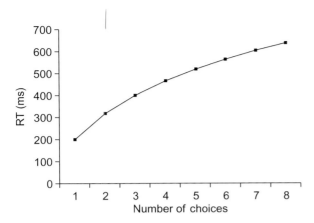

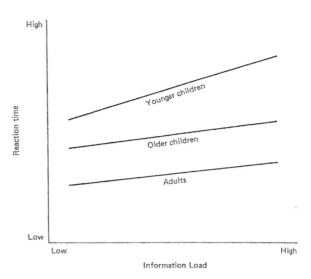

Fig. 3.2 Predicted reaction times (RT), according to Hick's law, for one- to eight-choice reaction time situations, based on a simple (i.e. one-choice) reaction time of 200ms.

Fig. 3.3 A general representation of increases in reaction time as information load increases.

needed to reduce 'uncertainty' by a half. Thus, one bit of information flows when two equally probable outcomes are reduced by a half: $\log_2(2)=1$ and likewise $\log_2(4)=2$. Hick added one to the number of alternatives because there is an added unit of uncertainty if participants do not know when the stimulus will appear. Reaction time scores predicted by Hick's law are illustrated in Figure 3.2.

The Dutch scientist Donders in 1868 (reprinted in 1969) tried to differentiate, within a reaction time, the decision processes of choice and discrimination. Donders' experiments were not totally successful, but a later series of experiments by Sternberg (1969, 1975) yielded a useful approach to discovering different decision processes within reaction time. Sternberg's experiments presented participants with a list of items followed by a single probe item. Participants had to determine if the original list contained the probe item, in effect, scanning their memory in order to compare the probe item with the items in the list. The time taken to respond increased linearly as the list lengthened, which led Sternberg to conclude that memory search proceeds in a serial order. Another finding was that it takes as long to decide that a stimulus is present as it does to decide that it is not. In other words, even if the item appears early in the list, an exhaustive search will still take place. Both Hick's (1952) and Sternberg's (1969, 1975) paradigms tell a similar story. Increase the number of choices, and the time for processing will increase; reduce the number of alternatives and processing time will decrease.

Children's reaction times have been measured in various situations, and the results have been reasonably consistent in the general patterns of change (Fig. 3.3). First, as expected, there are absolute performance differences, with children becoming faster as they grow older.

Second, Hick's law has been confirmed, with reaction time rising linearly as the amount of information to be processed increases. Third, the regression line defining the relationship of information load and reaction time for young children often has a steeper slope. Young children are not only slower in an absolute sense but also for higher information loads, as they also require more processing time. Additional data on the developmental aspects of reaction time are described in Chapter 6.

As children get older they increase their speed of processing, but processing speed is not a unitary factor because the rate (speed) of detection, recognition, and decision making may change at different rates over the course of development.

The most obvious way to reduce processing time is to *decrease uncertainty*, which in processing terminology is called *redundancy*. The less we know about incoming stimuli (*uncertainty*) the more processing time will be needed; if the stimulus is known or recognized, less processing time is needed. The consensus – with respect to processing speed – is that speed of responding improves rapidly with age, reaching an optimal level by the age of 16 years and maintaining that speed through the next five decades (Cerella and Hale 1994, Kail and Salthouse 1994).

Movement time
Processing time is measured as response time (i.e. the lag between a 'go signal' and the initiation of movement). Movement time is the time required to actually complete a movement. Also note here that reaction time + movement time = *response time*. Reaction time is a function of the

uncertainty related to the number of stimuli and response choices to be identified and organized. Movement time is a function of movement distance and movement accuracy, in that the variation in distance and accuracy requirements changes the information load related to the control of movement. The motor system's capacity to function under varying information loads has been studied extensively.

Fitts (1954) proposed that movement time varies in relation to movement distance and accuracy. His formula for this relationship has been tested and supported in many different contexts and under many different conditions. The data and analyses from studying Fitts' law are robust and have been of great benefit in studying processing requirements during rapid movements. Fitts' law is explained in Chapter 6, Box 6.5, along with two methods for measuring the motor system's capacity. Readers will note that the computations for the index of difficulty share the same logarithmic basis ($\log_2$) of Hick's law.

The findings from two studies (Salmoni and Pascoe 1978, Sugden 1980b) are presented in Table 3.1 to illustrate the differences in findings for younger children. The values for $1/b$ differ in the two studies because of the length of the trials and other procedural differences.

Both studies confirmed that older children and adults have similar slopes, which means that increases in processing load are not relatively more difficult for older children, even though their movement time is slower. Older children have a smaller capacity in an absolute sense, but they adjust to increases in their processing load in a manner similar to the way adults do. Capacity by age, expressed as index of difficulty/movement time is illustrated in Table 3.2. The general findings for the movement speed of children doing reciprocal and discrete tapping tasks are shown in Figure 3.4. As the figure illustrates, movement time is less for adults, and older children have faster movement times than younger children. Children's and adults' movement times increase as

TABLE 3.1

Capacity on a reciprocal tapping task as measured by rate of gain of information (1/b)

	Study	
Age (y)	Salmoni and Pascoe (1978)	Sugden (1980b)
6	7.6	8.9
8		8.1
10	10.6	8.6
12		8.9
14	11.0	
Adults	9.8	

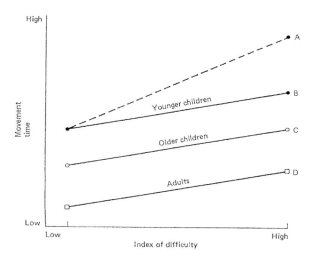

Fig. 3.4 General relationship of movement time and index of difficulty for different age groups (Sugden 1981).

TABLE 3.2
Capacity of children (index of difficulty/movement time) for reciprocal and single tapping

	Reciprocal tapping		Single tap	
Index of difficulty by bits of information	2.0	5.6	3.0	5.6
Age (y)				
6	3.0	5.4	8.1	9.3
8	4.4	6.4	8.5	10.3
10	6.8	7.5	10.7	12.3
12	7.5	8.4	12.8	14.7

Reproduced from data in Sugden (1981).

the index of difficulty increases because more information must be processed to control movement for a longer distance and/or accuracy to contact a smaller target. An important and unresolved question is whether children have relatively greater increases in movement time as index of difficulty increases. This is discussed further in Chapter 6.

KNOWLEDGE OF RESULTS

After completing a movement, movers can evaluate its quality and their success in achieving the intended movement objective in two ways. First, proprioceptive information is available as a consequence of the movement; second, error information as to the accuracy of the movement can be provided by the experimenter. This latter form of feedback is called knowledge of results. The evaluation of error information in the form of feedback provides information to be used in preparing for subsequent movements. Knowledge of results is a source of feedback, which provides both performance information and, to some degree, acts as a motivation for improvement. Both aspects have been studied with children and are interrelated because the more precise the error information the more time is required to process it. The level of precision of error information, however, may not be useful simply because the nature or form of the knowledge of results influences how useful it can be for the child learner. The consensus is that if the information is too general or too precise it does not assist children, regardless of the time available to process it.

The experimenter can control the processing time of knowledge of results in a number of ways. First, knowledge of results may be given immediately or may be delayed during the intertrial interval. Knowledge of results delay time becomes important when the delay is sufficiently long. A delay that is too great impacts on the value of the knowledge of results for future performance. Second, the time from receiving knowledge of results until the next trial begins is *post-knowledge-of-results delay*, which is the time available to process knowledge of results. We are concerned here with post-knowledge-of-results delay time because this time period may be too short for children to process knowledge of results adequately. This has been recognized as a difficulty for adults as well (Newell 1976).

The experimenter can also control the precision of error information when provided as knowledge of results, as well as the time when it is given during the intertrial interval. Knowledge of results may be too general to be useful in one situation but too precise or too complex in other situations. Post-knowledge-of-results delay time and precision of error information are also important and interactive conditions in studying the motor system's functional capacity.

As we might expect, younger children often need more time to process information, and their movement performance would be affected if they have insufficient time to prepare. A clear demonstration was provided by Gallagher and Thomas (1980), who varied post-knowledge-of-results delay time from 3 to 9 seconds on a curvilinear positioning task. Younger children (age 7) improved markedly as they were given more time, until they had a mean error score similar to that of older children (age 11) and adults. The performance of older children and adults did not change in relation to the time available to process knowledge of results. This means that we must decide whether younger children are unable to process information or merely do not have enough time to process it.

Barclay and Newell (1980) allowed participants to determine the length of the post-knowledge-of-results delay time on a linear positioning task by moving when they were ready. All of the participants cut their post-knowledge-of-results time interval as they became more familiar with the task, but the adults continued to use less time to process information. An optimal precision level of knowledge of results for improving movement performance was demonstrated by Newell and Kennedy (1978) to be a direct function of age. Different levels of knowledge of results were given to four groups of children (ages 6, 8, 10, and 14) performing a positioning task. A curvilinear relationship between knowledge of results and age was found: performance was poorer with extreme levels of very imprecise or very precise knowledge of results and the optimal level of knowledge of results became more precise with age. Newell and Carlton (1980) found that there were no differences among children at ages 9, 11, and 15 on a motor response recognition task, in contrast with a movement production task in which an intermediate level of knowledge-of-results precision was provided. However, 9-year-olds had larger mean errors than 15-year-olds when given extreme levels of very precise or very imprecise knowledge of results. Newell and Carlton suggest that developmental differences are more associated with planning and recall processes to produce movement rather than related to recognition. The precision of knowledge of results may also be task specific (Salmoni 1980), such as level of task difficulty, and later performance, when knowledge of results is removed. Thomas et al (1979) found that older children were better able to use more precise information on a difficult task and retain it for later use. The research on the developmental aspects of knowledge of results has changed little from the research completed in the 1970s and 1980s.

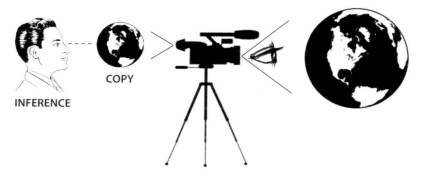

Fig. 3.5 Schematic representation of 'indirect perception', requiring a copy of the external environment to process perceptual information.

These selected studies give a flavour of the type of processing research that has been conducted across a range of ages. Although valuable information helps us to describe the way in which children get better with age, explanations about how and why development takes place have not been furthered in recent work employing these paradigms. In summary, the traditional information processing model has produced most of the motor learning and development research since the start of its role as a theoretical model in the mid-1960s. The specific contributions to motor development research have been limited to age effects and differences between TDC and those with some degree of intellectual disability and other children with atypical resources. This is not to minimize the contributions, but as we will now see, the alternative dynamic systems and ecological psychology approaches have produced more interesting additional insights into motor development and provided a very different theoretical perspective about the developmental trajectory of motor behaviour.

Alternative theories

Ecological Psychology
The traditional view of information processing requires the individual to 'work' on available sensory input in order to use it. Information processing theory assumes indirect perception; an alternative is that perception is direct (Gibson 1979). This view sees perception and action (doing) as directly linked without the need for complicated processing operations (see Fig. 3.5). Gibson argued that this coupled relationship between perception and action (movement) was a key element to his proposition that perception was direct and that it was via action that new information was detected that both guides and constrains future action. It was this perception–action link that contrasted dramatically and challenged the traditional information processing view of perception that required

translation or interpretation (processing) by the CNS in order to formulate an appropriate response. Earlier in this chapter we talked about the connection between mind and body and, without necessarily arguing in favour of this, we used it to illustrate the connection between action and cognition. Gibson's (1979) ecological psychology sees no need for an internal representation of the world; environmental information is rich and readily accessible by the perceiving organism. This is in stark contrast to the assumption that perception is indirect, as illustrated in Figure 3.5.

For Gibson it was through action that the individual directly perceived information from the environment by being sensitive to the invariant properties in the environment such as the ambient light, shadows, and the many other elements and contrasts that structure the world that we see. Gibson's theory of perception assumes that the performer is sensitive to opportunities for action in the environment. Gibson (1979) termed these opportunities 'affordances'. Thus, when viewing an object in the environment, the actor is sensitive to its inherent opportunities for action. For example, a cup may afford drinking, a spoon may afford eating, and a ball playful activity; a range of action possibilities may be drawn from viewing these objects. This action potential can, and often does, lead to an overestimation or an underestimation of the action opportunities an object might afford. These ideas have been developed alongside the continued adherence by many in cognitive psychology and cognitive neuroscience who continue to hold on to the information processing model. Neuroscience focuses more on the anatomy and fine analysis of neural activity in the brain, as it relates to simple motor skill activities in monkeys and small mammals and fish, and to a much lesser extent in individuals limited to small motor responses, constrained in large part by current limitations of magnetic resonance imagery. Information present in the environment (Gibson 1979) was labelled by Gibson as an 'affordance'. Figure 3.6

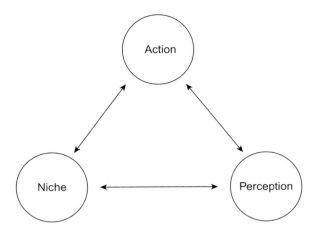

Fig. 3.6 Schematic diagram of the coimplicative relations among actions, perceptions, and the environmental niche. Reproduced from Michaels and Carello (1981).

depicts this relationship again in the form of a tripartite dynamic context.

From Figure 3.6 the implication is that no action can occur without considering the environmental context in which it takes place, and the specific location (niche) of the 'actor'. Gibson (1979) calls this the 'animal–environment' relationship. Thus a coordinative act must recognize the interrelationships among the action system, the perceptual system, and the environmental niche in which this takes place. These were the ideas exploited by Turvey and coworkers (Turvey 1977, Turvey et al 1978) to develop a theoretical perspective that minimized the need for internal representations, which in essence argued that the 'animal–environment' relationship required a set of internal 'devices' to interpret and make sense of the very world we inhabit.

THE PERCEPTION–ACTION LINK

Basic to any view of perception is the following question: What information is available to the individual? How is it obtained, and how is it used? Michaels and Carello (1981), in support of Gibson (1979), questioned the traditional information processing assumption that perception is indirect. First, they argue that if perception is indirect, then it assumes that the senses are engaging with an impoverished view of the world, thus processing or transformations are necessary in order to assign meaning to any environmental display. Second, because of this impoverished view of the world, the stimulus input from the environment must be processed. Perceptual and cognitive operations must therefore intervene constructively by detecting, selecting, attending, remembering, and making decisions. Third, perceiving is the sampling of sensory

input and is limited to one moment in time. Perception is in the present, and the present is a discrete moment, which creates the problem of how to relate one time sample to another. Indirect perception must perform this function, with memory as the internal mechanism. Fourth, perceiving and acting must be presumed to be separate or different entities if perception is indirect. The environment is seen, elaborated, and transformed by the individual to establish a basis for acting. The movement is then made by using any one of a number of control systems.

In questioning the traditional view that perception is indirect, Michaels and Carello (1981) are, in essence, questioning the idea that the environment in which we exist is somehow 'foreign' and 'unknown', thus requiring interpretation as to its meaning. This, they argue, is counterintuitive to the idea that organisms that have evolved in this environment cannot somehow directly interpret the precepts (meaning) embedded in it.

For Gibson, information represents complex structures of higher-order patterns of stimulation over time and comprises events rather than objects isolated in time and space. Stimulation specifies the environment and no elaboration is needed. From a direct perception viewpoint, perceptual richness comes with the structure (information), whereas with indirect perception, perceptual richness can be obtained only via elaborations performed by 'in the head' processing operations.

Perception is not limited to the present instant captured by a retinal snapshot, and the information and events that it specifies last over time. Thus, perception is defined as continuously knowing the environment. Michaels and Carello (1981) outline two differences in the concept of time between the direct-perception and the information-processing viewpoints. First, direct perception does not distinguish among past, present, and future. Perception is an unfolding of events, rather than snapshot instances, which blurs any distinctions between past, present, and future. Second, absolute time has little value to direct perception theorists. Events are the unit of analysis and they are determined by space and time. Perception is the continuous detection of information that can describe or specify an event of unlimited temporal extent. Figure 3.7 shows the distinction between indirect and direct modes of perceiving events and stimuli. An important consideration in direct perception is the assertion that, in order to study movement in the environment, the minimal system of analysis must be a coalition of mover and environment. This echoes our discussion in Chapter 1, in which we introduced a movement situation as the interplay of mover and environment to create a movement task and solution. Direct perception, however, does not involve the processing operations necessary in our analyses of

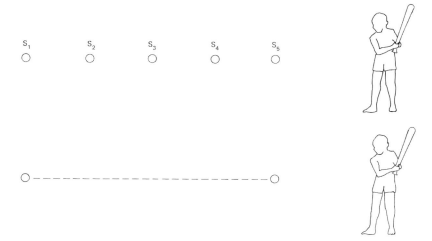

Fig. 3.7 *Indirect perception (upper image).* The ball flight is seen as a succession of occurrences, each with its own stimulus. The batsman must bring the separate occurrences together to form the total ball flight. *Direct perception (lower image).* The ball flight is seen as one event, such that information occurs over time and coexists with the event. The batsman has only to detect the event as specified by the environment.

movement situations. Two important concepts of invariants and affordances are offered in direct perception to explain the coalition of mover and environment.

If patterns of stimulation persist over time and space, and do not need embellishment, then stimulation will be invariantly tied to the environmental source. Invariants or stimulation patterns that do not change over time and space underlie the persistent properties of the environment that an individual knows. An example is the perceptual constancy – a phenomenon in which the perceived properties of an object, such as size, remain constant, even though the retinal image changes. An indirect approach says that the organism needs mediating processes to compensate for the changing image size. For direct perception, the answer lies in the properties of the stimulation, which has an invariance accompanying the objects' persistent properties. Within the changes in stimulation there are invariant patterns that provide the basis for perceptual constancy. Michaels and Carello (1981) state that 'Invariants come from the lawful relations between objects, places, and events in the environment…and the structure or manner of change of patterns of light, sound, skin deformation, joint configuration and so on' (p. 40).

Invariants specify objects, places, and events in the environment and are necessary for any information to be specified. However, environmental invariants are not sufficient without considering the individual. The individual is necessary because not all invariants are ecologically significant enough to permit or guide adaptive behaviour. Also, an individual's activities make available additional information. The integrating concept is that of

affordances to denote behaviour permitted by the environment. Affordances are what the environment means to an individual and describe an environment with reference to an individual. Gibson (1979) calls an affordance 'a specific combination of the properties of a substance and its surfaces with reference to an animal' (p. 67).

Affordances are what a situation offers to an animal or person. For example, when the properties of an object are seen as rigid, level, extended, and at 'knee height', an individual recognizes that the object affords sitting. The separate properties by themselves do not afford sitting; it is only when they are seen together that the affordance is recognized. This can be appreciated by changing only the property of 'knee height' so that the same object now affords leaning with the hands at shoulder level for a 3-year-old, affords crawling under for an infant of 9 months, and affords landing for a bird. The concept of affordances has been extended to a larger match of species and environment, called a niche. Humans fit into particular niches, which contain affordances relevant to humans. Other animals will fit into different niches; thus air affords flying for birds but not for humans. Gibson (1979) characterizes a niche as 'that into which an animal fits; it is that in relation to which the animal is habituated in its behaviour' (p. 129).

An example adapted by Walder (1981) from Turvey (1977) describes movement activity from a direct perception point of view. A soccer ball is passing a player and affords interception. In the player's field of view, the soccer ball is projected as a constantly changing pattern onto the optic array. The player's visual mechanisms detect those characteristics in the field of view that change over time and those that do not. The former specify the ball in terms of distance, speed, and projected path, and the latter identify the object as a soccer ball and as an object to be intercepted. To someone unfamiliar with soccer it might afford interception with the hands rather than the feet. Infants and young children would detect characteristics that change over time but probably less efficiently than older children and adults would. Invariant characteristics, however, might not afford interception.

DYNAMICAL SYSTEMS THEORY

The contributions of Bernstein's (1967) ideas on coordination dynamics and the constraining of the available degrees of freedom in the system formed the basis of what we now refer to as dynamical systems theory. Bernstein's ideas of coordination dynamics promote the self-organization of motor skills rather than the necessity for 'programmes' residing in the neurology to execute skilful intent. From a developmental viewpoint, the application of dynamical systems theory regards changes in the motor behaviour of the growing child as a function of the dynamic properties of the motor system (Kugler et al 1982). The 'motor milestones' viewed from a dynamical systems perspective see developmental change as an emergent process related to physical growth change; the development of a flexible skill set; and an understanding of how best to use that flexibility. Thelen and Ulrich (1991) and Thelen and Smith (1998) summarize a dynamical systems view of motor ability in the developing child as follows:

a) A preferred periodicity – motor behaviour is largely rhythmic in character.
b) The stability of the system can be maintained across a range of perturbations.
c) A capacity to reorganize at a different stable state if perturbations to the system become excessive.

In the terminology of dynamical systems, the above statements signify that an organism (child/adult) operating at a 'preferred' rate exhibits an 'attractor' state. The 'attractor' is the preferred rate at which the system maximizes stability and does not easily relinquish. At this rate the system can absorb some level of perturbation and maintain its stability (see statement b above). If the level of perturbation (some specified vector force) becomes too great, the system becomes unstable (briefly chaotic) and executes a phase shift to a new stable state (see statement c above). An example of this process would be to consider the stages of a horse's gait. Imagine we place a horse on a treadmill (such treadmills exist in veterinary schools): at a slow speed the horse will typically

walk; increase the speed and at some point the horse shifts (reorganizes its coordination) to a trot; add more velocity beyond stable trotting and the horse changes coordination again, producing a canter; finally, if the velocity of the treadmill continues to increase, the horse changes its gait pattern to a gallop. This is its final stable state, requiring maximum energy, and will last until fatigue makes it no longer possible to maintain. As a quadruped, the horse demonstrates four distinct gait patterns, which attain a stable state within a defined range of treadmill velocity. The horse can 'reorganize' its gait pattern in response to a treadmill speed that produces instability at the current gait. For the human biped, walk to run is the only shift in gait pattern available, but the system functions in the same way as a function of the velocity–speed vector. The example of the change in coordination is a good example of the 'self-organizing' principle of a dynamical systems approach to providing a relatively parsimonious account of motor skill expression. It obviates the need for specific programmes and separate input and output channels. A motor programme account for the above horse gait example would argue for a change in the GMP, from walking to trot, trot to canter, and so on. Such an account requires that the 'programme' be present in the neurology. There are examples of extremely novel coordination patterns arising where it would be hard to argue the presence of a programme. Such an example would be the experiments by von Holst (1939) on how fish spontaneously synchronized their fin motion to maintain stability in the water, when selected fins were removed! From these and other studies von Holst developed the idea of 'relative coordination', influenced by the coordinative properties of neuro-oscillators. These oscillators were capable of creating a large number of couplings to maintain stability of the system.

NEURONAL GROUP SELECTION THEORY

The 'neuronal group selection theory' (NGST) proposed by Sporns and Edelman (1993) contrasts the 'structural' view of traditional information processing, the ecological view that perception is direct, and dynamical systems theory to account for the processing of information. The traditional separation between perceiving and doing, distinguishing between the afferent and efferent streams of input and output, has given way to a more unified view of perception and action in the service of processing information. Edelman (1987, 1992), in proposing NGST, provides a 'brain science' rationale for the synthesis of perception. In much the same way that motor skills are now seen to 'emerge' as a function of exploration and selection by the developing infant, NGST provides a developmental account of brain development, building on the accepted

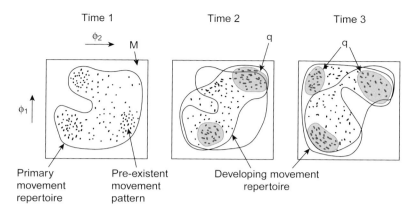

Fig. 3.8 Schematic of a developing movement repertoire. Movement within the space is specified by a combination of Φ_1 and Φ_2. Dot density represents movement frequency in a region of M. Time 1 represents pre-existent or innate movements. Time 2 and Time 3 represent evolving movement patterns, including previously unoccupied regions of M. On-going changes in both environmental and biomechanical constraints produce positive adaptations represented by θ. Reproduced from Sporns and Edelman (1993).

notion in contemporary neuroscience of brain plasticity; that is, brain development and change are seen as a function of experience.

Studying brain development at a finer level of analysis than gross anatomy reveals large variability with respect to cellular size and shape, as well as the range and type of neural connections. The NGST postulates that brain circuitry is not composed of rigid structures but develops as a function of the emergence of coordinated movement. In other words, the brain responds to the range and variability of the exploratory activities engaged in by the developing and increasingly active infant. Accordingly, NGST argues in favour of the development of neuronal 'groups' made up of interconnected neurons (synergies), which are a direct result of the unity of perception and action. This in turn produces a self-organizing neuronal process that is essentially a learning process engaged in by the developing brain. This is a radically different way of understanding how coordination and control emerge in the overall trajectory of motor development. These ideas incorporated into NGST provide common ground for both Gibson's (1979) ideas about direct perception and Bernstein's views of coordination and control. The process proposed by NGST is best illustrated in Figure 3.8.

Figure 3.8 depicts how movement repertoires expand from initial patterns of movement, over time, from birth (Time 1) to Time 2 and Time 3. Physical growth of the infant and the increasing number and variation of tasks bring about change in both the shape and density of the black dots, which represent the frequency of a particular set of movement patterns. Sporns and Edelman (1993) provide what is seen as a rapprochement between the

traditional information processing view and the more contemporary ecological and dynamical systems theorizing. It provides brain science rationale for how information is harnessed to promote overall development. Its value is that it provides an important role for the CNS, without labelling the CNS as the 'controller'. A good way of seeing this is to think of NGST as supporting the notion that 'the show runs the brain, the brain doesn't run the show' (TA Stoffregen, University of Minnesota, personal communication, March 2011). The Sporns and Edelman idea of NGST suggests that a rapprochement between traditional information processing perspectives and the more contemporary ecological and dynamical systems ideas is possible. This is a debate that will continue at a theoretical level for some time to come. A commitment to realism makes it unlikely that such a rapprochement will be possible without some realignment of the two views of perception.

The ecological view of information and how it might be interpreted sees as critical the perception–action link, especially in interpreting such traditional structural assumptions as memory. Certainly memory is a fact, irrespective of whether we distinguish between short-term or working memory and long-term memory. As we have already noted, the concept of a 'perception/action' cycle came into its own with the theoretical ideas of both Eleanor and James Gibson (JJ Gibson 1979, EJ Gibson 1982, 1988). Earlier, Piaget (1952) had noted the relationship between perceiving and acting in the context of the developing child's representational thought, but Piaget regarded sensorimotor activity as assisting in the development of 'structural' systems for cognition. The 'Gibsonian' view of this relationship is considerably more radical. First, as already noted, direct perception requires no 'in the head' transcription, which ascribes perception a powerful role with respect to movement and how the mover (actor) 'knows' or acquires information from their immediate environment. The key link here is the idea of an 'affordance' as described above.

Motor control and development

In Chapter 4, which covers the first 2 years of life, we shall see that the development of posture, reaching and grasping, and other *phylogenetic* skill sets are the foundation for, but different from, the development of *ontogenetic* skills, which reflect the motor tasks representative of our culture. The 'task' of mastering upright posture and independent locomotion is rather different from performing the plethora of laboratory tasks typically used and reported in the motor skills research literature, irrespective of its developmental orientation. We have devoted considerable space to the traditional information processing view of how we control and acquire motor skills: the centrepiece of this view is that symbolic movement plans are the primary influence. Very much in keeping with this information processing view, standard cognitive neuroscience seeks to locate where in the CNS these representations reside. It follows that practice is the mode for improving the optimization of these representations (motor programmes) in the CNS. Dynamical systems theory takes a very different view from this 'machine' view of traditional theory. The dynamical systems approach to skill acquisition has been referred to as a 'constraints-led approach' (Davids et al 2008).

Keogh and Sugden (1985) and Newell (1986), 25 years ago, promoted the notion that the dynamic relationship between *task performer* and *environment* were major constraints to any expression of skilled activity. This 'constraints' perspective has garnered substantial theoretical and empirical attention over the last 25 years. This is true with respect to the study of both motor learning and motor development. Newell et al (2001) proposed that

> There are potentially many indices of change in motor behaviour and many time scales over which the change in behaviour occurs. Nevertheless, theories of motor learning and development have been predicated predominantly on attempts to determine a single function of behavioural change across a range of task outcomes and context domains.
>
> (p. 57)

They (Newell et al 2001) promote the idea that there are multiple time scales that contribute to the learning and development of motor skills, rather than relying on a single function that accounts for change.

The topics and research discussed in Chapter 4 on the growing infant's journey of discovery and exploration, triggered by the ability to walk, are excellent examples of how dynamical systems theory has contributed to empirical research on motor development. The new terminology of dynamical systems theory allows the individual (child or adult) to explore what is called the *perceptual–motor landscape*, wherever that location might be; performing and learning a laboratory task, or exploring ways to climb a tree. The constraints placed on the individual to assemble a successful movement solution are a function of what is required (task demand); the context in which the movement is to be attempted (environment); and the abilities of the individual (performer). What transpires is a movement solution unique to the individual at that specific time and in that specific place, which may or may not be successful. In a sense this is 'trial and error' learning, which is much like the reported observations of infants learning to navigate down slopes of varying angles (Adolph 1995). As such, developing infants acquire a repertoire of responses to deal with an ever-increasing set of movement problems. This ever-changing perceptual–motor landscape reflects both the acquisition of new patterns of coordination and the physical development of the growing child. This idea was first proposed by Waddington (1957) but has been co-opted for its application to the dynamic aspects of motor development. This dynamic view of development is illustrated in Figure 3.9.

The principles outlined above stand in stark contrast to the traditional view that internal representations are needed to learn a skill rather than an ongoing exploration of the task demands from which a response *emerges* as a function of the actor's perception of the situation and what it *affords*. Thelen (1995), in discussing the developmental acquisition of motor skills, notes the contemporary emphasis as 'multicausal, fluid, contextual, and self-organizing nature of developmental change' (p. 297).

This approach to learning skills does not require computer-based terminology such as 'open and closed loop responding', 'modularization', or 'subroutines'. It is certainly possible to design laboratory experiments that require participants to respond as a 'closed' or 'open' loop system (e.g. slow movements vs fast [ballistic] movements), and the results of such research have contributed to a better understanding of how individuals use feedback, how performance improves over time, and what is retained as a measure of learning (permanent change). The message here is that, from a developmental perspective, how motor control and coordination arises is largely the *emergence* of self-organized movement patterns, both

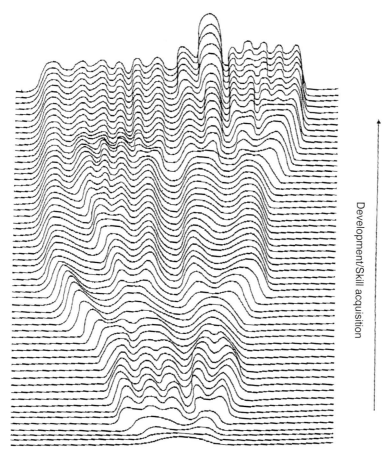

Fig. 3.9 As a learner's constraints change over time, the topology of the landscape alters to reflect the effects of development and new experiences as well as the acquisition of new skills. Reproduced from Muchisky et al (1996).

constrained and influenced by the task, environment and the individual performer's abilities. This latter constraint represents the variability present in humans as a function of such things as ethnicity, sociological and cultural background, and the resources available as they develop.

Summary

We have reviewed the major theoretical viewpoints regarding the acquisition of motor skill from a developmental perspective. We have noted differences between the evolutionary nature of movement skills (phylogenetic) and how these basic or fundamental skills support the variety of skill sets (ontogenetic) required to live in our cultural milieu. It is not necessary to directly compare the different theoretical views; rather, the true differences lie in the way in which skilled activity is organized and the differing viewpoints as to the role of the CNS. Clearly, the brain plays a key role in motor activity; the central question is whether the brain directly regulates the motor system ('run the show') or supports the regularity that

is a hallmark of human control and coordination. The essential difference is a question of the locus of control: is it a hierarchy ('top-down') or is it a heterarchy, a shared responsibility with other features of the system? Trauma to the CNS can be explained from either perspective. The brain is in reality a system regulated by its chemistry; changes in the chemistry produce observable changes in behaviour, both motor and social (i.e. drug induced), but behaviour can also change the brain chemistry – it is a two-way street! The traditional information processing approach has made major contributions regarding the learning of specific skills and the variables that mediate learning. From a developmental perspective, these differences relate primarily to age effects and levels of intellectual function. Both the ecological view that perception is direct and the dynamical systems approach to coordination and control, over the last 25 years, have had a major impact on promoting a better understanding of how the trajectory of change looks from a motor development perspective and how it is linked to overall cognitive development. This is reflected by the fact that not only has movement development research in the field of kinaesiology changed, but also developmental

psychology has 'rediscovered' movement development as a way of better understanding both perceptual and cognitive development.

REFERENCES

Adams JA, Dijkstra S (1966) Short-term memory for motor responses. *J Exp Psychol* 71: 314–318. http://dx.doi.org/10.1037/h0022846

Adolph KE (1995) Psychophysical assessment of toddler's ability to cope with slopes. *J Exp Psychol* 21: 734–750. http://dx.doi.org/10.1037/0096-1523.21.4.734

Barclay CR, Newell KM (1980) Children's processing of information in motor skill acquisition. *J Exp Child Psychol* 30: 98–108. http://dx.doi.org/10.1016/0022-0965(80)90078-8

Bauer PJ (2004) Getting explicit memory off the ground: Steps toward construction of a neuro-developmental account of changes in the first two years of life. *Dev Rev* 24: 347–373. http://dx.doi.org/10.1016/j.dr.2004.08.003

Bernstein N (1967) *The Co-ordination and Regulation of Movements*. New York: Pergamon Press.

Brown AL (1975) The development of memory: knowing, knowing about knowing and knowing how to know. In: Reese HW, editor. *Advances in Child Development and Behavior, Volume 10*. New York: Academic Press, pp. 103–152.

Brown AL (1978) Knowing when, where, and how to remember: a problem of metacognition. In: Glaser R, editor. *Advances in Instructional Psychology*. Hillsdale, NJ: Erlbaum, pp. 77–168.

Bruner JS (1970) The growth and structure of skill. In: Connolly KJ, editor. *Mechanisms of Motor Skill Development*. New York: Academic Press, pp. 63–91.

Cerella J, Hale S (1994) The rise and fall in information processing rates over the life-span. *Acta Psychologica* 86: 109–197. http://dx.doi.org/10.1016/0001-6918(94)90002-7

Connolly KJ (1970) Response, speed, temporal sequencing and information processing in children. In: Connolly KJ, editor. *Mechanisms of Motor Skill Development*. New York: Academic Press, pp. 161–192.

Conroy RL, Weener P (1976) The development of visual and auditory selective attention using the central-incidental paradigm. *J Exp Child Psychol* 22: 400–407. http://dx.doi.org/10.1016/0022-0965(76)90103-X

Davids K, Button C, Bennett S (2008) *Dynamic Skill Acquisition: A Constraints-Led Approach*. Champaign, IL: Human Kinetics.

Davidson PR, Wolpert DM (2005) Widespread access to predictive models in the motor system: a short review. *J Neural Eng* 2: 8313–8319. http://dx.doi.org/10.1088/1741-2560/2/3/S11

Diamond A (2000) Development and cognitive development of the cerebellum and frontal cortex. *Child Dev* 71: 44–56. http://dx.doi.org/10.1111/1467-8624.00117

Donders AF (1969) On the speed of mental processes. *Acta Psychologica* 30: 412–443. http://dx.doi.org/10.1016/0001-6918(69)90065-1

Druker JF, Hagen JW (1969) Developmental trends in the processing of task-relevant and task-irrelevant information. *Child Dev* 40: 371–382. http://dx.doi.org/10.2307/1127409

Dusek JB (1978) The effects of labeling and pointing in children's selective attention. *Dev Psychol* 14: 115–116. http://dx.doi.org/10.1037/0012-1649.14.1.115

Edelman GM (1987) *Neural Darwinism*. New York: Basic Books.

Edelman GM (1992) *Bright Air, Brilliant Fire: On the Matter of the Mind*. New York: Basic Books.

Elliott JM, Connolly KJ (1974) Hierarchical structure in skill development. In: Connolly K, Bruner JS, editors. *The Growth of Competence*. New York: Academic Press, pp. 135–168.

Fitts PM (1954) The information capacity of the human motor system in controlling the amplitude of movement. *J Exp Psychol* 47: 381–391. http://dx.doi.org/10.1037/h0055392

Flavell JH, Miller PH, Miller SA (2002) *Cognitive Development*, 4th edition. Englewood Cliffs, NJ: Prentice-Hall.

Gallagher JD, Thomas JR (1980) Effects of varying post-KR intervals upon children's motor performance. *J Motor Behav* 12: 41–56.

Gibson EJ (1982) The concept of affordances in development: the renaissance of functionalism. In: Collins WA, editor. *The Concept of Development: Minnesota Symposium on Child Psychology, Volume 15*. Hillsdale, NJ: Erlbaum, pp. 55–81.

Gibson EJ (1988) Exploratory behavior in the development of perceiving, acting and the acquiring of knowledge. *Annu Rev Psychol* 39: 1–41. http://dx.doi.org/10.1146/annurev.ps.39.020188.000245

Gibson JJ (1979) *The Ecological Approach to Visual Perception*. Boston, MA: Houghton Mifflin.

Goldberg M, Maurer D, Lewis TL (2001) Developmental changes in attention: the effects of endogenous cueing and of distractors. *Dev Sci* 4: 209–219. http://dx.doi.org/10.1111/1467-7687.00166

Hagen JW (1967) The effect of distraction on selective attention. *Child Dev* 38: 685–694. http://dx.doi.org/10.2307/1127246

Hagen JW, Fisch SR (1968) The effects of incidental cues on selective attention. Report no. 57, USPHS grant HD 03168. Ann Arbor, MI: Centre for Human Growth and Development, University of Michigan.

Hale GA, Alderman LB (1978) Children's selective attention with variation in amount of stimulus exposure. *J Exp Child Psychol* 26: 320–327. http://dx.doi.org/10.1016/0022-0965(78)90011-5

Harnishfeger KK, Pope RS (1996) Intending to forget: the development of cognitive inhibition in directed forgetting. *J Exp Psychol* 62: 292–315.

Hick WE (1952) On the rate of gain of information. *Q J Exp Psychol* 4: 11–26. http://dx.doi.org/10.1080/17470215208416600

von Holst E (1939) Die relative Koordination als Phaenomen und als method zentralnervoeser Funktionalyse. *Ergebnisse Physiol* 42: 228–306.

Kail R, Salthouse TA (1994) Processing speed as a mental capacity. *Acta Psychologica* 86: 199–225. http://dx.doi.org/10.1016/0001-6918(94)90003-5

Karniel A (2011) Open questions in computational motor control. J Integr Neurosci 10: 385–411. http://dx.doi.org/10.1142/S0219635211002749

Kelso JAS, Goodman D, Stamm CL, Hayes C (1979) Movement coding and memory in retarded children. *Am J Ment Deficiency* 83: 601–611.

Keogh J, Sugden D (1985) *Motor Skill Development*. New York: Macmillan.

Kreutzer MA, Leonard C, Flavell JH (1975) An interview study of children's knowledge about memory. *Monographs of the Society for Research in Child Development* 40: 1–60.

Kugler PN, Kelso JAS, Turvey MT (1982) On the control and co-ordination of naturally developing systems. In: Kelso JAS, Clark JE, editors. *The Development of Movement Control and Co-Ordination*. New York: Wiley, pp. 5–78.

Magill RA (2009) *Motor Learning and Control*. New York: McGraw-Hill.

Mandler JM, McDonough L (1995) Long-term recall of event sequences in infancy. *J Exp Child Psychol* 59: 457–474. http://dx.doi.org/10.1006/jecp.1995.1021

Michaels CF, Carello C (1981) *Direct Perception*. Englewood Cliffs, NJ: Prentice-Hall.

Muchisky M, Gerschoff-Stowe L, Cole E, Thelen E (1996) The epigenetic landscape revisited: a dynamic interpretation. In: Rovee-Collier C, Lipsitt LP, editors. *Advances in Infancy Research*. Norwood, NJ: Ablex Publishing, pp. 121–159.

Newell KM (1976) Knowledge of results and motor learning. In: Keogh JF, Hutton RS, editors. *Exercise and Sport Sciences Reviews, Volume 4*. Santa Barbara, CA: Journal Publishing Affiliates, pp. 195–228.

Newell KM (1986) Development of coordination. In: Wade MG, Whiting HTA, editors. *Motor Development in Children: Aspects of Coordination and Control, NATO ASI Series D, Behavioral and Social Sciences*. Dordrecht: Martinus Nijhoff, pp. 341–360. http://dx.doi.org/10.1007/978-94-009-4460-2_19

Newell KM, Carlton LG (1980) Developmental trends in motor response recognition. *Dev Psychol* 16: 550–554. http://dx.doi.org/10.1037/0012-1649.16.6.550

Newell KM, Kennedy HTA (1978) Knowledge of results and children's learning. *Dev Psychol* 14: 531–536. http://dx.doi.org/10.1037/0012-1649.14.5.531

Newell KM, Liu Y-T, Mayer-Kress G (2001) Time scales in motor learning and development. *Psychol Rev* 108: 57–82. http://dx.doi.org/10.1037/0033-295X.108.1.57

Piaget J (1952) *The Origins of Intelligence in Children*. New York: International Universities Press. http://dx.doi.org/10.1037/11494-000

Piaget J, Inhelder B (1973) *Memory and Intelligence*. New York: Basic Books.

Posner MI, Konick AF (1966) Short-term retention of visual and kinesthetic information. *Organizational Behav Human Performance* 1: 71–86. http://dx.doi.org/10.1016/0030-5073(66)90006-7

Reid G (1980a) Overt and covert rehearsal in short-term motor memory of mentally retarded and nonretarded persons. *Am J Ment Deficiency* 85: 69–77.

Reid G (1980b) The effects of memory strategy instruction in the short-term motor memory of the mentally retarded. *J Motor Behav* 12: 221–227.

Salmoni AW (1980) The effect of precision of knowledge of results on the performance of a simple line drawing task for children and adults. *Res Q* 51: 572–575.

Salmoni AW, Pascoe C (1978) Fitts' reciprocal tapping task: a developmental study. In: Roberts CG, Newell KM, editors. *Psychology of Motor Behavior and Sport*. Champaign, IL: Human Kinetics, pp. 288–330.

Schmidt RA (1975) A schema theory of discrete motor skill learning. *Psychol Rev* 82: 225–260. http://dx.doi.org/10.1037/h0076770

Schmidt RA, Lee TD (2011) *Motor Control and Learning: A Behavioral Emphasis*. Champaign, IL: Human Kinetics.

Schneider W, Pressley M (1997) *Memory Development Between 2 and 20*. Hillsdale, NJ: Erlbaum.

Shea CH, Wulf G (2005) Schema theory: a critical appraisal and reevaluation. *J Motor Behav* 37: 85–101. http://dx.doi.org/10.3200/JMBR.37.2.85-102

Simon HA (1972) What is visual imagery? An information processing interpretation. In: Gregg LW, editor. *Cognition in Learning and Memory*. New York: Wiley, pp. 164–203.

Sporns O, Edelman GM (1993) Solving Bernstein's problem: a proposal for the development of coordinated movement by selection. *Child Dev* 64: 960–981. http://dx.doi.org/10.2307/1131321

Sternberg S (1969) The discovery of processing stages: extensions of Donder's method. *Acta Psychologica* 30: 276–315. http://dx.doi.org/10.1016/0001-6918(69)90055-9

Sternberg S (1975) Memory scanning: new findings and current controversies. *Q J Exp Psychol* 27: 1–32. http://dx.doi.org/10.1080/14640747508400459

Sugden DA (1978) Visual motor short-term memory in educationally subnormal males. *Br J Educ Psychol* 48: 330–339. http://dx.doi.org/10.1111/j.2044-8279.1978.tb03019.x

Sugden DA (1980a) Developmental strategies in motor and visual motor short-term memory. *Percept Motor Skills* 51: 146. http://dx.doi.org/10.2466/pms.1980.51.1.146

Sugden DA (1980b) Movement speed in children. *J Motor Behav* 12: 125–132.

Sugden DA (1981) Dual task performance: a developmental perspective. *Information processing in motor skills: Proceedings of British Society of Sports Psychology*, pp. 13–32.

Thelen E (1995) Motor development: a new synthesis. *Am Psychol* 50: 79–95. http://dx.doi.org/10.1037/0003-066X.50.2.79

Thelen E, Smith LB (1998) Dynamic systems theories. In Lerner RM, editor, Damon W, Lerner RM, editors-in-chief. *Handbook of Child Psychology, Volume 1: Theoretical Models of Human Development*, 5th edition. Hoboken, NJ: Wiley, pp. 56–633.

Thomas JR, Mitchell B, Solomon MA (1979) Precision knowledge of results and motor performance: relationship to age. *Res Q* 50: 687–698.

Thomas JR, Thomas KT, Lee AM, Esterman E, Ashy M (1983) Age differences in use of strategy for recall of movement in a large scale environment. *Res Q Exercise Sport* 54: 264–272.

Tulving E (1985) How many memory systems are there? *Am Psychol* 40: 385–398. http://dx.doi.org/10.1037/0003-066X.40.4.385

Turvey MT (1977) Preliminaries to a theory of action with reference to vision. In: Shaw R, Bransford J, editors. *Perceiving, Acting and Knowing*. Hillsdale, NJ: Erlbaum, pp. 211–265.

Turvey MT, Shaw RE, Mace W (1978) Issues in the theory of action: degrees of freedom, coordinative structures and coalitions. In Requin J, editor. *Attention and Performance VII*. Hillsdale, NJ: Erlbaum, pp. 557–595.

Ulrich BD (1997) Dynamic systems theory and skill development in infants and children. In Connolly K, Forssberg H, editors. *Neurophysiology and Neuropsychology of Motor Development*. London: Mac Keith Press, pp. 319–345.

Waddington CH (1957) *The Strategy of the Genes*. London: George Allen & Unwin.

Walder P (1981) Contrasting theories of visuo-motor control with special reference to locomotion. University of Leeds. Unpublished PhD thesis.

Wickens CD, Benel DCR (1982) The development of time-sharing skills. In: Kelso JAS, Clark JE, editors. *The Development of Movement Control and Co-ordination.* New York: Wiley, pp. 240–253.

Wolpert DM, Flanagan JR (2010) Motor learning. *Curr Biol* 11: 467–472. http://dx.doi.org/10.1016/j.cub.2010.04.035

Wolpert DM, Ghahramani Z, Flanagan JR (2001) Perspectives and problems in motor learning. *TRENDS in Cognitive Sciences* 5, pp. 487–494. http://dx.doi.org/10.1016/S1364-6613(00)01773-3

Yan JH, Thomas JR, Thomas KT (1998) Practice variability facilitates children's motor skill acquisition: a quantitative review. *Res Q Exercise Sport* 69: 210–215.

4
EARLY MOVEMENT DEVELOPMENT: BIRTH TO 24 MONTHS

Introduction

At birth, infants appear to have minimal control of their arms, legs, and head; they cannot roll over, sit up, or move from a position and location in which they are placed. Their most distinct movements are specific reflexes, such as grasping and sucking, which are primarily necessary for survival. It was once thought that when infants initiate movements, rather than responding reflexively, their arms and legs moved seemingly at random, lacking both the precision and accuracy necessary to control posture, locomotion, and manipulation. We now know that these 'random' activities of prelocomotor infants in fact represent activity directly related to postural development and locomotion. By 24 months infants have developed sufficient postural control to cope with many basic postural adjustments; they can walk, explore their environment, and grasp and manipulate objects of a variety of shapes and sizes. Children at 24 months still cannot cope well with rapid self-movements and moving in relation to moving objects and other moving persons, and still require the assistance of others for a variety of motor activities. It is nevertheless a remarkable trajectory of development to think that in the short space of 24 months this newborn infant can progress and develop into an active inquisitive human being who has a clear understanding of what he or she wants and is rapidly acquiring the necessary skills to attain these 'wants' with an increasing degree of independence.

This begs the question: how helpless, really, is this newborn infant? Research in the early development of motor activity suggests that all of the ingredients are present for a range of motor skills, but the physical capacities to execute them are absent. In this chapter we track the changes in the developing infant from the appearance of early reflexive behaviour, through the ability to roll over and the commencement of crawling, to 'cruising' and experimenting with upright posture, to final victory over

gravity and embarking on independent exploration that comes with the ability to walk unaided. Research on the capacity to achieve these milestones suggests that much of the raw material is present at birth and a relatively simple set of constraints are all that prevent the young infant from achieving these important landmarks of motor development.

Movement activity in utero and at birth

GENERAL MOVEMENTS

The developmental neurologist Heinz Prechtl has devoted much of his research to qualitatively investigating the movements of the developing infant both in utero (up to 40 weeks' gestation) and in the ensuing 30 weeks post term. With a focus on what he termed ontogenetic adaptation, Prechtl (2001) reported on a series of studies that described three distinct categories of 'general movements' (Hopkins and Prechtl 1984, Prechtl and Nolte 1986). These are illustrated in Figure 4.1.

By analysing the qualitative descriptions of the general movements, Prechtl (2001) describes three distinct classes of movements, illustrated in Figure 4.1 and elaborated in Table 4.1:

* writhing movements
* fidgety movements
* voluntary movements.

All of these develop from essentially the 10th week in utero to the 20th week post term.

It is Prechtl's contention that a close observational analysis of these general movements reveals differences between typical development and abnormal general movements that signals in the latter a failure of ontogenetic adaptation, ideas he developed in subsequent research (Bruggink et al 2008). All of these studies speak to the

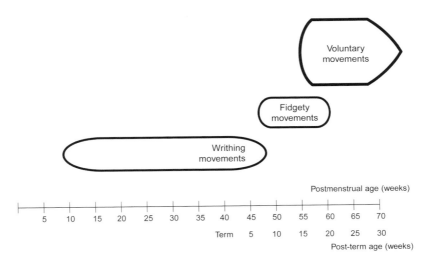

Fig. 4.1 Developmental course and general movements. Adapted from Prechtl (2001).

TABLE 4.1

Definition of general movements and their abnormal appearance officially agreed upon by the General Movements Trust

Age	Normal general movements	Abnormal general movements
Prenatal and preterm age	Gross movements, involving whole body. They may last from a few seconds to several minutes or longer. Variable sequence of arm, leg, neck, and trunk movements. Wax and wane in intensity, force, and speed, and have a gradual beginning and end. Majority of sequences of extension and flexion movements of arms and legs are complex, with superimposed rotations and often slight changes in the direction of the movement. These added components make the movements fluent and elegant and create the impression of complexity and variability	Poor repertoire of general movements: the sequence of the successive movement components is monotonous and the movements of the different body parts do not occur in the complex way as seen in normal general movements Cramped-synchronized general movements: these appear rigid and lack normal smooth and fluent character. All limb and trunk muscles contract and relax almost simultaneously
Term age until 8 weeks' post-term age	Writhing movements are characterized by small to moderate amplitude and by slow to moderate speed. Fast and large extension movements may occasionally break through, particularly in the arms. Typically, such movements are elliptical in form; this component creates the impression of a writhing quality of movement	Chaotic general movements: movements of all limbs are of large amplitude and occur in a chaotic order with no fluency or smoothness. They consistently appear to be abrupt
6–20 weeks' post-term age	Fidgety movements are circular movements of small amplitude and moderate speed and variable acceleration of neck, trunk, and limbs in all directions. They are continual in the awake infant, except during focused attention. They may be concurrent with other gross movements, such as kicking, wiggling/oscillating, and swiping of the arms or pleasure bursts. Fidgety movements may be seen as early as 6 weeks post term but usually occur around 9 weeks and are then present until 15 to about 20 weeks. This age range holds true for term as well as for preterm infants after correcting the age. Initially, they occur as isolated events (score: +); they gradually increase in frequency (score: ++) and then decrease once again (score: +)	Absent fidgety movements: fidgety movements are never observed from ages 6 to 20 weeks post term. Other movements can, however, be commonly observed Abnormal fidgety movements look like normal fidgety movements except that their amplitude, speed, and jerkiness are moderately or greatly exaggerated

Adapted with permission of the publisher from Prechtl (2001).

capacity to predict a degree of neurological dysfunction in young school-age children, which Prechtl argues is revealed by close examination of categories of general movements, a term he coined. Further, he claims these general movements have equal or greater reliability than more recent technological advances:

> As soon as a machine is between the patient and the examiner the method is considered as 'objective.' Forgotten is the fact that a visual analysis of an x-ray or EEG recording…are in no way more objective than straight forward observation.
>
> (Prechtl 2001, p. 841)

Hadders-Algra (2005) also studied the general movements of young children in the first 18 months of life, adding to Prechtl's research with respect to studying the spontaneous movements of the developing fetus both in utero and during the first 18 months of life. Hadders-Algra's research focused on both general development (Hadders-Algra 2001) and postural control (Hadders-Algra 2005). With respect to postural control, Hadders-Algra (2005) distinguishes between two functional levels of adjustment in the postural control of the developing infant. The first she refers to as 'direction-specific' adjustments whereby postural control does not respond to, or engage with, any situational demands from the surrounding environment. It is as if the first order of business is to maintain stability (as in sitting) by controlling both anterior and posterior variability. This Hadders-Algra refers to as 'primary variability'. By 6 months of age the infant exhibits what is referred to as 'secondary variability', when postural control becomes functionally active and situation specific. Postural adjustments take on a more sensitive degree of modulation, leading to anticipatory postural adjustments that occur at 13 to 14 months of age. By this stage of the development of postural control, the infant maintains both balance, that is stability within the support surface, and the capacity to generate a dynamic perception/action interface with the environment (Massion et al 2004).

It is interesting that the contributions of both Prechtl and Hadders-Algra are descriptive but clearly yield a different theoretical viewpoint from the early maturational contributions of Gesell and McGraw noted in Chapter 1. The video recordings of Prechtl's in utero infants (no date) and the electromyogram recordings of Hadders-Algra and coworkers (no date) have enabled a more expansive view of the early motor development of young infants and the implications it has for both atypical development and the critical role of posture in overall development. The outcome of this work gave credence to the proposition by Forssberg and Hirschfeld (1994) that postural control from a neural perspective was organized by a central pattern generator, which reflected the phylogenetic development of bipedal upright posture and locomotion. This idea with respect to posture, while not new, was further buttressed by the work of both Prechtl (2001) and Hadders-Algra (2005). As we have noted in Chapter 1, this solely neural explanation of movement development has been challenged by those promoting the view of dynamical systems theory, and we expand on the underlying reasons for this later in this chapter.

RHYTHMICAL MOVEMENT STEREOTYPIES
Most young infants move their limbs and body in many different ways that do not always seem purposeful or orientated to achieve a particular goal. They kick their legs, wave their arms, and rock their body seemingly at random and not to accomplish something. These responses appear to be both spontaneous and random movements, rather than reflexive, and seem general and diffuse. Few attempts had been made to formally describe them until Thelen (1979) made extensive observations of infants during their first year of life. Her observations provided an important starting point to study one aspect of change in spontaneous movements.

Thelen (1979) studied what are called rhythmical movement stereotypes: movements of parts of the body or the entire body for several repetitions at regular, short intervals. This excludes the single and non-repetitive movements that characterize most movement skills. Rhythmical movement stereotypes are abnormal in older children and adults; indeed, persistent rocking, swaying, and similar movement stereotypes at older ages are often associated with disturbed individuals. However, young infants engage regularly in rhythmical movement stereotypes, which they seem to enjoy, even though they seemingly achieve nothing beyond the movements themselves. She observed 20 infants for 1 hour every other week from 4 to 52 weeks of age in the home when the infant was awake and without changing the regular routine. She then analysed approximately 500 hours of observations. She reported a total of 47 different stereotypes. These movements were repeated at least three times at an interval of 1 second or less before they were counted as the occurrence of a rhythmical movement stereotype. Out of the 11 most frequently occurring stereotypes, which parents and others who have watched young infants will readily recognize, nine are shown in Figure 4.2. Thelen found few stereotypes present in the early weeks, but they increased from 6 to 8% of the observation time from 16 to 44 weeks. They then decreased to approximately

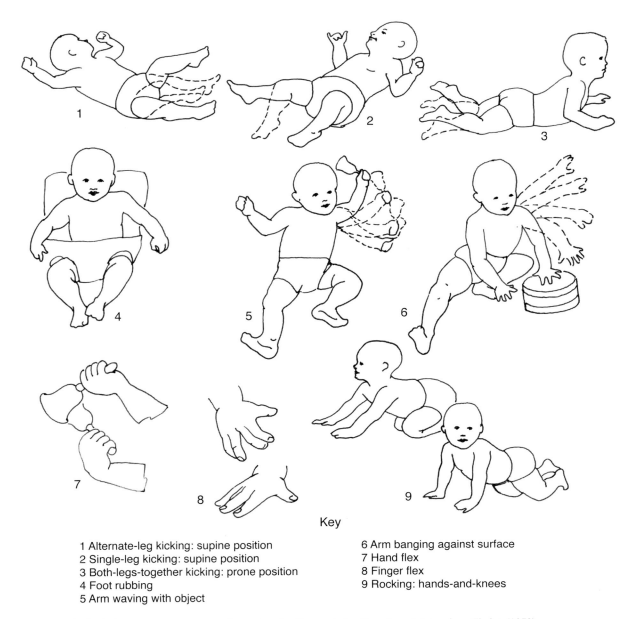

Key

1 Alternate-leg kicking: supine position
2 Single-leg kicking: supine position
3 Both-legs-together kicking: prone position
4 Foot rubbing
5 Arm waving with object

6 Arm banging against surface
7 Hand flex
8 Finger flex
9 Rocking: hands-and-knees

Fig. 4.2 Rhythmical movement stereotypes. Reproduced with permission from the publisher from Thelen (1979).

4% of the observation time during the last weeks of the first year. Thelen combined some of the movements into logical groups, such as different types of leg kicking, and found that the age at onset and the age at peak activity level varied for the different groupings. Thelen's (1979) study suggested that this pattern of development needs to be studied further; her data imply a relationship between the rhythmic kicking and the step reflex, which emerges once independent locomotion is achieved. Thelen (1979) proposed several other possibilities, which are discussed later in this chapter.

Newborn infants possess several movement reflexes that are movement responses elicited by a specific sensory stimulus, which can be light or sound, touch or pressure on a body location, or body position. Many reflexes present at birth typically disappear early in development and others remain throughout life. Reflexes present at birth and during the first months of life are evaluated with respect to intensity and quality, and are used as developmental indicators. Reflexes should be in an expected range of intensity, with too brisk or too soft a reaction being an abnormal or negative sign. Too much or too little activity may be a sign of distress, which suggests there is a desirable, perhaps even optimal, range of normal healthy activity. Extreme levels of activity become warning signs, whereas the midrange is satisfactory. The problem is to find the cut-off levels of too much and too little. It is important to note that more is not always better and that predictions can sometimes be made more accurately at the extreme levels than in the midrange. We may know that an extremely high or low value for a measure indicates poor achievement on another measure with a reasonable amount of certainty, whereas we predict achievement from a midrange value with a lot less certainty.

A lack of symmetry and incomplete reactions are qualitative signs of abnormality in some reflexes. Negative or abnormal signs are used as indications that specific aspects of the nervous system may not be sufficiently developed.

DEVELOPMENTAL INDICATORS

The newborn infant is evaluated in a number of ways at birth and in the days that follow in order to assess development status, particularly risk potential or possible developmental problems. Evaluation procedures of this type are used by medical personnel and psychologists as developmental indicators of problems that may require more detailed examination. Reflexes are tested, spontaneous behaviours are observed, and specific test situations are arranged, as illustrated by the Gesell and other developmental scales described in the next section. A scale devised by Apgar (1953) is discussed briefly to illustrate one type of developmental indicator.

The birth process, particularly the moment of emerging into a new environment, is a traumatic experience. The newborn infant must now breathe, which requires respiration movements to continue and constantly adjust to the oxygen demands of the internal systems. The womb's environment has given way to a larger and more complex environment.

The Apgar scale is often used at birth to determine whether a newborn infant may be at risk and need attention beyond normal birthing procedures. The five items listed in Table 4.2 are checked visually 1 minute after birth. Each item is assigned a numerical value of 0, 1, or 2, using criteria. If the total Apgar score is low, the newborn infant is considered at risk and action is taken to deal with the danger signals. The five screening items are identified by an acronym that spells APGAR.

Heart rate and breathing movements are basic indicators of a newborn infant's overall 'life'. Skin colour can signal jaundice and other disease conditions. Muscle tone, if too flaccid or too stiff, may reflect problems in neuromotor development. The newborn infant's facial grimace

TABLE 4.2
Test items in the APGAR scale

Item	General behaviour or characteristic
Activity	Muscle tone
Pulse	Heart rate
Grimace	Facial movements
Appearance	Skin colour
Respiration	Breathing movements

is the contraction of facial muscles when responding to stimulation and producing a newborn crying expression. Abnormal signs in facial movement mean a lack of contractions or extreme contractions and asymmetry, such as more movement on one side than on the other side.

The APGAR scale illustrates the type of initial movement development that is expected. Our example is limited because the scale's purpose is to identify life-threatening problems rather than assess movement development. We expect certain movement capabilities to be present and carried out within certain limits of the established movement pattern. Extreme differences in movement patterns and intensity may indicate problems in movement development.

REFLEXES

At birth, and in early life, various reflexes are evident and the ones listed in Table 4.3 are arranged in the order of their first appearance in utero. Each, except sucking, typically disappears during the first year of life. Rooting is a reflex that serves a functional purpose for a short period of time and then disappears when more adaptive means develop to provide a broader set of movement behaviours. The reflex can be elicited by pressure to the cheek resulting in rooting or movement of the head towards the pressure point. This serves as a direction finder to bring the mouth in contact with the breast nipple or bottle. Several months after birth, infants develop sufficient voluntary movement control to locate a breast or bottle and move their mouth into a position to feed, so this rooting reflex disappears. If it did not, we would respond with a rooting movement whenever we felt a particular pressure on our cheek! The point is that many early reflexes either disappear or are inhibited in order for voluntary and adaptive movements to develop.

Sucking is something of a compromise in that it will continue in our movement repertoire but will be under more voluntary control. Additional movements of the mouth are developed to enable us to drink, as well as suck in liquids, and chew and eat solid foods. Rooting and

TABLE 4.3
The appearance and disappearance of early reflexes[a]

Reflex	Gestational age of appearance (fetal months)
Rooting	2–3
Sucking	2–3
Palmar grasp	4–6
Tonic neck	6–7
Stepping	8–9
Placing	8–9

[a]Based on data reported by Taft and Cohen (1967).

sucking demonstrate the problem in discovering whether reflexes disappear, are suppressed, or become incorporated in voluntary movement control.

The noted 'disappearing' stepping reflex was addressed by Thelen and Fisher (1982) and in a later study by Thelen et al (2002). Rather than relying on a neurological explanation for the seeming disappearance of the stepping reflex, Thelen and her coworkers offered an essentially biomechanical explanation that took into account both the rapid growth rate and the differential changes that accompanied changes in muscle strength and mass of both bones and tissue. In the first study Thelen and Fisher (1982) made video and electromyogram recordings of both the kicking and stepping responses of 2-week-old infants. Essentially, the same muscle groups that trigger kicking also trigger stepping, which disappears after the first 2 months. Their 1982 study suggested the disappearance was a consequence of asynchronous development of muscle mass and bone length. The later study by Thelen et al (2002), in a series of three experiments, recorded a larger sample of infants measured at 2, 4 and 6 weeks. In addition to recording changes in body weight and frequency of stepping, Thelen et al manipulated limb mass by adding small weights to the infants' limbs and by negating the effects of mass by having the infants 'step' while their lower body was submerged in water. The overall conclusion of these innovative studies was that the disappearance and subsequent reappearance of stepping was a direct consequence of changes in both muscle strength and limb length. This finding poses a challenge to the traditional neuromaturational view and would support more a dynamical systems explanation.

PROGRESSIONS OF CHANGE
Early development follows a sequence that makes it possible to describe progressions of change. A progression of change is a list of specific achievements that lead to an important general achievement, such as standing upright, walking, or reaching. These progressions are intended to only describe patterns of change and are not meant to suggest whether they are fixed or invariant; although infants tend to follow the same general pattern of change, there is considerable variation among them.

Progressions of change were compiled for postural control, locomotion, and manual control from developmental scales prepared to assess individual infants and young children. A problem in using the data from these scales is that they are organized to analyse intellectual and personal–social development rather than movement. As movement behaviours are selected to represent other aspects of development, their observations and analyses are often insufficient to describe movement development. The Bayley Scales of Infant Development (Bayley 1969) and the Denver Developmental Screening Test (Frankenburg and Dodds 1967) are still in use for describing change during the first and second years of life.

More contemporary research by Karen Adolph and colleagues has challenged the traditional, presumed trajectory of developmental change as depicted by the Bayley and Denver scales. Adolph et al (2008), in an article entitled 'What is the shape of developmental change?', argued that sampling rates typically used in tracking developmental change may not be sensitive enough to detect patterns of variability and the shape of developmental change. This idea, which illustrates that the trajectories of different abilities are not linear but occur at different points in time and at different rates, has been discussed earlier (see Fig. 1.1 in Chapter 1 from Adolph et al 2008). This is much like the research presented by Thelen (1979) and others, discussed above, with respect to the step reflex.

Development of vision and visual perception
From birth, the infant, either lying on his or her back or propped more upright, is constantly faced with a changing visual array. This changing array has important effects on the development of both locomotor and manual skills, as the infant starts to explore his or her environment.

Vision is our principal and most comprehensive means of specifying our environment and provides a display to represent the part of the environment in our visual field. Reading the visual display becomes the general problem in visual–perceptual development. Individuals need to find and know specific objects and their spatial and temporal relationships. They need to perceive objects as parts and wholes and be able to combine them into larger configurations and patterns. They also must be able to see into the environment and perceive distance and depth and detect and follow movement. For example, we locate a chair as behind, in front of, or to the side of a table; we recognize that an object is either closer or further away; and we recognize that an object is bigger or smaller than another object. Vision provides spatial information with reference to the context in which the movement will take place. If objects or people are moving in the environment, vision provides temporal information about changes in locations as they occur and as they are predicted to occur. Vision is also used to monitor movements, especially when precision is required and when there is adequate time for such information to be used. Another use of visual information is after the completion of movements in order to observe the effects of movement (feedback) and determine whether the intended goals were achieved. Visual information helps specify the environment and control and evaluate movement. An extended description of vision is provided in Chapter 2 on biological influences and in Chapter 10 on visual impairment.

From the perspective of physical development the eye approximately doubles in size between birth and maturity, with considerable variability in the growth rate of different parts of the eye. The visual structures are intact at birth but many of them are immature. The fibres of the optic nerve at birth are myelinated but with a thinner nerve sheath than in adults. Estimates of the completion of the myelinization of the optic nerve range from 3 weeks to 4 months. The visual neural pathways and the visual cortex are functional at birth and continue to mature beyond birth (Cohen et al 1979). Visual acuity levels estimated for newborn infants are about 20 to 30 times lower than adult levels. However, this may not be as much of a handicap as it appears, as a high level of acuity is necessary only for tasks involving great distances or fractions of a millimetre, neither of which is of great importance to newborn infants. Vision is well developed by 2 months of age and infants begin to recognize faces that were previously undifferentiated, and they no longer attempt to grasp objects beyond their effective reach.

OBJECT PERCEPTION

Newborn infants see objects as things and do not see the space between them as things. That is, they extract objects for their visual attention rather than space from the visual display. When an object becomes known, it becomes recognizable as that object from whatever angle it is viewed. The shape of the object remains the same, even though the retinal image has changed. Constancy is established also for size and location. As we approach a stationary object in our visual field, the object retains the same shape, size, and location, even though our retinal image grows bigger and the object changes position on the retina.

Constancy

Constancy is an important perceptual attribute that applies to many, if not all, of our perceptual skills. We become able to recognize different sensory input as having the same perceptual meaning. In addition to perceptual constancy for the shape, size, and location of objects, perceptual constancy is an important prerequisite for kinaesthetic and other sensory input, such as recognizing an upwards movement of one's arm from different starting positions and recognizing one's name when spoken by different people. Position or location constancy is a complex and puzzling phenomenon, as an object will be projected onto different parts of the retina when the eyes move and the head is stationary, but the object is seen as staying in the same position in relation to the viewer.

Object relationships

Object relationships also become important in using parts of objects to construct and know more about objects and recognizing individual objects among many. This includes recognizing both the parts and the whole object, using part of the object to recognize the whole, extracting an object from a group, and organizing objects into a total picture. Object perception develops in relation to constancy and object relationships. Constancy provides the general perception of recognizing a visual feature as the same, even though it is projected differently onto the retinal image. Various object relationships enable us to organize visual pictures differently. Infants and young children seem to perceive more isolated features, as noted with object constancy, whereas older children and adults use more of the visual display's surrounding features. More flexibility in organizing our visual world is possible when not bound by specific features.

DEPTH PERCEPTION

Depth perception enables judgement of distance: recognizing that the glass of water is too far away to be reachable, the male is further away than the female, and the man is bigger than the dog, even though the man looks smaller because he is 200 yards further away. These various distance judgements require both absolute and relative judgements of distance. Throwing a ball to a partner requires an absolute judgement of distance, whereas determining whether a partner or an opponent is nearer is a relative judgement of distance. Absolute distance is used in many everyday tasks, such as reaching and grasping an object or tossing a ball to another person, and we do them quite easily and often with rather limited visual information. Performance errors may be caused by inaccurate distance perception or errors of coordinating or controlling the desired response. However, we know that infants at 4

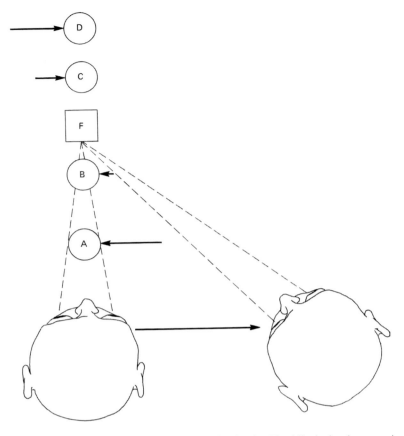

Fig. 4.3 Motion parallax occurs when the eyes remain focused on a fixed point (F) while the head turns or is moved. As the head is moved to the right, objects A and B, which are nearer to the head than the fixation point, move in the opposite direction (left). Objects C and D, which are further from the head than the fixation point, move in the same direction as the head (right). Objects further away from the fixation point (A and D) appear to move faster and further than objects nearer to the fixation point (B and C).

months are reasonably accurate in reaching and contacting both stationary and slow-moving objects (cf. von Hofsten 1979). A general expectation is that young infants know the absolute distance of objects within reasonable limits, but their motor control often lacks the necessary precision.

The ability to judge relative distance requires the use of a number of visual cues. One is a binocular parallax, which comes from possessing two eyes that are a distance apart. Each eye receives a slightly different retinal image, or visual picture. The visual system integrates the two retinal images into one visual picture, with the two retinal images providing distance and depth cues. A developmental consideration in binocular parallax is that adults' eyes are twice as far apart as newborn infants' eyes, which means that an ongoing recalibration is required throughout the growing years.

MOTION PARALLAX
Motion parallax is another visual cue in which objects on the retinal image are displaced or 'moved' when the head turns or is moved. The amount of retinal displacement of objects is a function of their distance and direction from the point of focus, as illustrated in Figure 4.3. The direction and rate of retinal displacement indicate the objects' relative distance. Motion parallax is not subject to the same growth problems as binocular parallax because changes in retinal image, as a function of head movement, are independent of physical growth changes.

OPTICAL EXPANSION
Another visual cue for distance is optical expansion (looming), which occurs whenever the distance between the perceiver and another person changes, as shown in Figure 4.4. If an object's retinal size increases by one-third as we approach it, we will know that the object is now one-third closer. Optical expansion (accretion), as well as optical contraction (deletion), specifies proportional changes from the starting point, rather than distance in absolute terms. This can also specify the ability to judge 'time to collision'. Relative distance can also be judged

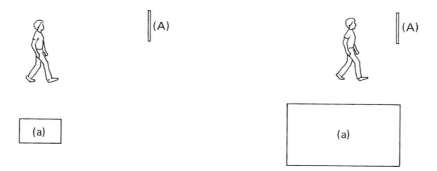

Fig. 4.4 The retinal image (a) of an object expands as a person moves towards the object itself (A).

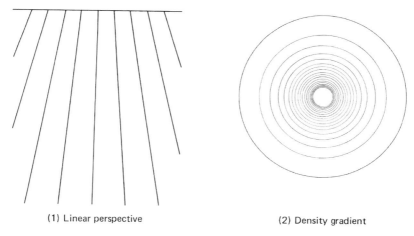

(1) Linear perspective   (2) Density gradient

Fig. 4.5 Relative distances shown by (1) linear perspective and by (2) density perspective.

by perspective, or what is called painter cues. Linear perspective and density gradient are shown in Figure 4.5 to illustrate the perspective cues that artists use to gauge distance and depth. There are similar perspective cues in our retinal images, which are important in judging distance and depth.

Binocular parallax is present in infants at 5 months and motion parallax is present at 2 months, perhaps earlier, and by the end of the first year differences of 5 inches can be discriminated. In 1960 Gibson and Walk conducted their now famous 'visual cliff' experiment. Infants from 6 to 14 months were placed on tables with a sheet of glass for the top. One-half of the table had a chequerboard pattern on the underside of the glass. The other half had the same kind of pattern several feet below the glass to create the illusion of depth. The infants were placed on the table and encouraged to crawl to their mothers, who were positioned on the opposite side of the 'cliff'. The infants would not crawl over the 'cliff', even with coaxing, and Gibson and Walk concluded that they could indeed see depth. Gibson and Walk (1960)

repeated this experiment with many different young animals and observed the same reluctance to move across the 'cliff'. An important finding is that depth perception is functional when human and other animal infants become mobile, presumably to help them avoid real cliffs and other places from which they might fall. This understanding of the 'cliff' was present in infants as young as 6 months (prewalkers), who would not cross the 'cliff' even when coaxed by their mother.

VISUAL PERCEPTION OF MOVEMENT: A CONTEMPORARY VIEW

The general case
The question of how young infants respond to approaching objects and the nature of the information used to make judgements such as 'time to collision', the 'blinking' response noted above, has been the focus of David Lee and colleagues.

In commenting on the importance of optical flow, Lee (1980) noted that 'the ecological stimulus for vision is a globally changing optic array or optic flow field...' (p. 169).

Animals and humans (in an awakened state) are constantly active and as they move around their environment they interact with objects and other living things. Whether sitting or standing they are never really 'still': they are always swaying (upright stationary posture elicits approximately 2Hz motion). This constant state of motion requires subtle control and as a result the head is always moving relative to the environment.

Irrespective of one's theoretical perspective (the classic view argues for internal perceptual representation) the fact remains that continuous perceptual regulation is a necessary and sufficient condition for purposeful motor activity. Such activity is spatial–temporal, as is the ecological stimulus that evokes such activity. Spatial–temporal information is detected via our perceptual apparatus, both intrinsic and extrinsic. For example, the control of posture has been studied in some interesting ways that suggest an interplay of vision and kinaesthesis in controlling movement. Lee (1980) outlined three types of information necessary for planning and controlling movement. First, exteroception is information that indicates external objects and events in the environment. It details the layout of the external environment so that an act can be planned accordingly. Vision is the main system in performing this function. Second, proprioception is information that specifies the positions and movements of the body parts in relation to the body. This information, which is traditionally called kinaesthesis, is used in the control of movements. Third is 'exproprioception', a relatively new term, which means obtaining information about body movement, position, and orientation relative to the environment. Exproprioception is used both in planning and controlling movement. Lee's proposal is different in that he introduces exproprioception to recognize the need for information about the environment and body in relation to each other, whereas exteroception and proprioception separate the environment and body. Lee summarized the functions of these three types of information as planning for exteroception, control for proprioception, and planning and control for exproprioception.

Lee argued that not only is vision the most powerful exteroceptive sense but it also functions as a proprioceptive and an exproprioceptive sense. Vision specifies the environment and then acts as an overseer in the control of movement by helping formulate patterns of action and tuning or preparing other perceptual systems. Vision acts as a proprioceptive check by intermittently monitoring to correct for drift in other sensory systems. Lee uses the example of playing a musical instrument such as a violin, which becomes an extension of the body. In the early

stages of learning, players use vision both exteroceptively to watch the teacher and proprioceptively to monitor their hand and finger movements. An accomplished player's movement control is taken over by mechanical proprioceptors (joints, muscles), which frees vision for reading music and planning the activity. Without vision, however, mechanical proprioceptive control tends to drift and is monitored intermittently by vision. Lee also presents anecdotes to illustrate the pervasive involvement of vision with other sensory systems. An everyday skill such as running over uneven ground is no problem during the day, but in the dark with limited vision it becomes a movement that jars the whole body. Vision in this case prepares the traditional proprioceptors to accept an irregular surface, as noted also by Turvey (1977).

The exproprioceptive functioning of vision is more difficult to conceptualize. The idea is that visual information plays a major role in planning and controlling movements that require an adjustment to the environment. Control of posture requires this type of adjustment and is the main way of examining this line of thinking.

Developmental research on visual perception
Lee and Aronson (1974) tested infants who had just started to walk in a room that could be moved forward and back in rhythmical and irregular patterns (see Fig. 4.6). When moving the room forward and back, they found that toddlers compensated by swaying with the room and they often fell over. The swaying of the room caused the toddlers to think that they were swaying (egomotion). Lee and Lishman (1975) extended this study by examining the relative effectiveness of vision and kinaesthesis in controlling balance in different types of stance. They used three different stances and found that vision was not only essential to each stance but that it also furnished more sensitive information compared with kinaesthesis, even in normal standing.

The moving of the room produces an optic flow field (pattern) on the retina, which provides information about the movement of the body relative to the environment. They further state that vision's exproprioceptive functioning prevails over vestibular and mechanical proprioception in infants who have recently learned to walk. Butterworth and Hicks (1977) ask whether this is because standing is so unstable for toddlers that their vestibular and mechanical proprioception are not powerful enough to maintain control, so that visual control develops with standing, or whether postural control, which occurs earlier than walking, also depends on vision. In other words, does visual exproprioceptive control come about with the unstable two-footed stance, or is it present earlier? Two experiments were performed using an apparatus similar

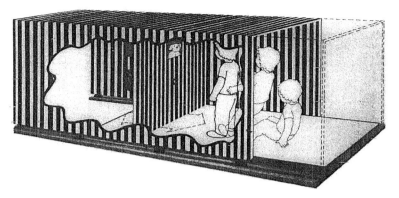

Fig. 4. 6 Schematic figure of moving room apparatus.

to Lee and Aronson's (1974) moving room. In the first experiment, standing stability was compared under two conditions of discrepant visual information in a group of infants who had recently learned to walk. The results replicated Lee and Aronson's, and the forward and back movement of the visual field produced a greater loss of postural control than its lateral movement.

In the second experiment, postural stability in a seated position was tested in an older group of infants (mean age=15.8mo) who could stand unsupported and a younger group (mean age=10.9mo) who could sit but could not stand unsupported. For both groups of infants, discrepant visual information produced a loss in stability of seated posture, but the amount of sway was less for the seated posture than for the standing posture. Butterworth and Hicks (1977) concluded that vision does not acquire its exproprioceptive function as a result of learning to stand. They also questioned Lee and Aronson's suggestion that postural control is the preference of one type of feedback over another. Rather, they suggest that postural control depends on a congruence among different indices of postural stability. As sitting seems to be a more stable posture than standing, the lesser effect of the moving visual field may indicate for a seated infant that a discrepancy between kinaesthetic and visual information is less critical in maintaining postural stability.

A more comprehensive study addressing some of the discrepancies discussed above was carried out by Bertenthal and Bai (1989). The central question they addressed was the issue of peripheral dominance. Bertenthal and Bai criticized both the Lee and Lishman (1975) and the Butterworth and Hicks (1977) studies based on several methodological issues: parents in the room; use of descriptive rather than statistical analyses; and a small sample size. In addition a study by Stoffregen et al (1987) confirmed that optical flow at the periphery (lamellar) induced more postural compensation than motion of the flow field induced by the front wall (radial

flow) of a moving room. Bertenthal and Bai (1989) in addressing the problem of peripheral dominance concluded that sensitivity to partial flow is present in infants as young as 9 months of age and developmental changes are ongoing between 5 and 9 months of age. Between 7 and 9 months infants appear to exhibit a substantial sensitivity to optical flow. Overall the infants' use of optical information to control posture seems not to develop all at once but '… the development of this action system is best characterized as gradual and self organizing … functionally driven by new tasks that emerge in conjunction with the development of new motoric processes' (Bertenthal and Bai 1989, p. 944).

A related question is whether focusing on a stationary object also provides visual exproprioceptive information for children, as Lee and Lishman (1975) reported that adults decreased their postural sway by focusing on a nearby object.

Even though Lee and Aronson (1974) found that anterior–posterior stability in 13- to 16-month-old children can be influenced by movement in the visual field, it seems that looking at a fixed visual target is not as useful for controlling anterior–posterior stability as for controlling medial–lateral stability. Developmental differences became apparent during the one-foot stance when older children can effectively use the visual target.

The cumulative findings from these studies support the case for the important role of vision in the control of posture, and the ability to use this information differs with age. Visual control of posture is present before an infant walks and changes qualitatively during childhood, and is a pervasive influence through adulthood. It is impressive how well and how early vision and kinaesthesis participate in the control of posture.

When objects start to move in the environment, children are faced with more and more visual problems to solve. They must detect, track, and predict the future locations of the objects. When an object is moving, they must also use all of the visual skills needed when the environment is stationary and do so more continuously. The object is no longer static but constantly changing and thus requires continuous visual–perceptual monitoring and updating relative to the child's position. Studies by von Hofsten (1979, 1980) and von Hofsten and Lindhagen (1979) (see below) support the idea that infants by 4 months of age are capable of tracking and predicting the path of a slow-moving object.

Individuals thus seem to devise knowledge rules, which guide their visual perception. We call these knowledge rules because individuals know things about their environment and themselves without needing to experience them directly and completely. An example is knowing that objects continue in motion, even though they disappear behind something. The object's speed and trajectory also are known and are used to anticipate when and where the object will reappear.

Knowledge rules related to the visual perception of movement are illustrated in a study by Bower et al (1970), who performed a series of experiments showing that infants at 3 to 4 months could identify a moving object from rules related solely to the object's movement speed, whereas older infants used additional rules related to other features of the object. In the first experiment, infants watched an object approach and then move behind a screen. When it was time for it to reappear, a different object emerged and continued on the same path at the same speed. Infants at 3 to 4 months continued tracking as if nothing unusual had happened, but infants at 5 months looked back for the original object. In the second experiment, the object moved behind the screen and then re-emerged but much sooner than expected if the speed had been kept constant. All of the infants made a rapid eye movement to catch up with the object, but they then looked back to the exit point on the screen.

The infants apparently thought that a different object had appeared. The change in speed in the second experiment apparently violated the rule that the object should have the same speed at exit as was seen at entrance. When the rule regarding movement speed was obeyed, as in the first experiment, only the older infants used the additional rule that the object should look the same at the entrance and at the exit. With increasing age, infants learn more about moving objects and their properties, and they begin to make accurate predictions based on these knowledge rules. The idea of knowledge rules can also be applied to other aspects of visual–perceptual development.

Vision and kinaesthesis: separate or global perception?
Visual and kinaesthetic development have traditionally been described separately; this has been done to not only

represent the traditional viewpoint but also to show, at a fundamental level, how each system operates. The more contemporary approach to sensory perception is to regard the different modalities not as separate but as essentially global perception. In other words, it is all perception and is detected by the animal and human as a direct consequence of the dynamic properties and constraints that relate to actor, task, and environment. True, the dominant modality is vision, but the haptic system is as, or perhaps more, important. The developmental literature is sparse regarding research on how growing children become sensitive to what Carello and Turvey (2004) refer to as 'muscle sense'. When movement occurs in almost any circumstance, both visual and kinaesthetic information are useful and usually necessary, as movement control depends very much on the development of an interplay between vision and kinaesthesis, as well as among other sensory systems to a lesser extent.

Newborn infants can clearly recognize intermodal equivalences, that is information gathered in one sensory modality is equivalent to information gathered in another (i.e. global perception), although there are serious methodological and design considerations that can confound the interpretation of findings (Meltzoff and Moore 1977). One way of testing the equivalence is to have 4-week-old infants suck on a pacifier that is either smooth or has small nubs on the protruding end and then remove it and observe the extent to which they attend to a picture of a smooth or a 'nubby' pacifier. Meltzoff and Borton (1979) found that infants attended more to the picture matching the pacifier they had been sucking. Thus the infants seemed to recognize the equivalence between visual information and the tactile information. In a different experiment, infants at 2 to 3 weeks were able to imitate adults' lip, mouth, and tongue movements (Meltzoff and Moore 1977). This is an impressive finding because the infants created a movement (for example tongue protrusion) to match what they saw, even though they could not see and probably never had seen their own 'matched' movement. This means that the visual information was perceived as equivalent to body movement with respect to both their own tongue movement and the visual information about the adult's tongue movements. Van der Meer et al (1995) published an important set of data in *Science*, providing empirical support for the importance ('functional significance') of arm movements in neonates, once dismissed as unintentional, purposeless, or reflexive. Their data provided support for the notion that arm movements indicate that newborn infants control their arm movements with respect to gravity soon after birth. This suggested that such coordination between body control 'cannot be represented in any preprogrammed, context-insensitive way' (van der Meer et al 1995, p. 693).

Their protocol permitted newborn infants to see only the arm they faced and the other arm on a video monitor, or neither arm. The infants responded to small forces that pulled on their wrist towards their toes. They opposed the pulling force with only the arm they could see directly or on the monitor to maintain it in their field of view. The 'take home message' from this study makes plausible that the seemingly 'random' spontaneous arm movements of newborn infants are not dissimilar to the findings of the research pioneered by Esther Thelen (1979) on newborn kicking: the conclusion of both studies supports the early development of a bodily frame of reference for future skilled action.

Much of the early research on vision and kinaesthesis (1960–1980) viewed each as separate systems (intermodal), rather than the more contemporary view that perception is global, albeit subject to differential levels of development as a function of age. What is clear is that, over time, children become more proficient at integrating global sensory information. This general capacity to integrate an ever-increasing array and variety of information suggests that the developing child has an increasing capacity to develop 'future-oriented control' (von Hofsten 2003, p. 253). This ability, which we address later in the chapter, is referred to as prospective control.

Locomotion

POSTURE AS A PRECURSOR TO LOCOMOTION
Postural control and locomotion both require stability of the entire body. The later development of body control cannot be observed in this simple control dichotomy. At older ages, it becomes necessary to look at changes in more specific types of tasks, such as running and jumping, which require the control not only of posture but other associated body segments. The early development of postural control and locomotion are described separately, although using many of the same or similar movement achievements to portray their progressions. Newborn infants lying on their back are supported by a surface, and can thus move their head and limbs without also having to control their postural position. However, when placed on their stomach, their facedown position limits what they can do with their head and limbs, and when held by another person, they are placed in a variety of postural positions depending on how they are held. Some held positions enable infants to move their head and arms, but other positions do not. An important achievement for infants is to control their own posture so that they can control other movements. A striking example is

when infants can control their posture and transition to an upright posture, and subsequently can move their legs in an alternating pattern to move forward, which demands postural control while moving forward. Postural control is the key element that underlines the control of all movements and thus influences all movements.

FROM SITTING TO STANDING
Postural control, irrespective of its orientation (sitting or standing) is a necessary and sufficient condition for a whole range of actions. A stable postural base in a variety of situations is a precursor for looking around, handling objects, or going somewhere (Stoffregen et al 1999). Until the infant can control a stable sitting posture, reaching for objects is not possible, as such activity requires that the head is stable between the shoulders and the trunk rigid. Prospective control of balance means that the infant must anticipate managing the reactive forces generated when reaching for an object in space. This has been well demonstrated by more recent research reported by Spencer et al (2000) and from earlier research by von Hofsten (1979). Collectively their studies demonstrated that postural support enabled young infants (younger than 3–4 months) to track and reach for objects. By 6 to 8 months of age infants can control their sitting posture and thus can track and reach independently.

An important achievement at 9 months is sitting down. Typically the focus has been on getting up, and we often overlook the problem of getting down in some manner other than falling down. Watching infants sit in a chair is an interesting movement to observe. The body must be lowered to a sitting position with the back to the chair, so infants will first climb into the chair and from there get into a sitting position. Griffiths (1954) observed infants' various approaches to chairs and noted that they seated themselves at 22 months in the conventional manner of having their back to the chair. Another way of getting down was observed in the Denver Developmental Test in which infants at 11 months could stoop to pick up an object and recover or return to an upright position. Sitting, stooping, recovering, and similar changes in body position reflect an increased flexibility in postural control.

Getting to an upright position was observed by Bayley (1935), who asked children lying on their backs to 'stand up'. She reported three different ways in which children responded to this request. Bayley observed that children at 14 months got up by first rolling over onto their stomach and then rising to a standing position; at 22 months they rolled onto their side before standing. The difference between rolling to a side position rather than to a stomach position probably indicates better postural control because the side position is less stable. Better postural control is needed to rise to a standing position from a side position. The third position was achieved at 32 months, when children stood straight up from sitting, without rolling to either side. The direct sit-up is more complicated and likely to reflect increased strength more than improved postural control.

Figures 4.7 to 4.10 illustrate the observable stages in the infants' progression with respect to postural control; righting reactions; locomotion; and homo- and contralateral patterns of creeping and crawling. It should be emphasized that the progressions and landmarks in postural control are difficult to observe directly and not always linear, beyond the first year, because postural control is both a precursor and an integral, and often inseparable, part of all movements.

Walking, running, and other locomotor movements all require considerable postural control, and in more subtle ways so do putting on trousers, using a spoon, and almost any other movements we can imagine. The control of all movements depends on the control of an upright posture while the movement is in progress. Infants at the end of their second year can walk quickly, run haltingly, generate many interesting variations of sitting and walking, and perform rudimentary examples of throwing and kicking. All of these achievements reflect a progression of overall postural control.

Postural control first involves the maintenance of a position, which ranges on a continuum from static to dynamic equilibrium; second, postural control involves the changing of positions, which ranges on a continuum from a single change to a continuing series or sequence of changes. The maintenance of a position in static equilibrium is our first developmental concern and is observed as the improved control of head position and the achievement of an upright posture to sit and stand. Infants then become able to change from one position to another, which includes rolling over, getting into standing positions, and sitting after standing. Then, as these movements become

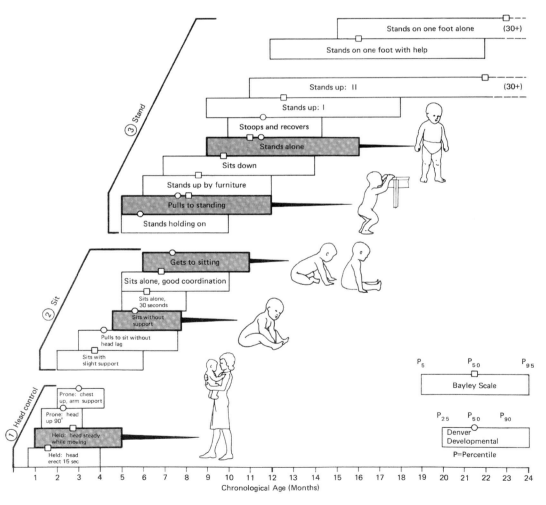

Fig. 4.7 Progression of change: postural control.

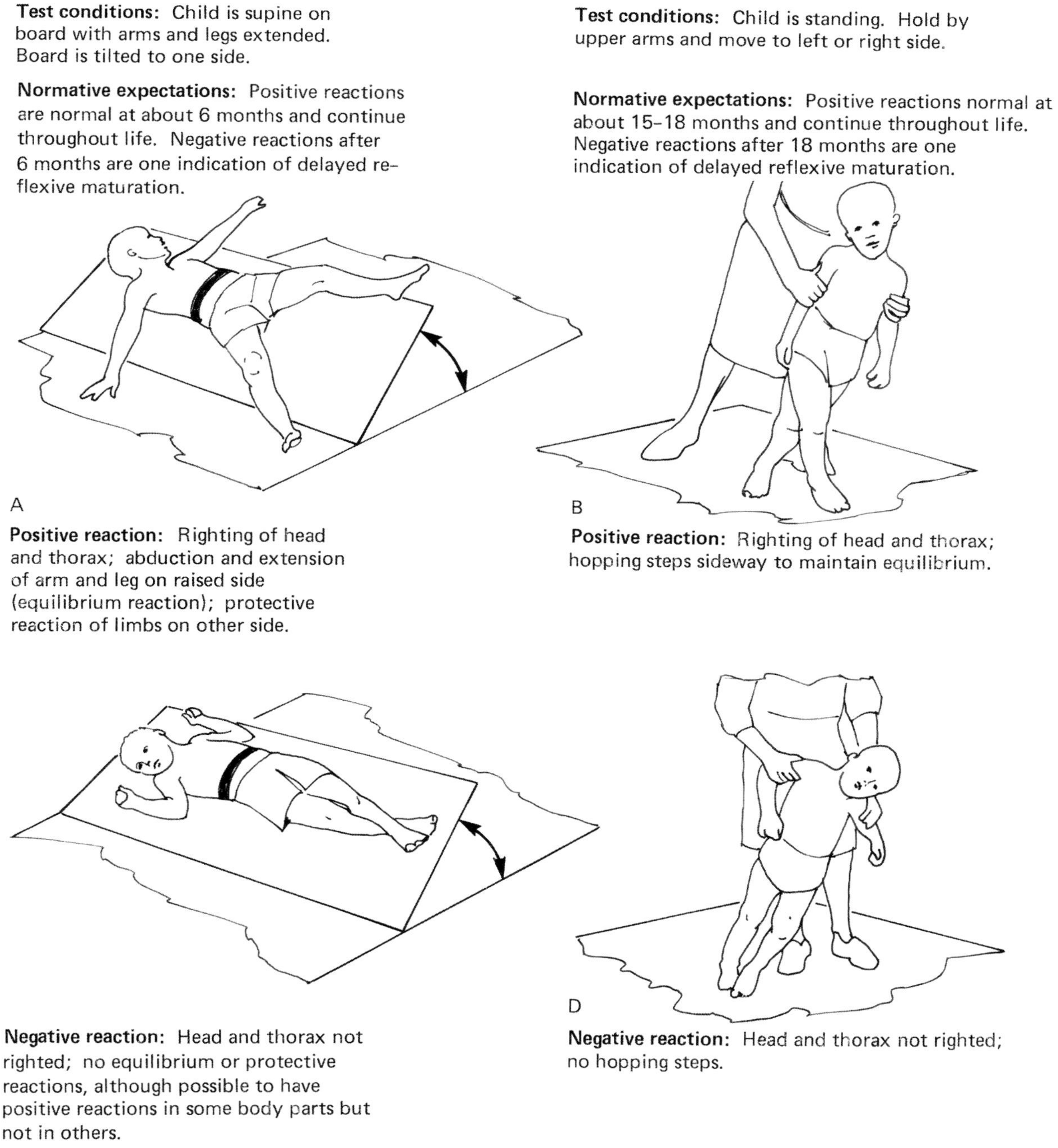

Test conditions: Child is supine on board with arms and legs extended. Board is tilted to one side.

Normative expectations: Positive reactions are normal at about 6 months and continue throughout life. Negative reactions after 6 months are one indication of delayed reflexive maturation.

A

Positive reaction: Righting of head and thorax; abduction and extension of arm and leg on raised side (equilibrium reaction); protective reaction of limbs on other side.

Negative reaction: Head and thorax not righted; no equilibrium or protective reactions, although possible to have positive reactions in some body parts but not in others.

Test conditions: Child is standing. Hold by upper arms and move to left or right side.

Normative expectations: Positive reactions normal at about 15–18 months and continue throughout life. Negative reactions after 18 months are one indication of delayed reflexive maturation.

B

Positive reaction: Righting of head and thorax; hopping steps sideway to maintain equilibrium.

D

Negative reaction: Head and thorax not righted; no hopping steps.

Fig. 4.8 Examples of positive and negative righting reactions.

a more continuous sequence of changes, dynamic equilibrium or motion stability is needed. Postural changes in a more continuous movement involve changes in body positions and locations while maintaining stability overall. Walking and running require a change in space while maintaining a general body position. Throwing and kicking involve a change in position to generate the necessary propelling and striking forces while maintaining an overall position of stability. The development of postural control beyond the first year, therefore, is the ability to make a sequence of changes while maintaining motion stability.

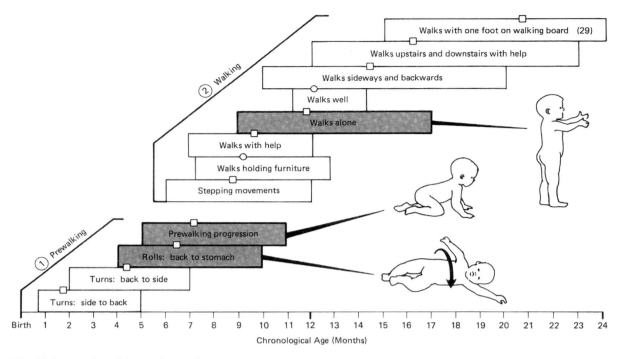

Fig. 4.9 Progression of change: locomotion.

CONTEMPORARY PERSPECTIVES ON SITTING TO STANDING

This important pioneering work describing the developmental changes in the infants' progress to independent walking is the focus of more recent research by Adolph and colleagues. They built on the rich description provided by the work of Shirley and others to generate important data that provide not only additional insight into Shirley's descriptive data but add important theoretical insights as to how more general cognitive development is triggered by the progression from crawling to independent locomotion.

In Chapter 1, we outlined the contributions of two key individuals who influenced contemporary theories of motor development, which support the theory of dynamical systems. First the notion that perception is direct, proposed by James Gibson in his theory of ecological psychology (Gibson 1966, 1979), and second the work of the Russian Nicolai Bernstein (1967).

The key assumption of direct perception is the importance of Gibson's idea of affordances. Affordances are described by Gibson as 'possibilities for action'. All individuals must determine which actions are possible and which are not present in the information contained in the affordance. Developing this theme of affordances as opportunities for action, we can quickly recognize that

action (movement with intent) is directly linked to perception, thus perception and action are bidirectional. We act to perceive, and perceive to act. It can be appreciated that locomotion, whether on all fours or bipedal (on two legs), provides rich opportunities for comprehending the world around us: this is especially true for the growing infant who achieves independence via walking. A series of studies by Adolph et al (1993, 1998, 2003) and Berger and Adolph (2003) not only produced impressive empirical support for Shirley's (1931) observations but added new important theoretical insights. This set of studies by Adolph and colleagues highlights the importance of independent locomotion not only as a biodynamical component of development but as a key feature of overall cognitive development. The connection between physical development and the child learning about the world he or she is discovering is a critical feature of development: 'The problem of perceiving affordances is complicated by the rapid, large-scale changes in the infants' bodies, skills and environments' (Adolph and Berger 2006, pp. 190–191).

The research of Adolph and her coworkers expanded the locomotion studies by the late Esther Thelen and colleagues discussed earlier in this chapter. Adolph's research brings into sharp focus the totality and the breadth of learning that independent locomotion makes possible for

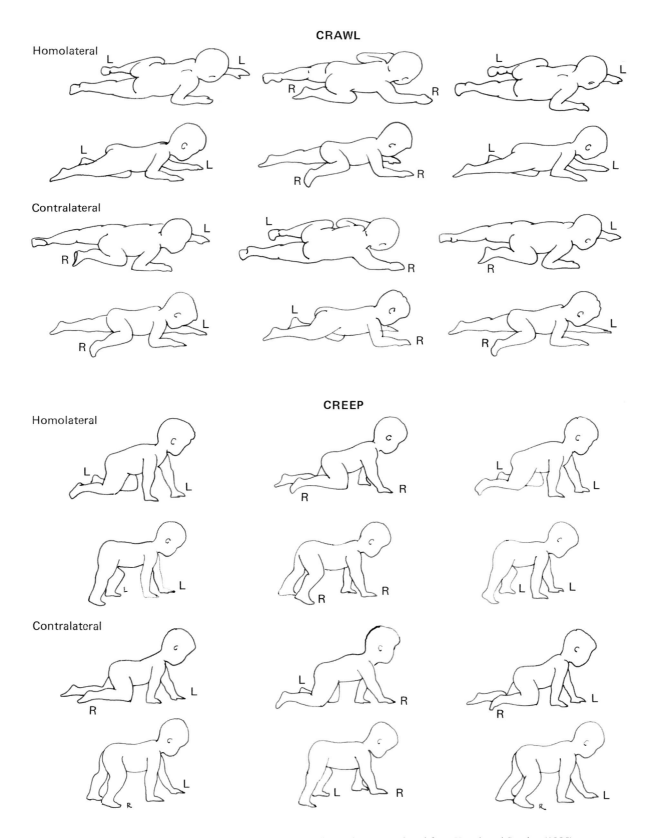

Fig. 4.10 Homolateral and contralateral patterns of crawling and creeping. Reproduced from Keogh and Sugden (1985).

the infant. The take home message here is that locomotion enriches not only the infant's observations of the environmental surroundings through which it moves but also the many opportunities to explore the objects, both animate and inanimate, that inhabit it. Movement changes the infant's perspective from a static, one-dimensional observation point (egocentric) to an ability to view the environment and what it contains from a dynamic (allocentric) perspective; this is truly an important milestone, to use the traditional terminology.

From Crawling to Cruising to Walking
By far the most important development for the young infant in many people's eyes is the capacity to first attain independent upright posture and subsequently locomotion. The stages through which the developing infant passes on the road to independent locomotion includes crawling (quadrupedal) and cruising (the transition from quadrupedal to supported bipedal locomotion). In Chapter 1 we discussed the ideas of the Russian physiologist Nikolai Bernstein (1967) with respect to a dynamical systems approach to understanding coordination and control from a developmental perspective. Bernstein opined how the many degrees of freedom present in the human musculoskeletal apparatus could be controlled or constrained to execute the many skilled activities displayed by humans. With respect to the transition from infants crawling to cruising this problem was addressed by Hael et al (2000). Bernstein (1967) suggested that initial coordination and control of movement was attained by 'freezing' (limiting) the available degrees of freedom in an action in order to attain initial success. Hael et al (2000) demonstrated that as infants transition from crawling to cruising, as a precursor to walking, the control of the trunk is the critical factor and infants exhibit 'just enough' control (but not actually 'freezing' their degrees of freedom) to accomplish successful cruising. A study examining some of these processes is described below in Box 4.1.

As can be seen from Figure 4.11, the belly crawlers did not use their multiple versions of belly crawling to refine belly crawling per se but exploited the variety of belly crawling patterns to hone their (quadrupedal) hands and knees crawling.

With respect to the transition from cruising to walking, Adolph et al (2003) investigated the relative contributions of changes in body dimensions, age, and walking experience. Since the early developmental research of the 1930s there has been general agreement that increases in strength and balance are the proximal causes for the onset of walking. However, as Adolph et al (2003) note, there is substantial disagreement as to the distal cause, in

part sparked by the appearance (in newborn infants) and disappearance (8 weeks post term) of the 'stepping reflex', followed by independent walking by the end of the first 12 months of life. Three candidates drive this theoretical argument:

- biomechanical factors
- neural maturation
- experience.

The substantial body of work reported by the late Esther Thelen and her coworkers has contributed to the biomechanical insights we have with respect to the development of walking (Thelen and Fisher 1982, Thelen 1983), especially those with a focus on leg fat and muscle mass as constraints on walking. Clearly biomechanical factors (the 'physics') play an important role when the infant begins to walk.

The second candidate, neural maturation, championed by the early maturationists – including Myrtle McGraw (1932) – found vigorous support from the work of Forssberg (1985), Zelazo et al (1989), and Zelazo (1998). They argued that the maturing cortex first suppresses the 'step reflex' and later permits the alternating leg pattern, once it is under cortical control along with the accompanying maturation of information processing capabilities. This maturing information processing capability in the child, claimed by Zelazo (1983), was challenged by Thelen (1983).

The third candidate is experience itself, or put in the language of motor learning we are talking about practice! Infants engage in a great deal of supported walking (cruising and assisted walking), which improves leg and torso strength. In their analysis Adolph et al (2003) concluded that experience was the overwhelming factor that contributed to the development of infant walking, rather than the contributions of body dimensions (biomechanics) or age (neural maturation). Their conclusions reflect not only their research but also the information analysed and reviewed by Campos et al (2000) in their article entitled 'Travel broadens the mind'. The impact of self-generated locomotion and the concomitant growth of experience cannot be underestimated. Both have important implications for the motor and cognitive development of both typically developing and atypically developing children.

Movement Biographies
An analysis of early development of walking made many years ago by Shirley (1931) described the progress and changes in 25 infants followed from birth to 2 years of age. This longitudinal study recorded medical, anthropometric, movement, and other data. Home visits were

Box 4.1 A closer examination

Crawling to walking: Adolph et al (1998)
Adolph et al (1998) observed 28 infants from their first attempts at crawling to when they began walking. They reported no adherence to a strict set of specific stages. Some crawled first on their bellies, whereas others skipped this stage and progressed directly to crawling on their hands and knees. What was interesting about this study was that the 'belly crawlers' were more proficient at crawling on hands and knees than the infants who skipped the 'belly' stage. The experience of first 'belly crawling' seemed to exert beneficial effects for subsequent hands and knees crawling. In other words 'experience' with an earlier form of movement benefits future actions. This is illustrated in Figure 4.11 (Adolph et al 1998).

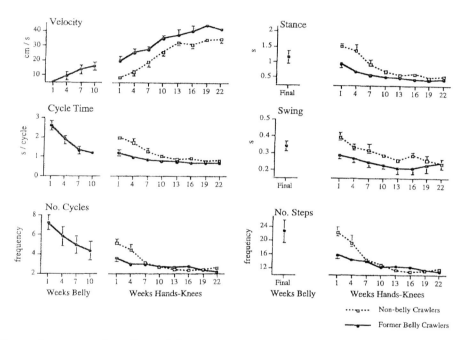

Fig. 4.11 Changes in measures of crawling proficiency over weeks on belly and weeks on hands and knees: overall velocity between marker posts, time to complete each crawling cycle, number of cycles between marker posts, stance duration, swing duration, and number of crawling steps between marker posts. Solid lines and solid symbols indicate former belly crawlers. Dashed lines and open symbols indicate non-belly crawlers. Error bars reflect standard errors.

made weekly during the first year and biweekly during the second year to make the necessary observations and measurements. Shirley made 6 to 10 home visits each day for 2 years. Her movement observations concentrated on walking, including the development of postural control, and prewalking locomotion, as preparation for walking. A graphic record of walking was made by having the infants walk or attempt to walk on a length of unglazed paper after putting olive oil or powder on the soles of their feet to produce footprints. A total of 743 walking records (approximately 30 per infant) were produced in this manner, with the infants held upright in earlier

prewalking months to make a record of their leg movements. Individual analyses were made according to walking age, rather than chronological age, by taking the age of walking alone as a zero point and counting the walking age as the number of weeks preceding (–) or following (+) the week when the child walked alone. This offers an interesting record of walking behaviour at comparable intervals preceding and following the achievement of walking alone, but this type of information is distorted when data points are averaged in relation to chronological age. Some examples are illustrated in a closer examination in Box 4.2.

Box 4.2 A closer examination

Movement biographies: Shirley

Shirley (1931) described the movement development of each of 25 infants in the form of individual movement biographies, which include many data from her observations along with her own extensive comments. Her interpretations and impressions are provocative and help us understand infants' movement development in the larger context in which movement occurs. Excerpts are provided without comment with the hope that this sample will encourage you to read the original.

> **Harvey**. At practically every test before he walked alone he stamped and patted most of the time. This trait fits in very interestingly with his other behavior; patting and slapping his stomach with good resounding smacks was a very favourite diversion with him before he was 3 months old, and swinging and banging and dangling toys was his characteristic reaction to the choice tests. At 72 weeks he inserted a hesitation step into his walking record; he stamped with his right foot, tossing his head and body to the left side, hesitated, stepped on his left foot, stamped with his right, and so on. Quite clearly this was not his method of walking to get somewhere but merely his way of jazzing up the dull old test. At 78 weeks he strolled leisurely; at 80 he ran to his brother; at 94 he fiddled along, making almost no progress; at 96, 98 and 100 weeks he slid, rubbed his feet on the paper, and refused to walk; and at 102 and 104 weeks he walked well. His record, more than that of any other child, reflects his mood of the moment and his general personality traits.
>
> (p. 87)

> **Virginia Ruth**. She was considerably advanced in motor development, Virginia Ruth was certainly the most independent child in showing off her accomplishments. If she were in the mood she rolled, crept, or walked with much enthusiasm. If she were not, neither love, in the form of her mother's coaxing, nor money, in the guise of enticing toys, could induce her to perform. She was an active baby, but, as her mother expressed it, she was a conscientious objector. Her chief objection was at being handled, and even the everyday processes of being dressed and undressed aroused her wrath, which she displayed by screams with vigorous motor accompaniments.
>
> (p. 152)

> **Winifred and Fred**. Fred compensated for his lack of motor skill by jabbering. So marked were these motor and vocal differences between the twins at 10 months that older children in the family nicknamed the pair 'Winnie Walker' and 'Freddie Talker'.
>
> (p. 156)

Shirley designated four stages of walking development based on analyses of the footprint data and related observations. Infants initially 'patted' the paper in the form of pseudo-steps while being held upright and neither stiffened their knees nor supported their weight. The second stage was standing with support. The age of onset correlated 0.8 to the age of walking alone. Shirley emphasized standing with support as the most important achievement in the progression to walking alone. The third stage was walking when led or supported by both hands and followed by the fourth stage of walking alone.

Numerous analyses of footprints were made after the infants could walk alone. The width between their footprints decreased from 12 to 5cm, and toe marks changed from toeing-out to a more parallel alignment. Stride length increased in 4 to 6 months to be approximately 20cm, which is similar to adults when considered in proportion to leg length. Infants at first walked very rapidly: 180 to 200 footfalls per minute, compared with approximately 140 for adults. The overall picture that emerges from Shirley's descriptive analysis is a change from short, rapid, toeing-out leg movements to longer (and fewer) strides, taken in line with the forward line of movement.

An unusual feature of Shirley's report was her descriptions of individual styles, such as the many walking variations observed in older infants who seemed to be playing by walking in 'fancy ways' (sideways, on tiptoe), and others who seemed bored and just walked off the edge of the paper. Shirley wrote a movement biography for each infant, describing individual walking progress (Shirley 1931, pp. 83–93) and what she calls motor play (gross motor activities observed during the home visits or reported by mothers) (Shirley 1931, pp. 148–164). These biographies are highly recommended reading for a better appreciation of individual differences. Excerpts are presented in Box 4.2 to illustrate her insight and charm in describing individual differences.

Manual control

DESCRIPTION

The achievement of upright posture together with the development of visual and kinaesthetic perception allows humans more effective use of their arms and hands for the manual control of objects and other limb manipulations. As arm and hand movements are used in such varied and complex ways, a general description of these movements is presented in Figure 4.12, which shows the development of manual control. The hand and arm work in unison but do have different functions as shown in Figure 4.12.

The first function listed for the arms is *support*, in which the arm linkage system is kept reasonably immobile in order to support the hand movements to manipulate an object. The second function of the arm is to *position the hand*, as when reaching to touch or grasp an object or when transporting an object held in the hand. The third function of the arm is to *generate and modulate force*. The first function listed for the hand is *grasp*, which includes picking up and holding an object. It can be picked up either with the fingers scooping up the object or the fingers opposing the thumb to pinch it, or with many variations thereof. When an object is held in the hand, we often describe the holding grip in terms of the functional control of the object. Holding an object, such as the handle of a hammer, in the palm of the hand is a power grip in which the handle is held tight to use the force in the arm linkage system to generate power in the hammer (Napier 1956). The holding of an object near the ends of the digits and away from the palm is a precision grip, which makes it possible to manipulate or change the object's position. A precision grip is useful in holding a pencil so that the digits can move it to write the letters of the alphabet. A second function of the hand is *manipulation*, in which fingers and thumb are used to change an object's position, as in using a pencil to write letters. The word dexterity is used often to indicate the degree of control of these digital movements. Manipulation is also involved when releasing objects, as digital movements are required to let go of the object. Release is seldom considered in the manipulation

of objects, but considerable control of digital movements is needed to release some objects in a skilful manner. Note that propelling an object requires releasing it, often with complex digital movements. This is particularly true when throwing to impart different types of spin on a ball.

Three movements illustrate the early development of manual control. They overlap in many ways because a true separation of arm and hand control, as we have emphasized, is not possible. The first progression focuses on hand control in the ability to grasp, hold, handle, and release an object. The second is arranged to show changes in the arm linkage system to achieve greater spatial accuracy in hand placement. The third is a more functional view in terms of the achievement of self-help skills, which are an extension of the basic manual control described in the first two progressions.

In the early weeks, infants often hold their fingers together in a fist but soon progress to having their hands open most of the time. They cannot accurately place either hand in a particular location and their random arm movements seem at times to be orientated towards objects, even though they cannot reliably make contact with them. They can bring their hands together at about 2 months, which is some indication that they can use arm movements to place their hands in a desired location. They can soon grasp and manipulate objects. A landmark achievement at 3 to 4 months is to be able to pick up a cube (included in the first two progressions), which is the first successful reach and grasp of an object. The first grasp of a cube is without thumb opposition, and so the cube rests against the heel, or ulnar, side of the palm, away from the thumb, and is held there by the fingers and not by the thumb (Fig. 4.13). Children at 5 to 6 months progress to thumb opposition, in which the thumb opposes the fingers to pick up a cube, with little or no contact with the palm. During the fifth and sixth months, other indications of manipulative dexterity can be observed. Children crumple or rattle paper in what Bayley (1935) calls an exploitive way, and they rotate their wrist, which increases their opportunities for manipulating objects. They also reach unilaterally rather than with both hands, and they transfer a cube from one hand to the other.

The grasping of smaller objects requires the opposition of the thumb with one finger. This is a landmark achievement at 9 to 10 months and is called a neat pincer grasp. This is preceded by raking or scooping up small objects and a partial finger prehension, or inferior pincer grasp, in which several fingers rather than one finger oppose the thumb. The importance of the neat pincer grasp and the complete thumb opposition in grasping larger objects is that a precision grip has been achieved and digital control of the object is then possible. The use

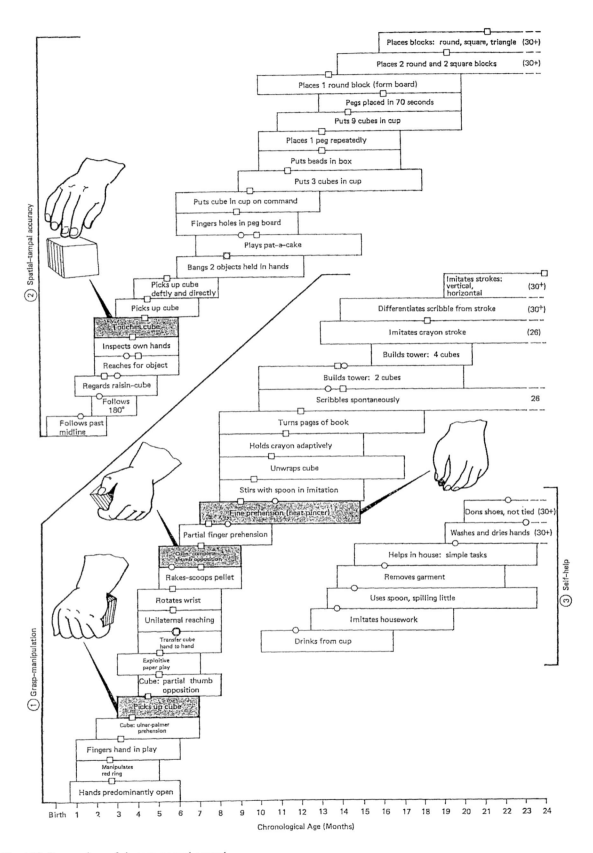

Fig. 4.12 Progressions of change: manual control.

of a palmar grasp, which is the only grasp younger infants can use, is limited to holding an object in the palm without any way to manipulate the object. The control of thumb opposition marks the real beginning of the development of manipulative dexterity.

Another landmark achievement in manipulating objects is the release of the object, which occurs at 8 months (Knobloch and Pasamanick 1974). This achievement is often overlooked, with the attention given to picking up and handling objects. The crude release at 8 months is little more than opening the hand and letting the object drop. Later development of manual control requires considerable dexterity in releasing objects, as noted earlier in tasks such as placing an object in a particular place and throwing a ball.

In addition, children by their first birthday have sufficient digital dexterity to stir with a spoon, unwrap a loosely covered object, hold a crayon in a position to scribble, and turn the pages of a book. During their second year, they can use a crayon to scribble and then make line strokes rather than scribbles. By their second birthday, they have sufficient control to make both horizontal and vertical line strokes. More precise control of hand movements is also observed at 13 to 14 months, in placing blocks on top of one another to build a tower of two blocks.

The second progression concentrates on manual control movements, using visual input to achieve greater spatial accuracy. Manual control clearly requires visual input to specify the environment and to participate in some aspects of monitoring and regulating arm–hand movements, as many arm–hand movements require considerable spatial accuracy. The visual and spatial aspects are heightened when arm–hand movements must be made in relation to moving objects, and thus such movements are known as eye–hand coordination. Our examples here are limited to movements in a stable environment.

Young infants can soon follow past the midline and through 180 degrees in tracking a slow-moving object. They regard or scrutinize their own hand and nearby objects at 2 to 3 months. They can reach and touch an object at 3 to 4 months, which was noted earlier as a landmark achievement. Infants soon can pick up a cube and transfer it from hand to hand. All of these achievements indicate that infants at 6 months can position their hands accurately and easily. Examples beyond 6 months merely reveal further progress in different types of situations. Infants at 8 and 9 months are spatially more accurate in banging two cubes together and in bringing their hands together successively to play pat-a-cake. By their first birthday, they can accurately place their finger in a hole on a pegboard and can put three cubes in a cup. During

their second year they can position pegs accurately and repeatedly and can place different shaped objects in their appropriate places in a form board.

The third progression is arranged to show the achievement of self-help skills. As these skills require some dexterity in hand control, few are observed during the first year. Young infants may be able to feed themselves a cracker and hold their bottle or spoon or other utensil but little else. When they acquire a precision grip, infants then have the movements to be used in feeding, dressing, and grooming. The skills listed in Figure 4.13 are merely some of those that may be expected. They may be more or less important and more or less taught in different child-rearing environments.

EXPLANATION

Halverson (1931) described infants' arm movements at 3 to 4 months as shoulder action, as the infants seemed to have very little movement in the elbow joint, thus making the arm more of a single unit directed by the shoulder. The back of the hand often faced the object because the wrist did not rotate to bring the hand into a more prone position. The path of the arm was also analysed by Halverson according to the arm's direction and height above the object. Infants at 6 months used a more circular path, or an arc, to approach the object and at 8 months had a more linear or direct route. Younger infants lifted their hand up and brought it down on the object; older infants slid their hand across the table surface or lifted it slightly while moving forward, as if taking off in an aeroplane. Infants at 9 months approached the object directly at a low height in a smooth and easy movement. Earlier accounts of the development of prehension described the changes in the styles of grip. Perhaps the best known is the study by Connolly and Elliott (1972). Their descriptions however did not analyse the dynamic relationship clearly evident between the object and the individual seeking to grasp it. This is a reflection of contemporary motor development research compared with the approach taken 30 years ago and earlier. Reaching has been described as changes in the approach, or path, taken to reach an object. Bower (1979) also noted that younger infants reach in a single, ballistic movement without correcting for the object's location, whereas older infants make corrections in the reach pathway. Younger infants start again if they miss the object, rather than correcting the ongoing movement.

The change from a palmar to a digital grasp was described by Halverson (1931) in a now-classic set of film analyses. Connolly and Elliott (1972) summarized these earlier analyses in a detailed review of hand function in primates and humans. Figure 4.13 is taken from their

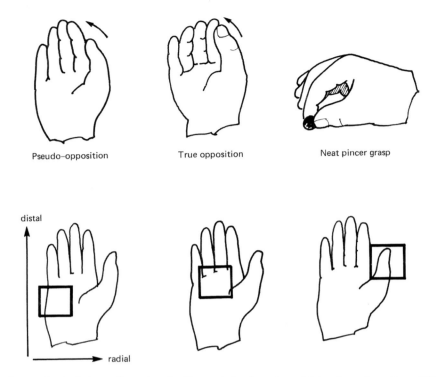

Fig. 4.13 Changes in grasping techniques. Reproduced with permission from the publisher from Connolly and Elliott (1972).

work to illustrate the hand and this change in grasping technique.

The thumb of the hand in humans can oppose a finger to bring the thumb tip in contact with the fingertip in what is known as true opposition. A pseudo-opposition is a limited version of opposition in which the thumb flexes against the side of the index finger and does not oppose the fingertip. Humans progress from no opposition to pseudo-opposition to true opposition. The hand can also be viewed as having a radial side (thumb side) and an ulnar side, which are named by the locations of the radius and ulna bones in the forearm. The palm of the hand can then be described as having a radial direction and a distal direction, as shown in Figure 4.13. When grasped, objects change in position to occupy a more radial and a more distal position. This places the object near the thumb and index finger rather than in the palm. The object is then not resting in the palm and can be handled better by the thumb and fingers. This shift in object position demonstrates the change from palmar to precision grip, which allows more intrinsic, or digital, movements of the hand to manipulate objects.

Infants before 6 months were not observed by Halverson (1931) to have thumb opposition in grasping a cube. The thumb opposition observed at 6 months was a pseudo-opposition but became a true opposition at 8

months. The size and shape of objects may alter the age at which these changes are observed, but the order is the same. As expected, the ability to pick up a raisin or other small object comes later. The initial thumb–fingers grasp of a raisin is noted in some developmental scales as an inferior pincer grasp (pseudo-opposition of thumb and opposition to several rather than one finger). The neat pincer grasp of the thumb up to the index fingertip is achieved at 9 to 10 months. As grasping shifts from palmar to digital, which is to a more radial and distal location of the object in the hand, the neat pincer grasp and general precision grip lead to more dexterity in handling and using objects. Wrist movements also contribute to the more precise handling of objects by rotation and flexion of the wrist in coordination with digital movements.

Infants at 52 weeks can easily and efficiently pick up small objects of different shapes and with some precision can transport them to a particular location. Reaching and grasping are now separate movements that can be combined in many ways, with grasping done with the fingers used in opposition to the thumb, which provides the base for manipulating objects. Above we have not only described these progressions but have also accounted for the progressions within a theoretical framework that seeks to connect motor development to the broader developmental progress of both perception and cognition – what we referred to as 'embodied cognition' in Chapter 1.

For adults, reaching and grasping objects of different sizes and shapes are skills that are regularly performed with ease. This is not so for the developing infant: as noted above, the developmental trajectory for the types of grips changes over time, especially over the first 24 months of life. As these different grasping skills develop, it begs the question: how does the infant 'know' how to reach for the variety of sizes, shapes, and distances reaching and grasping an object may require? Again the theoretical debate can attempt to answer this question in one of two ways: either the growing infant develops a set of reach and grasp programmes internally (information processing theory) or the infant uses his or her perception of the graspability of the object (an affordance) to scale both the distance and grasping technique to successfully acquire the target object.

Research by Claus von Hofsten (2003, 2004) favours a more ecological argument. From the onset of reaching at 3 to 4 months, infants show wide variability in when to use one hand (unimanual) or two hands (bimanual) when reaching for an object. Early reaching is visually guided whether objects are stationary or moving (von Hofsten 1979, 1980). The decision of whether to use a unimanual or bimanual reaching action fluctuates over the period of development, starting at 3 to 4 months of age. As we have noted above, this account differs from the more traditional developmental view, which reports an orderly and regular sequence (e.g. Gesell 1928, Halverson 1931, Connolly and Elliott 1972). This contrast in conclusion may reflect the sequence frequency of recorded data, a point raised by Adolph et al (2008) with respect to tracking the development of walking with the infrequent sampling of data often obscuring the patterns of variability and the shape of developmental change.

The decision by the infant of whether to reach with one or two hands indicates that the capacity to scale the reaching hand to the size of the object to be grasped can be quite variable during this period of development. This was the focus of a research study by Corbetta and Thelen (1996). This was a longitudinal study of three males and one female, seen every week from 3 to 30 weeks of age, and then every other week from 30 to 52 weeks of age. The data were recorded as kinematic data (i.e. portraits of the limb motion). The results for the four participants are presented in a closer examination in Box 4.3.

Clearly, across the range of both locomotor and manual development what is observed is an inherent variability that represents the infant discovering a range of coordination patterns, which are influenced by the opportunities for action present in the affordances of both animate and inanimate objects in the child's environment. Development at this stage represents the child's progression in scaling his or her motor response to the dynamic properties of the objects with which he or she wishes to interact. An important point to note is that, as is the case with the learning of all new skills, variability is highest at the start of the learning process and is progressively reduced over time, time being the ongoing experiential factor.

The development of more precise body scaling with respect to reaching for objects of varying sizes is well developed by the time the child reaches the age of 3 years. In a study comparing preschool children and adults, Newell et al (1989a) asked participants to reach and grasp cubes of different sizes (the sizes scaled as cube size/ the index finger–thumb range of motion). The results are presented in Figure 4.15.

The two graphs in Figure 4.15 depict the frequency of hand use (top graph) and the frequency of one- and two-hand reaching (bottom graph). The data plotted in absolute frequency against object/hand ratio are similar for both children and adults. The lower graph also shows a similar body-scaled switch from a one-hand grasp to a two-hand grasp. This study represents the relationship between task and the relative progression of prehension in the individual engaged in the task. This is an excellent example of the dynamic relationship of the three key elements (constraints) for all motor skills proposed by Keogh and Sugden (1985) and further elaborated by Newell (1986). The message is clear from a developmental perspective. The infant has to continually adjust an intended action by taking into account the task to be performed, the environment present, and the ability of the person performing the action.

INTERCEPTING, REACHING AND GRASPING MOVING OBJECTS

The early reports by von Hofsten (1979, 1980) and von Hofsten and Lindhagen (1979) document the early development of infants reaching and grasping objects via interception. The general picture is that infants at 4 months can track moving objects and can move an arm ahead of the target pathway to intercept the object; that is, they can anticipate the future location of a moving object and can lead the object to make an interception. The perceptual skill of specifying what the moving object is doing seems reasonably well developed by 4 months, but the control of the arm at 4 months is not well developed, in that arm movements are inefficient even when on target. This means that interception seems to improve as a function of better arm control rather than better perceptual development.

Box 4.3 A closer examination

Infant reaching and grasping: Corbetta and Thelen (1996)
This study investigated the fluctuating patterns of interlimb coordination associated with infant reaching and non-reaching over developmental time. Movement portraits were recorded for four infants – three males and one female. The four infants were monitored every week for the first year of their lives and were recorded reaching for an array of colourful toys, which the infants could easily grasp with one hand. The landscape portraits of spontaneous interlimb coordination for each infant are presented in Figure 4.14.

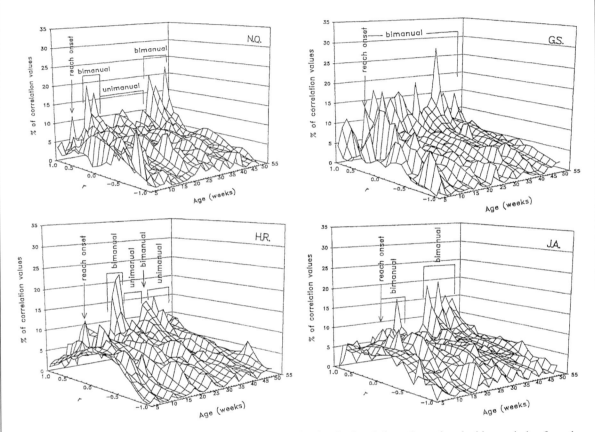

Fig. 4.14 Landscape portraits of spontaneous inter-limb coordination for four infants. Reproduced with permission from the publisher from Corbetta and Thelen (1996).

The peaks and troughs correspond to the emergence and disappearance of coordination tendencies in the non-reaching interlimb activity. The preference to reach bimanually occurred when a synchrony was evident in the infant's non-reaching interlimb activity; the preference to reach unimanually appeared when the synchrony decreased. What is readily apparent is the fluctuation (variability) between unimanual and bimanual reaching for each of the infants. These shifts in the movement patterns are evident not only in reaching data reported here by Corbetta and Thelen (1996) but also for supine kicking (Thelen and Fisher 1983) and in hand-to-mouth and object-to-mouth actions (Rochat 1992).

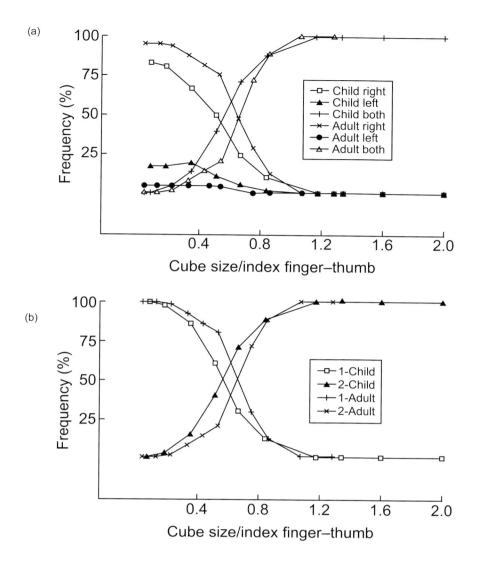

Fig. 4.15 (a) Frequency of hand use (right, left, both) as a function of age group and object/hand ratio. (b) Frequency of single- and two-hand use as a function of age group and object/hand ratio. Reproduced with permission from the publishers from Newell et al (1989b).

These three reports cover one study, in which the efforts of 11 infants to intercept a moving object are summarized (see A closer examination in Box 4.4). Observations were made of the object moving at three speeds and when stationary. Tested at 3-week intervals, the proportion of grasps continued to improve over weeks with only 10% of reaches missed throughout this time period. Infants could intercept the moving object at 15 weeks, but they could not also grasp the object until 18 weeks.

Prospective control

WHAT IS IT?

Prospective or anticipatory control is essentially the ability to link perception to action in an ever-broadening way. In Bernstein's (1967) view perception enabled the actor (developing child) to understand the impact of reactive forces present in a motor or movement problem that are not entirely predictable because of the number of degrees of freedom involved. Perception is an ongoing prerequisite in order to be able to guide our actions, von Hofsten (1993) noted

Box 4.4 A closer examination

The interception of moving objects by young infants: the von Hofsten study

The interception of moving objects by 11 young infants was studied by von Hofsten and described in three reports. The first report (von Hofsten and Lindhagen 1979) contains the procedures and basic analyses as well as the more general descriptions of interception accuracy. The second report (von Hofsten 1979) contains analyses of the number, duration, and direction of segments of arm movements during reaches. The third report (von Hofsten 1980) is concerned with the movement segments' spatial and temporal accuracy during reaches. The three reports should be read as a single study that we call the von Hofsten study.

An important aspect of the von Hofsten study is that each infant was observed at 3-week intervals. This provided a longitudinal look at interception of a moving object, rather than a cross-sectional look, which would be the observation of different infants at each age period. Longitudinal observations make it possible to trace an individual's change.

von Hofsten conducted his study because earlier studies of reaching had been limited to reaching for a stationary object. Additionally, he wanted to analyse reaching in a variety of ways that would show how young infants change. von Hofsten suggested that the interception of a moving object has three interrelated aspects. First, one must perceive motion. Second, hand motion must be coordinated with object motion, which means starting the hand motion in time to reach the intercept point. Third, the hand must move to an intercept point ahead of where the object is seen when the reach is initiated. von Hofsten used this perspective to identify the types of analyses he needed to make.

Participants

Eleven infants (six female and five male) were observed individually at 3-week intervals, beginning at an age of 12 to 24 weeks. The observations continued until 30 weeks and were followed by a final observation at 36 weeks.

Test apparatus

The infants sat in a chair in a slightly reclined position. The object to be intercepted was a wooden fishing lure (with hooks removed) attached to a metal rod, which moved horizontally in front of the infant at his or her nose height. The lure was colourful and attractive to them. Two TV cameras recorded two views of their movements and measurements were made on the video recordings at 100ms intervals to provide the data for von Hofsten's many analyses.

Experimental conditions

Eight experimental conditions were observed for each child at each test session. The object was moved at three velocities of 3.4, 15, and 30cm/s and was placed motionless in front of the infant. The object was varied to be 11 or 16cm from the infant's eyes when directly in front. Thus, there were four velocities (including rest=0cm/s) and two distances. The object was started randomly from one side and then moved horizontally back and forth until the infant grasped it or until three reaches had been made. If the object passed in front of the infant six times, it was stopped. The object was stopped in front of the infant at the end of each motion condition to let the infant reach for the object at rest.

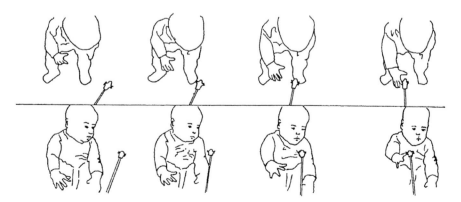

Fig. 4.16 Two views of a successful reach of a moving object (30cm/s) by an infant at 21 weeks. Reproduced with permission from the publisher from von Hofsten (1980).

Reaching

An elaborate system was used to classify the infants' movements as different types of reaching and non-reaching. Non-reaching movements were judged as not directed to intercepting the object and were included in the analyses only to find the proportion of reaching efforts among the total of all movements.

Movement segments

Reaching movements were analysed into units of movement labelled as movement elements, with an acceleration or deceleration within a single arm movement being called a movement element. If the arm changed acceleration at a particular point in a movement pathway, this indicated a change in the control messages, which can be considered as initiating a new element of the movement. A number of accelerations and decelerations were needed if the infant steered a variable course towards the target. This idea of adjustments in velocity was used to mark the beginning and ending of movement elements within the total reaching movement. Velocity was derived from the distance travelled by the base of the index finger from one reading to the next of the two video recordings at 100ms intervals. Acceleration was defined as the difference between two velocities.

Accuracy of movement

Separate movement segments were analysed in relation to their direction of movement and the location of the moving target. One measure was a simple observation of whether or not the movement segment was moving away from the path of the moving object. A second measure was a comparison of the hand's movement direction with the best interception point. These measures were used to examine the infant's effort to move ahead of the moving object rather than directly to its current position.

As can be seen in Figure 4.17 below, approximately 90% of the reaches at 15 weeks were successful, in that the moving object was touched. By 18 weeks, approximately 45% of the reaches were touches, and another 45% were grasps in which the infant got a hold of the object. The proportion of grasps continued to improve in subsequent weeks. An important point is that only 10% of reaches were misses throughout this time period. Infants could intercept the moving object at 15 weeks, but they could not also grasp the object until 18 weeks.

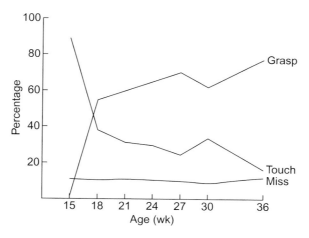

Fig. 4.17 Percentage of total number of reaches that require miss, touch, or grasp. Reproduced with permission from von Hofsten and Lindhagen (1979).

The von Hofsten study is important in providing a comprehensive set of observations and analyses to demonstrate that infants can intercept a moving object quite well by 4 months, providing that their sitting posture is stable. It also offers many ways to describe and analyse the changes occurring as reaching for a moving object becomes more accurate, both spatially and temporally, and demonstrates the importance of posture in such actions.

One may learn about properties that change and those that remain invariant during execution, depending on the posture of the body and how the movement is performed, and one may learn about problems that arise when coordination is linked to the external world.

(p. 255)

This ability or capacity is what we call prospective control. It is through actions that the developing child not only comes to understand the outside world but also his or her own action system. Repetition of skilled activities in different contexts (exploration) enhances both an understanding of their environment and an understanding of their own action system. Typically this ongoing exploration of the perceptual motor space produces in the developing child alternative modes of coordination and control to execute a skilled activity in a changing array of contexts or constraints. Every movement is slightly different from the last time it was performed because of the dynamic nature of the interactive forces at play (task, performer and environment). Piaget (1952) observed repetition in infants as essentially a way to form movement patterns. A more 'dynamic view' would be to see this repetitive activity as ongoing exploration of the 'task space'.

Is it a New Idea?
As noted above, the actual behaviour is not new. Piaget (1952) reported such activity in his observations of infants, but the interpretation of this activity has changed. Reed (1990) notes '...the importance of practice and repetition is not so much to stamping patterns of movement, but rather to encourage the functional organization of action systems' (p. 15).

The active child's exploration of the 'task space' serves to enrich not only perception but also motor and choice of actions in context. As such, prospective control argues more in support of the dynamic properties of the principle of 'self-organization' of motor abilities and less for the notion that motor skills are initially 'hard wired' and develop via maturing cognitive processing.

Summary
Movement development during the first and second years establishes the basic control of self-movements. Prior to the onset on any self-directed motion (e.g. crawling), the infant can usually only respond to the environment that may approach him or her; thus actions are by definition egocentric (self-referent). Once self-directed motion is possible, exploration of the environment produces actions that are allocentric (environmental referent). The first

months after birth are characterized by general movements and reflexes, in contrast with voluntary and adaptive movement control by the second birthday. The first and second years are when important movements are achieved and refined that provide 2-year-olds with an efficient movement repertoire for postural control, locomotion, and manual control. Movements by age 2 become more continuous rather than discrete, and movement coordination is impressive in its sequencing and timing (phasing) of the movement components. Force can be monitored and regulated within broad limits, but not to the level of precision achieved in later years. Difficulties are still encountered in controlling the movement momentum generated in making a movement and in responding to open-movement situations, so 2-year-olds can adjust to a variety of stable environmental conditions but are limited when the conditions are variable or changing.

For the young infant, striking a kinematic balance between refining his or her locomotor efficiency and at the same time reaching and grasping objects with either one (unimanual) or two (bimanual) hands presents a biomechanical challenge given both locomotion and efficient reaching and grasping are developing together. Corbetta and Bojczyk (2002) reported that, at the onset of independent walking, infants will often revert to two-handed reaching. They suggest that the interaction between mastery of upright posture and changing patterns of reaching may reflect critical periods of learning, as both neurological and behavioural reorganization is in progress. Reaching fluctuates back and forth between uni- and bimanual reaching actions as successive postural recalibrations occur. The acquisition and emergence of new skills are neither additive nor linear in their trajectories, but reflect ongoing reorganization and recalibration of the coordination dynamics required for an ever-increasing repertoire of skilled actions.

Basic postural control is established during the first year by means of several landmark achievements: keeping the head steady (without support) while being moved, sitting without support, getting into a sitting position, changing postural position, and standing alone. Postural control is such an inseparable aspect of all movements that further development of postural control can be inferred from achievements such as bending over, running, and riding a bicycle.

We presented a general perspective for thinking about postural control in which maintaining and changing positions were considered as a continuum ranging from static to dynamic equilibrium and single to continuing change. Motion stability in the form of maintaining dynamic equilibrium in a continuous sequence of postural changes, such as walking, is achieved to a limited extent by age

2, but infants have difficulty in controlling momentum generated when moving at a faster speed. The development of postural control beyond the first year is primarily improvement in controlling a continuous sequence of changes while maintaining motion stability.

The early development of locomotion was described in regard to two landmark achievements, rolling over and moving forward in a prone position, which precede the landmark achievement of walking alone. Obvious refinements in walking occur from 4 to 6 months after walking alone, in which the steps become more continuous and less widely spaced and the arms are lowered from a high-guard position and extended forward in unison with the extension of the opposite leg. The refinement of walking is seen in walking faster, changing directions, and performing fancy walks as well as in the functional activities of pulling or pushing a toy. Walking becomes more continuous and can be used in a variety of stable conditions, such as walking downhill and on different surfaces. Difficulties are still encountered in controlling momentum generated in walking faster and when environmental conditions are variable or changing.

The early development of manual control was described in regard to three similar but important landmark achievements: picking up a cube, forming a neat pincer grasp, and releasing an object. These achievements necessitate the accurate placement of the hand at a desired location and the control of fingers and thumb in several ways to grasp and manipulate objects of different sizes. We offered a framework for manual control to distinguish between the functioning of the arm and the hand (including fingers and thumb). An early achievement is in differentiating reach from grasp into separate but coordinated functions. Generally, spatial accuracy is achieved quite early. Digital dexterity soon follows in a shift from a palmar to a digital grasp and the achievement of a neat pincer grasp to pick up small objects. Digital dexterity improves rapidly when objects can be handled by the fingertips in opposition to the thumb. Infants at their first

birthday can easily and efficiently pick up small objects of different shapes and can transport them with some precision to a desired location. Functional asymmetry in bimanual control will also have been partially established. The second year is the refinement of primary manipulative achievements by attempting tasks of daily living.

The major achievements in the early development of movement control can be summarized in 6-month intervals. In the first 6 months of life the infant gains control of posture and can sit without support, with locomotion limited to rolling over and spinning on his or her stomach or back; grasping becomes voluntary but undifferentiated. In the next 6 months infants gain control of their posture and progress to sitting and standing and can move around on all fours or variations thereof, and can differentiate within a grasp to use their thumb in opposition to their fingers. The next 6 months (12–18 months of age) is a time of upright mobility and the initial use of utensils, and the final 6 months produces faster, more efficient, and more varied mobility as well as the initial start of dressing and similar self-help skills. How these important, and at times dramatic, progressions occur has been at the heart of the theoretical differences between traditional and contemporary views. The traditional views emphasize both the role of neurological maturation and the necessity for the development of 'programmes', which monitor and construct the information necessary for the motor responses. The more contemporary dynamical systems approach sees progress by the developing infant as a direct function of the physical development (neurological and physical) that permits a transition from a static to a dynamic capacity to move about and directly explore the environment and all it contains. It is this action ability that directly links to the perception of the child's rapidly expanding world. There is no need, say the contemporary theorists, for models or programmes; the developing infant perceives (sees, feels, smells, and tastes) all the properties of the environment directly and quickly comprehends their meaning and the consequences in their exciting entirety.

REFERENCES

Adolph KE, Berger SE (2006) Motor development. In: Kuhn D, Siegler RS, editors. *Handbook of Child Psychology, Volume 2: Cognition, Perception and Language*, 6th edition. New York: Wiley, pp. 161–213.

Adolph KE, Eppler MA, Gibson EJ (1993) Crawling versus walking infants' perception of affordances for locomotion over sloping surfaces. *Child Dev* 64: 1158–1174. http://dx.doi.org/10.2307/1131332

Adolph KE, Vereiken B, Denny MA (1998) Learning to crawl. *Child Dev* 69: 1299–1312. http://dx.doi.org/10.2307/1132267

Adolph KE, Vereijken B, Shrout PE (2003) What changes in infant walking and why. *Child Dev* 74: 475–497.

Adolph KE, Robinson SR, Young JW, Gill Alvarez F (2008) What is the shape of developmental change? *Psychol Rev* 115: 527–543. http://dx.doi.org/10.1037/0033-295X.115.3.527

Apgar V (1953) A proposal for a new method of evaluation of the newborn infant. *Curr Res Anesthesia Analgesia* 32: 260–267.

Bayley N (1935) The development of motor abilities during the first three years. *Society for Research in Child Development Monograph* 1, 1.

Bayley N (1969) *The Bayley Scales of Infant Development*. New York: Psychological Corp.

Berger SE, Adolph KE (2003) Infants' use of handrails as tools in a locomotor task. *Dev Psychol* 39: 594–605. http://dx.doi.org/10.1037/0012-1649.39.3.594

Bernstein N (1967) *The Co-ordination and Regulation of Movements*. New York: Pergamon Press.

Bertenthal B, Bai D (1989) Infants' sensitivity to optical flow for controlling posture. *Dev Psychol* 25: 936–945. http://dx.doi.org/10.1037/0012-1649.25.6.936

Bower TGR (1979) *Human Development*. San Francisco, CA: Freeman.

Bower TGR, Broughton MJ, Moore MK (1970) Demonstration of intention in the reaching behavior of neonates. *Nature* 228: 679–681. http://dx.doi.org/10.1038/228679a0

Bruggink JLM, Einspieler C, Butcher PR, Stremmelaar EF, Prechtl HFR, Bos AF (2008) Quantitative aspects of the early motor repertoire in preterm infants: do they predict minor neurological dysfunction at school age? *Early Human Dev* 85: 25–36. http://dx.doi.org/10.1016/j.earlhumdev.2008.05.010

Butterworth G, Hicks L (1977) Visual proprioception and postural stability in infants: a developmental study. *Perception* 6: 255–262.

Campos JJ, Anderson DJ, Barbu Ruth MA, Hubbard EM, Hertenstein MJ, Witherington D (2000) Travelling broadens the mind. *Infancy* 1: 149–219. http://dx.doi.org/10.1207/S15327078IN0102_1

Carello C, Turvey MT (2004) Physics and psychology of muscle sense. *Curr Directions Psychol Sci* 13: 25–28. http://dx.doi.org/10.1111/j.0963-7214.2004.01301007.x

Cohen LB, de Loache JS, Strauss MS (1979) Infant visual perception. In: Osofsky JD, editor. *Handbook of Infant Development*. New York: Wiley, pp. 393–448

Connolly K, Elliott J (1972) The evolution and ontogeny of hand function. In: Jones NB, editor. *Ethological Studies of Child Behaviour*. Cambridge: Cambridge University Press, pp. 329–383.

Corbetta D, Bojczyk KE (2002) Infants return to two-handed reaching when they learn to walk. *J Motor Behav* 34: 83–95. http://dx.doi.org/10.1080/00222890209601933

Corbetta D, Thelen E (1996) The developmental origins of bimanual coordination: a dynamic perspective. *J Exp Psychol* 22: 502–522. http://dx.doi.org/10.1037/0096-1523.22.2.502

Forssberg H (1985) Ontogeny of human locomotor control, volume 1: infant stepping, supported locomotion and transition to independent locomotion. *Exp Brain Res* 57: 480–493. http://dx.doi.org/10.1007/BF00237835

Forssberg H, Hirschfeld H (1994) Postural adjustments in sitting humans following external perturbations: muscle activity and kinematics. *Exp Brain Res* 97: 515–527. http://dx.doi.org/10.1007/BF00241545

Frankenburg WK, Dodds JB (1967) The Denver developmental screening test. *J Pediatr* 71: 181–191. http://dx.doi.org/10.1016/S0022-3476(67)80070-2

Gesell A (1928) *Infancy and Human Growth*. New York: Macmillan.

Gibson EJ, Walk RD (1960) The "visual cliff." *Scientific American* 202: 64–71. http://dx.doi.org/10.1038/scientificamerican0460-64

Gibson JJ (1966) *The Senses Considered as Perceptual Systems*. Boston, MA: Houghton Mifflin.

Gibson JJ (1979) *The Ecological Approach to Visual Perception*. Boston, MA: Houghton Mifflin.

Griffiths R (1954) *The Abilities of Babies*. New York: McGraw-Hill.

Hadders-Algra M (2001) Evaluation of motor function in young infants by means of the assessment of general movements: a review. *Paediatr Phys Ther* 13: 27–36. http://dx.doi.org/10.1097/00001577-200104000-00005

Hadders-Algra M (2005) Development of postural control during the first 18 months of life. *Neural Plasticity* 12: 99–108.

Hael V, Vardaxis V, Ulrich B (2000) Learning to cruise: Bernstein's theory applied to skill acquisition during infancy. *Human Movement Sci* 19: 685–715. http://dx.doi.org/10.1016/S0167-9457(00)00034-8

Halverson HM (1931) An experimental study of prehension in infants by means of systematic cinema records. *Genetic Psychology Monographs* 10: 107–286.

von Hofsten C (1979) Development of visually directed reaching: the approach phase. *J Human Movement Stud* 30: 369–382.

von Hofsten C (1980) Predictive reaching for moving objects by human infants. *J Exp Child Psychol* 30: 369–382. http://dx.doi.org/10.1016/0022-0965(80)90043-0

von Hofsten C (1993) Prospective control: a basic aspect of action development. *Human Dev* 36: 253–270. http://dx.doi.org/10.1159/000278212

von Hofsten C (2003) On the development of perception and action. In: Connolly KJ, Valsiner J, editors. *Handbook of Developmental Psychology*. London: Sage, pp. 114–140.

von Hofsten C (2004) An action perspective on motor development. *Trends Cogn Sci* 8: 266–272. http://dx.doi.org/10.1016/j.tics.2004.04.002

von Hofsten C, Lindhagen K (1979) Observations on the development of reaching for moving objects. *J Exp Child Psychol* 28: 158–173. http://dx.doi.org/10.1016/0022-0965(79)90109-7

Keogh JA, Sugden DA (1985) *Movement Skill Development*. New York: Macmillan.

Knobloch H, Pasamanick B, editors (1974) *Gesell and Amatruda's Development Diagnosis*, 3rd edition. New York: Harper & Row.

Lee DN (1980) The optic flow field: the foundation of vision. *Philosophical Transactions of the Royal Society London B* 290: 169–179. http://dx.doi.org/10.1098/rstb.1980.0089

Lee DN, Aronson E (1974) Visual proprioceptive control of standing in human infants. *Percept Psychophys* 15: 529–532. http://dx.doi.org/10.3758/BF03199297

Lee DN, Lishman JR (1975) Visual proprioceptive control of stance. *J Human Movement Stud* 1: 87–95.

McGraw MB (1932) From reflex to muscular control in the assumption of an erect posture and ambulation in the human infant. *Child Dev* 3: 291–297. http://dx.doi.org/10.2307/1125356

Massion J, Alexandrov A, Frolov A (2004) Why and how are posture and movement coordinated? *Prog Brain Res* 143: 13–27. http://dx.doi.org/10.1016/S0079-6123(03)43002-1

van der Meer ALH, van der Weel FR, Lee DN (1995) The functional significance of arm movements in neonates. *Science* 267: 693–695.

Meltzoff AN, Borton RW (1979) Intermodal matching by human neonates. *Nature* 282: 403–404. http://dx.doi.org/10.1038/282403a0

Meltzoff AN, Moore MK (1977) Imitation of facial and manual gestures by human neonates. *Science* 198: 75–78. http://dx.doi.org/10.1126/science.198.4312.75

Napier JR (1956) The prehensile movements of the human hand. *J Bone Joint Surg* 38B: 902–913.

Newell KM (1986) Development of coordination. In: Wade M, Whiting HTA, editors. *Motor Development in Children: Aspects of Coordination and Control, NATO ASI Series D, Behavioural and Social Sciences*. Dordrecht: Martinus Nijhoff, pp. 341–360. http://dx.doi.org/10.1007/978-94-009-4460-2_19

Newell KM, Scully PV, Baillargeon R (1989a) Task constraints and infant grip configuration. *Dev Psychobiol* 22: 817–832. http://dx.doi.org/10.1002/dev.420220806

Newell KM, Scully DM, Tenenbaum F, Hardiman S (1989b) Body scale and the development of prehension. *Dev Psychobiol* 22: 1–14. http:/dx.doi.org/10.1002/dev.420220102

Piaget J (1952) *The Origins of Intelligence in Children*. New York: International Universities Press. http://dx.doi.org/10.1037/11494-000.

Prechtl HFR (2001) General movement assessment as a method of developmental neurology: new paradigms and their consequences. *Dev Med Child Neurol* 43: 836–842. http://dx.doi.org/10.1017/S0012162201001529

Prechtl HFR, Hopkins B (1986) Development transformations of spontaneous movements in early infancy. *Early Human Dev* 14: 233–238. http://dx.doi.org/10.1016/0378-3782(86)90184-2

Prechtl HFR, Nolte R (1984) Motor behavior of preterm infants. In: Prechtl HFR, editor. *Continuity of Neural Functions from Prenatal to Postnatal Life. Clinics in Developmental Medicine Number 94.* London: Mac Keith Press, pp. 79–92.

Reed ES (1990) Changing theories of postural development. In: Wollacott M, Shumway-Cooke A, editors. *Development of Posture and Gait Across the Lifespan*. Columbia, SC: University of South Carolina Press, pp. 3–24.

Rochat P (1992) Self-sitting and reaching in 5- to 8-month old infants: the impact of posture and its development on early eye-hand coordination. *J Motor Behav* 24: 210–220. http://dx.doi.org/10.1080/00222895.1992.9941616

Shirley MM (1931) *The First 2 Years: A Study of Twenty-Five Babies*. Minneapolis, MN: University of Minnesota Press.

Spencer JP, Vereijken B, Diedrich FJ, Thelen E (2000) Posture and the emergence of manual skills. *Dev Sci* 3: 216–233. http://dx.doi.org/10.1111/1467-7687.00115

Stoffregen TA, Schmuckler MA, Gibson EJ (1987) Use of central and peripheral optical flow in stance and locomotion in young walkers. *Perception* 16: 113–119. http://dx.doi.org/10.1068/p160113

Stoffregen TA, Smart LJ, Bardy BG, Pagulayan RJ (1999) Postural stabilization of looking. *J Exp Psychol* 25: 1641–1658. http://dx.doi.org/10.1037/0096-1523.25.6.1641

Taft LT, Cohen HJ (1967) Neonatal and infant reflexology. In: Hellmuth J, editor. *Exceptional Infant, Volume 1*. Seattle: Special Child Publications.

Thelen E (1979) Rhythmical stereotypies in normal human infants. *Animal Behav* 27: 699–715. http://dx.doi.org/10.1016/0003-3472(79)90006-X

Thelen E (1983) Learning to walk is still an 'old' problem: a reply to Zelazo (1983). *J Motor Behav* 15: 139–161.

Thelen E, Fisher DM (1982) Newborn stepping: an explanation for a 'disappearing reflex'. *Dev Psychol* 18: 760–775. http://dx.doi.org/10.1037/0012-1649.18.5.760

Thelen E, Fisher DM (1983) The organization of spontaneous leg movements in newborn infants. *J Motor Behav* 15: 353–377.

Thelen E, Fisher DM, Ridley-Johnson R (2002) The relationship between physical growth and a newborn reflex. *Infant Behav Dev* 25: 72–85. http://dx.doi.org/10.1016/S0163-6383(02)00091-7

Turvey MT (1977) Preliminaries to a theory of action with reference to vision. In: Shaw R, Bransford J, editors. *Perceiving, Acting and Knowing*. Hillsdale, NJ: Erlbaum, pp. 211–265.

Zelazo PR (1983) The development of walking: new findings and old assumptions. *J Motor Behav* 15: 99–137.

Zelazo PR (1998) McGraw and the development of unaided walking. *Dev Rev* 18: 449–471. http://dx.doi.org/10.1006/drev.1997.0460

Zelazo PR, Weiss MJ, Leonard E (1989) The development of unaided walking: the acquisition of higher order control. In: Zelazo PR, Barr RG, editors. *Challenges to Developmental Paradigms*. Hillsdale, NJ: Erlbaum, pp. 139–165.

5
MOTOR DEVELOPMENT OF YOUNG CHILDREN: 2 TO 7 YEARS OF AGE

This chapter examines a 5- to 6-year period from age 2 to approximately age 7, following young children from preschool to their early school years. At the start of this period a child will have acquired some basic locomotor and manual skills, which are supported by improving sensory–perceptual abilities. The child will be able to walk and run and pick up and manipulate objects to a certain degree, but the more advanced locomotor skills and manual activities are not present. However, there is a strong argument that by 6 or 7 years of age a child will be able to perform all of the naturally developing fundamental motor skills to some degree. Children will have sufficient control of their body movements to perform many fundamental play-game skills and many functional hand skills, although they will be limited in more open movement situations with changing and unstable contexts. Beyond this period they will continue to improve their control of body and limb movements by increasing their level of performance and their repertoire of movement skills to cope with personal desires and situational requirements and conditions.

Here there is a concentration on the description of developmental change in two large global categories of movements: those involving movements of the whole body and those involving manual control. Within both of these categories, various activities are described and examined as examples of the changes that occur. Following these, there is a short section on control of limb movements, which combines movements from these two global categories. In addition to this description of change, here, as in other chapters, there are also examples of potential reasons why change occurs. Thus, in addition to the description of change, within each movement category, examples of potential causation or explanations of changes are presented and include themes from ecological psychology and the more traditional information processing theory.

Descriptions of change

GENERAL ACHIEVEMENTS

This chapter follows on from Chapter 4 by looking at general achievements in motor skills between the ages of 2 and 7 years, during which time many new skills develop and others are refined and varied, with improved movement control being shown by varying it or using it in different ways. For example, while pedalling a tricycle, children might

* go faster
* pedal with one leg
* wave to friends
* ride to school or navigate in and out of obstacles in a playground.

Pedalling a tricycle has been mastered to a point that the movement problem is no longer to make the tricycle go in the proper direction at a manageable speed, but pedalling can now be varied and used in other movement situations. This is a recurring theme in development and happens at all ages. For example, at a later age a child may begin to text messages on a mobile phone and with age and experience become more proficient, becoming able to do this faster and while walking. It is in tasks such as this that the twin concepts of development and learning interact and overlap. The progression from mastery of a skill to being able to use it flexibly in different situations is seen in both development and learning, and with children who are in the developmental period, it is often complex to determine the contribution of each process. Many of the variations are clear indications of increased movement control, and the many uses of the movement in different situations are more subtle indications. Although the different variations and uses do not represent an orderly and sequential progression of change, they are useful indicators, especially in relating developing movers to different movement contexts.

MOVEMENT MECHANICS

Specific movement tasks during early childhood have long been analysed and reported by authors such as Wickstrom (1977) to trace changes in movement mechanics for angular relationships among body parts, accelerations and velocities of body parts, and similar measurements. More recently, Watkins (2008) proposed a dynamical systems framework to describe many of the variables involved in the development of biomechanical change. These analyses show phases (sometimes labelled as stages) in the development of a movement skill. Phases in the development of play-game skills, such as running and throwing, indicate what certain body parts or segments are doing and the changes expected in each phase. An example is that children first walk with their feet wide apart and then progress to walking with their feet more in line. Roberton (1977) emphasizes that change, however, does not necessarily proceed at the same rate in all parts of the body, and although there may be an orderly sequence of phases, there is probably considerable variation in the relationship and order of changes among the body parts. Roberton (1977) noted, using throwing as an example, that movement changes in the trunk can precede or follow changes in the legs or throwing arm. These descriptive analyses of movement mechanics document smaller and more precise amounts of change in body movements, and although these analyses are descriptive tools, they have also been employed to provide clues to the causal mechanisms, with multiple interacting factors being the rule rather than the exception.

MOVEMENT COMPONENTS

Describing movement components is another way to trace changes in the development of movement control. Each movement can be defined according to the parts or components that must exist regardless of the level of achievement. When picking up a coin and placing it in a cup, the large movement components are

- picking up the coin
- carrying it to the cup
- releasing it.

Changes in each movement component can be broken down and measured in different ways to find similarities and differences among groups of children for each component. Older children may pick up the coin differently and in less time than younger children, whereas they may carry and release it in the same way. This would point to

change in a particular aspect or component of the movement, which in this example would indicate improved control of digital movements. If the differences were that younger children took more time to get their hands lower and closer to the cup at the point of release, this might suggest a difference in movement strategy. This could be combined with *movement mechanics* to provide a more detailed examination of the components. These have been studied as separate components, but more recently a holistic approach has been taken with the interrelationships and dynamics of the situation analysed with more multiple variables examined (Adolph et al 2003).

Many movements are now analysed in more sophisticated ways, with factors being examined using detailed biomechanical methods. Jensen (2005) proposes that using this type of analysis is akin to having a window on motor development, particularly with regard to four questions.

- What is the definition of competence?
- What is the mechanism of change?
- Where is the source of movement skill?
- What happens when there are perturbations?

She likens these questions to the ones asked about language and communication by linguists, but the techniques for answering them are very different.

The different forms of description, however, are alike in many respects, particularly in that similar observations and measurements are often used but for a different purpose. General achievements focus our attention on the total achievement, such as standing upright or riding a bicycle, and are quite visible indicators of change. Observations are extended to movement variations and different uses of a movement, as we make more functional analyses of developing movers in everyday movement situations. Analyses of movement mechanics can be used to discern detailed patterns of movement changes, and analyses of movement components discover where changes occur in different aspect of a movement.

Body control

The control of body movements was described in Chapter 4 as postural control and locomotion. In this chapter there are descriptions of six movement tasks, which represent the development of body control during early childhood. The six tasks are the following:

- walking
- running
- jumping
- hopping and skipping

- throwing and catching
- posture and balance.

At the end of these whole-body control tasks there is a short section on *moving slowly and quickly*, which examines the differences between maximum performances in each.

Descriptions of movement skills such as the following six have been commonplace and involve a more traditional approach, mostly stemming from the classical and detailed information that was obtained by early researchers such as McGraw, Gesell, Shirley, Rarick, and Keogh and illustrated in many developmental texts. This tradition is carried on here but with samples rather than a comprehensive coverage of descriptions being presented to show the various progressions in skill development. Much of the work is well established, stemming from the years when researchers had access to large-scale longitudinal data. In all descriptions of development, we are aware of the cautionary note by Adolph et al (2008), who advise that multiple sampling on many occasions should be used to obtain a true perspective of a child's development. They show convincingly that means or averages of behaviours are not sufficient to determine the whole developmental story and that multiple samples are necessary, often even over a short period of time. It is with this cautionary note that we present descriptions of motor development in the six skills.

Currently, researchers are turning their attention beyond descriptions towards trying to explain these changes, while recognizing that there is not always a clear boundary line between detailed description and explanation. In Chapter 1 we showed different explanations for the developmental changes, detailing maturational, ecological, and information processing viewpoints. Adolph et al (2003) argue that experience is a major determining factor in development, having a greater influence than maturation or specific factors such as biomechanical changes due to growth. Experience provides the child with different contexts comprising a variety of visual and other sensory arrays, such as different surfaces to run on, for example, which all contribute to a richness of potential motor outputs. The child is provided with a range of potential modes of motor responses, which link with the environmental contexts. These multiple explanations, often self-organizing, present a logical fit within a child resources–task–environmental model. We have chosen the six tasks because walking is our basic means of locomotion; running, jumping, hopping, and throwing and catching are fundamental play-game skills; and balancing is a means of assessing one aspect of postural control and crucial to the previous tasks. Other movements could be

included, but much of the available descriptive information pertains to these six tasks. At selected occasions in the developmental descriptions of these six tasks, studies are presented that offer explanations of the developmental changes. These explanations are not simply from the development of the motor system but include sensory–perceptual factors that underpin, support, and often guide the choice of movement at various stages of the child's development.

In all of these six tasks, limbs and body parts must be properly coordinated in sequencing, timing (phasing), and spatial relationships. Appropriate force must also be generated to make the movements, and a related concern is the need to move fast enough to make the movement easier, without going too fast and thus decreasing the time available to start subsequent portions of the movement sequence. Children must not only execute the movements, but also control the momentum they generate, while moving fast enough to maintain their inertial advantage. This complex trade-off is seen in running, in which sufficient speed is needed to avoid coming to rest and having to overcome inertia to continue the forward movement. However, running faster means more body control problems when turning or stopping. The development of body control thus requires postural control and the coordination of the limbs and body parts in relation to the speed that can be maintained.

In addition to the obvious changes in motor coordination, visual and kinaesthetic processes are improving, particularly with respect to the interaction of these two modalities. Vision is our major source of obtaining information from the environment, enabling our movements to link with and match the contextual demand. Kinaesthesis provides us with information about our activity before, during, and after any movement and links with the sensory environmental information. These developing resources influence how a child approaches a given task within the environmental context, how it is controlled and the type and accuracy of any feedback that is generated.

WALKING

Description

Young children can walk by the age of around 12 months, but walking becomes further refined in movement mechanics as the child develops. The legs and arms are alternated and the feet are placed more in line to provide a less stable but more efficient walking pattern. Walking, however, does improve in ways that can be noted in general terms. Walking becomes more automatic, so children can walk and talk or walk while manipulating something in their hands. Walking can be done in different environmental

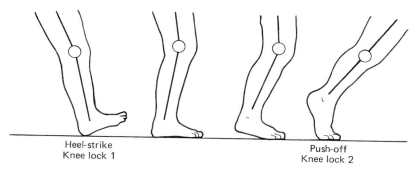

Fig. 5.1 Knee lock at beginning and end of stance phase when walking.

conditions, such as walking up or down a steep slope, on slippery surfaces, and in the wind. Walking can be done at faster and slower paces and in step with another person.

Within a 2- to 3-month period around the end of the first year or life, most human infants will take their first independent steps. During the second year, they become increasingly proficient, and as well as solving the challenge of remaining upright while moving forward, they also control intralimb coordination (Clark and Phillips 1993). In this second year, the infant starts to resemble the adult in such variables as per cent of the walking cycle spent in double-time support, stride frequency, and thigh–shank limit cycles, with the possibility that strength and posture may be deciding factors in the move towards mature walking (Thelen 1985, Clark and Phillips 1993).

There are detailed descriptions of changes in walking movements. Statham and Murray (1971) observed seven infants as they progressed from supported to independent walking. Their increase in stride length was small, but the infants walked faster and spent less time with one foot in contact with the ground. They also acquired more consistency in their overall movement pattern and in the component parts of each step cycle. Scrutton (1969) observed children, ages 13 months to 5 years, stepping into talcum powder before walking across the room and then measured their footprints in several ways in relation to their line of walk. Toeing out faded with age, with the heel–toe line of the foot becoming more parallel to the line of walk.

Wickstrom (1977, 1983) summarizes other important changes in walking development, including a change from a flat-footed contact to a heel-strike at contact, followed by a toe push-off and a decrease in hip flexion, which prevents the thigh and heel from rising as high. He stresses the achievement of a double-knee lock involving extension–flexion–extension during the contact period, as shown in Figure 5.1. The knee extends (lock 1) at heel-strike, followed by plantar flexion of the foot and knee flexion until near mid-stance, and finishing with knee

extension (lock 2) and heel-raise during the push-off. The double-knee lock pattern assists the child in achieving a full range of leg motion. Generally, patterns in walking are quite noticeable up to the age of 5 or 6, but after that more detailed analysis is required to detect the more subtle changes.

Recent data from the Movement Assessment Battery for Children (Movement ABC; Henderson et al 2007) presents norms for slight modifications in walking. For example, children are tested on walking a line with their heels raised for up to 15 steps with seven being the number at the 50th centile for 3- to 4-year-olds, rising through 14 steps at 4 to 5 years of age indicating that this task has a ceiling effect at between 4 and 5. Although these data are useful, there is little indication of the development of quality of walking, which we know includes such actions as an increase in coordination of oppositional arm swing with the movement of the legs and improved balance with a reduction of forward trunk lean. In addition, tests such as these only provide an end-product score with limited qualitative information and say little about how information in the form of sensory–perceptual accuracy and sensitivity influences the movement.

Stair climbing presents a modified form of walking when one uses alternating steps to go up or down stairs and is a movement task that illustrates how children adjust their walking pattern to environmental demands and how the control of their walking pattern improves. Children first walk up and down stairs without support by marking time. They move one foot forward to the next step, then bring the other foot to the same step, and repeat the cycle of one step at a time. This soon becomes alternate stepping for going upstairs, but with the support of a handrail or the hand of another person. Descending stairs by marking time occurs at about the same time as marking time to ascend stairs, but the differences between ascending and descending stairs with alternating steps is minimally 15 months. Children can walk upstairs earlier, around 30 months with alternating feet, than downstairs, which is up to 4 years, a considerable difference that is interesting to examine (Bayley 1935, Wellman 1937).

In order to walk downstairs with an alternating step pattern, one leg must be moved forward while the weight-bearing leg flexes to lower the body. The stepping leg reaches the step to become the weight-bearing leg, and the other leg must be moved from behind the body to go forward and down. If this sequence of movements is not controlled properly, the mover will fall forward. When walking upstairs, a similar movement sequence is used, except that the weight-bearing leg is in a flexed position and the back leg starts up and forward. The weight-bearing leg then extends, and the sequence continues in this manner. Walking downstairs is probably a more difficult movement to control because of the flexion of the

weight-bearing leg to balance the body, and also walking downstairs carries with it the possibility of falling.

Explanation
The causal explanations for walking have been long debated with authors such as Hamilton (1992) and Hirschfield and Forssberg (1992) suggesting that neural maturation is the decisive factor in ambulatory behaviour. However, for those subscribing to a dynamical systems explanation this would only be part of the answer, with the work of Thelen and colleagues (Thelen and Fisher 1982, Thelen et al 1984, Thelen 1985, 1995, Thelen and Smith 1994) being prominent over the last 20 years, particularly in the infancy stage. In Box 5.1 there is a closer examination of a study in a similar vein.

Box 5.1 A closer examination

Anticipatory adjustments during gait initiation in young children: Ledebt et al (1998)
Ledebt et al (1998) analysed anticipatory adjustments during gait initiation in children aged 2 years and 6 months and 4, 6, and 8 years of age, noting that anticipatory behaviour is crucial in the build-up of the feedforward mechanisms so important for motor control. In previous work, Bril and Breniere (1992) suggested a two-stage walking progression. The first, which only lasts a few months after the onset of walking, they label a process of 'integration', which involves the biomechanical properties of the system; this is followed by a period lasting up to 7 years of age that involves a period of tuning of walking. Anticipatory behaviour is lacking in the first stage, but they proposed that it develops in the second stage with fine tuning of the postural and locomotor components of gait.

Method
Using a force plate, the children walked a number of step sequences with around two to three steps. Each sequence on the force plate was followed by a few steps on the walkway just off the plate. The acceleration of the centre of mass and the displacements of the centre of foot pressure were both measured. Their measure of anticipatory behaviour was the construction of the feedforward control of gait.

Results
When anticipatory behaviour first appeared, with backward and lateral shift of the centre of pressure, it was spasmodic and not organized, even though it was present in all age groups. Systematic backward anticipation was found in all but the youngest group, whereas lateral anticipation was absent in the two youngest groups and started at 6 years of age. The amplitude of any backward shift did not relate to the upcoming velocity in children, as it did in adults. An interesting finding was that growth of foot length permitted a greater backward shift, thus leading to increased velocity at the end of the first step. They concluded that there was anticipatory behaviour even in the youngest groups, but it was only later that this was finely tuned to the characteristics of the forthcoming movement.

Comment
They made the important statement that '…one need no longer interpret the discrepancies between early and mature-gait anticipatory behaviour as a consequence of immature neural functioning' (Ledebt et al 1998, p. 16).

The conclusion was that other variables such as growth in foot length are influencing factors in anticipatory behaviours, thus presenting arguments for a dynamical systems explanation. This examines all transacting variables and proposes that neural maturation is not the only influential factor relating to walking.

Work of two of the authors, Breniere and Bril (1998), examined children during their first 5 years of independent walking for a total of 457 step sequences. They also invoke a dynamical systems perspective that views walking as a multidimensional activity, with components of gait that can be locomotor, postural, or anticipatory in nature, and the developments of these components do not always coincide. They first examined the postural requirements of gait, noting that the strength demands of gravity forces in the hip are considerable during the one-leg stance phases of walking, and secondly they analysed the developmental progression of this capability. Four males and one female were examined longitudinally from the onset of walking and for the following 5 years. They were measured while walking naturally on a force plate and for several steps beyond. They proposed the value of the centre of mass vertical acceleration at the point of contact of the foot as a developmental index of the postural capacity of the child to control gravitational forces. They confirmed first that this reflects hip kinematic behaviour. Second, they found that during the one-leg stance in the walking phase, the global index used takes 3 to 4 years after independent walking to control the gravity forces and more than 4 to 5 years – making the children 5 to 6 years of age – to reach a level that is seen in adults.

A constraints dynamical framework explanation has also been used by other workers in the field. Adolph et al (2003) analysed walking behaviour in infants (1–2y), young children (5–6y), and adults by calculating the relative contribution to the walking process of a number of variables. These included neural maturation (from chronological age), height, weight, leg length, head circumference, crown–rump length, and practice (number of days from first step). The interesting results showed *practice* to be the single most important factor and neither neural maturation nor morphological features on their own could account for improvements in walking skill. It was noted that variability in experience and intrinsic constraints combine to promote the development of postural control and walking and provide empirical evidence of behavioural flexibility.

Sensory–perceptual variables, such as estimation of slope and texture of the surface, also make contributions to variations in the development of walking. The work of Wann et al (2011) outlined in the throwing and catching section of this chapter equally applies to walking in different environmental contexts such as on a busy pavement or crossing a road. As one would expect, perceptual factors also play a substantial role in the development of stair climbing. It has long been well established that a common perceptual parameter in stair climbing is the use of the ratio between the height of the stair and hip height as

a body-scaled invariant – first proposed by Warren (1984) with college students. This has been extended by researchers such as Cesari et al (2003) who propose the parameter of the angle of the ratio between the height of the stair and the distance taken from the feet to the top edge of the stair before the initiation of the movement. This angle was the same for both children and adults despite the different kinematics of the action. Thus children perceive environmental invariants that are body-size scaled, illustrating the importance of sensory–perceptual information in actions such as stair climbing, and regardless of age and differences in ability, individuals utilize common perceptual variables to guide the action.

RUNNING

Description

Walking can become running in that arm–leg movements are used in a similar pattern to move the body forward. The principal difference is that while running the mover is sometimes airborne (when both feet are off the ground), whereas while walking one foot is always in contact with the ground. A normative description of running is as follows: some children begin to run at 18 months and most run by 24 months. Clark and Whitall (1989) and Whitall and Getchell (1995) report that running starts to occur about 6 to 7 months after children begin to walk. Children attain a reasonably good running form by ages 4 to 6 (Fortney 1983), and after that the interest is in how fast they can run and how well they can use running in play-game activities. In addition there have been detailed analyses of the movement mechanics of running, particularly to discover the movement parameters of high-level adult performers (Dillman 1975). Classic work by Wickstrom (1977) summarized a number of important changes in the movement mechanics of young runners, and this will be used as the basis for our review.

The changes in running described by Wickstrom (1977) in Figure 5.2 were based on cinematographic analyses, which are presented by comparing a beginning runner, Child A, with a more experienced runner, Child B. In Figure 5.2 the side view of Child A compared with that of Child B shows the increase in length of stride and the longer period of non-support that characterize development in running in Child B. The support leg, the leg in contact, of Child B becomes extended at take-off in a forward direction, which places the body further forward than the centre of gravity. The leg now loses contact with the ground and must be brought forward as the recovery leg to regain contact with the ground. Analyses have also followed the path of the centre of gravity, which decreases in fluctuations up and down to

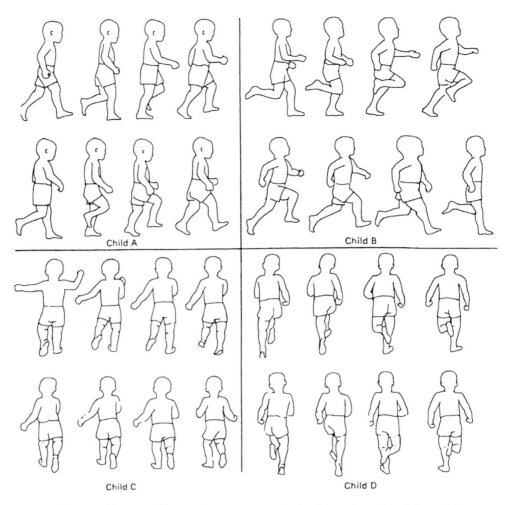

Fig. 5.2 Sequence of pictures to illustrate differences in movement mechanics for running. Adapted from Wickstrom (1977).

become a smoother forward motion. Arms and legs fairly soon coordinate with the opposite arms and legs to move in unison. Individuals, however, establish idiosyncratic arm motions in running that are not useful in describing the general development of running form. With the developing child, the time characteristics of running change to have less time in contact with the ground, more time in the airborne or non-support phase, and faster leg movements. The foot of a beginning runner's support leg contacts the ground with the full sole, which changes to heel–toe contact and then to contact with only the forward portion of the foot when running fast. An additional change is that the forward thrust of a leg produces a rotary motion in the body's vertical axis, which with development is countered by the forward thrust of the opposite arm.

There is also a limited range of movement in the beginning runner's arms and legs, often with the arms held higher and not used in a forward–backward motion.

With development the arm movements become better synchronized with the leg movements to produce a pattern in which the opposite leg and arm extend forward and backward together. In the rear view of a more experienced runner, Child D, the arms stay closer to the body, which can be observed by following the movements of the elbows. Following the movements of one segment of a limb is often very informative and helps focus one's observations. In general, watching from the side helps to trace the leg movements, trunk lean, and arm–leg coordination, and watching from the rear helps to trace the movements of the elbows and heels.

When running, the action is very much influenced by perceptual factors, which specify the environmental context. In Chapter 2 we described the proposal by Lee (1980) that tau, the rate of change of an optic variable, can control the approach and deceleration towards an object or person. As environmental objects and texture change, the rate of dilatation on the retina equates to the reciprocal of the time left until contact with the object. Wann et al (1993) examined this in preschool children (3–5y) by comparing them with adults in a task that required running as fast as possible to touch a target with the hand or with a stick, like a baton used in relay running, and running back after the touch. Tau was calculated to estimate how well they coordinated the deceleration to the target. When asked to touch the target with the hand, the preschool children in some ways showed a similar profile to the adults. They had a constant tau in the approach phase and a comparable kinetic energy when contact was made with the target. However, when running with the stick the children did not adjust their approach strategy appropriately and had a much higher kinetic energy when they hit the target surface, suggesting that they had no real strategies for the changing conditions of the task. They did not take into account the extra length of the baton. This and other studies show that the development of running is influenced not only by mechanical and morphological changes but also by perceptual variables that are attuned to the environmental context.

The explanation of the development of running follows similar lines to that of walking. The proposal is that the action develops in a dynamic manner with several transacting variables operating in a system that is self-organizing. There is still some way to go in controlling running when contexts are changing, with different task requirements showing the limitations of children at this age. As the child develops further, described in the next chapter, he or she not only becomes much faster but is also able to flexibly use running appropriately in more complex and demanding environmental contexts, and experience becomes a crucial variable in this ability. In addition, the child is moving faster than when walking and thus the perceptual variables, particularly vision, have to be utilized more quickly and compared with ongoing kinaesthetic feedback.

JUMPING

Description

Jumping in the simplest sense is a single, discrete movement in which the body is propelled by the legs off the ground for a brief period of time. A jump may start with either a one-footed or a two-footed take-off, and the landing may be on either or both feet. Jumping in various forms becomes part of play-game activities, for example when children jump to avoid a ball hitting their feet in dodge ball, jump over a hurdle, or jump to rebound a basketball. Jumps may also be part of a movement sequence in activities such as jumping rope.

The specific age of achievement for a particular jumping task varies across different studies, but the general pattern is consistent. Some of the variation is related to the test conditions and whether the age of achievement was calculated as a mean or median or by some other method. Becoming airborne briefly when stepping down from a step, which has been observed at 18 months (Hellebrandt et al 1961), is usually the first type of jump to be executed. However, a more important achievement, as well as a more sensible way to consider the beginning of jumping, is the two-foot take-off from the ground. This starts as jumping up and down rather than forward or over an obstacle. The two-foot take-off is a landmark achievement, which can be achieved in rudimentary form near the second birthday and is the basis for the many jumping variations. By 3 years of age a child will jump a distance of around 51cm, and this rises to around 107cm by 6 years of age (Keogh and Sugden 1985).

The standing long jump (standing broad jump) is a good movement for observing the development of body control. The general task is to jump forward with a two-foot take-off and make a two-foot landing. This is a discrete movement requiring a well-coordinated summation of forces to propel the body forward and to maintain postural control sufficiently when landing. Picture sequences of children making a standing long jump are shown in Figure 5.3. Although their goal was to jump as far as possible, the concern here is with observing how they used their body parts to summate forces and to control the resulting movements of their body. The standing long jump has been tested more than any other task involving total body movement, thus providing a great deal of performance data and related movement analyses in published studies (see Chapter 6).

Table 5.1 describes Child A's jump to illustrate the analysis of movement and body parts. Child A's jump has an adequate form to summate force, propel the body off the ground, and land under control. The legs are flexed and the arms are drawn back when preparing to jump. The arms are brought forward as the legs extend to form a straight body line at take-off. However, the head does not stay up in midflight, and the arm and leg movements are not completely symmetrical. The legs are extended somewhat in preparation to land, and there is hip flexion to 'sit down' when landing. The overall jump shows a coordinated sequence of movements with minor points of asymmetry and some incomplete movements.

Child B's jump in Figure 5.3 is a mixture of movements that is often characteristic of young children's jumping. Child B goes into an extreme crouch with arms withdrawn to a point far behind the body. Leg and trunk extensions at take-off are well coordinated and forward,

Preparation   Action

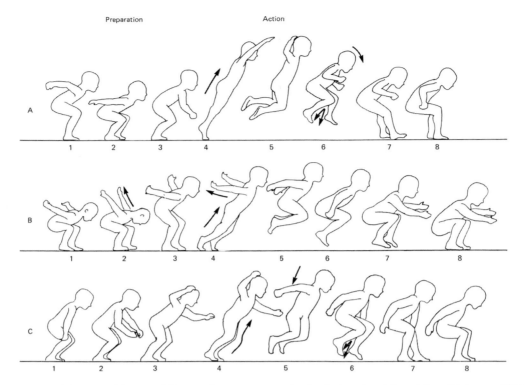

Fig. 5.3 Sequence of pictures to illustrate differences in movement mechanics for jumping. Adapted from Wickstrom (1977).

TABLE 5.1
Analysis of movement mechanics for Child A in Figure 5.2

Body part	Movement phase		
	Preparation (pictures 1–3)	Action (pictures 4–6)	Completion (pictures 7–8)
Arms	Retracts and extends	Swings forward and extends to midline overhead, flexes and brings down	Remains in flexion and brings slightly to rear of midline
Legs	Moderate knee flexion	Complete knee extension at take-off, quick flexion with feet to rear, some asymmetry of legs (pictures 5 and 6)	Moderate knee flexion
Trunk and head	Forward lean of trunk, head somewhat upright (picture 2)	Forward lean of trunk, head goes from upright to slightly down (picture 6)	Moderate forward lean of head and trunk

but the arms remain behind the body. The legs are flexed in flight without extending, as if preparing to sit down while in midair. The arms come forward on landing, perhaps more with the forward momentum than as a purposeful movement. Overall symmetry is generally good and the child seems to be making a great effort yet is not effective in getting the arms involved and is overflexing the legs and hips.

In contrast, Child C made an incomplete jump and did not put enough force into it. Preparation for the jump starts with a lean forward and the arms forward rather than back.

The legs are not fully extended at take-off, and the trunk is drawn up and back rather than forward. The arms rotate up and back while in midair and then come down by the time of landing. The feet are not far off the ground, and the legs are flexed for landing soon after take-off.

Jumping tasks are used in the assessment of motor abilities and in the Movement Assessment Battery for Children (Henderson et al 2007); this involves jumping into square mats with two feet for a maximum of five jumps. The tasks change slightly for 5- and 6-year-olds, requiring better form and continuous jumps with no alterations between jumps. For 3- to 4-year-olds, the 50th centile is three jumps and this rises to five by the time the child is over 4 years of age, indicating that 5 years is the median age for the accomplishment of this task. This task requires perceptual linking to the movement, as the child has visual targets and has to perform the jumps in relation to these constraints. Thus it is reasonable to assume that the coordination of jumping into visual targets is a more difficult task than a simple two-footed jump, and the improvement as the child moves from 3 to 5 years old may be partially the result of the increasing competence of reacting to visual information from the environmental context to coordinate the jumps.

Explanation

There any many types of jump, making any single explanation for age-related changes difficult. Biomechanical analyses have attempted to provide explanations with more detailed examinations of the jump itself. For example, various studies on jumping in children between 3 and 7 years have examined the temporal coupling of hip/knee or knee/ankle reversals or the temporal delay of peak extension velocities in the vertical jump (Clark and Whitall 1989). No age differences in these variables were found, but there are related changes such as distance jumped, take-off angle, and use of upper limbs. Some variables remain constant and others change, leading Jensen et al (1994) to make the distinction between measures of coordination and those of control. The former is how degrees of freedom are synchronized into coordinative structures with invariance being a regular feature. The latter, on the other hand, refers to metric parameterisation such as speed, amplitude and displacement, and adjustments to control variables, which tune the performance in relation to the context and thus can be variable.

Jensen et al (1994) tested the hypothesis that coordination has invariant features and control varies with context with three groups of participants: young children aged 3 years and 6 months and a group of adults. The children's group was divided into two, according to whether their take-off trajectory was high or low, giving three groups altogether. The results showed that all three groups, despite different ages and angles of take-off, displayed the same temporal coupling such as hip–knee–ankle reversals, and timing relationships among peak extensions of lower extremities of joints again were the same across the three groups. The coordinative structures appeared to show invariance despite age and performance differences. However, the novice jumpers (young with low-angle take-off) had different control parameters from the other two groups. They tended to fall or not correct a stumble; they had postural limitations; and they were generally poorly controlled jumpers because of their inability to adjust the movement to the task demands. Thus it would appear that, as Adolph et al (2003) suggests, the role of experience or practice is an important causal factor in jumping.

Jumping improves with age from the child's first attempts, and this improvement continues in various guises through puberty. There are changes in maximum performance and in the manner in which the jumper performs, with a refinement of the jumping action determined by a number of factors such as body and limb size, strength, and other intrinsic constraints such as coordination. In addition, the jump is also moderated by a perception–action link, involving extrinsic constraints such as task demands, which would differ between a horizontal and vertical jump and would probably be developmental in nature.

HOPPING AND SKIPPING

Description

A hop is a one-legged jump that children use in many play-game activities, such as skipping, galloping, and playing hopscotch. A hopper becomes airborne when one leg is flexed and then extended to lift the body off the ground. The same leg is used to contact the ground as the body comes down, and the sequence is repeated. Hopping is a series of discrete movements, which are difficult to make continuously because the body is always propelled by the same leg. This means that the body comes somewhat to rest while the leg is being flexed in preparation for extension. Very good hoppers can minimize the time in contact with the ground to make the movement more continuous.

When first hopping, children often propel their bodies too high by pushing too hard off the ground, as if unable to exert the appropriate amount of force. However, propelling the body too high makes the landing recovery difficult, and the children then cannot prepare for the second hop without putting down the non-hopping leg for support. When first able to hop successfully, the non-hopping leg tends to be held forward, with the upper body leaning back as if providing some equilibrium in the overall postural control. The arms tend to be held high away from the body and extended somewhat, similar to arm use when first walking, and are often moved up and down as if flapping wings. Movement mechanisms change to having the non-hopping leg flexed, with the knee pointed to the ground and the heel to the rear. The arms are flexed and at the side, although this may vary. In addition, less force is used, with the hopping foot coming barely off the ground.

Hopping forward appears to be easier than hopping in place, as the momentum generated by each hop can be partially dissipated by moving forward. When first hopping forward, children often hop very quickly, as if trying to make as many hops as possible before they lose postural control and need to put down the other leg for support. This is another example in which too much force seems to be used, thus creating too much to be controlled.

Children at 3 years and 5 months can make a single hop on either leg, and hopping soon becomes part of other locomotor movements such as skipping and galloping. Most children can skip at age 5, with some skipping quite well at age 4. Galloping is pretending to ride a horse, in which one leg remains the lead leg. The child steps forward on the lead leg, jumps into the air with both feet, lands on the back leg, and steps forward to continue the cycle. Galloping is an interesting coordination of leg movements, and most children can gallop at age 5.

Males tend not to do hopping tasks of any kind as soon or as well as females (Keogh 1968, 1969). This is one of the most distinct sex differences in movement development before age 6. As an example, Keogh (1968, 1969) found that, at age 5, 80% of females compared with 67% of males could hop five times in place on either foot; also 91% of the females could skip five successive cycles, compared with 53% of the males. In addition, females are quicker to skip and hop smoothly and continuously, whereas males are often more discrete and use more force in making jumping and stomping movements (Keogh and Sugden 1985). Similar results were reported by Loovis and Butterfield (2000) who investigated the influence of age, sex, and static and dynamic balance on mature skipping in males and females from 4 to 14 years of age. By Grade 1 (7 years old) 95% of children showed mature skipping patterns, whereas in kindergarten this was 83% for females and 74% for males, indicating a step change at this age. Skipping is a more complex variant of hopping, involving both a hop and a step, which are merged to form a skip. A classic and well-proven way of teaching a child to skip is to break it down into these two distinct parts and gradually increase the speed such that they become the one skill of skipping.

Whitall (2003) notes that developmental changes in some locomotor skills show similarities in that they require the continuous adaptation to balance and bilateral coordination, with the different skills showing great similarity in the developmental progression of coordination. For example, both running and galloping progress from flat-foot to heel–toe movements and from stiff arm and leg movements to full leg motion with arms assisting. Hopping and skipping progress from one-sided jerky movements, with arms inactive or used inconsistently, to smooth and rhythmic leg action with reciprocal arm support.

Explanation

Hopping and skipping, like walking, running, and jumping, will be influenced by a number of factors which combine to produce the finished product, whether skilful and controlled or otherwise. The development of balance and the coordination of the upper and lower limbs combining with stabilizing perceptual factors in the visual display all influence the final product. Classic longitudinal information on hopping in seven children was presented by Roberton and Halverson (1988) after collecting filmed data over a minimum 15-year period and a summary is shown in Box 5.2.

Roberton and Halverson (1988) in Box 5.2 viewed the child's hopping leg like a mass spring or an inverted pendulum, distally fixed when the foot is on the floor. As a pendulum of constant stiffness oscillates at a given rate for a given displacing force, changes in children's mass or leg length will change the oscillation rate. Thus as the child becomes older, hopping frequency could slow down because of increased mass and leg length and not simply due to underlying neural substrates. They suggested that muscle stiffness, and the need to reduce it to allow a softer landing thereby reducing risk of injury, may be an important variable. Also they proposed that the stiffness of the hopping leg may reach a value that is critical for the movement to be reorganized to ensure safety and functionality. This reorganization would involve swinging the non-hopping leg to produce greater flexion in the hopping leg or spread the flexion over a longer period of time, both of which would soften the landing, that is, reduce stiffness.

Getchell and Roberton (1989) took this further to propose that a change in the hopping leg action would still be accompanied by a reduction in the stiffness of the hopping leg, even after the mass and leg length were controlled. In addition, they tested the notion that children with a more advanced technique could simulate a lower level by not swinging their non-hopping leg and this would increase the stiffness of the hopping leg. Their results confirmed the earlier work by Roberton and Halverson (1988) in that stiffness does decline between two defined developmental levels. At the lower level, children had difficulty adjusting stiffness levels, thereby hindering a safe and soft landing and thus stressing the musculoskeletal system. At the higher developmental level, children could set a lower stiffness level prior to hopping, thus enabling a soft landing and suggesting a reorganization of the system. In addition, engaging children at the higher developmental level to simulate the lower level by not swinging their non-hopping leg only accounted for a small amount of stiffness, leading the authors to conclude that it was the hopping leg itself that affected muscle stiffness. They

---

Box 5.2 A closer examination

Hopping: Roberton and Halverson (1988)

The purpose of the study was to examine relative timing in changes children experience in their hopping move-ment. The authors did this by describing timing changes within and between leg action and changes in the dynam-ics of leg action. Each child was individually filmed four times a year from ages 3 to 4, every 6 months from 5 to 7, and yearly up to their 16th or 18th birthday. Here the concentration is on data up to 7 years of age. They begin by describing qualitative changes in hopping over the period.

Results

From age 3 to age 5, the predominant changes in leg action were using the hopping leg from flexion to lift the leg off the floor to extension to push it off, and the change in the non-hopping leg from immobility to the start of a swinging motion. Arm action changed from both arms moving together in an upwards and forward manner to leg and arm opposition beginning. With respect to timing, they found a number of timing invariants (intralimb) that remained up to adulthood. These occurred in the hopping leg irrespective of what was happening in the rest of the body. These invariants included the 'landing invariant', accounting for 13 to 17% of the time and being the amount of time needed to dissipate the downwards force while simultaneously beginning upwards force.

Comment

The authors suggested that the hopping leg could be modelled on a simple vibratory system, with the resultant restoring force proportional to the distortion. The authors interpreted the data in the then growing movement towards dynamical systems explanations, with a tentative proposition of vibratory systems as explanatory analo-gies for the changing relationships of the growing parts of the body.

---

summarize their work by noting that body stiffness causes a reorganization of children's hopping movements, allow-ing for a more functional and safer landing.

THROWING AND CATCHING

Throwing and catching have been linked together even though they are clearly different skills requiring different subcomponents. Throwing is a ballistic action that can vary from performing it in the thrower's own time or in time with someone else's action, such as trying to run out a batter in cricket or baseball. Catching, on the other hand, involves continuous tracking and the act is always in response to someone else's time, unless the thrower is throwing to him or herself.

Both throwing and catching require sensory–percep-tual information in order to achieve a movement goal. In throwing the layout of the environment has to be deter-mined and the accuracy of the throw is directed to this. In the case of a moving target, it becomes more complex when the thrower has to determine when the receiver will reach a certain required destination and judge the throw accordingly. Thus, prediction and anticipation loom large in this action. In catching, the catcher always has to predict when the object will reach him or her and coordinate their actions in time with the approaching object. Throwing and catching are often seen together, being involved in many of the activities and games that children play.

Throwing

Throwing is a general movement pattern used to propel objects. Throwing can be accomplished in so many ways with so many objects that it is difficult to isolate a basic pattern. Throwing can be a full-arm motion in an over-hand, underhand, or side-arm movement, or can be a partial arm–hand motion to toss or flip an object. Objects vary in size, weight, and configuration and can be held and thrown differently, and the goal of throwing may be to achieve accuracy, force, distance, special flight char-acteristics, or a combination of these effects. Throwing possibilities and variations, which are almost limitless, are probably influenced as much by our social–cultural environment as by our biological make-up. Here throwing is limited to the single-arm, overhand throwing motion used to propel balls and similar small objects. Very little descriptive information is available to trace changes in other types of throwing motions.

The overhand throwing motion is a discrete rather than a repeated movement. The primary concern in the initial development of throwing is to achieve a general accuracy so that the object will land in a desired location, often in order for someone else to catch it. The thrower must summate enough force through the arm linkage system and the trunk to impart force on the object; a proper direction and flight path must be imparted on the object, and the thrower must maintain general postural control. If the location, either an object or a person, is moving, the thrower has to predict how this will affect the throw, thus creating a good example of a perception–action link.

If we observe young infants as they approach their second birthday, they can propel an object in a manner that resembles an overhand throw, but the object does not often go to the intended location and is often thrown too hard for a nearby partner to catch. They have the rudiments of an overhand throwing motion, but they do not have enough control to propel an object to a desired location at an appropriate speed. Young children by age 3 can propel an object in the general direction of a target and for a distance of 1.52 to 3.05m, but they have difficulty in adjusting or modulating the force sufficiently to make it easy for a partner to catch their throws. Even at 7 years of age, a child finds it difficult to throw a ball accurately enough so that a moving person can catch it. Both perceptual and motor variables would appear to play a part in this type of skill.

The throwing form can be described as the early development of control of the throwing motion. (Accuracy, distance, and other performance outcomes will be considered later in Chapter 6.) Four general phases in the development of the overhand throwing motion are shown in Figure 5.4, which is based on classic analyses by Wild (1938) of 32 children from ages 2 to 12. These should not be viewed as a fixed progression.

Young children first throw with the arm only, as seen in the forearm extension to phase 1. The feet remain in place, the trunk does not rotate, and the body makes little forward movement, probably to minimize trunk and leg movements in order to maintain postural control. Fewer body movements make it possible to throw in the intended direction, as fewer forces have been generated to disrupt the release.

Young children soon rotate their trunk, which means that the shoulder and hip turn to the rear on the side of the throwing arm and then come forward with the forward motion of the throwing arm (phase II). The feet remain in place. Wild's phases III and IV include, first, a forward step with only the right leg during a right-arm throw and, second, a step with the left leg raised and extended forward during arm withdrawal and the right leg coming forward after the forward motion of the arm has been completed. Phases III and IV show a much fuller involvement

of trunk and legs, indicating that the children can contain the force they are generating. The step with the opposite leg provides a wider rotation to the rear by the shoulders and hip, which will lead to more force production and more stability at the end of the throwing motion. The follow-through of the throwing arm and leg on the same side provide a way to dissipate the force generated in the throwing motion. Flexing the opposite leg on the follow-through in order to lower the body is also important in maintaining postural control at the end of the throwing motion. Phase IV figures represent a more effective and thus more mature throwing motion in terms of generating force and maintaining postural control. The throwing arm will eventually be drawn more to the rear, perhaps even into full extension, and the arm collapses as it comes forward to accelerate the speed of the object held in the hand. The movements of the wrist and fingers just before and during the release can be used to determine the extent of object rotation and to influence the direction and velocity. Looking at these pictures one can easily invoke a dynamical systems explanation, with the more mature throwing position showing a freeing of the rather rigid degrees of freedom that are illustrated in the younger child.

Roberton (1977, 1978) reported a more elaborate set of analyses that led her to suggest that the development of the component parts of throwing and other movements may proceed at different rates. This means that a movement's components also may not change at the same rate among different individuals, so it may be useful to identify these components in order to trace the changes in them. She states that 'development within component parts may proceed at different rates in the same individual or at different rates in different individuals' (p. 55).

Roberton calls arm movements and pelvic–spinal movements *components of the throwing motion*. Based on previous research, she then suggests five categories of change in the arm component and eight categories of change in the pelvic–spinal component. Roberton limited her analysis to a group of first-grade children (ages 6 and 7), which limited the number of movement categories she might have seen, as younger and older children would need to be included to observe a full range of movement categories.

A total of 73 children (42 males, 31 females; ages 6, 7, and 8) were filmed from two locations while doing 10 overarm throws. Each throw was analysed to describe movements of the two components: arm and pelvis–spine. Categories were identified to mark changes in movement mechanics in each component. Roberton found that some children were consistently in one arm category but were more variable in the pelvic–spinal categories. This indicates some consistency in what a child's arm movements

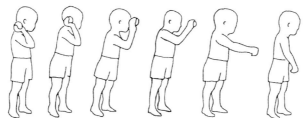

Phase I: The ball is thrown primarily with forearm extension. The feet remain stationary, body does not rotate, and there is a slight forward sway.

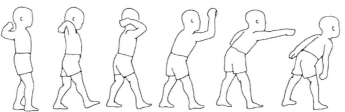

Phase II: Rotatory movement is added. The hand is cocked behind the head during the preparatory movement and the trunk then rotates to the left. The throwing arm swings around in an oblique-horizontal plane.

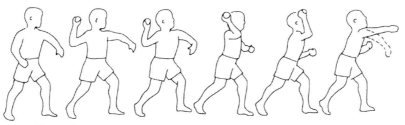

Phase III: A forward step with the right leg is added in a righthand throw. The step produces additional forward force for the throw.

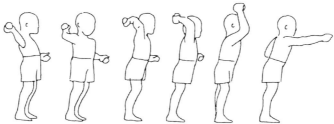

Phase IV: Throwing arm and trunk rotate backward during preparation. A contralateral step moves body weight forward.

Fig. 5.4 Sequence of pictures to illustrate differences in movement mechanics in four phases proposed by Wild (1938). Adapted from Wickstrom (1977).

will look like, whereas pelvic–spinal movements may be more variable in a series of throws. Roberton then described the total body configuration according to the category for each component.

Roberton's explanation of the variations in combinations of component categories is that each component develops at a different rate, and the variations noted in her analyses support this. Control in one component category may also permit the use of that component in another category. Postural control is needed before pelvic–spinal rotation can be done without disrupting the body position, and pelvic–spinal rotation in some form is needed before the arm can be withdrawn. That is, there may be some mechanical considerations determining arm movement, whereas other developmental constraints, such as postural control, may limit one or more components. Throwing can

119

also be broken down into different components, such as withdrawing the ball, bringing it forward, and releasing and following it. These components focus on the movement pieces and their order, rather than on the anatomical parts of the arm and pelvis–spine.

Sugden and Soucie (2008), commenting upon the development of the throwing action in young children, note that the young child limits the throwing action to one from the elbow and does not fully engage in the transference of body mass during the throw. If the young child tried to use a more mature throwing posture by releasing more degrees of freedom he or she would probably end with the action being uncontrollable. Thus, in the early stages of throwing, the degrees of freedom are frozen to enable effective control, embodying a self-organizing system that continuously adapts to the internal and external constraints that are present. This adaptation involves the progressive release of the degrees of freedom, providing more flexibility in the throw, bringing in more movement of the hips and non-throwing arm, for example, and a new category of movements emerges: 'The child's movements are being tuned to their ever evolving resources' (Sugden and Soucie 2008, p. 193).

Catching
Catching is usually included when throwing is mentioned because of the social aspects of games and recreational activities, but it does involve a very different set of processes to throwing. An important feature of catching is that the child has to move to someone else's timing. In throwing, the child can choose when and, to a certain extent, where to throw. However, in catching the child has to respond to the speed and location of the approaching object and react accordingly; he or she is no longer in control of all of the variables.

Descriptions of types of catching or skills that underlie catching in the first months of life from the work of researchers such as Claes von Hofsten in Sweden are presented elsewhere in Chapters 1 and 4, with the concentration here on ages 2 to 7 years. From the age of 3 children begin to catch in the traditional sense of stopping and controlling an aerial ball with the hands. At first there are large body and trunk movements, with the later stages characterized by more refined hand and finger movements. At 3 the children hold their arms stiff and straight at the elbows and catching begins by 'trapping' the ball, usually involving the trunk, arms, and hands. At 4 the children open their hands even though the arms are still stiff and at 5, as the skill develops, children have a more relaxed position: the arms are lowered with the elbows flexed and the hands positioned in anticipation of the arrival of the ball (Wellman 1937). Later this becomes

quite sophisticated, with the hands 'giving' as the ball arrives, but this rarely happens by the age of 7. Normative data is available from the Movement ABC 2 (Henderson et al 2007), with the task being to catch a bean bag thrown underhand from a distance of 1.8m. At 3 to 4 years of age the 50th centile is 5 caught out of 10 and this rises to 8 or 9 by the time the child is between 6 and 7 years of age.

Explanation
Strohmeyer et al (1991) chronicled the progression of catching skills in 5- to 12-year-old children, with the youngest group fitting in the 2- to 7-year-old range of this chapter. The children were tossed a ball to three different locations: directly to the body; at the forehead; and a selection of other locations. The authors used the categories of prelongitudinal developmental screening procedure (Roberton et al 1980), involving arm preparation, arm reception, hands and body readiness. They found that younger children had advanced skills when the ball was thrown directly to the body and less advanced skills when the ball was tossed to other locations. They discussed this from a constraints perspective, noting that tosses to various other locations did not result in predictable patterns of catching behaviour and that this is in keeping with the result of any constraints being non-specific and non-prescriptive. Small changes in the demands of the task result in small and non-dramatic changes in catching behaviour, but when a critical point was reached in the form of a very different throw, there was a dramatic change in performance.

Savelsbergh et al (2003) interpret this catching development in a Bersteinian perspective as a progression from 'freezing the degrees of freedom' in the first instance to 'freeing' them in the later stages and finally exploiting them. This is shown in Box 5.3 as a closer examination.

Catching is usually dependent on the timing of another person and as such involves skills of anticipation and prediction, all to be performed in a finite window of time. It is predictable that children's catching skills improve as they get older, and in the period from the upper end of this chapter (6/7 years of age) until the teenage years great improvements are made, often because of improvements in flight prediction, a shorter reaction time, and an ability to use shorter ball viewing time. With development, the child becomes more adaptable through the progressive releasing and exploiting of controlled degrees of freedom, enabling successful participation in activities and games where variable and unpredictable requirements are made.

Both of the skills of throwing and catching include some degree of anticipation and prediction, which involve relying on perceptual, usually visual, judgements. This

---

Box 5.3 A closer examination

Catching: Savelsbergh et al (2003)

Savelsbergh et al (2003) report from their work that from early in childhood children seem to be using what they call 'informational constraints', being similar to adults in the grasp component in a one-handed catch. They propose a theoretical model of catching based on this informational constraints model in which the progression in catching moves through the following three stages.

- *Freezing the degrees of freedom* involves both a coupling between information and action emerging to fit the task, with the movement tuned to the information. This coupling, while limited in its repertoire of responses (different circumstances will disrupt the coupling), is strengthened by successful practice. Catching is limited to fairly rigid conditions, with a ball caught that is thrown directly to the catcher.
- *Freeing the degrees of freedom* involves a different form of coupling, enabling a whole repertoire of responses to be generated without having to learn the task from scratch. This enables the catcher to be flexible, adapting to changing conditions and being able to deal with balls coming in different directions and speeds.
- *Exploiting the degrees of freedom* allows the catcher to engage in the potential of different information couplings, with information tuned to one movement being used in a different one. Thus the coupling for catching can also be used for heading or striking (Savelsbergh et al 2003).

---

judgement helps us locate a moving object whether it is approaching us or moving in a different direction altogether. In order to catch we require this information to estimate the point of contact for us to close our hands/fingers around the object. In throwing this information allows us to predict where the object will be to coincide with the throw.

POSTURE AND BALANCE

Description

A strong argument can be made that balance in early childhood is an extension of postural adjustments in infancy, which tend very often to be precursors to locomotion and in particular the onset of walking. As part of this progression to gait initiation, a variety of postural adjustments are required. This progression was examined by Assaiante et al (2000) who studied postural adjustments in infants aged 1 to 4 months and 9 to 17 months of walking experience, children aged 4 to 5 years, and adults. Previous work had shown that muscular response patterns associated with walking continue to mature up to 5 to 7 years of age (Berger 1992), and this age range appears to be important for the maturation of postural muscle responses. Assaiante et al (2000) investigated the kinematics of the upper portion of the body (head and trunk) during gait initiation in children and adults together with the muscular response patterns in children. Using kinematic and electromyographic analysis they found that anticipatory postural adjustments (APA), although varying by age,

were present in all of the groups evidenced by an anticipatory lateral tilt of the pelvis and the stance leg, enabling the child to unload the opposite leg before the swing phase. An interesting finding was that APA did not appear consistently until 4 to 5 years of age, with refinement of muscle activation latencies at this age with shorter onset latencies for trunk flexors and extensors.

These measures along with others led the authors (Assaiante et al 2000) to conclude that 4 to 5 years of age is a turning point in postural stability and locomotor skills, with other measures also prominent at this age such as steady-state velocity during the first step. Big improvements have taken place by the time the child reaches 3, and further improvements take place up to 7 years of age, but the slope of change is shallower, and 4 to 5 years of age appears to be an age that indicates a significant change.

Balancing tasks are used at about 30 months to monitor changes in a child's ability to control a stationary and a moving body position. Children are asked to stand on one foot in various postures or to walk on a line or a balance beam, and they can stand briefly on one foot by their second birthday, but not until they are 3 years and 2 months can they stand for 5 seconds. Children at 23 months can walk on a line on the floor with their footsteps astride rather than on it, and at 27 months they can walk backwards on the line in the same way. They can walk a circular path forwards at 3 years and 1 month, with each footstep touching the line. Walking heel–toe is more difficult and is achieved only partially at 3 years and 5 months walking forwards and 4 years and 8 months walking backwards (Keogh and Sugden 1985).

In summary, children at 24 months cannot hold a one-foot position more than momentarily, but they can walk astride a straight line. By their third birthday, or soon after, they can stand on a walking board and take several alternating steps, and they are nearly 4 years old before they can walk heel–toe to follow a line on the floor. DeOreo (1976) suggests qualitative levels of achievement in performing some beam-walking tasks, with the more adept children alternating their steps in walking the beam, whereas less adept children will shuffle or slide their feet without alternating them and will need the support of stepping off with one foot or taking the hand of another person. Observations of the kind suggested by DeOreo are useful in describing performance on balancing tasks.

A set of seven balancing tasks outlined in Box 5.4 was used with young schoolchildren in a classic study by Keogh (1969) to represent four types of activities involved in keeping a position in place whether during holding, controlling, travelling, or explosive movements.

More recent data on achievements is available from the Movement ABC (Henderson et al 2007). The balance task in this instrument is trying to hold a one-legged stance for up to 30 seconds. Between 3 and 4 years of age the 50th centile is 4 seconds, rising to 9 seconds between 4 and 5 years of age, through 15 to 20 seconds at 5 to 6 years, and around 28 seconds at 6 to 7 years of age, showing a steady, almost linear, progression on this task. A critical comment that could be made here is that 30 seconds is a long time for any young child, and the task may be confounded by such variables as motivation and not understanding the length of time required, with the result that more than balance is being tested.

Balancing tasks such as those described in this section are useful through age 5. After that, these tasks offer little information, except that children can do them for longer periods of time while in unrealistic postures, such as standing like a stork for 30 seconds with one foot on the knee of the standing leg and the hands held on top of the head. It would appear more appropriate to consider postural control rather than more variations of balancing tasks, and one could argue that posture and balance become not skills in themselves but more synergistic resources that underpin a range of movement activities. This can be seen in activities such as children standing with one leg on a scooter or skateboard and using the other leg to push, riding a bicycle, dodging a playmate, diving into a swimming pool, and other play-game skills in which the control of body posture and balance is an important part of a movement skill.

Explanation

Obvious candidates for the development of posture and balance would be motor aspects such as neural development and strength variables together with anthropometric changes. In addition, it has long been recognized that somatosensory information has a strong effect on the developing postural control in infants and children. Early studies by Lee and Aaronson (1974) showed using a 'moving room' that moving the surrounding visual environment disrupted infants' upright posture and balance. Other studies confirmed the importance of visual linking, with proprioceptive information on both standing and sitting posture and balance (Butterworth and Hicks 1977, Stoffregen et al 1987, Higgins et al 1996).

To investigate how somatosenory influence changes with development Barela et al (2003) employed an experimental paradigm examining the coupling of body sway to dynamic somatosensory information in children and adults. More specifically, there was an examination of gain and phase responses to sinusoidal information at different frequencies, while touching an oscillating contact surface. Four groups of 10 males were examined with children of ages 4, 6, and 8 years and adults. The participants were required to touch the centre of a touch plate, which moved at three randomly assigned frequencies, and their responses to these frequencies were measured through body sway using centre of mass in the medial lateral direction. The authors characterized the dynamic behaviour between postural sway and touch by an examination of response sensitivity (sway) and response timing (phase). The results showed that a light touch to a moving touch pad induced postural sway in all participants, which appeared to be developed by 6 years of age, but overall focused postural coupling to the different sensory frequencies was not as well developed in children as in adults. The children's responses were more generic to the different frequencies and more variable, with the authors suggesting that this variability may arise not from a sensory feedback process but from the children's inability to accurately estimate an internal model of body orientation. These results are different to previous studies and may arise from the different presentations requiring either fast (Woollacott et al 1987) or relatively slow (Barela et al 2003) reactions to somatosensory information.

The development of posture and balance involves a complex set of resources, which change with age and influence the final product with great gains being demonstrated in functional tasks between the ages of 2 and 7. The continued development of the neural system, the gain in strength, and changes in anthropometric variables all contribute to this development. Of equal importance appears to be the development of how the sensory information is

Box 5.4 A closer examination

Analysis of body control tasks: Keogh (1969)

Young schoolchildren's ability to control their limb and body movements was tested in relation to a framework in which, first, movements were made in place or at least in a limited space (Keogh 1969). The body position was held, or a controlled or an explosive movement was followed by a held position. Holding a position is like the more traditional tests of static balance. The controlled and explosive movements both change and regain the body position, which is like our description in Chapter 2 of achieving and maintaining static equilibrium. Second, movements were made to maintain dynamic equilibrium while moving or travelling. This type of balancing task is used often in measuring dynamic balance. The tasks with a controlled or an explosive movement combine the traditional categories of static and dynamic balancing tasks.

A total of 270 children (ages 5, 6, and 7) were tested individually in a test session, which took 15 to 25 minutes. Children were barefooted, which tends to make balancing more difficult than when wearing shoes, were allowed to keep their eyes open, and were allowed to move their arms and body, as long as the foot or feet in contact with the ground were not displaced or moved out of position.

The heel–toe stand and one-leg stand had to be held for 10 seconds. The heel–toe touch required the children to touch the forward foot with both hands, return to an upright posture, and hold both hands on top of their heads for 3 seconds. The ring over foot required children to stand on one foot, place a 6-inch wooden hoop over the foot of the free leg, and not move the support for 3 seconds. The jump–turn and hop–turn items involved jumping in the designated direction with a two-footed take-off, landing with two feet, and holding the landing position for 3 seconds. The heel–toe walk comprised 10 steps, heel to toe, while keeping both feet on the line.

Two points were given for passing the first trial, and one point was given for passing the second trial after failing the first. A maximum of 32 points could be scored by receiving two points for each of the 16 items. The passing percentages for males and females of age 5 are listed in Table 5.2. The total mean scores are plotted by age and sex in Figure 5.5.

TABLE 5.2
Body control framework and percentage passing at age 5

Position		Task	Males	Females
In place	Hold	Heel–toe stand		
		(R)	78	83
		(L)	83	87
	Controlled	Heel–toe touch		
		(R)	61	67
		(L)	52	70
	Explosive	Jump–turn		
		Backwards	80	80
		90°	85	91
		180°	50	57
		Hop–turn		
		Forwards	78	78
		Backwards	13	46
		90°	53	52
Travelling		Heel–toe walk		
		Forwards	65	87
		Backwards	7	15
		Total mean score (SD)		
		Age 5	16.2 (5.6)	18.6 (6.4)
		Age 6	21.9 (4.5)	24.8 (4.7)
		Age 7	26.0 (3.1)	27.8 (3.5)

R, right; L, left; SD, standard deviation.

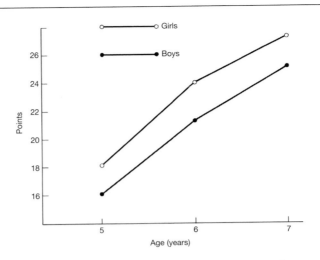

Fig. 5.5 Total mean score for body control tasks by age and sex.

All of the test items, except the two involving walking backwards, were passed by at least 50% of the males and females at age 5. The passing figure increased to at least 75% at age 6, except for walking backwards, and only 58% of the males successfully jumped and turned 180 degrees. Females had a significantly better mean score at age 5, as shown in Figure 5.5, and had a higher percentage of passing on nearly every task, as shown in Table 5.2.

utilized in the various balance tasks. This has been shown in studies using visual and proprioceptive information. How this development affects the final movement product does appear to be a function of the type of task that is being utilized and the measures employed. What is certain is that, while there is improvement between the ages of 2 and 7, the development at 7 is not yet complete, with more changes to come particularly with respect to more complex tasks such as those demanding speed of response. This would appear to articulate with other different, yet linked, changes beyond 7 when a child has to react to moving people or objects; these changes are substantial from 7 through puberty.

CONTROL OF SLOW AND FAST MOVEMENTS
An important and generally overlooked indicator of improved movement control is moving slowly, that is making a movement slowly rather than more rapidly and more forcefully. Initial efforts in making most movements tend to be too rapid and too forceful, with subsequent adjustments made to lessen the amount of force. Moving slowly also requires a high level of movement control and is another indicator of improved movement control. Following this general line of thinking, Gipsman (1973) worked with two groups of children (mean ages of 4y 6mo and 6y 10mo) who performed six movement tasks

quickly and then slowly. She used the difference between the fast and the slow times to calculate a mean range of movement rate (RMR) for each task in order to measure the ability to control or vary the movement rate. The six tasks were walking a 9.1m curved path, rolling a large ball on the path, riding a tricycle on the path, drawing a line on the path (reduced to fit on a piece of paper), alternating hands to touch crayons in a line of boxes ('walking your crayons down the page'), and winding a 60cm fishing line onto a reel.

The older children had higher RMR mean scores on all of the tasks, as shown in Table 5.3, but the mean differences were not significant for rolling the ball and riding the tricycle. The RMR mean scores more than doubled for the other tasks. Interestingly, there were no sex differences. The mean fast times improved, but only by a small amount compared with the much larger increases in the mean slow time. Thus, the increases in the RMR mean scores were primarily a function of improved control in making slower movements. The correlations of RMR scores for each pair of tasks ranged from 0.4 to 0.8, indicating something of a general ability to control movement rate. Other studies involving walking slowly and drawing slowly support the statement that children improve markedly from age 4 to age 9 in moving slowly (Maccoby et al 1965, Constantini and Hoving 1973, Constantini et al 1973).

TABLE 5.3
Range of movement rate scores for two groups of children[a]

Task	Younger (mean age=4.5y)		Older (mean age=6.8y)	
	Mean	SD[b]	Mean	SD[b]
Walking	8.1	9.6	20.9	18.3
Rolling a ball	12.3	9.2	22.6	16.1
Riding a tricycle	12.4	9.7	18.9	13.7
Drawing a line	6.1	6.6	25.9	20.9
Walking the crayons	2.0	1.5	6.3	7.1
Reeling a fishing line	13.2	11.9	25.4	18.2

[a]Based on data from Gipsman (1973). [b]Standard deviations (SDs) are large in proportion to mean scores, indicating that there are some extremely high scores because low scores cannot be less than zero.

These studies are interesting, but considerable care is needed in selecting the tasks to study moving slowly, as illustrated in Gipsman's observations (1973). When walking slowly, some older children shuffled while making sounds, as if they were imitating trains, and others made high, exaggerated stepping movements while taking small steps. These children continued to move rapidly or move a great deal, rather than making the same movement more slowly. That is, their strategy for moving slowly was to take small steps. These children simply found a different way to solve the movement problem, without having to move slowly. The movements are more fixed for riding a tricycle, drawing a line, and reeling a fishing line and provide a better test of moving slowly.

The sizeable changes in moving slowly occur in such a short age period that they probably involve more than just an improvement in the neuromotor control system. The stepping strategies used in walking show that children solve this problem by altering the task and not really moving slowly. The children also improved greatly in drawing a line and reeling a fishing reel when made to do the same movement. Moving slowly seems to be a movement problem that includes improvement not only in neuromotor control but also in the manner in which the child constructs the context and makes adjustments accordingly, thus articulating a dynamic system.

COMMENTS ON BODY CONTROL

The developmental progressions made by children in body skills, as illustrated by the selected examples, are quite profound during the years 2 to 6 or 7. At 2, these skills are either absent or have just emerged and are performed at a rudimentary level. By 7, these skills are mastered, particularly in closed situations in which the environment is predictable, but there is still much development to occur to enable the child to engage proficiently in activities that demand predication and anticipation of moving objects or persons. Much of the increase in performance from age 2 to 7 is due to the child learning through experience to adapt to the constraints set by the environment, the task, and his or her own personal resources. A good example of this is the changes children make to their movements when asked to move slowly. A second involves the progression from freezing degrees of freedom in the early stages of development to progressively and selectively freeing them as the child becomes more proficient, thus enabling the activity to be performed in a more adaptable manner. In order to progress the attainment of more open tasks, the child engages in more efficiently utilizing the perception–action match, as described in the following chapter.

Throughout this section we have included perceptual as well as motor constraints as these are a determining factor in the final movement product. The child with development between the ages of 2 and 7 will be better able to predict the features of the environment and also to recognize that a moving object will require a different action in order for such an object to be caught, thrown, or anticipated so that someone else can catch or intercept it. It is also clear that this attribute is not complete by the age of 7 and children are still at a learning stage at this age. There is little information on how the progression of motor abilities such as the recruitment of coordinated structures links with the perceptual development so often needed in a task. In experimentation we are caught between two almost conflicting paradigms: if we measure motor and perception separately, we are in danger of not presenting realistic situations, yet if we measure them in a classic perception–action task, it is difficult to determine where the development is taking place, save in the performance of the whole task.

Manual control

By their first birthday, children are reasonably proficient in separating reaching and grasping movements, and they can readily pick up objects by means of a power or precision grip. By their second birthday, they have well-coordinated movement sequences in the arm linkage system, are quite accurate spatially in placing a hand where desired, and are more dexterous in manipulating objects. In succeeding years, children become progressively more able to care for themselves, in feeding, dressing, and grooming themselves, which are often considered self-help skills. Children also use objects and materials to construct larger and different objects, as well as using tools of various kinds, including pencils and similar writing–painting tools, in addition to saws, hammers, screwdrivers, and wrenches. Normative data for self-care skills and construction tasks, including using particular tools, vary extensively because initial achievement in these movements is affected greatly by opportunity and expectations. For example, many of these movement tasks are considered social functioning and thus are observed as part of children's social development. Social expectations probably influence how a cup or spoon is held, and holding a cup or spoon in an expected or a different way probably influences the personal–social response, exemplifying a mover–environment transaction in which both mover and social environment will change.

Hand movements are used in such varied and complex ways, as noted in Chapter 4, that it is difficult to describe systematically their changes in control; we shall use the framework and terminology presented in Chapter 4 to analyse changes in manual control from ages 2 through 7, with normative data included when available. Manual movements require control of an arm linkage system and digital manipulations in unimanual and bimanual form. The hand grip may be power or precision, with the precision grip offering more dexterity in manipulating an object. In addition, they require the appropriate sensory–perceptual abilities that allow them to perform the movements in context. Possible explanations for the changes in achievements are presented at various locations in the text.

SELF-CARE SKILLS

Dressing, grooming, and feeding require many types of movements, as shown by the self-care skills listed in Table 5.4. Frankenburg and Dodds (1967) report the general observations in the Denver Developmental Screening Test that children can dress with supervision at 32 months and without supervision at 3 years and 6 months, but they do not indicate when children can use specific dressing skills. Knobloch and Pasamanick (1974), using data from Gesell's earlier findings, name 4 years as the age when children can dress and undress with supervision. They also note that children can pull on a single garment at 4 years. The normative differences in these two reports reveal the range in age of achievement expected for such general skills. Some of the differences among these observations may be in the types of clothing and the extent of parental involvement and societal expectations.

Putting on garments is a dressing task that requires matching the garment to the proper body parts in an appropriate spatial relationship of garment and mover.

TABLE 5.4
Age of achievement of self-care skills

Task	Age (mo)	Study
Pulls on a simple garment	24	Knobloch and Pasamanick (1974)
Puts on shoes	36	
Laces shoes	48	
Unbuttons accessible buttons	36	
Distinguishes fronts and backs of clothes	48	
Dresses and undresses with supervision	48	
Buttons up	36	Frankenburg and Dodds (1967)
Dresses with supervision	32	
Dresses without supervision	43	
Washes and dries hands and face	42	Knobloch and Pasamanick (1974)
Brushes teeth	48	
Handles cup well	21	Knobloch and Pasamanick (1974)
Inhibits overturning of spoon	24	
Feeds self, spills little	36	
Pours well from pitcher	36	

Knobloch and Pasamanick (1974) report that children can distinguish the fronts and backs of clothes at 4 years. Children at an earlier age may be able to hold and manipulate garments but not be able to arrange the proper spatial relationship between the garments and themselves. If the proper spatial relationships can be arranged, well-modulated movement control will be needed to place the body part into the garment with proper force and accuracy. This is seen in the difficulty in getting an arm to the end of a sleeve or a foot into a tight-fitting shoe. Putting on garments is a self-paced task that is usually bimanual and requires very little digital dexterity. The problem of putting on garments includes spatial relationships as part of the movement control. Thus perceptual development concerning directionality, size, and form will greatly affect this task.

Buttoning and tying a garment is quite a different task. Children are expected to button and unbutton at 36 months. Dexterous control of the fingers and thumbs are required to get a button in or out of a hole and make the many movements to tie laces properly. Snaps, zippers, and similar garment closures also involve a fairly high level of bimanual dexterity. Buttoning tasks not only differ by size of button but also whether vision is involved. If the button is high on a shirt or blouse, then the task becomes almost purely kinaesthetic; if the button is on the sleeve, the child has the added advantage of vision, although fine-grained manipulation is still required.

Grooming is another self-care task, but one that uses implements such as towels, brushes, and combs. Children can wash and dry their face and hands at 3 years and 6 months and brush their teeth at 4 years. The movements are often serial or repetitive, such as rubbing or brushing for several strokes. Some dexterity of the fingers and thumb is required, as when using a bar of soap, but they mainly involve arm–hand movements, with the implement held in one position in the hand. Some movements are unimanual and others are bimanual.

Feeding is a self-care skill that varies depending on the utensils to be used and social customs. Children at 24 months have some general control of holding a glass or cup and also can use a spoon to feed themselves, including preventing the spoon from turning over when bringing it to their mouths. Feeding activities of this kind are only generally successful. There is some spilling of food, a great deal of attention is required, and the movements are made in rather slow motion. Children at 36 months can feed themselves, again, at a basic level of using different utensils, pouring into a cup, and the like. Data are not available regarding control of more intricate movements, such as using a knife to spread butter or cut while holding the food with a fork. Rosenbloom and Horton's observations (1975) in watching young children (ages 1 to 4) use teapots to pour into cups exemplify the type of movement analyses useful in describing the development of feeding skills. The older children were able to minimize shoulder and trunk movements when lifting and pouring. However, the younger children moved their entire body, and the arm and hand not holding the teapot made associated movements. The teapot's path became a more direct and more continuous movement towards the cup and less a discrete set of movements to lift the pot high, bring it down to the cup, and then pour from it.

Many of the movements in feeding are unimanual and illustrate the development of control in one hand. The use of a spoon to eat cereal or soup illustrates the development of unimanual control: the spoon must be picked up, placed in the bowl, filled with cereal or soup, transported towards the face, and placed in the mouth. Placing the spoon in the bowl is not difficult, but the spoon must be gripped so that it can be filled. A natural and comfortable way to hold the spoon in the bowl is with the handle flat against the palm or the inside of the fingers in a power grip, which means that the wrist must be moved to place the bowl of the spoon in a horizontal position to enter the cereal dish. It is more efficient to use a precision grip in which the fingers and thumb control the spoon and provide various ways to

change the position of the bowl of the spoon. When the spoon is filled, the next problem is to keep it level until it is in the mouth. As the spoon comes up and towards the mouth, the body posture and arm–hand position must be adjusted to keep the spoon level. Children eventually learn to bring the spoon to their face while adjusting their fingers and thumb to compensate for the movement of their arm towards their face. The final problem is to place the spoon in the mouth, which cannot be seen by the eater. Using a spoon is a complicated movement task requiring careful timing (phasing) of the hand's movements with the movements in the arm linkage system. Spoon use, like most eating tasks, is unimanual and self-paced; the principal problem is to control and coordinate an extended sequence of arm and hand movements.

Much of the observational work on self-care and tool use has a historical, though distinguished, character to it, but more recent analysis and examination of children learning spoon use was conducted by Van Roon et al (2003), using the constraints framework of Newell (1986). They take the term 'constraints' from Newell to mean limiting the possible number of solutions to a movement task. They specify organismic constraints, which include morphological and neurological features of the child such as the child with cerebral palsy; environmental constraints, which include gravity and the optical array and are not usually manipulated in these kinds of experiments; and task constraints, which include the goal of the task, the implements, or equipment used and any rules that may constrain.

By 2 years of age Van Roon et al (2003) report that the young infant has progressed from movements of the shoulder to movements of the wrist joint when filling the spoon and an increased use of flexion during the movement of the spoon to the mouth. In addition, the whole movement is more fluent and smooth, and different types of grip configuration are beginning to be used.

Between 2 and 4 years of age the dominant grip is the transverse digital radial grip, allowing more precise control. The adult grip comes along at around 4 and this grip is not so much for more control but for greater degrees of flexibility according to task demand. The progression to this again takes a classic Bernsteinian sequence with a rigid grip in the first instance (freezing the degrees of freedom) to a looser grip allowing more flexibility (freeing the degrees of freedom) and adapting to the goal of the task and less spillage of food. This type of analysis goes beyond surface-level descriptions and brings the observations into a more dynamic framework.

In a similar vein, an examination of the manipulation of implements was undertaken by Steenbergen et al (1997) in children aged 2 to 4 years with six types of

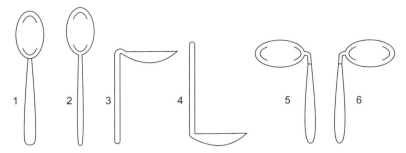

Fig. 5.6 The spoons used by Steenbergen et al (1997) and adapted by Van Roon et al (2003). Reproduced from Van Roon et al (2003) with permission from the publisher.

implements (see Fig. 5.6 as adapted by Van Roon et al 2003). In all cases the concave surface of the spoon was used for scooping up the rice, but children varied the grip according to the shape of the spoon and some of the grips reverted to being more rigid, thus restricting/freezing the degrees of freedom. This shows that the physical implements can change the seemingly natural progression from freezing to freeing the degrees of freedom and especially in the younger children, who often changed to inappropriate grips, whereas the older 4-year-olds simply used a more rigid grip and stuck to it. The task and context may also demand that freezing to freeing may be different for different body parts (Konczak et al 2009). In a similar and related vein, Van Roon et al (2003) describe the non-physical, such as cultural, rules that may affect the development of spoon use, with the authors tracing this in European cultures from the 18th century and noting that children are bound by culture through imitation and copying and being corrected by parents to move from a fist type grip to one that is generally recognized as the adult grip, using three fingers.

Lockman (2000) examined the processes by which children use environmental information to direct their actions, noting in particular the advances made in perception–action coupling to direct the efforts. He addresses three major issues in the development of tool use:

- child variability
- detecting and relating affordances
- action patterns in early tool use.

Individual infants show great variability in how they use a spoon, for example, at a given age, and it may be a while before they settle on one grip. Lockman (2000) believes this variability is the rule rather than the exception and that children are using variability to promote stability and efficiency, exploring how they can satisfy adaptive demands of a particular task. He proposes that within-participant variability scores are just as important

and probably more so than mean scores of age of achievement and may provide clues as to when children are attaining stable forms of tool use or when changes are about to occur.

The second point he makes is that tool use is a problem of affordance detection, that of seeking potential relations between objects directly perceived in context, rather than some objective of constructional representation. He provides the example of work surfaces affording different use of tools, with 3-year-olds choosing to use a paint brush for wet surfaces and not choosing a pencil. It is not the construction of what they wish to achieve that drives this behaviour, but the interface between the work surface and tool. It is the young child's efforts to detect and act on the affordances that the context provides. Lockman (2000) continues to propose that the detection of affordances is not enough and that tool use also requires an environmental frame of reference. As objects do not occupy fixed positions, the young child has to master many different frames of reference from which to detect potential affordances. Instead of researchers examining outcomes of tool use, such as when a particular tool is used, the emphasis should be changed to processes such as how infants align surfaces for tool use and how the task influences this process that incorporates both cognitive and motor abilities.

Finally, Lockman (2000) proposes that precursors of tool use are found earlier in infancy in often repetitive behaviours, and do not suddenly appear during the second year of life. This is consistent with the idea that tool use is a much more continuous development than has previously been supposed, and consistent with tool use being exploratory behaviour involving the detection of affordances and similar to direct manipulation in younger infants. Tool use in infants in their second year is embodied and based on actions that have been practised in the first year.

The Lockman, Steenbergen, and Van Roon studies are indicative of the type of research that is ongoing in motor development. They are not simply examining ages and stages of children's achievements, but looking at both how the child performs the task and what causal factors are involved. Invariably the answer to the last question includes explanations from a framework involving sensory–perceptual development as well as the development of motor control within a child–environmental–task context.

CONSTRUCTIONAL SKILLS

Developmental scales usually include tasks in which children must handle objects and materials in various ways to build or construct something. Children at 36 months can build a block tower that is 9 or 10 blocks high and at 3 years and 6 months can use three blocks to build a bridge (Knobloch and Pasamanick 1974). Children at age 5 can do a more delicate bridge-building task, by placing a Cuisenaire rod across two upright Cuisenaire rods, which are narrow and not very stable (Keogh 1968). Construction tasks of this type are self-paced and often require some dexterity in holding and manipulating the objects and materials to put them in place. The release of objects becomes important in more delicate tasks, such as using blocks or Cuisenaire rods to build towers or bridges.

Tools are involved in many construction activities. A tool must be held correctly, and a particular spatial relationship must be maintained between the tool and an object. Children can use some toy tools by 24 months, and tools are included in instructional activities in the early school years. No formal testing of these skills is usually reported, except as single items or anecdotal reports. Tool use is often a unimanual skill, although the other hand is sometimes used to hold or support the object or material. If the tool is used to create force, a power grip is used and the arm linkage system generates the necessary force while controlling the movement. A series of somewhat continuous strokes is usually needed, as when sawing or pounding. Errors in each stroke may create progressively greater correction problems for later strokes in the series. The force used when sawing must be enough but not too much, or the saw will bind in relation to the material. Screwdrivers and wrenches are somewhat different in that they must be held in a proper relationship to the object being turned, and the turning movements are often discrete but are repeated rapidly. Construction tools require considerable accuracy in the arm linkage system's overall control of movements. Digital dexterity is needed only when using minimal force to make delicate adjustments and when using scissors and similar tools that require dexterity to control their moving parts.

For tool use and construction skills, learning to coordinate load and grip forces is a crucial developmental progression. Forssberg et al (1992) found that very young children mainly use a feedback strategy with a sequential rise in grip and load forces and a stepwise increase of load force, but from 2 years of age onwards the grip and load forces start to occur in parallel. The early large grip forces may occur to keep a safety margin for such activities as carrying cups and plates to lay a table. Gordon et al (1992) showed that children from 2 years and 6 months could scale load and grip forces according to a change in size of an object and between 3 and 7 years of age started to do this as well as adults. When perturbations occur in lifting objects, 2-year-olds respond with an increase in grip force, and this steadily improves but is not mature until 10 years of age (Eliasson et al 1995).

WRITING AND DRAWING

Perhaps the most common tool uses are in writing and drawing, which involve holding an instrument to make marks on paper or similar material. The task is unimanual and requires considerable dexterity. The movements are often repetitive initially, as when scribbling or colouring, but eventually become more continuous in drawing figures or writing words. In a recent review of handwriting, Feder and Majnemer (2007) noted the continued importance of handwriting despite the rise in other written communication modes, as provided by various forms of information technology. It is essential for success at school, with poor handwriting hindering higher-order abilities such as spelling and story composition; it is important for self-esteem and many everyday life skills still require legible and often rapid handwriting. In secondary schools a child who cannot write legibly and quickly is at a disadvantage in tasks such as recording actions to perform, taking down homework, and writing examinations, and lower marks are often given to those with poor handwriting despite similar context to those who write well.

Lines and figures

Children at 24 to 30 months can make vertical and horizontal lines that go in the appropriate direction but are quite variable in quality, and circles by 3 years of age (Griffiths 1954, Knobloch and Pasamanick 1974, Beery and Butenika 1967). The order of difficulty tends to be that curved lines can be drawn before up-and-down lines, which come before horizontal or back-and-forth lines. Children first draw lines haphazardly and do not copy the lines shown to them, whereas schoolchildren can draw letters, which requires considerable digital dexterity. A pencil or pen is first used with arm movements, whereas letters are written more precisely with movements of the digits and wrist; the manual control of a pencil is reasonably good by the early school years, when children can trace a pathway of one eighth of an inch (Keogh 1968).

Copying simple figures is a standard test item in most developmental scales and intelligence tests for young children. The general progression, with the approximate age expectancy in parentheses, is first to draw a circle (36mo), a cross (48mo), a square (54mo), a triangle (60mo), and then a diamond (72mo) (Knobloch and Pasamanick 1974, Beery and Butenika 1967). Infants at 12 months can distinguish squares, triangles, and circles and by age 2 can fit them into form boards (Maccoby and Bee 1965). Children can make separate lines to draw these figures (Connolly 1968) and can use matchsticks to construct them (Landmark 1962, Wedell 1964) before they can draw them. The use of matchsticks is interesting because children begin with one matchstick and shift the position of the second until it is in place. The matchstick can be moved and checked again and again. Drawing with a pencil does not offer the opportunity to change line relationships except by erasing. The problem seems to be translating from perception into representation and not controlling the basic directional movements. Feder and Majnemer (2005) note that handwriting develops rapidly in 6 and 7-year-olds and then slows down but starts to become more automatic by ages 8 and 9, when it is used to develop the child's ideas rather than being an end in itself.

Speed and legibility are the two most important measurable elements in handwriting and are influenced by other qualities such as spacing, slant, size, posture, and grip. Speed is required in most schools and can be varied by the child according to task demands and context, and legibility is always a required quality whether by the child or another person reading the work. Speed develops almost linearly in primary school but also continues after the age of 11. A test of speed of handwriting, the DASH, is a welcome addition to measure this ability (Barnett et al 2007).

Feder and Majnemer (2005) break down the skill of handwriting into several intrinsic components, which include fine motor control, in-hand manipulation, bilateral integration, motor planning, visual motor integration, and sustained attention. They also note that extrinsic factors, which are environmental or biomechanical, also have an effect. These include sitting position and posture, height and angle of desk and chair, and type of paper used and how it is placed on the table. A further influencing factor is the type and length of instruction used, with much variation in these two factors being present.

Whenever drawing and writing are taking place, there is a strong sensory–perceptual process influencing the final outcome. In Box 5.5 there is a closer look at one such study.

Various ways of examining line drawing and copying have been used in assessment instruments. For example, in the Movement Assessment Battery for Children (Henderson et al 2007), there are clear progressions in the age range from 3 to 6 years on a tracing task that involves staying between two lines that outline a figure, with the error count at the 50th centile reducing from six to zero between these two ages. The Beery Test of Visual Motor Integration (Beery and Butenika 1967) is a standard instrument for examining some of the underlying processes involved in handwriting. Developmental improvement on instruments such as these will be a function of the increasing coordination skills of the children together with the refinement of sensory–perceptual abilities, which accurately specify the context and monitor the ongoing movements.

Grips

Grips have been described with respect to activities such as using a spoon, and another common use of grips is with pencils, pens, and paintbrushes. Children at 16 to 18 months can hold a pencil or crayon and by age 4 have a large repertoire of holding grips. Changes in holding a pencil to draw were described by Saida and Miyashita (1979), who distinguished the four grip styles shown in Figure 5.7. A power grip of some form was the first style, as expected, in which the pencil was held across the palm and the arm linkage system was used to make the drawing movements. That is, the hand held the pencil, and the arm was used to move the pencil. Neither the elbow nor the wrist was in contact with the paper. The children then changed to a tripod grip with three styles noted.

The tripod grip is holding the pencil by the thumb, index finger, and middle finger. The tripod grip in any style is a precision grip that enables control of the pencil's movements by digital manipulation and wrist movements rather than arm movements. The first version of the tripod grip, in which the pencil is often held between two fingers rather than between the thumb and the index finger, is called an incomplete tripod. It has many variations but does not fully meet the requirements of a tripod grip. The second version is a proper tripod grip without digital movements; here wrist movements do not include the concurrent use of digital movements. This version is labelled a tripod posture because the tripod grip is used to hold but not to move the pencil. The third version is the dynamic tripod with tripod grip and digital manipulation of the pencil.

The dynamic tripod grip marks the achievement of pencil control by the hand without using the arm linkage system to move the pencil. The Japanese children observed by Saida and Miyashita achieved a dynamic tripod grip at age 4. English children also achieved this landmark in manual control at age 4, but several months

---

Box 5.5 A closer examination

Visuomotor representations and line drawing: Contreras-Vidal et al (2005)

Contreras-Vidal et al (2005), when studying visuomotor representations in hand movements of children as they were drawing, asked the questions of how visuomotor representations of children change with age and how children adapt when the visual feedback is distorted.

Three groups of males and females aged 4, 6, and 8 years were asked to draw a line on a digitizing tablet by looking at an image on a computer screen. Direct vision of the arm and hand was prevented with only the image on the screen being visible. The children started from a point on the screen and drew a line to four different and randomized targets located at 45, 135, 235, and 325 degrees. The instructions were to move as fast and as straight as possible. The experimental session involved three procedures: first with normal visual feedback with the pen tip movement shown on the screen in real time (20 trials pre-exposure); second, with the pen's movement shown with a 45 degree rotation (60 trials during exposure); third, the last 20 trials, under the normal visual feedback conditions in real time and space (post exposure).

In the pre-exposure trials the older children produced lines that were smoother, straighter, and performed faster than the younger children. During the exposure trials all children decreased their error scores in planning and execution, indicating that they could use the visual feedback to improve over trials. After the exposure only the older group of 8-year-olds were able to keep the gains made under the exposure trials to use during the post-exposure stage, with the authors suggesting that only this group had effectively learned an internal model of the distorted environment. This led to speculation that the younger groups relied on broader, less acute models of internal representations and that this development had yet to be honed through visuomotor experience.

The development of line drawing and other such abilities in young children relies upon a number of characteristics. Contreras-Vidal et al (2005) suggest poorer performance of younger children is probably due to a combination of poorly developed visuomotor representations and an inadequate model of internal limb dynamics. The interaction of these variables produces the final movement product and again the complexity and nature of the task would appear to be a strong influence on performance, with factors such as combinations of eye, hand, and trunk, complexity of movement, as indicated by the number of degrees of freedom, and target location all playing an important role.

---

later than the Japanese children did (Rosenbloom and Horton 1971). Japanese females were approximately 6 months ahead of Japanese males. Many variations of a tripod grip are possible, such as holding the pencil against the first knuckles of the index and middle finger rather than the fingertips. Some variations offer a wider range of motion than others, but the important consideration is that these variations enable intrinsic hand movements rather than arm movements to control writing or drawing tools.

Another analysis of holding grips was made by Connolly and Elliott (1972), who observed 3- and 4-year-old children using a paintbrush. The children were standing and using a brush to paint on paper attached to an upright easel. The paint brushes were 30cm long and 1cm in diameter. The larger size of the brush and drawing in a vertical plane make this task somewhat different from using a pencil to write on a horizontal desk top. The findings for using a paintbrush are similar to those for using a pencil. The children used a tripod grip 75% of the time but

used arm movements to control the brush's movements. Only 12% of the movements with the paintbrush were made with the wrist and digital movements in a dynamic tripod grip. It may be that the children by using arm movements were freezing the wrist and digits in order to make the difficult and unusual posture a little easier.

The grips observed by Connolly and Elliott are presented in Figure 5.8. The adult digital grip was noted in 75% of the observations with only the adult digital and transverse digital grips being precision grips. The others are power grips in which the paintbrush is fixed in the hand so that arm movements are needed to control its movements. The oblique and transverse palmar grips are more obviously power grips because the paintbrush rests across the palm. The ventral, ventral-clenched, and adult-clenched grips do not rest in the palm, but the digits are clenched or fixed in a manner that precludes intrinsic hand movements. The thumb in these three grips is in pseudo-opposition, although closer to being in opposition for the adult clenched grip.

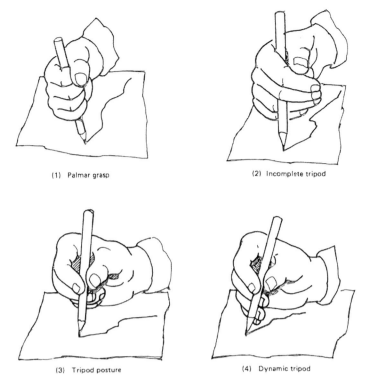

(1) Palmar grasp (2) Incomplete tripod

(3) Tripod posture (4) Dynamic tripod

Fig. 5.7 Grip variations leading to dynamic tripod grip. Drawn to represent grip variations observed by Saida and Miyashita (1979). Reproduced with permission from the publisher from Saida and Miyashita (1979).

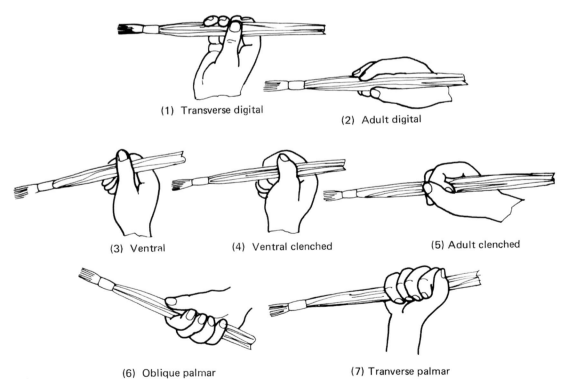

(1) Transverse digital

(2) Adult digital

(3) Ventral

(4) Ventral clenched

(5) Adult clenched

(6) Oblique palmar

(7) Tranverse palmar

Fig. 5.8 Grip variations of 3- and 4-year-old children when painting on an upright easel. Reproduced with permission from the publisher from Connolly and Elliott (1972).

Connolly and Elliott's observations (refined by Moss and Hogg 1981) display a variety of anatomical configurations, but the function of the grip for power and precision may be a more important distinction than the anatomical configuration. That is, the power and precision distinction may tell us more about the nature of manual control than a description of different anatomical configurations of grips.

Rosengren and Braswell (2003) describe the well-known changes in children's grips as noted above but challenge the seemingly underlying assumptions that, first, the development of these is maturationally determined and, second, there is a stable progression of grip configuration through to more complex and efficient ones. They propose that variability within and across children is more characteristic than stability and this variability is an important driver in developmental change. Their approach is based on constraints of environment/organism and task, again using the model of Newell (1986), and they show how each of these constraints is related to variability in grip configuration. For example, organismic constraints would include the biomechanics of the fingers, arm, and hand as well as cognitive factors such as the development of abstract concepts, and the latter of these two would be influenced by the wider context of culture. They report on their own work on the effect of task constraints on stability of grips, noting that children actually changed grips on average 12 times during a 10-minute drawing session. Their results from this and other studies lead them to conclude that grip configuration is not as stable as previously thought, and task and drawing implement are factors that contribute to producing variability. They conclude by proposing that the constraints are interactive, with cognitive constraints driving one part of a drawing or writing and biomechanical constraints influencing another, and one often overriding the other, illustrating the complex ways in which the constraints interact in a dynamic manner to produce the final result. Often the problem is planning and organization, not executing the movements, and Rosengren and Braswell (2003) propose that cognitive constraints have an impact on shape drawing, which in turn may be influenced by culture and practice, and moderated by other constraints such as morphology of the fingers, hand, and arm linkage. One could also add that perceptual factors such as visual information and how it is used are also determining factors in the progressive development of these skills.

Reaching and Grasping

Reaching and grasping, skills we perform every day without thinking, involve specifying the location of the object followed by the act itself. The act of reaching and grasping demands skilled perception–action linkages with the object location, size, texture, and rigidity all having to be anticipated a priori from visual information. The single act of reaching and grasping contains two motor components, that of spatial positioning of the arm, involving the proximal muscles of the shoulder and elbow joints, and the pre-shaping of the fingers to the size and shape of the object, involving more distal muscles. For efficient prehension these two components must be precisely coordinated. It is the linking of the visual–perceptual information to the context of the to-be-reached object that provides the information for the motor act.

By the age of 2 years children have developed reasonably effective reach and grasp actions but there is still some way to go before a mature state is reached (Konczak and Dichgans 1997). A number of variables involved in reaching and grasping were examined in a series of papers by Kuhtz-Buschbeck et al (1996, 1998a,b), with the data overlapping between this chapter and the next one and more detail provided in Box 6.1 in the following chapter. Kuhtz-Buschbeck et al (1998a) used kinematic analysis to examine reaching and grasping in children aged 4 to 12 years of age with the experimental procedure and setup scaled to the body size of the individuals. The movement duration did not change significantly with age, and peak spatial velocity remained relatively similar. However, the coordination between reaching and grasping improved by 12 years of age, with the younger children opening their hand wider than the older ones, providing a larger safety margin, and also appearing to rely more on vision during the movement, as only the older children could accurately scale the hand opening to the size of the object when vision of the movement was absent. The youngest children often missed the target, with the authors suggesting that these two groups were unable to maintain a mental image of the target location, rather than blaming erroneous proprioception of the hand position in space.

Figure 5.9 shows the kinematic profiles of prehension in three children aged 4, 7, and 12, with hand velocity plotted against grip aperture on repeated prehension trials. The distinctive feature of these three profiles is the decreasing variability over trials with age, showing that by age 12 the performance is more automated.

In the second article, Kuhtz-Buschbeck et al (1998b) compared 6- and 7-year-olds to adults under different experimental conditions of reaching and grasping involving distance, size of target, and visual feedback during the movement. Similar results were obtained with the finding that mature grip formation is not complete in 6- or 7-year-olds and they rely more on visual feedback than adults do in the act of reaching and grasping. Again, as in the first study (Kuhtz-Buschbeck et al 1998a), intra-individual variability was very much higher in the children.

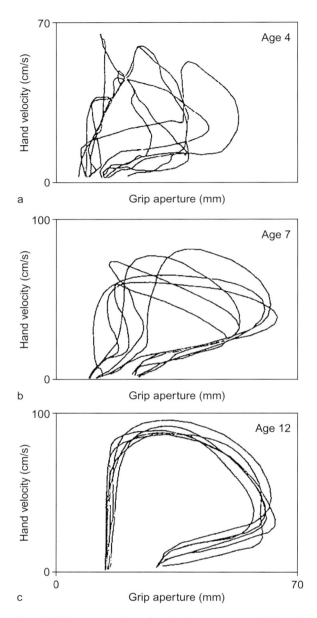

Fig. 5.9 Kinematic profiles of prehension at the ages of 4, 7, and 12 years. The hand velocity is plotted against the grip aperture in three children of different ages. Six trials are superimposed for each participant (visual condition). Reproduced with permission from the publisher from Kuhtz-Buschbeck et al (1998a).

The authors suggest that with repeated practice, or what they term 'perception–action cycles', errors are reduced and more consistent accuracy is achieved. This notion of practice or experience is in agreement with proposals by Adolph et al (2003), who suggest that experience is the dominant variable in the development of motor competence. (More detail of this work is presented in Box 6.1 in the following chapter.)

Body-scaled ratio has been proposed as a control parameter in the development of prehension in children, noted in Chapter 3 with the work in infants (Newell et al 1989). A similar finding was reported by van der Kamp et al (1998) in reaching and grasping in 5- to 9-year-old children. Their work involved children aged 5, 7, and 9 years who were required to grasp and lift 14 cubes of different sizes. They found that at all ages the shift from a one-handed to a two-handed grasp occurred at the same body-scaled ratio between cube size and finger span. This replicated Newell et al (1989) and gives support to the proposition that perceiving and acting are guided by body-scaled ratios and these are invariant over development with differences in body sizes. This body-scaled ratio of hand size and object size appears to be a control parameter for switches in prehensile action.

In different tasks, the importance of vision during reaching and grasping appears to change during the developmental period. In some instances, it can be argued that this importance decreases because the action becomes more automated. However, this may depend on the task to be accomplished. Smyth et al (2004a,b) when testing children aged 5 to 10 years of age and adults found that all participants were able to use visual information about the size of the target to form and scale grip opening. However, when vision of the hand was removed, this had little effect on the younger children (5–6-year-olds), whereas it did have an effect on the older ones and the adults, who were faster with vision of the hand and increased maximum grip aperture when vision of the hand was removed. This suggests that, although younger children are using vision, they are not fully utilizing all the advantages it provides in different contextual situations. By 10 years of age this has improved considerably but is not yet at the level of adults. When examining the use of vision in children, it seems to be dependent upon not only the resources of the child but the kinds of task contexts and movement problems that the child is being asked to solve. As a task becomes more demanding, complex, and difficult, the use of vision changes and the developing child will show progressions in response to these demands.

BIMANUAL CONTROL

Most of the time we use both hands, often asymmetrically, in our activities of daily living such as drawing, using a ruler, taking the top off a jar, and using a knife and fork, with both hands working together in time and space. Steenbergen et al (2003) use the concept of constraints to examine these movements, with space and time being the more obvious ones and most actions including both. They give the example of using a knife and fork and how the two implements in different hands have to be coordinated in space and time and the manner in which this is done, particularly when they start at different points and different distances away and yet have to meet to complete the task.

In line with our view on intrinsic and extrinsic constraints, the development of bimanual coordination is influenced by the intrinsic neural constraint of interhemispheric cooperation and inhibition. It is notable that the corpus callosum, the major bundle of fibres connecting the two hemispheres, is late in completing myelinization. Generally, it is more difficult to move fingers or hands together in the same direction, that is parallel movements (both moving clockwise or both moving counter clockwise), than to move them together in the opposite direction (mirror movements). This has been demonstrated many times both with adults (Kelso et al 1979) and also with different samples of schoolchildren (Jahoda 1976). Different explanations have been proposed for this phenomenon. Fagard et al (2001), examining performance on a bimanual task in children between 3 and 10 years of age, found increasing improvement in interhemispheric coordination with age. In an earlier study Fagard (1987) showed that, when children were asked to rotate with the same velocity, better performance was obtained with mirror than with parallel movements, and this difference decreased with age until at 9 years of age they were equally competent in both movements. The maturation of the corpus callosum does seem to be a development that is important to bimanual coordination because, in order to perform a bimanual movement with parallel movements, the children must inhibit mirror movements and resisting the attraction to in-phase movements is related to interhemispheric connections (Steenbergen et al 2003).

Robertson (2001) examined groups of individuals in an age range from 4 to adulthood, performing unimanual and bimanual continuous circle drawing to investigate natural development of bimanual control in young children. She found that in the bimanual tasks 4- to 7-year-olds produced larger circles with longer movement durations than the older groups; that the 4- to 7-year-olds had higher variability; and stability increased with age. The causes of the instability in the younger children she proposed were the variables of the attention of the person and the speed demands of the task. She also concluded that the switching of in-phase and antiphase transition in the bimanual task was consistent with a dynamical systems view.

An important type of bimanual control is the functional asymmetry noted by de Schonen (1977), in which the two hands make different movements in a coordinated and complementary manner. While one hand holds a piece of fruit, the other controls a knife to peel or cut it. Adults have a stable lateralization in this type of manipulation, as when one hand is used to hold a box of matches and the other strikes the match (Annett 1976). Additionally, the pattern of hand use is similar across adults, with more than 80% using the same hand for the same function. Children at ages 4 and 5 have established some stability in their lateralization of functional asymmetry, both across tasks and for individuals (Auzias 1975).

Some bimanual tasks may vary as to which hand performs which function, and it is not unusual for the left hand of an otherwise right-handed person to control the more precise aspect of the task. This occurs in dealing cards, in which the left hand slides one card forward on the top of the deck and the right hand grasps the card in a fixed digital position, with arm and wrist action used to distribute it. One can demonstrate this by reversing the hands in dealing cards: note that the main problem is sliding a single card forward out of the deck. Grasping and distributing the card generally can be done with either hand.

An interesting type of functional asymmetry is tying shoelaces, because the laces are soft, flexible objects that do not offer an externally consistent source of reference (de Schonen 1977). In tasks such as this, both hands must adjust continuously in relation to the other hand's position and movements, whereas many manipulative tasks involve objects or tools that provide some regulator or reference information. As an example, scissors are fixed to some extent in the range and direction of their movement, and their firmness is a constant. De Schonen (1977) notes that, although apes can do many of the manipulative tasks that humans can and have been taught to untie laces, they have not learned to tie them. Untying provides some constant locations and pressures of materials, whereas tying is a much more open problem in the relationships between the two hands. Young children also have difficulty tying soft laces. They seem to lack some of the manipulative control needed in the hand's intrinsic movements, as well as the spatial and perceptual organization needed to coordinate the changes in hand position.

A classic study by Elliott and Connolly (1974) in Box 5.6 offers some interesting analyses of the development of manual control before they present their study of bimanual coordination to observe movement sequences to analyse how children solve a movement problem.

GENERAL COMMENTS

The anatomy of our hands limits what we can do but does not totally define their functions. Many anatomical configurations can be used to produce movements that will differ somewhat, yet will have the same functional effect, and environmental circumstances will determine to some extent what we need to do and will do. Movement,

Box 5.6 A closer examination

Observations of bimanual control: Elliott and Connolly (1974)
A group of 24 males and 24 females (ages 3, 4, and 5) were tested on a marble board game modified into the board layouts illustrated for Tasks 1 through 6 (see Fig. 5.10). One knob tilts the board on one axis, and the other tilts the board on a second axis, arranged at a right angle to the first. Each knob can be turned right or left and separately or together in eight combinations of hand movements. For example, in Task 1 turn the right knob to the right, and the board will tilt in that direction to move the marble in direction R. Starting again with the marble in your corner, move it in direction L by turning the left knob to the left. To get the marble to move from the far corner in the diagonal direction you must simultaneously turn the right knob to the right and the left knob to the left.

The eight hand movements can be divided into four *separate movements* and four *simultaneous movements*. The separate movements are merely the movement of the right knob to the right or left and the left knob to the right or left. The four simultaneous movements are the two opposite or mirror movements of both hands turning out or turning in and the two movements in the same direction with both hands turning right or both turning left. A series of movements can be made by combining hand movements into a movement sequence.

The board can be modified to create different movement problems, ranging from the open board in Task 1 to the pathways to be followed in Task 6. The movement problem can also be changed by placing the marble in a different location. Task 6 has railings to mark a square path with holes at each corner. Successive movements must be made and timed to avoid the corner holes. The complete movement sequence is 'right knob right, left knob left, right knob left, left knob right.' Task 6 requires precise control of knob movements to keep the marble from rolling too fast, as well as making movement changes from one knob to the other at the appropriate time.

Older children used simultaneous movements more often than younger children did when exploring the open board in Task 1 and in doing the diagonal marble roll in Tasks 2 and 3. Older children were better able to use a simultaneous (bimanual) movement, whereas younger children turned the knobs separately as successive (unimanual) movements. Opposite direction or mirror movements were easier for children of all ages, just as such movements were easier for both children and adults in turning handles in the Jahoda (1976) study. This can be seen in comparing Tasks 2 and 3. A simultaneous movement is needed in both tasks, but the hand movements are mirrored (both turn out) in Task 2 and are in the same direction (both turn left) in Task 3. More children did Task 2 with simultaneous movements, whereas many children did Task 3 with successive movements to roll the marble to a near corner before rolling it to the opposite corner (for example, the right knob turned left and then the left knob turned left).

Task 6 was very difficult, as expected, because the task requires continuous movements and cannot be done successfully with discrete movements, whether successive or simultaneous. Children must anticipate when to make the next hand movement, and if they do not complete the movement in time, the marble will fall in the hole rather than turn at the corner. Older children, as expected, were better able to anticipate and time the change in movements.

like language, is generative with the same outcome being produced in different ways according to the internal and external constraints that are present. Children in some societies do not need to use writing or drawing instruments, but if they do, many grip variations that provide a satisfactory outcome are possible, with digital grips being better suited to precision outcomes. Detailed observations and analyses of grips according to anatomical configurations will show how children handle an object, but our observations and analyses will be incomplete without analysing what is to be accomplished, which involves information about the task and the environmental array for

which sensory–perceptual information is vital and plays a major part in change with development.

A second point is that children develop *rules* and *strategies* in making movements and the movements then must be selected for the effect desired. *Movements cannot be made without being aware of the consequences.* In order to do this the child has to show competence in prediction and anticipation, as obtained through visual–perceptual information. Thus the development of rules and strategies is strongly influenced by visual–perceptual information and how the child uses this information to plan the movements. Movement strategy is demonstrated

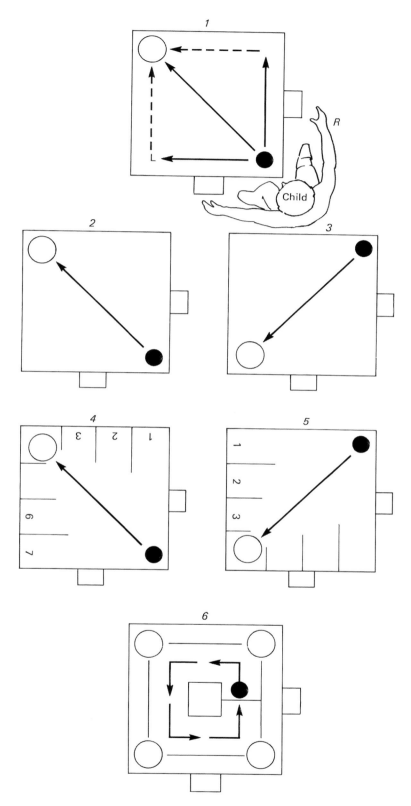

Fig. 5.10 Marble board layout. Reproduced with permission from Elliott and Connolly (1974).

in an analysis of Task 6 of the Elliott and Connolly study (1974), which requires accurately anticipating when to execute the next hand movement. If not done in time, the marble will fall into the hole. If done too soon the marble will hit the railing and not go around the corner. Older children, as expected, were better able to time the change in movements. The movement sequence could be executed in different ways and again older children will show superiority in the range of approaches they have at their disposal. Again the combined influence of these two factors, anatomy of the hands and rules and strategies governed by perceptual and cognitive information, are good examples of intrinsic constraints in our model.

Control of limb movements

LIMB MOVEMENTS

Another way to think about the development of movement control is to study the control of all limb movements working together. The examination of the coordination of limb movements brings together the two previous sections on body and manual control. Arm and leg movements are used to move the body and control objects, given that the control of the trunk and head help in postural control. The focus is on the general accuracy of control and not on speed and force, and improved control of limb movements is another indicator of the development of movement control. This general line of thinking was used in organizing a project to study the control of limb movements of children, ages 5 through 9, and is shown in Box 5.7 below (Keogh 1968, 1969). The main focus of Keogh's (1969) work was on control rather than speed and force so that children could work at their own pace without the need for fast or forceful movements.

The explanation of sex differences in the development of limb movement control may be that females are biologically more mature than males. Females reach puberty earlier and are more advanced in skeletal development and other indicators of biological maturity. Another possibility is that these movements are culturally influenced and that females are more likely to practise them. This might be true for children several years older; whether it is true for females younger than age 5 is open to debate. Females are generally able to hop sooner than males, which supports the findings from the wider range of limb movement tasks. This is despite the fact that hopping is a gross body movement that is often claimed to be something males do better.

It is important to note that the differences among age–sex groups remained similar from the first to the second testing. Individuals maintained like positions within their age groups, as indicated by correlations of approximately 0.8 within age–sex groups. That is, the

group means increased from the first to the second test session, but the high correlations indicate that high scorers on the first day were again high scorers on the second day and that low scorers remained low scorers, although their scores did increase. Sex differences remained in the second testing, in that both males and females increased by a similar amount.

Movement errors

Observations of children's movement errors are a useful way to study movement problems to be resolved. A good time to observe movement development is when children can first approximate the movement so that we can observe their efforts to solve the movement problem. Children at this time are not often successful, according to test criteria, but they make movements that can be analysed in relation to the desired outcome. This allows us to analyse what Bruner (1970) calls the morphology of failure or what a person does when not quite able to perform a task.

In the Keogh study (1969) the examiners commented on unusual and interesting movements, whether unsuccessful or successful, and how children made a movement successfully but in a less elegant fashion. An important observation is that, whereas some children seem to know that an error has been made, often indicated by comments or stopping to start over, other children do not seem to recognize movement errors and keep moving until an examiner says 'OK' or they stop because they think they did it correctly.

An effort was made to identify problems in performing the 2–2 hop by looking at the types of errors made and modifying the task to determine which parts of the task could be done (Keogh 1970). A total of 106 males were tested within 3 months of their seventh birthday (at two different times, generally 2 days apart) on the 2–2 hop. Only 21% of the males did the 2–2 hop on the first day. Another 15% were successful on the second day, which is also consistent with other findings and indicates that some males merely need some practice. A third group of 22 males (21%) did the 2–2 hop on the second day, but only when holding the back of a chair for support. The remaining 46 males (43%) did not successfully do the 2–2 hop, even though given additional practice and support trials on the second day.

Overall, the females were much better than the males, to the extent of being about 1 year in advance. For example, 46% of the 6-year-old females could do the 2–2 hop, which is the approximate percentage for the 7-year-old males.

Limb movements must be coordinated into a correct sequence with an appropriate temporal or phasing

Box 5.7 A closer examination

Study of limb movements: Keogh (1968, 1969)

Two technical reports (Keogh 1968, 1969) analyse individual test items used to measure the control of limb movements. A framework was formulated for a variety of limb movement tasks and is outlined in Table 5.5, with the tasks listed as representing the limbs and body position used when performing them. Limb movements were selected to be repetitive, continuous, and self-paced, not made in relation to external temporal–spatial requirements and not requiring strength or stamina. These criteria eliminated tasks such as tapping for speed or in synchrony with an external beat, movement of hands and body to stay in target areas, and imitations of movements or gestures. The 1968 report explored many test items to learn how well and in what ways children controlled their limb movements. A group of 300 children (ages 5 through 9) from a school district in the Los Angeles area was tested in the 1968 test programme. Another 270 children (ages 5 through 7) from a different school district in the Los Angeles area were tested in the 1969 test programme. The data summarized in Figure 5.11 are for 450 children from the two school districts and cover only ages 5, 6, and 7. The children were within 3 months of their mid-year birthday.

More than 80 separate test items were initially used to find a suitable set of movements to observe the control of limb movements. The limb movements for arms and hands included touching each finger separately with the thumb of the same hand, opening and closing the hands together and alternately, and clapping the hands and slapping them on the thighs at the same time and alternately. Tapping tasks were used, with children holding a pencil and tapping the edge of a desk and tapping their toes with their heels on the ground. Tapping was done with a single limb and in several combinations of hands and feet together and alternately. The children hopped in place and moved forward and also skipped. They made stride jumps to move their feet out and back as if doing a jumping jack and then added arm movements to do a jumping jack. Another form of stride jump was to start with one foot forward and the other foot back and then change foot positions while staying in place. Each movement was carried out for five cycles, such as tapping five cycles of once with the right and once with the left.

An important outcome of this study was the observation of movement errors collected as part of the performance record for each child on each test item. These observation notes commented on the nature of movement problems in controlling limb movements. Children from age 5 through 7 greatly improved their control of these limb movements, and females were quantitatively and qualitatively better than males. Performance data for 18 test items are summarized in Table 5.6 and Figure 5.11 to show these performance changes.

TABLE 5.5
Limb movement framework

Limb(s)	Body position		
	Seated	Standing	Travelling
Arm–hand	Finger touch		
	Hands open–close		
	Hands clap		
Leg	Feet tap	Hop in place	Hop forward
		Stride jump: legs	Skip
Arm–leg	Feet–pencil tap	Stride jump: arms–legs	Walk–clap

Age and sex differences are clearly seen in Figure 5.11. Both males and females improved markedly from year to year with the females' mean performance approximately 1 year better than that of the males'. The females were also qualitatively better than the males, as noted in the examiners' observations. The females did not look at their movements very much, whereas the males often looked at their movements, as if needing to see what they were doing and to think about the order of their movements. The females generally were softer in their movements, whereas some of the males splintered their pencils when tapping, slapped their hands when clapping, and pounded the ground when hopping. The males more often jumped too far out in the jumping jack and then jumped their feet back together to collide in midair and upset themselves. The females maintained an easier and quicker rhythm in their movements, and the males made more discrete and halting movements.

TABLE 5.6
Passing percentages and total mean scores for 18 limb movement tasks

Task	Pattern	Boys			Girls		
		Age 5	6	7	Age 5	6	7
Open-close hands	Separate	29	56	71	37	74	79
	Together	22	47	78	43	62	83
Clap-slap hands/thigh	2–1	38	73	86	70	90	91
	R/L	39	63	81	66	90	91
Feet tap	2–2	45	73	79	55	79	94
Tap pencil and foot	Right	46	78	90	59	86	93
	Left	57	67	83	46	77	84
	1–1	24	56	75	47	77	71
	2–2	3	5	14	14	18	34
Hop in place	Right	83	97	100	97	97	100
	Left	80	97	99	91	99	100
	2–2	3	10	48	16	45	69
Stride jumps	Out-back	34	77	86	75	92	94
	Jumping jacks	8	42	62	30	55	97
	Forward-back	17	40	70	74	86	94
Skip		61	88	89	86	91	98
Jump-clap	One	83	96	97	88	97	99
	Two	29	78	97	30	71	84
Total points	N	76	73	77	76	78	70
	Mean	11.5	20.2	25.0	18.0	25.4	28.6
	SD	5.4	6.4	6.0	7.0	6.4	5.5

Source: Keogh (1968, 1969)

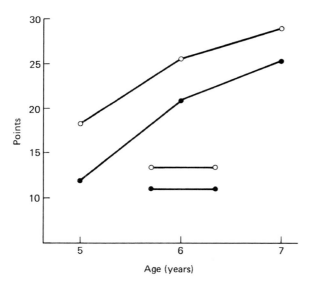

Fig. 5.11 Mean scores for males and females for selected limb movement test items (Keogh 1968, 1969).

relationship. Children can sometimes initiate the appropriate movement sequence but cannot maintain the sequence beyond two or three cycles, with all of their resources seemingly being needed in this first approximation of the task. Their movements tend to be discrete rather than continuous, and the children often look at the task as if they are consciously trying to organize each part of the sequence. They may be unable to maintain the movement sequence beyond two or three cycles because they 'lose time' with each repetition and eventually do not have enough time to execute the next movement in the sequence. The movement sequences need to be organized and executed as a larger movement unit rather than as a series of discrete movements.

The amount of force must be appropriate, as excessive force creates additional movement problems. Too much force in one part of a movement requires a sizable correction in the next part of the movement, which

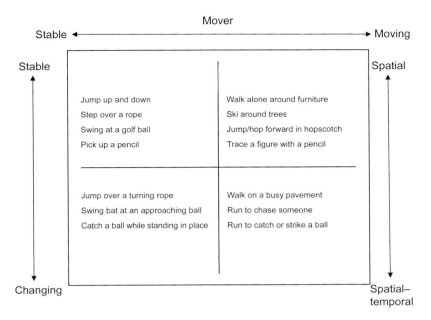

Fig. 5.12 Movement situations in relation to mover–environment conditions and spatial–temporal requirements (Keogh and Sugden 1985).

eventually leads to disruption or failure. Too much force may also create problems in postural control, and the problem initially may be how force can be inhibited either partially or totally. Inhibition in this sense may be the fundamental problem in movement development. Inhibition may be difficult to achieve in early development and may be the key to the early development of movement control, but much of this will be context dependent with variations seen across tasks and environments.

Summary

The manner in which we study developmental progressions has changed from classic studies, giving us rare detail and descriptions of this development. With technological advances we have been able to study the biomechanics of these actions, providing even more detail about the movement components and mechanics. We are now in a position where these detailed changes are being supplemented by explanations from theoretical positions mined from studies involving variables such as body-scaled parameters, perception–action sequences, development of visual control, and the role of experience.

Young children develop good control of self-movements and have a large repertoire of movement skills by the time they finish the early school years. By age 7 they can perform most fundamental motor skills in some manner; the children may not be elegant or able to use these skills effectively in changing environmental conditions, but the basic fundamentals are there. During the period between 2 and 7 years of age, children's movements become more continuous and appear to be easier and smoother. They make fewer extraneous movements and go through a fuller range of motions. Their movements are more consistent, efficient, and effective. Simple observations of changes in walking, running, and many manipulation movements illustrate these general descriptions of change, as do the analyses of many movement skills. Young children also become able to do more things simultaneously and achieve intended outcomes in many different ways. Sex differences begin to be noticed in both the quantity and quality of achievement.

To illustrate how far children have progressed in their motor development, Figure 5.12 is used as a guide both here and in the next chapter. The interplay of mover and environmental conditions creates spatial and temporal requirements, with both being either stable or changing. If the mover remains stable by not moving into the environment, there will be fewer external requirements for spatial–temporal accuracy than when moving into the environment. The conditions of stable and moving are not separate but are on a continuum from stable to moving into the environment. The same is true for environmental conditions and spatial–temporal requirements, each of which forms a continuum, as shown in Figure 5.12. These ideas were originally from Gentile et al (1975) and have since been elaborated.

The examples in the upper left-hand corner of Figure 5.12 are movement situations in which the mover remains in place and objects and other people in the environment are stable unless acted upon by the same mover. Jumping up and down, stepping over a rope, and swinging at a golf ball keep the body in the same location without any need to adjust to the moving of objects and other persons. By 6 or 7 years of age children are quite competent in many of these skills, although, as shown in studies on reaching and grasping, for example, they are still quite variable in their responses over repeated trials.

Keeping the environment stable and having the mover move into it are more *open* movement situations and, as shown in the upper right-hand corner of Figure 5.12, the mover creates additional spatial–temporal requirements by moving. For example, walking alone through a room or with other people standing still requires navigation around a series of obstacles. There are more spatial–temporal requirements than when walking in an empty room, but the increase is not sizeable unless the task requires a high level of movement speed and accuracy, such as when skiing fast downhill around trees, which demands making rapid adjustments to avoid obstacles in the environment. From 2 to 6 or 7 years of age children improve considerably on these types of tasks, but they still find difficulty in moving at speed or when a high level of accuracy is required in their response.

In the lower row of Figure 5.12, in which objects and people are moving in the environment, the mover must now move in relation to the environment's temporal requirements. Movers may remain in place to jump a turning rope, or may move into the environment to walk in a crowd of moving people, run to catch a ball, or return a tennis shot on the run. Spatial accuracy is required in each movement situation, but in addition the speed of the ball, rope, and other people determines when the mover must move. When engaging in manual control, body movements must be considered a part of the manual control movements, as they provide either a stable or a moving support structure from which the arm linkage system can function. Again children improve markedly between 2 and 6 or 7 years, but they are still at a relatively immature stage and much improvement will be seen on tasks of this type between the end of this stage and puberty. Skills such as striking a fast-approaching ball, ones that require accurate and speedy perception–action links and match, are very demanding at this age and are not performed well by the majority of children.

A stable environment requires varying degrees of spatial accuracy with few temporal requirements, unless more are created by moving faster. The mover determines the temporal requirements in self-paced movement situations. Fast movements by the mover can produce more temporal requirements, as when skiing fast downhill. A changing environment can have the same requirements for spatial accuracy as a stationary environment, but temporal accuracy is now imposed by moving objects and other persons. The mover can also influence the context by changing movements, causing others to modify their actions. The mover, through experience and the development of intrinsic constraints, improves the perception–action match, leading to more competent movement outcomes. As the tasks become more complex and/or difficult, the variety of experiences the mover engages in enables them to interact appropriately with new and differing environmental demands.

Despite children at the end of this period still being far from mature in skills involving a changing environment, they have made significant improvements in a wide range of skills and abilities. For example, in this age period force control is developing, as children become more proficient at modulating and varying force production in movements. They can then make more delicate and precise movements and can adjust to task and situation requirements, such as needing to move slowly. They become more proficient at generating force more effectively by using movements to summate and transmit force, for example in throwing. They also improve their postural control to control the forces generated in movements, which has the reciprocal effect of enabling more forceful movements. This also leads to some movements becoming less difficult, as additional speed provides motion stability.

Manual control improves markedly during the preschool and early school years. Children at age 7 have a good repertoire of manual movements, including grip variations and numerous ways to combine arm and hand movements. They can form letters and are producing writing that can be read. The intrinsic movements of each hand provide dexterous control in handling objects, as when using drawing instruments. Older children can make power and precision movements with the same tool, whereas younger children are often limited to power movements. Functional asymmetry is well established in providing a wide range of collaboration between the two hands. The simultaneous release of objects is difficult for children to do, which brings our attention again to release as an important part of manual control. Some general neuroanatomical constraints may limit manual control skills, as noted in the difficulty encountered by children and adults in making bimanual movements in the same direction. Children do quite well in self-paced manual movements, but they will improve considerably over the next 10 years in movement speed and in timing their manual movements to external task requirements. Cultural skills such as handwriting are present and in most cases legible, but there is much improvement in both legibility and speed in the coming years.

We have presented much evidence to show that sensory–perceptual qualities improve during this period, such as in predicting movements in time and space, but again these are not fully developed and improvement of these attributes continues into puberty. There is also development of movement rules and movement strategies, which seem essential to the adequate development of movement control. Rules and strategies remind us that task and situation requirements, including knowledge of movement consequences with a specific task within a particular context, must be considered in the production of movement, along with the intrinsic constraints such as the neuroanatomical structures and systems.

Movers encounter difficulty when the task and situation requirements exceed their resources. Young children become 'overmatched' when they must move too rapidly and must do too much in too little time. This occurs particularly when executing a longer movement sequence, even when the movements are repetitive, and when doing several things at the same time. They also lack the resources for moving in relation to more variable conditions and the movements of objects and other persons. However, this is not only true for young children; it is a comparative statement as all movers will have difficulty when the task and environmental demands exceed the mover's resources. What we do know about this critical period of 2 to 7 years of age is that by age 7 typically developing children can accomplish relatively advanced coordination patterns in most locomotor skills and fundamental manual activities. The development seen between 2 and 7 years of age involves the acquisition of a large repertoire of movement skills, which are performed with increasing control of force and are smoother and more effective on a wide range of tasks involving both total-body and manual activities. The explanatory factors for this development are multiple, involving both intrinsic and extrinsic variables, with the amount and range of experience and practice being crucial. The child at 7 has progressed massively from the age of 2, but there is much development to come and the changes that occur from the end of this period to puberty are detailed in the next chapter.

REFERENCES

Adolph KE, Vereijken B, Shrout PE (2003) What changes in infant walking and why. *Child Dev* 74: 474–497. http://dx.doi.org/10.1111/1467-8624.7402011

Adolph KE, Robinson SR, Young JW, Gill-Alvarez F (2008) What is the shape of developmental change? *Psychol Rev* 115: 527–543. http://dx.doi.org/10.1037/0033-295X.115.3.527

Annett M (1976) A coordination of hand preference and skill. *Br J Psychol* 67: 587–592. http://dx.doi.org/10.1111/j.2044-8295.1976.tb01550.x

Assaiante C, Woollacott M, Amblard B (2000) Development of postural adjustment during gait initiation: kinematic and EMG analysis. *J Motor Behav* 32: 211–226. http://dx.doi.org/10.1080/00222890009601373

Auzias M (1975) *Enfants Gauchers, Enfants Doiters*. Paris: Delachaux et Niestle.

Barela JA, Jeka JJ, Clark JE (2003) Postural control in children: coupling to dynamic somatosensory information. *Exp Brain Res* 150: 434–442.

Barnett A, Henderson SE, Scheib B (2007) *The Detailed Assessment of Speed of Handwriting (DASH)*. London: Pearson.

Bayley N (1935) The development of motor abilities in the first three years. *Monographs of the Society for Research in Child Development* 1.

Beery K, Butenika N (1967) *Developmental Test of Visual–Motor Integration*. Chicago, IL: Follett Education Co.

Berger W (1992) Normal and impaired development of children's gait. In: Forssberg H, Hirschfield H, editors. *Movement Disorders in Children*. Medicine and Sports Science, volume 36. Basel: Karger, pp. 182–185.

Breniere Y, Bril B (1998) Development of postural control of gravity forces in children during the first 5 years of walking. *Exp Brain Res* 121: 255–262. http://dx.doi.org/10.1007/s002210050458

Bril B, Breniere Y (1992) Postural requirements and progression velocity in young walkers. *J Mot Behav* 24: 105–116. http://dx.doi.org/10.1080/00222895.1992.9941606

Bruner JS (1970) The growth and structure of skill. In: Connolly KJ, editor. *Mechanisms of Motor Skill Development*. New York: Academic Press, pp. 63–94.

Butterworth G, Hicks L (1977) Visual proprioception and postural stability in infants: a developmental study. *Perception* 6: 255–262.

Cesari P, Formenti F, Olwarto P (2003) A common perceptual parameter for stair climbing for children, young adults and adults. *Human Movement Sci* 22: 111–124. http://dx.doi.org/10.1016/S0167-9457(03)00003-4

Clark JE, Phillips SJ (1993) A longitudinal study of intralimb coordination in the first year of independent walking. *Child Dev* 64: 1143–1157. http://dx.doi.org/10.2307/1131331

Clark JE, Whitall J (1989) Changing patterns of locomotion: from walking to skipping. In: Woollacott MH, Shumway-Cook A, editors. *Development of Posture and Gait Across the Lifespan*. Columbia, SC: University of South Carolina Press, pp. 128–151.

Connolly KJ (1968) Some mechanisms involved in the development of movement control. *Aspects Educ* 7: 82–100.

Connolly KJ, Elliott J (1972) The evolution and ontogeny of hand function. In: Jones NB, editor. *Ethological Studies of Child Behaviour*. Cambridge: Cambridge University Press, pp. 329–380.

Constantini AF, Hoving KL (1973) The relationship of cognitive and motor response inhibition to age and IQ. *J Genetic Psychol* 123: 309–319. http://dx.doi.org/10.1080/00221325.1973.10532690

Constantini AF, Corsini DA, Davis JE (1973) Conceptual tempo, inhibition of movement and acceleration of movement in 4-, 7- and 9-year-old children. *Percept Motor Skills* 37: 779–784. http://dx.doi.org/10.2466/pms.1973.37.3.779

Contreras-Vidal JL, Bo J, Boudreau JP, Clark JE (2005) Development of visuomotor representations for hand movement in young children. *Exp Brain Res* 162: 155–164. http://dx.doi.org/10.1007/s00221-004-2123-7

DeOreo KL (1976) Dynamic balance in preschool children: quantifying qualitative data. *Res Q* 47: 526–531.

Dillman CJ (1975) Kinematic analysis of running. In: Wilmore JH, Keogh JF, editors. *Exercise and Sports Science Reviews, Volume 3*. New York: Academic Press, pp. 193–218.

Eliasson AC, Forssberg H, Ikuta K, Apel I, Westling G, Johansson R (1995) Development of human precision grip. V. Anticipatory and triggered grip actions during sudden loading. *Exp Brain Res* 106: 425–433.

Elliott JM, Connolly KJ (1974) Hierarchical structure in skill development. In: Connolly KJ, Bruner JS, editors. *The Growth of Competence*. London: Academic Press, pp. 135–168.

Fagard J (1987) Bimanual stereotypes: bimanual coordination in children as a function of movements and relative velocity. *J Motor Behav* 19: 355–366.

Fagard J, Hardy-Leger I, Kervella C, Marks A (2001) Changes in interhemispheric transfer rate and the development of bimanual coordination during childhood. *J Exp Psychol* 80: 1–22.

Feder KP, Majnemer A (2007) Handwriting development, competency and intervention. *Dev Med Child Neurol* 49: 312–317. http://dx.doi.org/10.1111/j.1469-8749.2007.00312.x

Forssberg H, Kinoshita H, Eliasson AC, Johansson RS, Westling G, Gordon AM (1992) Development of human precision grip. II. Anticipatory control of isometric forces targeted for object's weight. *Exp Brain Res* 90: 393–398.

Fortney GE (1983) Kinematics and kinetics in the running pattern of two-, four- and six-year-old children. *Res Q Exercise Sport* 54: 126–135.

Frankenburg WK, Dodds JB (1967) The Denver developmental screening test. *J Pediatr* 71: 181–191. http://dx.doi.org/10.1016/S0022-3476(67)80070-2

Gentile AM, Higgins JR, Miller EA, Rosen BM (1975) The structure of motor tasks. *Mouvement* 7: 11–28.

Getchell N, Roberton MA (1989) Whole body stiffness as a function of developmental level in children's hopping. *Dev Psychol* 25: 920–928. http://dx.doi.org/10.1037/0012-1649.25.6.920

Gipsman SC (1973) Control of range of movement rate in primary school children. Master's thesis, University of California, Los Angeles, CA, USA.

Gordon AM, Forssberg H, Johansson RS, Eliasson AC, Wrestling G (1992) Development of human precision grip. III. Integration of visual cues during the programming of isometric forces. *Exp Brain Res* 90: 399–403.

Griffiths R (1954) *The Abilities of Infants*. New York: McGraw-Hill.

Hamilton ML (1992) Effect of optokinetic stimulation on gait initiation in children ages four and ten. Woollacott MH, Horak F, editors. *Posture and Gait: Control Mechanisms, Volume II*. Portland, OR: University of Oregon Press, pp. 255–258.

Hellebrandt FA, Rarick GL, Glassow R, Carns ML (1961) Physiological analysis of basic motor skills: I. Growth and development of jumping. *Am J Phys Med* 40: 14–25.

Henderson SE, Sugden DA, Barnett A (2007) *Movement Assessment Battery for Children 2*. London: Pearson.

Higgins CI, Campos JJ, Kermoian R (1996) Effect of self produced locomotion on infant postural compensation to optic flow. *Dev Psychol* 32: 836–841. http://dx.doi.org/10.1037/0012-1649.32.5.836

Hirschfield H, Forssberg H (1992) Development of anticipatory adjustments during locomotion in children. *J Neurophysiol* 68: 542–550.

Jahoda G (1976) Rapidity of bilateral arm movements: a cross cultural study. *Psychologia Africana* 16: 207–214.

Jensen JL (2005) The puzzles of child development: how the study of developmental biomechanics contributes to the puzzle solutions. *Infant Child Dev* 14: 501–511. http://dx.doi.org/10.1002/icd.425

Jensen JL, Ulrich BD, Thelen E, Schneider K, Zernicke R (1994) Adaptive dynamics in the leg movement patterns of human infants: I. The effect of posture on spontaneous kicking. *J Motor Behav* 26: 366–374. http://dx.doi.org/10.1080/00222895.1994.9941686

van der Kamp J, Savelsbergh GJP, Davis WE (1998) Body-scaled ratio as a control parameter for prehension in 5- to 9-year-old children. *Dev Psychobiol* 33: 351–361. http://dx.doi.org/10.1002/(SICI)1098-2302(199812)33:4<351::AID-DEV6>3.0.CO;2-P

Kelso JAS, Southard DL, Goodman D (1979) On the nature of interlimb coordination. *Science* 203: 109–131. http://dx.doi.org/10.1126/science.424729

Keogh JF (1968) Developmental evaluation of limb movement tasks. Technical report 1–68, University of California at Los Angeles, CA, USA.

Keogh JF (1969) Analysis of limb and body control tasks. Technical report 1–69, University of California at Los Angeles, CA, USA.

Keogh JF (1970) A rhythmical hopping task as an assessment of motor deficiency. In: Kenyon G, editor. *Contemporary Psychology of Sport*. Chicago, IL: Athletic Institute, pp. 499–506.

Keogh JF, Sugden DA (1985) *Movement Skill Development*. New York: Macmillan.

Knobloch H, Pasamanick B, editors (1974) *Gesell and Amatruda's Developmental Diagnosis*, 3rd edition. New York: Harper Row.

Konczak J, Dichgans J (1997) The development toward stereotypic arm kinematics during reaching in the first 3 years of life. *Exp Brain Res* 117: 346–354. http://dx.doi.org/10.1007/s002210050228

Konczak J, Velden HV, Jaeger L (2009) Learning to play the violin: motor control by freezing not freeing degrees of freedom. *J Motor Behav* 41: 243–252. http://dx.doi.org/10.3200/JMBR.41.3.243-252

Kuhtz-Buschbeck JP, Boczek-Funcke A, Stolze A, Heinrichs HH, Illert M, Stolze H (1996) Kinematic analysis of prehension in children. *European Journal of Neuroscience Supplement* 9: 131–141.

Kuhtz-Buschbeck JP, Stolze H, Johnk K, Boczek-Funcke A, Illert M (1998a) Development of prehension movements in children: a kinematic study. *Exp Brain Res* 122: 424–432. http://dx.doi.org/10.1007/s002210050530

Kuhtz-Buschbeck JP, Stolze H, Boczek-Funcke, Johnk K, Heinrichs M, Illert M (1998b) Kinematic analysis of prehension movements in children. *Behav Brain Res* 93: 131–141. http://dx.doi.org/10.1016/S0166-4328(97)00147-2

Landmark M (1962) Visual perception and the capacity for form construction. *Dev Med Child Neurol* 4: 387–392. http://dx.doi.org/10.1111/j.1469-8749.1962.tb03194.x

Ledebt AS, Bril B, Breniere Y (1998) The build up of anticipatory behaviour: an analysis of the development of gait initiation in children. *Exp Brain Res* 120: 9–17. http://dx.doi.org/10.1007/s002210050372

Lee DN (1980) The optic flow field: the foundation of vision. *Philos Trans R Soc Lond B Biol Sci* 290: 169–179. http://dx.doi.org/10.1098/rstb.1980.0089

Lee DN, Aaronson E (1974) Visual proprioceptive control of standing in human infants. *Percept Psychophys* 15: 529–532. http://dx.doi.org/10.3758/BF03199297

Lockman JJ (2000) A perception-action perspective on tool use development. *Child Dev* 71: 137–144. http://dx.doi.org/10.1111/1467-8624.00127

Loovis EM, Butterfield MS (2000) Influence of age, sex and balance on mature skipping by children in grades K–8. *Percept Motor Skills* 90: 974–978. http://dx.doi.org/10.2466/pms.2000.90.3.974

Maccoby EE, Bee HL (1965) Some speculations concerning the lag between perceiving and performing. *Child Dev* 36: 367–377. http://dx.doi.org/10.2307/1126463

Maccoby EE, Dowley EM, Hagen JW, Degerman R (1965) Activity level and intellectual functioning in normal preschool children. *Child Dev* 36: 761–770. http://dx.doi.org/10.2307/1126921

Moss SC, Hogg J (1981) Observation and classification of prehension in preschool children: a reliability study. *Res Q Exercise Sport* 52: 273–277.

Newell KM (1986) Constraints on the development of coordination. In: Wade MG, Whiting HTA, editors. *Motor Development in Children: Aspects of Coordination and Control.* Amsterdam: Martinus Nijhoff, pp. 341–361. http://dx.doi.org/10.1007/978-94-009-4460-2_19

Newell KM, Scully PV, Baillargeon R (1989) Task constraints and infant grip configurations. *Dev Psychobiol* 22: 817–832. http://dx.doi.org/10.1002/dev.420220806

Roberton MA (1977) Stability of age categorizations across trials: implications for the 'stage' theory of overarm development. *J Human Movement Stud* 3: 49–59.

Roberton MA (1978) Longitudinal evidence for developmental stages in the forceful overarm throw. *J Human Movement Stud* 4: 167–175.

Roberton MA, Williams K, Langerdorfer SJ (1980) Prelongitudinal screening of motor development sequences. *Res Q Exerc Sport* 51: 724–731.

Roberton MA, Halverson LE (1988) The development of locomotor coordination: longitudinal change and invariance. *J Motor Behav* 20: 197–241.

Robertson SD (2001) Development of bimanual skill: the search for stable patterns of coordination. *J Motor Behav* 33: 114–126. http://dx.doi.org/10.1080/00222890109603144

Rosenbloom L, Horton ME (1971) The maturation of fine prehension in young children. *Dev Med Child Neurol* 13: 3–8. http://dx.doi.org/10.1111/j.1469-8749.1971.tb03025.x

Rosenbloom L, Horton ME (1975) Observing motor skill: a developmental approach. In: Holt KS, editor. Movement and Child Development, Clinics in Developmental Medicine, no.55. Philadelphia: JB Lippincott.

Rosengren KS, Braswell GS (2003) Learning to draw and to write: issues of variability and constraints. In: Savelsbergh G, Davids K, van der Kamp J, Bennett S, editors. *Development of Movement Coordination in Children.* London: Routledge, pp. 56–74.

Saida Y, Miyashita M (1979) Development of fine motor skills in children: manipulation of a pencil in young children aged 2 to 6 years. *J Human Movement Stud* 5: 104–113.

Savelsbergh G, Rosengren K, van der Kamp J, Verheul M (2003) Catching action development. In: Savelsbergh G, Davids K, van der Kamp J, Bennett S, editors. *Development of Movement Coordination in Children.* London: Routledge, pp. 191–212.

de Schonen S (1977) Functional asymmetries in the development of bimanual coordination in human infants. *J Human Movement Stud* 3: 144–156.

Scrutton DR (1969) Footprint sequences of normal children under five years old. *Dev Med Child Neurol* 11: 44–53. http://dx.doi.org/10.1111/j.1469-8749.1969.tb01394.x

Smyth MM, Katamba J, Peacock KA (2004a) Development of prehension between 5 and 10 years of age: distance scaling, grip aperture, and sight of hand. *J Motor Behav* 36: 91–103. http://dx.doi.org/10.3200/JMBR.36.1.91-103

Smyth MM, Peacock KA, Katamba J (2004b) The role of sight of the hand in the development of prehension in childhood. *Q J Exp Psychol* 57A: 269–296.

Statham L, Murray MP (1971) Early walking patterns of normal children. *Clin Orthopaed Related Res* 79: 8–24. http://dx.doi.org/10.1097/00003086-197109000-00003

Steenbergen B, van der Kamp J, Smitsman AW, Carson RG (1997) Spoon handling in two- to four-year-old children. *Ecological Psychology* 9: 113–129.

Steenbergen B, Utley A, Sugden DA, Thieman PS (2003) Discrete bimanual movement coordination in children with hemiparetic cerebral palsy. In: Savelsbergh G, Davids K, van der Kamp J, Bennett S, editors. *Development of Movement Coordination in Children.* London: Routledge, pp. 156–176.

Stoffregen TA, Schuckler M, Gibson EJ (1987) Use of central and peripheral optical flow in stance and locomotion in young walkers. *Perception* 16: 113–119. http://dx.doi.org/10.1068/p160113

Strohmeyer HS, Williams K, Schaub-George D (1991) Developmental sequences for catching a small ball: a prelongitudinal screening. *Res Q Exercise Sport* 62: 257–266.

Sugden DA, Soucie H (2008) Motor development. In: Armstrong N, Van Mechelen W, editors. *Paediatric Science and Medicine.* Oxford: Oxford University Press, pp. 188–197.

Thelen E (1985) Developmental origins of motor coordination: leg movements in human infants. *Dev Psychobiol* 18: 1–22. http://dx.doi.org/10.1002/dev.420180102

Thelen E (1995) Motor development: a new synthesis. *Am Psychol* 50: 79–95. http://dx.doi.org/10.1037/0003-066X.50.2.79

Thelen E, Fisher DM (1982) Newborn stepping: an explanation for a 'disappearing reflex'. *Dev Psychol* 18: 760–775. http://dx.doi.org/10.1037/0012-1649.18.5.760

Thelen E, Fisher DM (1983) The organisation of spontaneous leg movements in newborn infants. *J Motor Behav* 15: 353–377.

Thelen E, Fisher DM, Ridley-Johnson R (1984) The relationship between physical growth and a newborn reflex. *Infant Behav Dev* 7: 479–493. http://dx.doi.org/10.1016/S0163-6386(84)80007-7

Thelen E, Smith LB (1994) *A Dynamic Systems Approach to the Development of Cognition and Action.* Cambridge, MA: MIT Press.

Van Roon D, van der Kamp J, Steenbergen B (2003) Constraints in children learning to use spoons. In: Savelsbergh G, Davids K, van der Kamp J, Bennett S, editors. *Development of Movement Coordination in Children.* London: Routledge, pp. 75–93.

Wann JP, Edgar P, Blair D (1993) The use of time to contact cues in the locomotion of adults and pre-school children. *J Exp Psychol* 19: 1053–1065. http://dx.doi.org/10.1037/0096-1523.19.5.1053

Wann JP, Poulter DR, Purcell C (2011) Reduced sensitivity to visual looming inflates the risk posed by speeding vehicles when children try to cross the road. *Psychol Sci* XX: 1–6.

Warren WH (1984) Perceiving affordances: visual guidance of stair climbing. *J Exp Psychol Hum Percept Perform* 10: 683–703. http://dx.doi.org/10.1037/0096-1523.10.5.683

Watkins J (2008) Developmental biodynamics: the development of coordination. In: Armstrong N, Van Mechelen W, editors. *Paediatric Exercise Science and Medicine*. Oxford: Oxford University Press, pp. 169–185.

Wedell K (1964) Some aspects of perceptual-motor development in young children. In: Loring J, editor. *Learning Problems of the Cerebral Palsied*. London: Spastics Society, pp. 146–149.

Wellman BL (1937) Motor achievements of preschool children. *Child Educ* 13: 311–316.

Whitall J (2003) Development of locomotor coordination and control in children. In: Savelsbergh G, Davids K, van der Kamp J, Bennett S, editors. *Development of Movement Coordination in Children*. London: Routledge, pp. 251–270.

Whitall J, Getchell N (1995) From walking to running: using a dynamical systems approach to the development of motor skills. *Child Dev* 66: 1541–1553. http://dx.doi.org/10.2307/1131663

Wickstrom RL (1977) *Fundamental Motor Patterns*, 2nd edition. Philadelphia, PA: Lea & Febiger.

Wickstrom RL (1983) *Fundamental Motor Patterns*, 3rd edition. Philadelphia, PA: Lea & Febiger.

Wild MR (1938) The behaviour patterns of throwing and some observations concerning its course of development in children. *Res Q* 9: 20–24.

Woollacott M, Debu P, Mowatt M (1987) Neuromuscular control of posture in the infant and child: is vision dominant? *J Motor Behav* 19: 167–186.

6
MOVEMENT DEVELOPMENT OF YOUNG CHILDREN: 7 YEARS TO PUBERTY

In the preceding chapter, it was noted that by the age of 7 years a typically developing child will be able to perform, at some level, a full range of fundamental motor skills. These will involve walking, running, jumping, hopping, skipping, climbing, throwing, catching, striking, kicking, writing, drawing, and other manipulation skills. From the age of 7 years through puberty a number of developmental changes take place, and these are reflected in the three major sections of this chapter.

- The first section covers the child developing the capacity to adapt to the spatial and temporal requirements of the environment, moving in response to non-stationary others and objects. This had been occurring in the ages up to seven, but after this age, more complex environmental demands are becoming prevalent in the child's life.

- Second, the child starts to engage in play-game activities for which normative comparisons in maximum performance are made.

- The third section examines how the abilities of children can be measured in clusters such that more global pictures of a child's profile can be presented.

A specific task illustrating spatial and temporal demands

Many everyday tasks involve moving our whole body or specific body parts in relation to the location and movements of other objects and other people. We move to chase or dodge another person, catch a ball and take a dish of food as it is being handed to us. When driving vehicles, from scooters and bikes to automobiles, the vehicle must be controlled to stay in unison with or avoid others, whether it is other vehicles or other people. Moving in a changing environment is such a multifaceted problem that no one movement task will capture the many aspects we

need to observe and study. However, a general sense of the development of movement control in more variable and unstable movement situations can be obtained by tracing the development of performance in rope jumping, a common play-game skill that progresses from the most basic performance of moving over a rope lying on the ground to successive jumps over a fast-moving rope. Several variations are shown in the movement sequences in Figure 6.1.

Young children trying to step over a rope lying on the ground will often step on it. When asked to run and jump over the rope, some children will run and stop and then will move up and down without lifting a foot off the ground, as if trying to jump. Other children will continue running while crossing over the rope, perhaps with exaggerated movement of arms, trunk, and head, again as if trying to jump, and will often step on the rope or sometimes make an exaggerated lift of the back leg after the forward leg has landed. Even when moving in a stable environment, seemingly minimal environmental constraints will influence the type and quality of movement.

Another variation is for two people to move the rope slowly back and forth, but not overhead, requiring children to jump over the rope at the appropriate time. If running to jump over it, young children often run through the rope or stop and try to step over it. Also, occasionally they will sway forwards and backwards in time with the rope. As it moves towards them, they will bend back, and then forward as it moves away.

Eventually, children will master a single jump over a rope slowly swinging through a full rotation, though they will have difficulty in making successive jumps. A problem in making a second jump is that the rope is now behind them and cannot be used as a visual signal or cue for making the next jump. Children soon learn to stand sidewise to the rope, enabling them to keep it in sight, but jumping is now different and probably more difficult

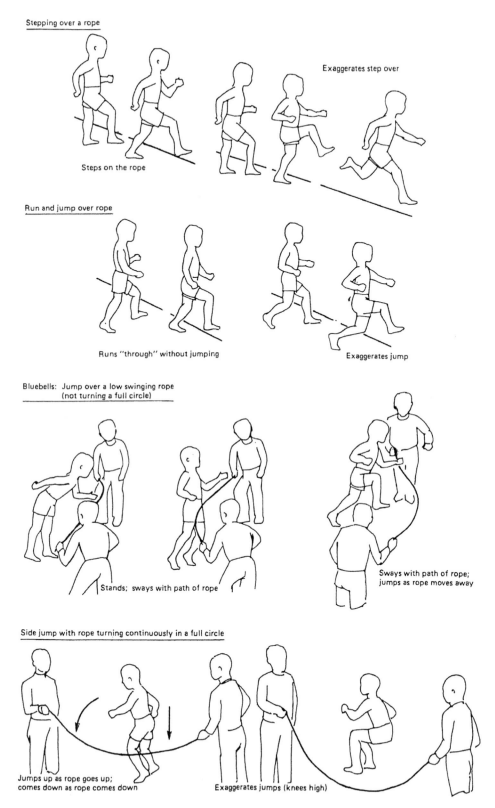

Fig. 6.1 Movement variations in performing different rope-jumping tasks (Keogh and Sugden 1985).

because the rope approaches from the side. Several single, discrete jumps may be made in succession with this side-wise strategy, but it is difficult to make more than three or four single jumps without being caught by the rope. The single jumps generally are large and do not leave enough time for the next jump. Jumping must become a more continuous set of smaller jumps, with a pace that matches the speed of the rope. Children often add an even smaller jump between two jumps over a rope in order to continue the movement.

Children finally become able to maintain a continuous set of jumps over a swinging rope, and thus accomplish two things. First, they gain better control of their own movements in order to make smaller jumps in a more continuous and rhythmical manner. Second, they know what the rope is doing without constantly watching it, which is critical for continuous jumping with a fast-moving rope. A jumping rhythm must be established to coincide with the rope's spatial and temporal path: a stationary rope creates spatial accuracy requirements and a moving rope creates temporal accuracy requirements.

This example illustrates many of the challenges children face when moving from a predictable to an unpredictable situation where it is no longer sufficient simply to control their own movements. They now have to move in response to moving others and objects, which restricts their choice of when and where to make the movement.

Modelling mover and environmental conditions

We concluded the previous chapter by illustrating the interplay of the mover and the environment with a modification of a model by Gentile et al (1975) elaborated by Keogh and Sugden (1985). This was shown in Chapter 5 (Fig. 5.12) and is reproduced below in Figure 6.2.

The figure shows how the requirements of a movement problem are influenced by the state of the mover, whether he or she is stationary or moving and whether the environmental context is stable or changing. We noted that in 2- to 7-year-olds, the addition of a changing environment, whether objects or persons, presented demands that were often too much for their capabilities. From 6 or 7 years onwards, the child is faced with more unpredictable environmental contexts that require anticipation, coincidence and predication in order for them to successfully accomplish tasks of daily living. These may involve recreational activities such as sports or everyday functional skills such as crossing a road or walking on a busy pavement. These are actions that all take place in constrained time and space and often these variables are outside of the mover's control.

Spatial accuracy

Spatial accuracy is required in all movements because the whole body or certain body parts must be moved to a particular spatial location and sometimes along a particular

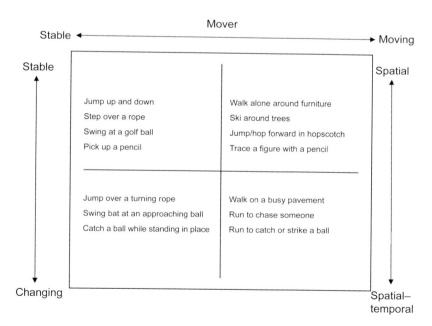

Fig. 6.2 Movement situations in relation to mover–environment conditions and spatial–temporal requirements (Keogh and Sugden 1985).

spatial path. The whole body or body parts also must be moved in an appropriate direction and for an appropriate distance, often with an appropriate amount of force and speed.

PLAY-GAME SKILLS

Most play-game skills involve both spatial and temporal demands, but it is possible to isolate spatial accuracy in many play-game skills; for example, single movements to strike and propel stationary objects and movements of the whole body into a stable environment. The striking and propelling of stationary objects are movement situations in which the mover and the environment are stable according to the general framework in the upper-right corner of Figure 6.2.

One of the most basic of these movements is striking a stationary object, which can be done by using the leg to kick or the arm to swat or by holding an implement to strike an object. Children must control the sequence of movements in the arm or foot linkage system and bring the limb or implement to the object's spatial location. Throwing is another way of propelling an object, yet is different from striking a stationary object, in that striking involves a visible point of contact on the object as the movement target, whereas throwing involves no visible release point at the movement target. The sequence of limb segment movements, however, is similar in approaching the point of contact or point of release. Movement errors in both are similar and involve releasing the object too soon or too early, which is like missing the point of contact when striking.

When striking or throwing a stationary object, children need to control the sequence of their limb segment movements while controlling their overall posture. They must move their limb in a direction and path that will contact the object in the desired position or reach the desired release point. They must coordinate the sequence of limb segment movements in order to finish at the time of contact or release. Finally, the object must be propelled a particular distance or at a particular rate, the mover must modulate the amount of force generated in the limb movement and imparted to the object (Keogh and Sugden 1985). It is useful to break down a movement in this manner; however, in practice these all come together in a perception–action sequence when the total movement is a direct consequence of the environment–child match.

Children encounter similar situations when their whole body moves into a stable environment, except they generally try to avoid rather than contact or propel objects involving the skill of navigation. For example, walking must be directed spatially to avoid furniture, pass through door openings, and generally navigate in the environment. Running has the same spatial accuracy demands, except that the body moves faster, thus limiting the time to change directions and correct movement errors. As children develop, through experience, they acquire more capability, allowing them to competently solve more complex and difficult movement problems. In Chapters 7 to 12 of this book we shall describe how some children, through lack of experience and different typical personal resources, such as blindness, heighten the difficulties they face in navigating even stable environments.

MANUAL CONTROL

A fundamental manual skill movement is reaching and grasping, and we have seen in Chapters 2 and 3 how this facility develops in the early years. However, although it would appear that children have relatively mature reaching and grasping skills by 7 years of age, development does not stop, with progressions that show more sophisticated strategies becoming evident. A progression to smooth coordinative reaching and grasping is a continuous process, with Konzack et al (1995) and Konzack and Dichgans (1997) showing that, with development up to the age of 3 years, there is kinematic evidence of increasingly smooth muscular production, but there are still differences between young children and adults. During the period from 7 years of age, children are able to exploit reaching and grasping in much more complex environmental contexts and adjust their movements accordingly.

The development of this was examined by Kuhtz-Buschbeck et al (1998), who looked at reaching and grasping in children aged 4 to 12 years and analysed how changing the task and environmental demands changed the outcomes. With increasing age children performed with a smoother, more consistent performance and had a more accurate grip formation, yet the movement duration remained roughly constant. The detail of Kuhtz-Buschbeck et al (1998) is shown in a closer examination in Box 6.1.

Temporal and spatial accuracy

External requirements for temporal and spatial accuracy are created when the environment and/or the mover moves at increasing speed with increasing complexity of both play-game skills and manual skills. Temporal accuracy means timing self-movements to the place and time of external events, coinciding the self with objects and other people to stay in unison or to intercept or avoid them. Examples are trying to stay in time with a partner and the music while dancing, trying to intercept or tag another player, and trying to avoid being tagged by another player. We present various examples of spatial–temporal

Box 6.1 A closer examination

Reaching and grasping: Kuhtz-Buschbeck et al (1998)

Design and methods

Fifty-four children aged 4 to 12 years were analysed repeatedly when reaching for a cylindrical object, with the trajectory of the reach and the hand shaping monitored using kinematic analysis. In the first experiment object sizes and distance travelled were kept constant and the body was scaled to each individual to try to obtain parity between age groups. This follows the work of researchers who have shown that changing the nature of the task and/or environment changes the movement accordingly, often to a totally different action (Newell et al 1989). In the second experiment, object sizes and distance travelled were varied to examine adaptability. Trials were carried out with and without the visibility of both hands and object.

Results

In these age groups of 4 to 12 years, the kinematics of hand transport improved, with better and smoother bell-shaped velocity profiles and a decreasing number of movement units per reach and more linear trajectories. This was illustrated in Chapter 5 (Fig. 5.9) and is reproduced here in Figure 6.3, which displays velocity–grip size profiles of repetitive trials of the three different ages. The variability decreased with age with the authors proposing that this indicates a more automated performance. All children showed appropriate scaling of movement velocity to movement amplitude when distance was varied.

Second, anticipatory action in the form of grip formation was present in all children, with the youngest opening their hand wider in relation to the object size than older children. Grip formation did improve with age and developed into a consistent pattern with a single peak that was in synchrony with the deceleration of hand transport.

Third, when visual control was examined, all children scaled their hand transport velocity to the distance to travel, even in the non-visual mode. However, the 4- and 5-year-olds often missed the target in the first instance, which indicates that younger children have a greater dependence on visual guidance. This could have been the younger children's lack of ability to keep a mental image of the target location. Movement time was almost constant in the visual condition with a slight decrease from around 850ms in 4- to 5-year-olds to around 700ms in 12-year-olds. In the non-visual mode the 12-year-olds stayed relatively the same, at around 750ms, but the 4-year-olds took much longer (1600ms), indicating again their much greater reliance on vision. In the middle groups (6- to 8-year-olds) this reliance on vision had reduced substantially.

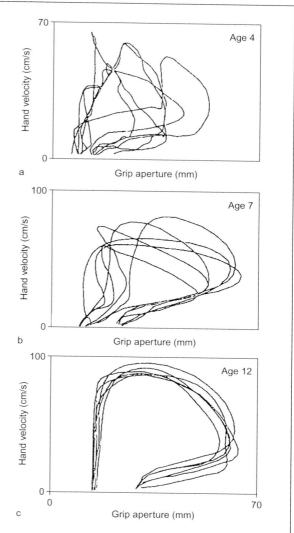

Fig. 6.3 Child moving to where ball will land. Reproduced with permission from the publisher from Kuhtz-Buschbeck et al (1998a).

Discussion

This reliance on vision can be interpreted in a number of ways. A processing view would talk of the lack of good internal representation in the absence of vision, whereas from a dynamic systems viewpoint, the difficulty could be explained by a lack of an appropriate perception–action match and not enough experience to compensate and construct in other ways. By the start of the age range in this chapter (6–7 years), when the task was adapted to correspond with the size of the child, he or she could make the appropriate movements but there was still further improvement with age through to 12 years. The older children were found to be more adaptable to changing experimental conditions.

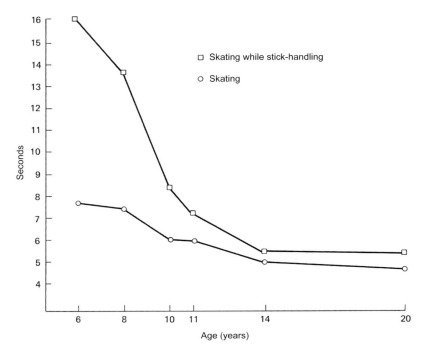

Fig. 6.4 Time to skate a 15m course (Keogh and Sugden 1985). Drawn from data reported by Leavitt (1979).

situations to illustrate the developmental changes in later childhood from 6 to 7 years of age.

BODY CONTROL

Improvement in the total body dealing with increases in temporal accuracy requirements is demonstrated in a study by Leavitt (1979), who measured the speed of males when ice-skating through a 15m course with pylons placed at 3m intervals. These ice-hockey players, aged between 6 and 20 years, were timed; first, for skating as fast as possible on alternate sides of the pylons and, second, for skating as fast as possible while stick-handling a hockey puck without losing control if it. Figure 6.4 summarizes the mean performance times by age for the two skating conditions. The speed of skating improved by age groupings, and the 6- and 8-year-olds were alike, but they were slower than the 10- and 11-year-olds, who were alike but slower than the 14- and 20-year-olds, who were alike. As expected, the mean time for each age group was higher when stick-handling because the moving skater had to stay in contact with the moving puck. The important finding is that the stick-handling mean times for younger males increased much more than those for the older skaters, showing the impact on the younger males' performance when the task was changed to require them to deal with moving objects.

Skating for speed among the fixed pylons is a movement situation in which the mover enters into a stable environment, as illustrated in the upper-right corner of Figure 6.2. As the mover goes faster, the requirements for temporal accuracy increase because less time is available to make each change in direction. These requirements again increase when a puck must be moved and handled while skating among the pylons. The movement situation now is more open in the sense shown in the lower-right corner of Figure 6.2, with the task having the two demands of skating fast and controlling the puck. Younger males probably cannot control the puck well enough, making it difficult to cope with the high levels of spatial–temporal requirements. We can see something of the magnitude of their difficulty by looking at the size of the difference in mean times when comparing skating only and skating while stick-handling. Younger males took 6 to 8 seconds longer and essentially doubled their time when stick-handling; older males added less than 1 second to their mean time. Figure 6.4 shows that the major changes take place between 6 and 11 years of age, with the time decreasing by 8 seconds in the stick-handling condition compared with a 2- to 3-second decrease between age 11 and adulthood.

At first, performing two tasks at once leads to different demands. Skating only may lead to arm movements made in coordination with leg movements, whereas

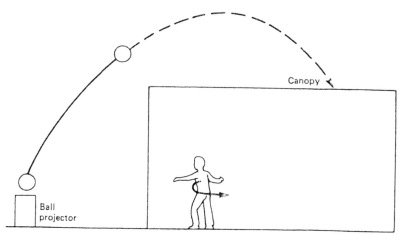

Fig. 6.5 Representation of ball projected to land on overhead canopy with child moving to where s/he thinks ball will land (Williams 1973, Keogh and Sugden 1985).

stick handling requires that the arms be used separately to control the stick and puck, so that they reach and turn separately from the legs. The ability to do both at once in a competent manner appears to develop between the ages of 6 and 11 years.

When children are asked to adapt their movements to different environmental and task demands, we see developmental differences as the children have a different set of resources and experience that allows more or less appropriate adaptation to the task. Changes in moving to intercept a moving object when vision was limited were studied by Williams (1973). She had children stand under a large canvas 'roof' and watch a ball projected in the air by a tennis ball boy, as shown in Figure 6.5. They could see the ball's initial flight path until the canvas blocked it, and it landed silently in a net above the canvas. They were asked to move quickly to the spot where they could catch the ball if it came down. All of the children moved in the correct direction, but the younger children (grades 1, 2, and 3) had a mean error of 7m in locating the projected landing spot, compared with the older children (grades 4, 5, and 6), who had a mean error of 76cm. The younger children moved very quickly in the correct direction of the ball's flight, but well beyond where it would have landed. The fourth graders were very good in locating the probable landing place, but they took a long time to make the judgement and they would not have arrived in time to catch it. The fifth graders were a little less accurate than the fourth graders, but moved quickly to the probable landing place. The sixth graders were both quick and more accurate.

It is impressive that older children and adults can perform adequately in movement situations that are far more complex and demanding than anything we have described and analysed. Developmental change occurs through an improved perception–action match with the environment, and children using their knowledge of and experience with different tasks and environment arrays to cope with increasingly complex movement situations.

WHOLE BODY AND MANUAL SKILLS
Temporal accuracy in controlling hand and arm movements can be divided into coincidence timing and keeping time.

- *Coincidence timing* is matching a mover's position to the changing position of an object or another person. The task may be to intercept or avoid the object or other person or to match its movements, and is always concerned with moving in relation to the moving of others.
- *Keeping time* is maintaining a temporal pattern in a continuous set of movements. The temporal pattern may be regular or irregular and can be established by the mover or might match an imposed temporal pattern.

Keeping time and coincidence timing are different aspects of the problem of coping with temporal accuracy requirements. Keeping time is a more limited and regular set of movements, without the unpredictability of coincidence timing. Keeping time, also, is the ability to maintain a temporal pattern in a movement, often in relation to an imposed temporal pattern, whereas coincidence timing is the ability to move in relation to others' moving.

Coincidence timing

Coinciding one's own movements with the movements of an object or another person occurs in two ways. First, the mover tries to intercept a moving object or another moving person; second, the mover tries to match self-movements to movements in the environment.

- *Interception* involves a single coincidence point, and so the mover or an object propelled by the mover comes to a place occupied by a moving object or another moving person. For example, ball skills require interception, such as catching a ball, passing a ball to a running partner, and kicking a moving ball.
- *Continuous matching* has the mover maintain a consistent position in relation to the ongoing and changing movement path of a moving object or another moving person. Examples are dancing with a partner or guarding an opponent in sport.

The important distinction is that the interception is a single coming together, whereas continuous matching is the ongoing maintenance of a moving, spatial relationship. The distinction is somewhat artificial, but it is useful in tracing the development of movement control in more open movement situations.

Interception

Many movement situations involve moving a limb, usually an arm or hand, to intercept a moving object. This is done directly to intercept a moving object and indirectly to propel an object, such as a ball, at a moving target. Bard et al (1981) offers some descriptive information about other aspects of spatial and temporal accuracy when throwing at a target. Children aged 6 to 11 stood 2m away from a target apparatus that produced a stationary or a moving target (coming from right to left and travelling 75 or 150cm s^{-1}). Spatial and temporal accuracy were measured for three test conditions: (1) throwing at a stationary target, (2) pressing a button to intercept a moving light at a designated point, and (3) throwing at a moving target. As expected, the children were spatially more accurate when throwing at a stationary target, but their mean performance in throwing at a moving target was only slightly worse. The pattern of mean improvement with age was also strikingly similar for both target conditions. The temporal error for intercepting a moving target was markedly less for pressing a button than for throwing. Children at all ages were more accurate in knowing when a moving object was nearing a given location (button pressing), but they were slightly less spatially accurate in throwing at a moving target than at a stationary target. This provides some confirmation

of perception–action links and how environmental and task requirements afford various actions, and often are different with differing ages.

An everyday task is reaching for a moving object when either stationary or walking. A number of studies have used this paradigm invoking an optic variable, called the bearing angle, which can aid us in understanding the interception of a moving object. In the Netherlands, a group involving Savelsbergh, Lenoir, Rickens and Cohan has examined children's interception of moving and stationary objects using bearing angles. In adults it has been shown that by using the head as the angle centre, the angular position of the ball remains constant with respect to the interception point (Lenoir et al 1999, 2002). The advantage of this in an interception task is that only one piece of information is required to aid interception by the mover maintaining a constant bearing angle (CBA) throughout the task to intercept at the appropriate time. Work with adults suggests that the bearing angle remains constant during the locomotion part of intercepting a moving object but at the point of interception it breaks down and the bearing angle of the wrist takes over and makes final finer adjustments. There are also deviations from a CBA according to the size of the angle of approach (Chohan et al 2006). Work with children seemed a natural progression from adults examining the developmental trends, and results showed that they lengthened the deceleration phase of their reach and recruited more trunk and arm movements when intercepting the ball. Chohan et al (2008) extended this work by allowing children to approach and intercept an object from a defined distance and direction. This work is elaborated in Box 6.2.

The study of variables such as the CBA with manipulations using curvilinear paths can help shed light on what visual information children use to intercept objects and how this ability to use the information develops. This is a relatively new area but it does appear that clear differences are being found between younger (5- to 7-year-old) and older (10- to 12-year-old) children. An exciting way forward on this would be to employ learning experiments and analyse whether, with experience, the younger children start to employ the same strategies as the older ones.

There is evidence that, when navigating complex environments, even older children use different anticipatory control strategies to adults. Vallis and McFadyen (2005), who studied 10-year-olds and adults, found that in preparing anticipatory behaviour the 10-year-olds were later than adults in changing foot placements as they approached an obstacle. For adults, the task appeared to comprise a unitary sequence, whereas the children seemed to divide it into two parts. The first part involved steering

Box 6.2 A closer examination

Children's use of the bearing angle in interceptive actions: Chohan et al (2008)

The bearing angle is the angle produced at the point of observation by the current position of the ball and current direction of displacement. By actively keeping the bearing angle constant, the catcher can arrive at the point of interception at the same time as the object, and this strategy reduces any computational burden. The catcher does not have to know the final position point of the ball in advance; he or she merely needs to keep the bearing angle constant. In adults, the angle of locomotion was a key variable to a constant bearing angle (CBA) strategy. Chohan et al (2008) used a freely adjustable walking task with the purpose of exploring the use of bearing angle in children through the manipulation of ball velocity and angle of approach.

Method

The children were in two age groups: 5- to 7-year-olds (eight males and two females) and 10- to 12-year-olds (six males and four females). A tennis ball was placed on a platform that moved along a track with light-emitting device (LED) markers on the ball and on the children's wrists, hips and heads, all monitored by a motion analysis system. Two 4-m paths were marked and the children walked (running not permitted) as soon as the ball started moving with the object of intercepting the ball with their preferred hand at three ball velocities.

Results and discussion

Adhering to a CBA strategy required the children to maintain a near-constant walking velocity throughout the approach. Both groups showed a fluent movement with a steep acceleration before decelerating as they approached the target, with all children successfully attuning walking to the approach of the ball. Older children's velocity profiles plateaued more than the younger children, with a more pronounced bell shape exhibited by the younger children, but were more like the older children when at the lowest velocity. The authors suggested that the younger children accelerated and decelerated more quickly depending on the speed of the object, with older children having a more stable and consistent strategy no matter what the speed.

There were both similarities and differences between the two age groups when adhering to a CBA strategy. Both groups, like adults, had deviation patterns that were coupled to ball velocity; they deviated from the CBA strategy when they approached the track from the larger angle and for faster balls deviation occurred later than at the two lower velocities. However, younger children deviated more from the CBA strategy than older children, with the latter more like adults, suggesting that more time is required for the younger children. They deviate earlier for slower than for faster balls with older children, like adults, not differentiating between ball speeds but keeping the bearing angle as constant as possible.

head and trunk with proactive movements and the second involved making adjustments to the gait trajectory and being more dependent on visual information. Again, it would be interesting to employ learning studies to determine the role of experience on tasks such as this.

These studies, and the study on catching in Chapter 5, illustrate how interception develops such that the child can catch or collide with an object. Another temporal ability that involves this prediction and anticipation judgement is the one that involves avoiding contact with an upcoming object. This ability to detect, intercept, and/or avoid looming objects has been examined in different fields showing developmental trends. Box 6.3 describes one such study.

This study has real implications for road safety in younger children who are not accurate in their predictions of vehicle speeds, showing that the neural mechanisms for looming are not fully developed until adulthood. It also has implications for other activities where approaching objects are present, such as in catching or the ability to predict the motion speed of another person such that an object can be thrown to be intercepted and caught. It is probably safe to assume that developmental progressions in this age group are present with predictions and anticipation of motion being crucial to the skills of throwing and catching and other activities for which these abilities are required.

Two laboratory tasks, both of which involve ballistic rather than continuous movements, show a different type of interception task. One task is pushing a metal doughnut down a rod to intercept and knock down a cartoon figure

---

Box 6.3 A closer examination

Wann et al 2011: Visual looming in children to moving vehicles

Wann et al (2011), noting that pedestrian accidents are the third leading cause of death in 5- to 9-year-old children, examined looming in children under different presentation conditions and converted these data into speeds that would show the limits of children's ability to estimate the speed of approaching vehicles. Looming involves the change in the size of an object on the retina as it moves towards or away from a person, and so allows us to make predictions about speed, size, and point of contact.

The ages of the children employed in this study overlap the ages in this and the previous chapter across three developmental groups: 6 to 7 years, 8 to 9 years and 10 to 11 years, plus an adult group. Four conditions of visual simulation of approaching vehicles were presented: two in foveal (central) vision and two outside this range. The children were asked to indicate whether they thought an image of an approaching car in the simulation changed size or stayed the same size.

The detection of looming showed an age effect with no difference between the 6- to 7-year-old and 8- to 9-year-old groups, but this was poorer than in the 10- to 11-year-old group, with adults being better than all three groups of children. This effect was seen in both central (foveal) and extrafoveal presentations. In addition, the responses to extrafoveal presentations were poorer than the foveal ones, indicating that viewing movement from the side caused more difficulties than head on. Differences between adults and children were evident in the foveal condition, with the object expanded isotropically; when there was additional lateral translation adults could reliably detect vehicles moving towards them at a speed of almost 40mph whereas young children were only able to do this if the car was travelling at less than 25mph. In the extrafoveal conditions, 6- to 9-year old children were unable to detect cars approaching at speeds over 30mph, often a speed limit in urban areas.

---

moving at right angles to the rod (Wade 1980). The other task is intercepting a moving dot on an oscilloscope by moving a handle that controls a cursor or an interceptor dot (Dorfman 1977). Movement direction is fixed in both situations because the doughnut is fixed on the rod and the lever moves horizontally in a fixed position. Spatial accuracy requirements were minimized in order to focus on temporal accuracy. In the Wade study, there were three age groups (7–9y, 9.5–11y, and 12–14y); in the Dorfman study, there were six age groups covering a range of 6 to 19 years.

The interception task in the two studies is similar: making a quick, and probably ballistic, movement to intercept the moving target. Little, if any, adjustment can be made in the movement once either the metal doughnut or the hand lever has been pushed. However, the movements are different. In the Wade study, the movement was to propel an object to intercept, whereas in the Dorfman study the movement involved the limb to intercept.

Another feature of the Dorfman task is that it is not a direct interception of a moving object. The hand guides a lever that moves a dot on a screen, and the distance moved by the lever in this type of task often is not the same distance moved by the guided dot, although there is a proportional relationship of four units of lever distance for one unit of guided dot distance. Younger

children may have had difficulty with this translation, showing more difficulty in relating the hand movement to the movement of an object on a screen or in similar display modes.

The general finding for the two studies was a steady decrease in interception error as the children grew older. Children of all ages in both studies improved their performance with practice, as noted by a decrease across trials in both absolute error and variable error, again suggesting that experience is a crucial variable in the development of skilled performance. From ages 6 to 9, the males were better than the females in the Dorfman study; Wade did not report any male–female comparisons.

Wade found that younger children were quite early in intercepting the moving target, in contrast with older children, who intercepted later. Dorfman reported that all of the children were late, with the older children being less late or closer to intercepting the target. The mean reaction time to start moving the lever after seeing the target dot first appear is ≥300ms for the younger children, in contrast with 200ms for the older children and adults. It seems likely that the children in the Dorfman study were late to the interception point because they did not have enough time to catch up with the target dot, whereas the children in the Wade study had to delay their response until the target was approaching the interception point.

The conditions in the Wade study appear to provide a better test of whether or not children are early or late in arriving at the interception point.

The target's speed was varied by Wade, with the expectation that the slower speed of 30cm per second, which provided 5 seconds of viewing time, would be the easier task and would produce smaller errors and less variable performance than would the faster speeds of 90cm per second (1.7s of viewing time) and 1.5m per second (1s of viewing time). But the children were less accurate and more variable at the slower target speed, with their performance generally better at the middle target speed. Wade speculated that there may be an *optimal target speed* for children in a coincidence–interception situation that slower or faster target speeds may not match as well with their perceptual abilities. A developmental possibility is that there may be a shift in the optimal target speed for coincidence–interception functioning and/or a widening of the range of optimal target speeds. Again, this provides support for perception–action links that are tuned by the experience of the environment–body resource interaction.

In a similar vein, Shea et al (1982) support an optimal or desired speed of moving targets. They also measured changes in the speed of the intercepting limb during the interception task in order to describe differences in adjusting the limb to the target speed. They found the expected result that interception accuracy improved with age for the three test groups, which consisted of 5-year-olds, 9-year-olds, and adults. Overall, accuracy tended to decrease as velocity increased. However, the curve for the younger children was U-shaped and indicated poorer accuracy at slower and higher velocities, with better accuracy at a moderate velocity. This is the pattern of performance suggested by Wade (1980); that movers may be better tuned to or more compatible with a particular range of target speeds. As children develop, experiencing a larger variety of environmental arrays, they may expand their compatibility range to deal equally well with multiple target speeds, again confirming the proposal by Adolph et al (2003) that practice and/or experience is probably a more important factor than other variables such as neural growth, processing ability, or biomechanical constraints.

Continuous matching

A continuous matching, or a coincidence of the hand and the moving target rather than a single interception of a moving target, is our second type of coincidence timing and has been a favourite with researchers over a number of years. The pursuit rotor apparatus, often used with children, requires the continuous tracking of a moving target, whose path can be varied in speed and shape. Time on target (TOT) is a standard performance score, but other scores can be obtained to show when a person is on target, as a means of determining movement strategies.

An early study by Ammons et al (1955) demonstrated a consistent increase in TOT from age 9 to age 18. A rather fast speed of 60 revolutions per minute (1 per second) was used, and the percentage of time on target was less than 10% for younger children. Males had a better mean TOT than females, with small differences at earlier ages, compared with means that were more than double those of females at ages 17 and 18. Females peaked at age 15 and levelled off, whereas males had a linear increase from age 9 to age 18. Children at all ages improved with practice.

Younger children, ages 5 to 10, have been tested with slower speeds of 15 to 45 revolutions per minute (Davol et al 1965, Davol and Breakell 1968, Horn 1975). TOT increased with age and was better for the slower speed of 33 revolutions per minute. College students tested at 33 revolutions per minute had a mean TOT of 530 seconds out of a possible 600 seconds, compared with third-grade children (approximately age 8) who had a mean TOT of less than 60 seconds.

The inability of younger children to stay on target for even 10% of the total test time of 600 seconds is a dramatic illustration of child–adult differences when continuously tracking a moving object. Adults approach 90% on-target time at a slower speed of 33 revolutions per minute. Target speed again raises the issue of whether certain speeds are more compatible with the movement capabilities of different ages. We presently know that younger children do not perform well in matching their movements to a continuously moving target compared with older children, but we do not know much detail about the level of speed at which they can function more adequately and how they try to stay on target. Again, the match between the task and the child resources appears crucial.

Zanone (1990) found that younger children aged 5 years relied mainly on feedback information to track, whereas 15-year-olds used visual feed forward cues to correct their movements. Van Roon et al (2008) elaborated on these data in their study, which is shown in Box 6.4.

Studies involving keeping time with rhythmical movements have found increased accuracy and decreased variability in performance from ages 6 and 7 through puberty (Wolff and Hurwitz 1976). In an alternate finger tapping test to a metronome, 5-year-olds were found to have large deviation scores, to be quite variable in trying to keep a steady pace, and were very disrupted by the built-in interference. Deviation and variability scores decreased (improved) steadily from age 6 to age 16. In both tapping conditions, females to age 10 and sometimes beyond were more accurate than males in matching the

Box 6.4 A closer examination

The development of feed forward control in a dynamic manual tracking task: Van Roon et al (2008)
This study required children and adolescents to manually track an accelerating target. They used a digitizing tablet upon which participants had to move an electronic pen to track a target moving in a circle presented on a computer monitor, with the target accelerating as it was successfully tracked. This task requires the participants to use a predictive model of the target's motion but also to keep updating this model as the target accelerates. At lower speeds the low speed velocities enabled feedback control to be employed but as the target increased in speed, feed forward control had to be employed. The authors' question was how feed forward control and predictive behaviour on this type of task developed during childhood and adolescence.

Participants
A total of 62 females and 55 males took part, distributed as shown in Table 6.1.

TABLE 6.1
Background data on participants

Age group (years)	Male/female	Mean age
6–7	10/13	7.1
8–9	15/12	9.1
10–11	12/9	11.1
12–14	11/15	13.6
15–17	7/13	15.11

Adapted from Van Roon et al (2008). MABC, Movement Assessment Battery for Children.

Using the Movement Assessment Battery for Children, no child was identified as motor impaired, with none scoring below the fifth centile.

Task and procedure
The participants were required to track a red dot on a computer monitor by the use of a wireless electronic pen on a white sheet of paper. As the dot was successfully tracked the speed increased in small discrete steps. The children were told that the dot was a villain and the cursor a policeman. Two conditions were presented with the dot moving in a circular path of diameter 3cm or 10cm.

Results and discussion
The number of circles and maximum target velocity were higher in the older children and the number of velocity peaks and stops decreased with age. From this the authors concluded that with increasing age the children were more likely to be using feed forward rather than feedback strategies. All children were able to track the target at some speed but the younger ones (6- to 9-year-olds) could track successfully only at the lower speeds. At these lower speeds they used a 'stop-and-hold' strategy, which is feedback-based and can be used only with lower velocities. This strategy decreased with increasing age.

Based on these results the authors suggested three phases in tracking skills:

- learning to stay on target;
- anticipating the movement of the target to track at higher velocities; and
- relying less on visual feedback with fewer submovements.

The age-related differences were firstly attributed to using more and better feed forward processes, enabling smoother movements. Second, the authors discuss the contention that increased speed of information processing may have played a role with the possibility that this may allow the older children to still use feedback information at higher speeds. However, they concluded that the motor delay on the task was too short, leading them to favour the feed forward explanation. They also discussed the possibility of decreasing variability with age, the improvement of visual pursuit and the increased ability with age to perceive acceleration. Overall, they conclude that the increased performance on this task with age was due to the older child's ability to more fully exploit feed forward control.

expected beat, and females were better in holding a steady or less variable beat. This task did not have any spatial accuracy demands.

Smoll (1974, 1975) included and measured both temporal and spatial accuracy in repeating movement, although the spatial demands were minimal, with the arm moving a lever to shoulder height in response to a visual or auditory signal. He found that children improved steadily from age 5 to age 11 in both spatial and temporal accuracy with both constant and variable error reducing with increasing age. Children performing on the Smoll apparatus showed a steady, linear increase with age in their ability to stay in unison with an external event.

SUMMARY OF CHANGES IN SPATIAL AND TEMPORAL PERFORMANCE

Improvement of movement control in open movement situations is striking during the elementary school years, with even casual observations indicating the better performance of children aged 10 to 12 in comparison with that of children aged 5 to 7. Laboratory measurements confirm the magnitude of the improvement on different types of coincidence-timing tasks. Children continue to improve beyond these early school years, and based on performance data presented in the next section, it is reasonable to propose that young people at age 14 are similar to adults in their mean performance levels in many open movement situations. The general picture is that there are very large improvements from ages 6 to 10 and 11, which continue at a slower rate to age 14, when mean performance levels approximate those of young adults. This statement applies only to those open movement situations in which strength and endurance are not involved significantly.

Some sex differences have been reported, indicating that young females keep time better and at a steadier pace. A similar finding was reported in Chapter 5 for young females making repeated limb movements better than young males, but we do not know whether these differences continue beyond the early school years. Younger and older males are better on some coincidence-timing tasks in which children intercept a moving object or continuously match the position of a moving object. All of these findings regarding sex differences in open movement situations are tentative and should be interpreted cautiously, because male–female comparisons are not reported in many studies, and we do not have the number and variety of descriptive data needed to deal with this very broad issue.

Moving adequately in an open movement situation requires the mover to read the internal and external surrounds and to produce movements that relate to these readings. As described in Chapter 4, the rudiments of responding to moving objects and persons are present early in life but later in the ages described in this chapter; children are exposed to contexts where the external demands become greater. Young children encounter difficulties in moving in open movement situations when they are rapid and continuous and involve multiple movements. They may be able to make the same movement if done in separate parts at their own rate, which would indicate that they can read their surrounds and respond adequately if the spatial–temporal accuracy is appropriately matched for their developmental level. As time becomes more limited or movements need to be made simultaneously and continuously, their resources may not be adequate for coping with higher levels of spatial–temporal requirements. This occurs even when, as adults, we try to do too much in too little time, and it is even seen in high-level performers, such as when a bowler in cricket or a pitcher in baseball propels the ball at a faster speed than the batsman can deal with. Very often the movement patterns become dysfunctional when the demands of the task are not met by an increase in the resources of the individual. Again, this is confirmation of the model that is consistently shown throughout the text that outcomes are a function of the transactions among the child resources, the environmental demands, and the specific task instructions and requirements.

It is likely that younger children, like older children and adults, are, in many circumstances, time constrained in their actions, and that a natural developmental progression is being able to deal with a higher temporal demand set in a particular spatial context. This developmental progression appears to be highest between the ages of 6 and 10 to 11 with less of an improvement from 11 to 14 where achievements close to adult levels are achieved. We note and stress consistently that practice and experience are such crucial variables in acquiring these skills, and there are rather obvious conclusions and implications to be drawn from this for education, in particular the primary school curriculum in physical education and other subjects where motor skills play a part.

Development of maximal performance: normative comparisons

Movement development beyond the early school years often is traced through normative performance data. Children and young adults have been tested in different movement tasks to establish norms and to make age- and sex-related comparisons. These comparisons provide general descriptions of change for movement tasks that require maximal performance in closed movement situations.

The influence of participation experiences pertains to what individuals are allowed and encouraged to do, that is the nature, extent, and quality of involvement in movement activities. Some quite young children may swim, and others may ride horses, ski, or participate in other sports. Some children may be very active, but not in organized movement activities, and others may not be active at all. Social values, as transmitted through family members, peers, and others, will influence what an individual does and the way it is done. Social influences may come directly through parental rules and guidelines and less directly, but very powerfully, through sex roles. Again the influence of experience and practice are seen to be crucial variables.

Our review of normative change is a description of age- and sex-related changes. Age-related changes are related to age only through the agents of change functioning over a period of time: age is only the passage of time in months and years and not an agent of change; it is the change agents that produce the development. Similarly, *sex differences* reminds us that being female or male is only a designation, just as age represents only the passage of time. Normative sex differences often are found when comparing the mean performances of females and males on closed movement tasks requiring maximal force production. Biological differences following puberty provide

males with more potential for force production, and differences in participation experiences also still favour males, who are encouraged and rewarded for maximal force production. But with increasing opportunities and support for females to more fully develop their potential in these movement tasks, future data may provide a different picture.

PLAY-GAME SKILLS

As a continuation from Chapter 5, we have chosen the three play-game skills of jumping, running, and throwing to further demonstrate performance changes with age and, where appropriate, differences between males and females. Composite curves from a number of studies for the mean performance scores of males involving data from several European studies and other American studies show that similar patterns of change for males and females across ages have been found in different regions and in different time periods. The following composite performance curves for jumping, running, and throwing for a 10-year period from ages 7 to 17 years were developed by Keogh and Sugden (1985) and are presented in Figures 6.6 to 6.8.

Jumping

The mean values for the standing broad jump of males and females in Figure 6.8 increase by 8 to 12cm per year from age 7 through age 11, and the males jump 8 to

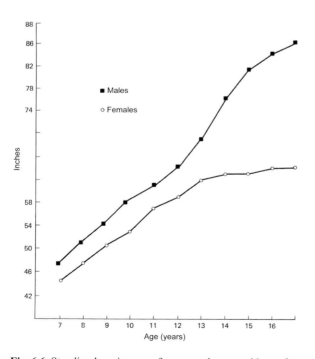

Fig. 6.6 Standing long jump performance changes with age for males and females aged 7 to 17 years based on composite mean values (Keogh and Sugden 1985).

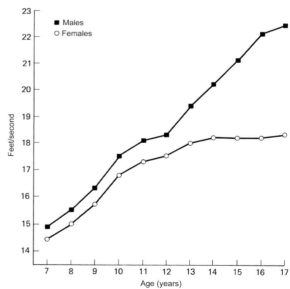

Fig. 6.7 Performance changes with age on timed dashes for males and females, aged 7 to 17 years, based on composite values (Keogh and Sugden 1985).

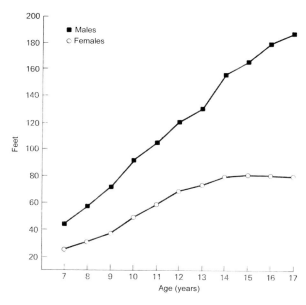

Fig. 6.8 Performance changes with age in throwing for distance for males and females, aged 7 to 17 years, based on composite mean values (Keogh and Sugden 1985).

12cm further, on average, than the females do, at each age. Performance on the standing long jump improves steadily during these years, with the males' mean values approximately 1 year ahead of the females'. The pattern of change after age 11 is quite different. The females' mean scores level off, whereas the males' continue to increase until age 15 and somewhat beyond. The mean difference between males and females increases from 8cm at age 12 to 48cm at age 15 and 56cm at age 17. Individuals may continue to improve with intensive and specialized instruction, but the general performance differences for the age and sex groups will be the same.

Another way to look at performance changes across ages is through the relative amount of percentage of change in a particular time period. Both males and females improve by approximately 45% on their mean performance on the standing long jump during the 5-year period from age 7 to age 12. The curves for the males and females are parallel and increase at a similar rate, even though the males have higher mean scores at each age. The percentages of change are quite different for the 10-year period from age 7 to age 17 when males increase by 83% and females by 49%, the differences being between the ages of 13 and 17.

Comparisons among mean performance scores sometimes may be misleading if we do not consider how much *overlap* exists among the groups being compared. At age 11 and age 13 the males had a higher median score than the females, but there was a considerable overlap of the two distributions at each age. There is also a considerable overlap when comparing children between the two age groups. Many of the 11-year-olds jumped as far as the median distance of the 13-year-olds, even though the 13-year-olds had a higher median score. However, there is a minimal overlap between distributions when comparing 17-year-old males with 17-year-old females and 17-year-old males with 11-year-old males. We can say that most 17-year-old males jumped further than did most 17-year-old females and most 11-year-old males.

Graphic and tabular summaries describe group (mean/median) performance but do not indicate individuals' performances. The general expectations for ages 7 to 11 are that mean performance will increase steadily each year and that males will have higher mean values than females at each age. However, some individuals at these ages perform more like children of the opposite sex or children who are older or younger by 1 or 2 years. The males' mean performance continues to increase up to age 17, in contrast with the levelling off of the females' mean performance. Few young women jump as far as the young men of the same age. Few males at age 11 jump as far as any young adult males do, whereas many females at age 11 jump as far as the mean distance for young women.

Running

The speed of running a dash has been measured in a number of studies. Composite curves for the mean performance scores of males and females are presented in Figure 6.7 to cover ages 7 to 17. The length of the dashes varied from 27 to 46m. Times were reported in tenths of a second and have been converted to feet per second as a common basis for comparison. Although it is preferable to use a running start and eliminate initial reaction time and acceleration, a standing start was used in most studies. Mean performance data from different studies naturally cannot be meaningfully compared unless the same timing procedure is used.

The general patterns of change for the timed clashes are similar to those for the standing long jump. The increase up to ages 11 or 12 is essentially linear, followed by a levelling off for females and a continuing increase for males. Males consistently have better mean performances than females do up to ages 11 or 12, with a considerable overlap in distributions at each age. The mean difference between males and females at age 17 is sizable, with very little overlap in distributions. The composite means at age 17 are 7m per second for males and 5m per second for females. Transforming these figures to time for a 46m dash, the mean times at age 17 are 6.8 seconds for males and 8.3 seconds for females. The mean times for a 46m dash at age 11 are 8.3 and 8.7 for males and females, respectively. It is obvious that the mean time differences at age 11 are much smaller than those at age 17. Also, the mean time for males at age 11 is the same as that for females at age 17.

Both males' and females' performances increased by 23% during the 5-year period from age 7 to age 12. Males continued to improve and had an increase of 49% in the 10-year period from age 7 to 17, whereas females had only a slight improvement beyond age 12. The change for both males and females averaged just less than 1 foot per second per year from age 7 to age 12.

Throwing

The general skill of throwing has been measured most often as the distance that children can throw. There are many problems in obtaining distance scores that can be compared across studies because procedural differences can bias throwing performance. Procedural considerations are the size of the ball, style of throw (underhand or overhand), and starting position (stationary or running up to the throwing line). But the differences between age and sex groups are so large that the procedural differences do not affect the general pattern of change summarized in Figure 6.8. Males begin at age 7 with a composite mean distance that is greater than the females' and increases progressively to be more than double the females' mean throwing distance at age 17. The overall patterns of change for males and females are similar to their jumping distance and running speed, in that males increase until age 16 or 17, whereas females level off at an earlier age. The patterns of change are different, as male–female differences became greater at each age, in contrast with a constant difference in the early years for jumping distance and running speed.

The percentage of change across ages is somewhat misleading for throwing distance, as males begin at age 7 with a much larger mean score. Both males and females increase threefold in their mean throwing distance from age 5 to age 12. These proportional changes are very large compared with jumping distance and running speed. Females as well as males increase relatively more in throwing distance than in other skills. Males increase by approximately 18m in throwing distance beyond age 12, whereas females level off with a small mean increase of 3 to 5m. Group variability increases noticeably from early to later ages, which indicates that some children have even greater increases with age than noted for their sex groups and that others have quite small increases.

Throwing skill also has been measured for accuracy, but test procedures vary so much that the data cannot be summarized across individual studies. The pattern of

change cannot be described beyond the general statements that children improve with age in throwing accuracy and that males generally are more accurate (Peacock 1960, Keogh 1965, Gardner 1979). One important limitation is that an increased distance to a target creates a strength problem for younger children, but is too close for older children. Another problem is that a large number of throws are needed to obtain a reliable estimate of an individual's level of performance.

Rippee et al (1990) examined accuracy as part of a study involving 6- to 10-year-olds throwing a baseball for velocity, distance, and accuracy, and showed that even after adjusting for size on distance, older children were more accurate. Burton and Rogerson (2003) investigated throwing accuracy and velocity in 7-, 9-, and 11-year-olds and adults in throwing a baseball at three different target distances of two, three, four, and six times an individual's height. At the longer distances the 11-year-olds and adults have significantly lower error scores than the other groups. Also, at the longer distances the velocity did not vary in all groups (75–83% of maximum), but at the shorter ones, the older children and adults threw relatively slower than the younger groups, seemingly being able to better control the velocity to the requirements of the task. Burton and Rodgerson (2003) attributed age-related changes to accumulated practice and experience together with myelination of the corticospinal tract. They are invoking both intrinsic and extrinsic constraints for this improvement and encourage the use of Newell's (1986) constraints model to examine throwing with a particular emphasis on the conditions set by the context and the task.

Balancing tasks

A variety of tasks have been used to measure balancing skill. Walking on a beam and maintaining a balanced position on a stabilometer are the two tasks that have been used most often and that we shall use to show the general patterns of change in balancing skills. Both tasks require maintaining equilibrium; first, while walking on a narrow path and, second, while standing on an unstable platform. Tests such as the Movement ABC have incorporated balance into the range of tasks assessing children's motor performance (Henderson et al 2007). In this instrument Age Band 2 examines children from 7 to 10 years of age and has three balance tasks, one static and two dynamic. The static task involves balancing on two foot-sized balance boards with a raised rim of 3cm width on which to balance for up to 30 seconds. At 7 years of age the median time for the balance on the favoured leg is 16 to 19 seconds and by 10 years of age is 27 to 29 seconds. On the other leg the times are 6 to 7 seconds and 10 to 16 seconds for the favoured and other leg, respectively. It is possible

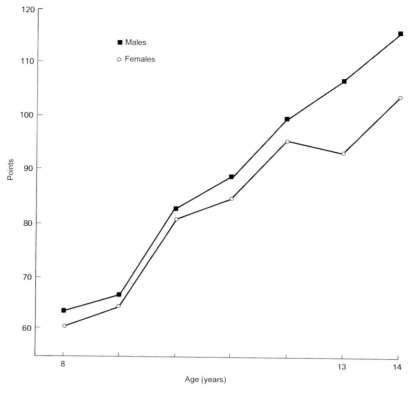

Fig. 6.9 Beam walking performance as a function of age (Keogh and Sugden 1985). Drawn from data reported by Heath (1949) and Goetzinger (1961).

that a test such as this is confounded by motivational variables as well as overall competence.

Walking beams of different widths have been used to measure this type of balancing skill. Variations in test procedures have influenced performance scores with differences between wearing shoes or not and, additionally, there are no standards for length of beams, number of trials, and scoring system. Data from the studies of Goetzinger (1961) and Heath (1949) are combined in Figure 6.9 to show the general change in beam walking from age 8 to age 14. The same beam widths and test procedures were used in both studies and the results were similar in the two samples. Males and females had a similar pattern of improvement with age, except that females' mean performance did not increase from age 12 to age 13. The overall pattern of change was uneven from year to year, with smaller mean increases from age 8 to age 9 and age 10 to age 11. Keogh (1965) also found a similar pattern of uneven change from age 5 to age 11. The mean differences between males and females were small in these studies, with the males slightly better in Heath's and Goetzinger's studies and the females slightly better in Keogh's study. The overlap between the distribution for

males and females is large at all ages, indicating that any differences are minimal.

Bachman (1961) tested eight males and eight females at each age from 6 to 26 using a stabilometer and reported their mean scores for 2-year intervals, beginning with ages 6 and 7 and continuing to ages 24 and 25. Each individual did 10 trials. Work-adder mean scores (where high is a poor score) were reported only for trial 1 and trial 9 and are plotted for males and females, with each age group improving markedly from trial 1 to trial 9. The grand mean score for all performers was approximately 60 on trial 1 and decreased to approximately 20 on trial 9. There were no significant sex differences in this overall improvement and individuals of all ages improved their stabilometer performance in a small number of trials. One of Bachman's more important findings is that balancing skill, as measured by performance on the stabilometer, did not improve with age, which is contrary to performance on walking beams and the play-game skills reviewed earlier in this chapter. Although Bachman does note the older children's poorer performance, this contradictory and confusing finding has been accepted without comment in other reviews of movement development. The trend of lack of improvement in older children's stabilometer performance was replicated when Eckert and Rarick (1976) found no age and sex differences among children aged 7, 8, and 9 years.

The older children's lack of improvement on the stabilometer probably is due to their heavier weight, because a heavier child will cause the platform to move more rapidly, thus creating a more difficult movement problem to resolve. Anooshian (1975) obtained a correlation of 0.36 for age and work-adder score, indicating that older children tend to have higher (poorer) work-adder scores. When weight was partialled (removed mathematically from the calculation), the correlation of age and work-adder score was –0.51. This indicates that older children tend to have lower (better) work-adder scores if their weight is held constant. The task of maintaining an in-balance position on an unstable platform must be similar for each performer before age, sex, or other performer characteristics can be compared. Anooshian's analyses indicate that stabilometer performance improves with age, which seems reasonable, but performance data are required on a stabilometer adjusted for apparatus stiffness and performer weight to determine age–sex differences more completely.

Performance data for beam walking and stabilometer do not present a clear picture of the balancing skills of males and females from ages 7 to 17. It seems unlikely that balancing skills deteriorate or do not change during this 10-year period, as shown with some stabilometer data. Performance on walking beams increases during this age range, which is a better general indicator of change in balancing skills. But performance data for walking beams are quite limited, whereas performance data for the stabilometer can be gathered in a variety of ways and can be separated to analyse performance components.

The scoring procedures and analyses that Anooshian (1975) used indicate some of the possibilities. He was able to trace continuous changes in platform movement to demonstrate what each performer was doing, rather than being limited to a single outcome measure of amount of total board movement (work-adder score) or time in balance. Anooshian found two different movement strategies of (1) quick alternations in platform direction and (2) leg opposition for braking the platform's movement as it moved in one direction. Quick alternations is a movement strategy similar to the quick alternations of hand movements used to control a marble moving through a maze, as used by Elliott and Connolly (1974) and discussed in Chapter 5. Stability and control can be produced by keeping the platform in motion, whereas braking is an effort to achieve minimal movement by having the force in one leg counteract the force in the other. Wade and Newell (1972), using similar procedures and analyses, found another strategy in which performers seemed to be trying to keep the platform at an angle rather than having their feet at the same level. This could be to provide a discrepancy to work against rather than to bring the balance information to zero. We are limited by measurement problems in equating the levels of task difficulty, but we do know that the nature of the task is an important variable to consider when the development of balance is being considered.

In a review of balance in children, Assaiante (1998) proposes a model showing multiple interactions that describe the development from birth through adulthood. This development involves the improvement in preparatory adjustments and the gradual mastery and control of the redundant degrees of freedom. Such activities as stabilization of the head appear to be task dependent whereas pelvic stabilization is a more intrinsic operation. These are part of the multiple frames of reference that allow for appropriate balance development that is attuned to contextual demands. Assaiante (1998) argues that such is the complexity of the many parameters, the development of balance continues well into and through adolescence.

SPEED OF MANUAL MOVEMENTS

The speed of manual movements has been measured in various ways, ranging from the time needed to do specific tasks or skills, such as stringing beads or moving pegs, to the time needed to respond to single or multiple stimuli. We shall describe three patterns of change in the speed of manual movements:

1. specific movement tasks or skills requiring manipulation to sort or construct objects;
2. tapping a single digit or hand; and
3. reaction time and movement time in making a limited movement.

This progression will take us from a broader look at speed in doing a movement task to a narrower view of limb movement speed.

Manipulation tasks

Tasks involving manipulation can be picking up an object and placing it in a container or on a peg and putting objects together to construct a larger unit. Objects are manipulated, rather than just held, and both unimanual and bimanual movements are included. Examples of functional tasks are picking up matchsticks or pennies and placing them in a container, picking up washers and placing them on a peg, and stringing beads on a shoelace.

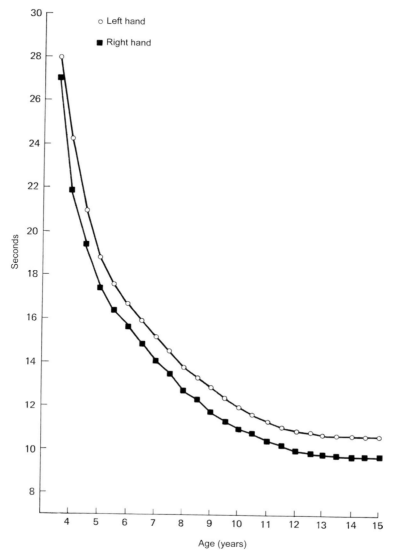

Fig. 6.10 Speed of moving pegs. Reproduced with permission from Annett (1970).

The speed of moving pegs from one row to another is described in Figure 6.10 for children from ages 3 to 15 (Annett 1970). These performance data illustrate a basic pattern of change seen in studies using similar tasks. Gains are larger during the earlier years, with quite small changes beyond age 10.

A limitation of most performance data is that a single score is obtained that represents total achievement without indicating how the performer produced the outcome. Connolly (1968) analysed several performance components for children doing a peg task to study change beyond the knowledge that children improve in speed as they grow older. Connolly had children, aged 6, 8, and 10 years, move 12 pegs from one row to a parallel row

of 12 target holes 20cm away. Four sizes of target holes were used so that the task could be changed from having the peg just barely fit to having it fit easily. Connolly measured the total time to move the 12 pegs and also four component times: (1) grasp, (2) carry, (3) release, and (4) return.

1 *Grasp time* – the time from when the peg was touched to when it was pulled away from contact with the positioning hole.
2 *Carry time* – the time from leaving the positioning hole to contact of the peg with the target hole.
3 *Release time* – the time from initial contact with the target hole to release of the peg in the target hole.

4   *Return time* – the time from release of the peg in the target hole to contact with the next peg to be transferred.

As expected from what we know from other studies, the older children were faster in overall time, and all of them were slower as the size of the target hole became smaller. Connolly looked beyond these findings to find out where the changes occurred within the four component times. Grasp time was significantly faster for 10-year-olds than for 8-year-olds, who were significantly faster than 6-year-olds. Grasp time did not change as the size of the target was changed. Connolly observed that the younger children sometimes readjusted their grip as if their initial effort was not adequate for carrying and releasing the peg. The faster grasp time for the older children indicates that manipulative skill in the form of digital dexterity helped them improve their performance speed.

Carrying time decreased with age and target size, but there were no significant differences between the 8- and 10-year-olds, who both had significantly lower mean scores than the 6-year-olds. Younger children lifted the peg up, moved it over the hole, and seemed to 'bomb' the peg down to the hole in discrete movements, in contrast with Connolly's observation that older children made a more continuous movement in the form of an arc.

The release and return times are less clear-cut and are somewhat confusing. The older children were much better than the young children, with the 8-year-olds and 10-year-olds often not significantly different from each other. Connolly also reported that individual release times were quite variable and that group mean comparisons were erratic across target and trial conditions. It is interesting that 10-year-olds increased their release times from day 1 to day 5, perhaps in trying different ways to resolve a difficult part of the movement task. Connolly's component analyses and related observations suggest some interesting ways to look beyond the total performance score.

Tapping speed

Speed of tapping is often used as a measure of maximum performance of manual skill. The increase is reasonably linear in contrast with the speed of moving pegs (Annett 1970), in which there were larger increases for younger children and levelling off after age 10, and few sex differences have been found. The mean differences between hand and foot speed were significant, but quite small in size to favour hand speed. The correlations of speed of dominant hand and dominant foot for two different test sessions were 0.58 and 0.70. The slightly slower foot speed and moderately high correlation between foot and hand speed has been found in other studies of movement speed. Denckla (1973) measured digital speed in another way by having younger children, ages 5, 6, and 7 years, repeatedly touch their thumb to their index finger and successively touch each finger to their thumb. She found an increase in speed with age and found that females were faster in successive finger–thumb touches. The pattern of change for tapping speed and digital speed is a steady increase to at least age 15, with a similar level of speed expected for arm and leg tapping.

Movement strategies for the development of speed were suggested by Connolly et al (1968) in a study of tapping speed. Children, ages 6, 8, and 10 years, tapped back and forth between two circles with a 2.5cm radius and centres 13cm apart. The females tapped faster than the males did, and the older children tapped faster than the younger children did. All of the children improved with practice, but the older children (ages 8 and 10) improved more than the younger children did. The children making the fewest taps were described as 'wasting time' in two ways: they lifted their pencil in a high arc when moving between circles, and they tended to look from target to target in time with the pencil's movement. They seemed to treat the task as a series of discrete movements, whereas the children with the larger tapping scores watched one circle and moved the pencil in a low arc.

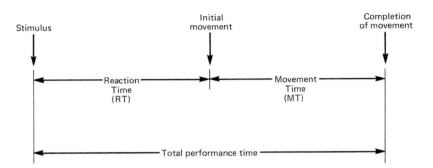

Fig. 6.11 Division of total performance time into reaction time and movement time.

Reaction time and movement time

Much of what has been reported in the previous two sections is dependent upon speeds of reaction and movement. Figure 6.11 shows how these relate to each other. The total performance time to make a movement includes both the time needed to prepare for the movement and the time that the limb or body part actually is moving. The reaction time is the preparation time, and the movement time is from when the movement can first be measured up until the movement task is completed. The total performance time is the sum of reaction time and movement time.

Reaction time and movement time are usually measured by having a signal or stimulus to indicate when an individual should make a movement. Reaction time is the time from the signal's appearance to the initial movement, which often is lifting a finger off a key or switch. Movement time is the time from the movement's onset to its completion by reaching to touch a plate or turn a switch. A general introduction to these topics is found in Chapter 3.

Reaction time

Reaction time varies according to the task. At a basic level reaction time is called either simple reaction time or choice reaction time; simple reaction time is responding only to one signal, and choice reaction time means that one or more of several signals can appear. Reaction time will increase as more choices are involved and uncertainty increases. Data from an early study by Thomas et al (1981) report on the general pattern of developmental change, with males moving from over 350ms at age 7 to around 300ms at age 11 and 250ms at age 13. Differences appear in the developmental data because of the variety of experimental conditions employed, but the general pattern of change is a proportionately large decrease in simple reaction time during early childhood. We can expect that children aged 6 or younger will have a simple mean reaction time of at least 350ms in many studies, decreasing to around 240ms at 12 and 13 years of age and 200ms in adults. Procedural differences in warning or alerting signals and the stimulus signal may explain some of the mean differences among the studies, but the simple reaction time for young children is much greater than that for older children and young adults. This is an important child–adult difference, because young children in many movement situations simply may not have enough time to respond and to process information in correcting and changing movements.

In the Thomas et al (1981) study there is a consistent sex difference, with males approximately 2 years ahead of females, but Fulton and Hubbard (1975) did not find a sex difference from age 9 to age 17, and Hodgkins (1962,

1963) did not find a sex difference among young children. Standard deviations are large at earlier ages, which means that there is a great deal of overlap, even in the male–female differences reported by Thomas et al (1981). Young adult males seem to have lower mean simple reaction time values than young adult females, but the mean differences are only 10 to 30ms and are not important in most movement situations.

Connolly (1970) investigated reaction time in adults and children using a card-sorting task to vary the information loads. Hick's law was confirmed, and the slopes of the regression lines were typically steeper for the younger age groups. Connolly found two transition ages when large performance differences were observed: from age 6 to age 8, and from age 14 to adults. He suggested that selective 'filtering mechanisms' were poorly developed (if such 'mechanisms' exist in the brain) in younger children, because irrelevant stimuli had less effect on older children. Connolly also argued that more than one mechanism is involved and that many simultaneous developmental changes take place to produce a faster processing speed.

Surwillo (1977), using differences between simple and choice reaction times, estimated that 5-year-olds take nearly three times as long as 17-year-olds to process 1 bit of information. On his card-sorting task, Connolly (1970) measured processing speed by dividing the amount of information per card by the decision time per card. This varied from 1.69 bits per second for 6-year-olds to 4.07 bits per second for adults, to approximate the relative size of the difference that Surwillo reported.

Kerr et al (1980) investigated the ability of children and adults to use the information that one item provides about the most probable subsequent event in a partially predictable reaction item sequence. The results showed that children used the sequence probability information quite successfully and in parallel with other processing, but recorded larger recovery times when the expected event did not occur. Although the children performed more slowly than the adults, their processing trends were the same, with the exception that the unexpected event affected children more than it did the adults.

Movement time

Movement time will vary according to the movement task. If the movement must cover a long distance, movement time will, quite naturally, be greater if the speed of the body part is the same for the shorter and the longer movement. The actual speed of the movement also depends on the degree of control required to make the movement. If more accuracy is required during the movement or as an end product, the movement speed will decrease and movement time will increase.

Box 6.5 A closer examination

Fitts' law and the capacity of the motor system: Fitts (1954)

Adults' movement time was determined by Fitts (1954) to vary in relation to movement distance and movement accuracy. Fitts' law states that more movement time is needed to move further and touch a small target than is needed to move a shorter distance and touch a larger target. Its formal statement is movement time=a + b log(2*A*/*W*), where *A* is movement amplitude (distance) and *W* is target width (accuracy). The terms a and b in Fitts' law are constants, with a being where the equation line crosses the *y* (vertical) axis and b being the slope of that line. Recall that the amount of information in reaction time is $\log_2 N$, where *N* is the number of choices. The amount of information in Fitts' law is defined by $\log_2 2A/W$. Distance to travel (*A*) and width of the target (*W*) are the variables that determine the amount of information present in the execution of a movement task. Another way to express Fitts' law is that movement time varies linearly with the logarithm of the index of difficulty ($\log_2 2A/W$). Index of difficulty is the information load for a movement that has been shown to vary in relation to movement amplitude and target width.

Different combinations of amplitude (*A*) and width (*W*) are listed in Table 6.2 to illustrate how the index of difficulty changes in relation to changes in *A* and *W*.

TABLE 6.2
Index of difficulty in relation to amplitude and width

A	W	2A/W	Index of difficulty
8	4	16/4 = 4	2
4	2	8/2=4	2
8	2	16/2=8	3
8	1	16/1=16	4

The index of difficulty is 2 when *A* is 8 and *W* is 4, because 2*A*/*W* = 4 and $\log_2 4 = 2$. If *A* is reduced to 4 and *W* to 2, the index of difficulty will not change. A smaller target width of 2 will increase the movement time, but this is counterbalanced by reducing the movement distance. The index of difficulty increases to 3 when *A* increases to 8 and *W* remains at 2. The index of difficulty is further increased to 4 by keeping *A* at 8 and decreasing *W* to 1.

Movement time is a function of movement distance and movement accuracy, in that the variation in distance and accuracy requirements will change the information load related to the control of movement. The motor system's capacity to function at different information loads has been studied extensively in regard to movement time. Fitts proposed in 1954 that movement time varies in relation to movement distance and accuracy. His formula for this relationship has been tested and supported in so many conditions that it now is called Fitts' law. A detailed description of Fitts' law is shown in Box 6.5.

It would be expected that with development children would improve in their performance on such tasks, and the general findings for the movement speed of children doing reciprocal and discrete tapping tasks are shown in Figure 6.12. The index of difficulty is the part of Fitts' law representing the extent of difficulty in changes in

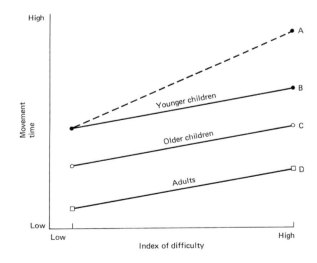

Fig. 6.12 General relationship of movement and index of difficulty for different age groups.

TABLE 6.3
Capacity of children with intellectual disability on serial (reciprocal) and discrete (single) tapping tasks

Age (y)	2		3		3.6		4		4.6		5		5.6	
	Serial	**Discrete**	**Serial**	**Discrete**	**Serial**	**Discrete**	**Serial**	**Discrete**	**Serial**	**Discrete**	**Serial**	**Discrete**	**Serial**	**Discrete**
6	3.0		4.8	8.1	5.3	8.5	5.4	7.3	5.5	7.3	5.4	7.8	5.4	9.3
8	4.4		5.6	8.5	6.3	8.8	6.0	9.7	6.5	9.5	5.9	9.9	6.4	10.3
10	6.8		6.9	10.7	7.4	10.9	7.7	11.3	8.4	10.9	7.3	10.9	7.5	12.3
12	7.5		8.9	12.8	9.9	13.1	8.9	14.1	9.3	14.3	8.6	14.9	8.4	14.7

Based on data from Sugden (1980) and Keogh and Sugden (1985).

movement amplitude (distance) and target width (accuracy). Movement time, as expected, is less for adults at any level of difficulty, and older children have smaller movement times than younger children. Children's and adults' movement times increase as difficulty increases, because more information must be processed to control movement over a longer distance and/or control movement accuracy to contact a smaller target.

Two ways of defining and measuring the motor system's capacity are described in Box 6.5. The first measure of capacity is the amount of information used per unit of time, which is the index of difficulty divided by movement time. Younger children clearly have less capacity in this absolute sense of information used per second, because their movement time is larger at each level of difficulty. Sugden's (1980) findings are listed in Table 6.3 to show the increase in capacity with age for both serial (reciprocal) and discrete (single) tapping tasks. There was little overlap between ages, and each group stayed within a narrow range on both tasks. Twelve-year-olds at their maximum capacity values overlapped the adults' minimum levels on both discrete and serial tasks, as reported by Fitts (1954) and Fitts and Peterson (1964).

The second measure of capacity is the reciprocal of the slope of the regression line, or 1/b. This is the capacity to adjust to increases in processing loads, which addresses the important and unresolved question we posed earlier. A larger value of 1/b indicates a greater capacity for adjusting to increases in processing loads. The findings from two studies (Sugden 1980) are presented in Table 6.3 to illustrate the differences in findings for younger children. The values for 1/b differ in the two studies because of the length of the trials and other procedural differences. The important concern is the value of 1/b among the groups in each study. Group values are quite similar in Sugden's study, indicating that the slopes of the regression lines are similar.

Group values also are similar in the Salmoni–Pascoe study, except that 6-year-olds have a much lower 1/b value and thus a higher slope, as shown by Group A in Figure 6.12. Kerr (1975) reported no slope differences for children to support the Sugden findings, whereas Hay (1981) found slope differences to support the Salmoni–Pascoe findings. There is no obvious and simple explanation for the discrepancy represented by Groups A and B in Figure 6.12. The tapping tasks and related procedures are similar and do not suggest any explanations. Salmoni and Pascoe tested only females, but Hay studied both males and females. We suggest that the findings from these studies be interpreted in two ways. First, they both agree that older children and adults have similar slopes, which means that increases in processing load are not relatively more difficult for older children, even though their movement time is not as good. Older children have a smaller capacity in an absolute sense, but they adjust to increases in their processing load in a manner similar to the way adults do. The second concern is the capacity of younger children who have a smaller absolute capacity and may or may not adjust as well to increases in their processing load. The latter may be that the capacity to adjust is marginal for younger children, and so we find a difference in one study and not in another. If there is a difference, we need to examine how younger children adjust. Sugden (1980) suggested that, as they grow older, children may programme movements more effectively to function more efficiently with greater information loads. This suggestion formed part of a study by Smits-Engelsman et al (2006), who examined cyclic and discrete aiming movements in 6-, 8-, and 10-year-old children. Two discrete aiming tasks were used in a Fitts task paradigm to examine developmental speed accuracy effects. All children performed the task appropriately and the speed–accuracy trade-off was similar across groups but with performance increasing with age as expected. All

TABLE 6.4
Information load conditions with eith amplitude or width held constant

A held constant			W held constant		
A	W	Load	A	W	Load
8	4	2	2	1	2
8	2	3	4	1	3
8	1	4	8	1	4
8	0.5	5	16	1	5
8	0.25	6	32	1	6

children showed differences between cyclic and discrete movements with the former being faster and more ballistic. They suggested that the younger children's slower movement speed was the result of their limited ability to use open-loop control. As with other differences between younger and older children in this age group it would be interesting to explore whether these differences could be minimized through experience and practice. Group B is one possibility in which younger children are slower, but the increases in processing requirements are not relatively more difficult for them. Group A is a second possibility in which increases in processing requirements are relatively more difficult, as if younger children are less able to adjust to the larger processing loads. That is, their motor system may be limited so that larger processing loads become increasingly more difficult for them (possibly geometric rather than linear) than for older children and adults.

Younger children clearly have less capacity in this absolute sense of information used per second, because their movement time is longer at each level of index of difficulty. The older children (Group C) also used less information than the adults (Group D) at each level of index of difficulty. Sugden (1980) found an increase in capacity with age for both serial (reciprocal) and discrete (single) tapping tasks, with little overlap between ages, and each group stayed within a narrow range on both tasks. Twelve-year-olds – at their maximum capacity values – overlapped the adult minimum levels on both discrete and serial tasks, as reported by Fitts (1954) and Fitts and Peterson (1964).

The second concern is the capacity of younger children who have a smaller absolute capacity and may or may not adjust as well to increases in their processing load. The latter may be that the capacity to adjust is marginal for younger children, and so we find a difference in one study and not in another. If there is a difference, it would be important to examine how younger children adjust. Sugden (1980) suggested that as they grow older, children may execute movements more efficiently. Some

children may also need to use more visual information, which will increase movement time. Adjustment to increases in processing load may be in transition, which would identify an important time of change.

Lastly, changes in distance and accuracy might differentially affect movement time as load increases (Welford et al 1969). Salmoni and Pascoe (1978) tested this possibility with children by having nine load conditions arranged in two sets to keep either A or W constant (Table 6.4).

Note that the middle condition (8, 1 + 4) of each set is the same, thus providing nine rather than 10 load conditions. There were no significant differences in performance between the load sets, which means that distance and accuracy did not differentially affect the movement time as the load increased. This supports the robustness of Fitts' law and also tells us that children perform in a manner similar to that of adults, although at a lower absolute level of performance. The consensus with respect to processing speed (both reaction time and movement time) is that speed of responding improves rapidly, especially after age 6 years, reaching an optimal level by 16 years of age, maintaining that speed through the next five decades (Kail and Salthouse 1994). Smits-Englesman et al (2006) reported differences in speed–accuracy trade-offs when comparing a cyclic (rapid reciprocal) task with a discrete task. The advantages of cyclic tasks over discrete tasks, reported by Smits-Englesman et al (2006), are not dissimilar to the resilience to forgetting of continuous tasks compared with discrete tasks, and the findings of Spencer et al (2003), with regard to forms of timing when executing both discontinuous (discrete) and continuous tasks. The type and structure of the task clearly plays a role across the developmental spectrum, and reflects the broad application of Fitts' law.

STRENGTH

Strength is an important consideration when studying maximal performance, and it is covered in more detail

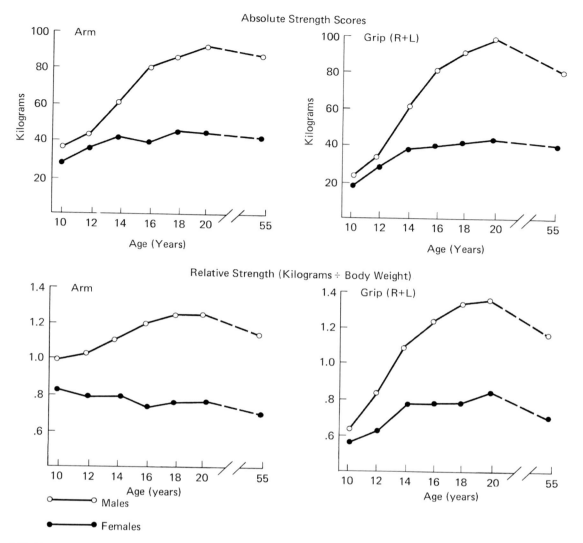

Fig. 6.13 Absolute and relative strength of males and females in the Tecumseh (Michigan) study. Drawn from tabular data reported by Montoye and Lamphiear (1977).

in Chapter 2. Here, selected measures are shown to demonstrate some of the changes in strength that take place in the years through puberty. Early movement development is gaining control of the motor system to achieve a particular movement, and sufficient strength usually is available. The problem is to control the force that can be generated. Later development is generating and controlling the high levels of force needed to move faster and further. Children's strength at older ages helps increase their levels of achievement, but it is difficult to relate strength to levels of achievement, in particular movement skills. A high level of strength does not necessarily mean that it can be used effectively to produce a higher level of achievement.

Strength usually is measured with dynamometers and tensiometers to record the force output of isometric contractions. Individuals push or pull to exert force on a fixed plate or wire, such as squeezing a hand dynamometer or trying to extend a leg constrained by a wire. Measuring muscle tension in this way does not indicate the extent to which a person can summate force to produce more functional strength in jumping, throwing or similar movement tasks. The summary of strength changes during the 10-year period from age 7 to age 17 is limited to isometric force production.

Grip and arm strength are summarized in Figure 6.13 for age and sex, based on testing 82% of the residents in Tecumseh, Michigan, between 1962 and 1965 (Montoye and Lamphiear 1977). Notice that the changes in *relative strength* and *absolute strength* (strength divided by body weight) were quite similar for arm and grip strength. For grip strength, males initially had slightly higher absolute mean scores, with sex differences pronounced from age 14 onwards. Men at age 20 had an absolute mean grip score that was more than twice the mean score for women. Mean grip strength scores relative to weight show the same difference between men and women, beginning at about age 14. The absolute scores for men were more variable by age 14, but there was very little overlap in distributions between men and women at age 20. These results are typical of other findings, except that the absolute values may differ from study to study depending on sample differences and instrument or test-procedure differences. The mean values for females may be equal or slightly higher than those for males for ages 9 to 11, as females are entering puberty but males are several years away from it. Greater mean strength scores also have been reported for newborn males on measures of grip and a prone head reaction taken at approximately 30 hours after birth (Jacklin et al 1981).

An extensive study of strength in childhood was part of a longitudinal project conducted by Clarke (1971) in Medford, Oregon. The Medford study was limited to males and included a wide range of anthropometric and performance measures. Changes in age were measured on a cable tension strength test that incorporated shoulder flexion, shoulder inward rotation, hip flexion, knee extension, and ankle plantar flexion. The strength measures for younger males were made at yearly intervals for 44 males from age 7 to age 12 (Jordan 1966). The strength measures for older males were taken at yearly intervals for 111 males from age 12 to age 17 (Bailey 1968). The mean strength score more than doubled (132%) between age 7 and age 12 and then doubled (101%) again between age 12 and age 17, making an increase of 362% from age 7 to 17. Similar proportional increases were reported for left grip and back lift (312% from age 8 to age 17) and for right grip strength (393% from age 7 to age 17).

Strength increases threefold to fourfold for males in the 10-year period from age 7 to age 17. Although fewer data are available to describe strength changes for females, they probably double their strength from age 7 to age 12 and have a substantial increase beyond age 12. Males have higher mean strength scores, presumably from birth, with mean differences increasing by age 20 so that there is little overlap between men's and women's strength scores. The strength changes described here include only measures of isometric strength, without any measures of strength as part of movement skills. Strength is quite variable within

individuals and among groups, can increase greatly with training, and can decrease with inactivity.

SEX DIFFERENCES

Sex differences in favour of males have been found in many of the normative maximal performance comparisons reviewed in this chapter. These sex differences have been traditionally viewed as being due to both intrinsic and extrinsic constraints such as biological make-up, practice, societal influences, and participation experiences, as well as the type of tasks that have been tested and are subject to constant change. The point we make about differences, whether they are due to sex or to some atypicality, is that the differences are clearly not due to some unidimensional construct, but are the result of the transactional effects of intrinsic and extrinsic constraints. To illustrate this point we want to present two examples of the potential impact of one of these constraints: participation experiences as related to sex roles.

Our first illustration concerns the effort that individuals must make when attempting to produce a maximal performance. Fleishman (1964) conducted an extensive study of movement abilities, including a national sample of adolescents who were asked to make a maximal performance on a number of strength and skill tasks and summarizes the mean performance scores of males and females on two strength measures. Grip strength changes were linear for males and females from age 13 through age 18; males had higher mean scores at each age and increased at a more rapid rate. This finding is similar to the normative strength changes noted earlier. An important point is that females doubled their mean strength score during this 5-year period. However, a different picture emerges when examining the mean score changes for holding a half sit-up. Males maintained a steady figure of approximately 60 seconds, whereas females decreased steadily from almost 60 seconds at age 13 to just 20 seconds at age 18.

How can we explain this decrease in females' strength for one task and their increase in another task? In a half sit-up, the upper body is raised off the ground and is held in that position as long as possible. Why would an individual's ability to do this decrease? One possibility is a loss of strength in the abdominal muscles, but everything we know indicates that individuals become stronger during these years, as seen with grip strength and other strength tasks. A more reasonable explanation is that during these years it becomes less important to females to do this task; it is simply boring to them. The motivational state is sex-related and is probably a product of experiences occurring in the context of our society's sex roles. This illustration is obvious, whereas others are not, but we must consider that many sex differences are greatly influenced by sex-related experiences.

Our first example points to negative influences that serve to increase sex differences. The opposite consideration is to offer females participation experiences similar to those for males and see if the sex differences decrease. Although we cannot do this in controlled experiments, we can look at sex differences during time periods in which participation experiences change. This means that we must look in retrospect at differences in normative comparisons across an extended time period. As females are offered more participation opportunities and the activities become more important to them, so the differences in maximum performances between the sexes are decreasing in many areas.

INDIVIDUAL CHANGE

Descriptions of change in movement development are primarily descriptions of group patterns of change and the main problem is that movement development data are mostly cross-sectional, whereas longitudinal data are needed to chart individual patterns of change. Longitudinal studies are time consuming and are limited by many methodological considerations, including loss of participants, effects of retesting, cost, and problems in analysing gain scores in changing distributions. Nonetheless, several longitudinal studies have been made of performance on the play-game skills included in this chapter.

The results from the five longitudinal studies are used to describe individual change in several play-game skills. Children were tested in each study for at least 3 years, with intervals between test sessions varying from 6 months to 1 year. Each study included a test of throwing distance or velocity, and all but one (Halverson et al 1982) included a timed dash and a standing long jump. The studies of Glassow and Kruse (1960) and Keogh (1969) started with more than one age group, which extended the age range but meant that each child was tested for only part of the age range indicated focused on the early and middle school years. Also, Rarick and Smoll (1967) and Halverson et al (1982) held a final test session after a 5-year interval to provide a longer age interval between the initial and final test sessions.

Individual change for the children in these studies is outlined here in two ways. First, the stability of individual performance is determined by the correlations between the test sessions. The higher the correlation, the more stable the relative level of performance of individuals for the time period. Second, and only for the studies of Espenschade (1940) and Keogh (1969), individual patterns of change are described by plotting separately

individual children's performances, rather than plotting the group's mean performance. The correlations provide a statistical summary of stability, which is a group average and conceals individual patterns of change. Each way of looking at individual change is useful, but each is limited in relation to what the other provides.

Stability

The stability of individual performance is the extent to which an individual maintains the same relative position for two test sessions, even though others increase, perhaps even decrease, in absolute performance score. An individual maintains the same relative position when changing the same amount as the group mean change. If most individuals maintain approximately the same relative performance level for two test sessions, the correlation will be higher than when many individuals change their relative performance level. However, a correlation is a summarizing statistic, and some individuals may be more or less stable than indicated by the size of the correlation. This again means that some will be more stable and others will be less stable than indicated by a correlation or a group of correlations.

Two groups of correlations have been taken from the longitudinal studies on jump, throw, and dash. First, the correlations between adjacent test sessions (e.g. test sessions 1 and 2, 2 and 3, and 3 and 4) are summarized showing a short-term view of stability. Second, the correlations between early and late test sessions are summarized as a long-term view of stability. Short-term stability, for test intervals of 6 and 12 months, showed that, as expected, the correlations generally are high because only a small amount of change takes place in such a short time period. From large numbers of studies correlations are listed for jump and throw combined, with more than 40% of the correlations being 0.8 or larger and only around 10% being less than 0.6 (Keogh and Sugden 1985). The general picture is that children maintain similar relative performance levels on these tasks over a short time period, but the size of correlation for type of task and sex group varied among the studies.

Long-term stability for test intervals of 3 to 10 years has data from the study of Rarick and Smoll (1967), which has the most comprehensive coverage in terms of early data from age 7 to age 12 and a final test session at age 14. Again, the correlations vary considerably in size among studies, which means that a number of studies are needed to compile a general picture of long-term stability. The standing long jump has the most consistent set of correlations, with all but a few values in a range from 0.5 to 0.7. The correlations for females are slightly higher overall, but males have similar or higher values in many comparisons.

The correlations for throw and dash range from quite large to quite small, with many contradictions in sex comparisons among the studies. The correlations for the throw are low for the males and females in the Rarick and Smoll study (1967), high for the females in studies by Espenschade (1940) and Halverson and colleagues (1982), and above 0.6 for the males in Espenschade's (1940) and Keogh's (1965) studies. The correlations for the dash are high for the females in the Rarick–Smoll (1967) and Glassow–Kruse (1960) studies and low for the males in the Rarick–Smoll (1967) and Espenschade (1940) studies and are above 0.7 for the males in the Keogh (1965) study.

The general picture for long-term stability is that correlations can be quite high across reasonably long time periods, but it is not unusual to find low correlations and quite different correlations among studies. There may be methodological considerations that contribute to the rather variable pattern of results for long-term stability. It is not easy, however, to sort out the effects of different examiners, different scoring procedures, and the like without conducting a series of longitudinal studies. The best we can do at the moment is recognize that we do not have a clear picture of stability of movement performance over an extended time period.

Individual patterns of change
Individual patterns of change have seldom been documented systematically, and there are many problems in compiling such a representation. One problem is that there are no conventional procedures, particularly to summarize individual patterns of change into similar types of groups. General impressions of individual change have been recorded in comments about individual children, and some detailed records and comments are available, as illustrated by the classic studies in Shirley's (1931) movement biographies and the analyses of changes in movement mechanics (Halverson et al 1982). Espenschade (1940) prepared what is probably the most extensive set of individual descriptions of changes in movement development. Her descriptions were organized according to biological maturity, with extensive comments about relationships to other aspects of the development of the males and females who were part of the adolescent study conducted at the University of California.

Data and analyses from Keogh (1969) show individual patterns of change and some of the difficulties in studying them. Individual change includes both absolute (raw score) gain and alternations in relative level or position within a group. Individual children generally increase

or gain in absolute level of performance score over several years, but the amount of change between test sessions may vary considerably. The pattern of change for an individual also should be viewed in relation to that of other children in the appropriate age, sex, or regional group. A child might have a steady rate of absolute improvement, though not matching the pattern of group change. Stability, therefore, can be viewed from different and sometimes conflicting perspectives.

Individual change in movement performance was studied as part of the Santa Monica project (Keogh 1965). The first year of the project was a normative test programme conducted in the school year of 1963–64, with 13 movement tasks and 1171 children in kindergarten to the sixth grade (Keogh 1965). The subjects for a longitudinal test programme to examine individual change were selected from all 6- and 8-year-olds. The children were ages 6 years 0 months to 6 years 11 months or 8 years 0 months to 8 years 11 months at the first test session, and 9 years 6 months to 10 years 5 months or 11 years 6 months to 12 years 5 months at the eighth and final test session. The four tests used for describing individual change were standing long jump, ball throw for distance, 15m hop for time, and grip strength (hand dynamometer; sum of right and left grips). Group data were used to calculate correlations for each test across all combinations of the eight test sessions, and the correlations show group stability (the extent to which individuals maintain a relatively similar level of performance in the group during a designated time period).

A simple procedure was used to measure individual stability in the range of standard scores across the test sessions. Each performance score for each child was converted to a standard score so that one standard deviation was 10 points and the mean score was 0. The range of standard scores for each task was converted to a stability score by calculating the difference between the lowest and the highest standard score after the most discrepant standard score was removed. The stability was increased by excluding the most discrepant score and limiting the standard scores to a range of –20 to +20. The purpose was to determine the general level of stability over time and not to predict individual scores.

A stability score was calculated to find the width of the range of standard scores, or the width of the relative level of achievement, on a task across the eight test sessions. On each of the four tasks many children had stability scores of 12 or less, which indicates that the width of their general level of achievement was 1.2 or fewer units of standard deviation. A few children were more variable than this, but many were less variable, as approximately 50% of the stability scores were less than 10. The problem remains to decide what should be used as a criterion level or cut-off for identifying stable and unstable. A stability score of 5 seems quite stable, and an argument could be made for 10, as a general level of achievement (good, average, poor) probably includes a range of one standard deviation. How much further should a stability criterion be extended? Our opinion is that many children were quite stable in relative performance level on individual tasks, but others might not view a stability score of 12 as stable. Stability of individual performance can be quite high for both short and long time periods, but there can be considerable variation from one study to the next. Individual stability for shorter periods of time is likely to be quite high because only a small amount of change is expected. Females tend to be more stable than males, although contradictions to this general statement are easy to find, and results within some tasks vary in different studies. In later chapters, the changing nature of the conditions over time is analysed, occasionally detailing children's experiences in formal intervention.

SUMMARY

Normative data for a variety of movement tasks were presented to trace changes in movement proficiency from the early school years to and through puberty. The general picture is that movement performance improves markedly during these years, meaning that mean scores will double and even quadruple or will decrease by similar proportions for tasks in which proficiency is measured by a decrease in the performance score. The absolute amount of improvement is greater in the earlier years up to ages 10 or 12 for reaction time and many manual movements. The mean changes in play-game skills and strength continue to later ages, particularly for males. Changes in the components of performance scores were described as a way to study the nature of change in these movement tasks. Changes in movement strategies can be inferred from changes in component scores, as demonstrated by alternating and braking strategies in stabilometer movements and discrete and continuous strategies in moving pegs.

Males' and females' mean performance differences do not follow a consistent pattern across the normative data reviewed. Small and occasionally significant mean differences on manual movements and balancing tasks favour first one and then the other. The mean reaction times clearly are smaller (faster) for young adult males and perhaps for young male children, but the mean differences are fairly insignificant for most recent movement tasks. Young males have small and significantly better mean performance scores on play-game skills. These differences become quite large during adolescence when the mean performance scores for females tend to level off, though they continue to improve for males. A similar pattern of mean differences is expected when comparing the strength of males and females, except that the females' mean scores continue to improve during adolescence, but at a lesser rate than the males'.

An important qualification for the many statements about age and sex comparisons is that distributions sometimes overlap to the extent that many individual children perform more like the comparison group than like their age or sex group. However, male–female mean differences on strength and some play-game skills become sufficiently large by late adolescence that few females score better than any but the lower-scoring males. This is a constantly changing situation as experiences by sex varies. Individual patterns of change are more difficult to describe and analyse and we have only individual 'pictures' of change. Individual change also should include change across different types of movement achievements, and perhaps we need to make even more detailed descriptions of individual change and link change to what individuals do to be competent in their environments.

Movement abilities

This final section takes a brief look at movement abilities that are thought to underlie aptitudes that suggest general traits or qualities. These traits are thought to determine the level of performance in similar movement situations and function throughout an individual's lifetime. We all think and speak of abilities when we use terms such as agility, coordination, dexterity, rhythm, speed, and balance, and we often describe people in terms of ability, such as having good eye–hand coordination or poor dynamic balance.

An ability is an inference derived from observing performance consistencies across similar kinds of movement tasks. This means that an individual consistently performing at the same level on several movement tasks indicates that a basic trait or quality is responsible for the consistent level. Ability can be quite broad, as when stating that an individual is athletic, or can be more limited, as when saying that an individual has poor arm speed. An ability or a combination of abilities should predict levels of performance across a number of movement tasks, as described in more detail in Chapter 1.

Two issues are involved in studying the development of movement abilities. One is identifying children's movement abilities, and the other is the extent of changes in these abilities. Identification obviously must be accomplished before changes can be studied.

FACTOR ANALYSIS

The basic approach to identifying abilities and testing related predictions uses factor analysis, which is a mathematical procedure for determining the extent of commonality or similarity among tests. Each cluster or grouping of similar tests is viewed as representing a factor or ability. The process begins with the investigator preparing a tentative list of what seem to be important movement abilities, with several movement tasks being selected to represent each ability. A sample of people is tested on each of the movement tasks; all combinations of performance scores are correlated and the correlations are analysed to see how the tasks cluster or group. Each cluster is a factor identified by the nature of the clustered tasks, and is labelled by the investigator. A factor analysis leads to identifying those factors that represent abilities.

There are many ways to calculate a factor analysis, depending on the particular mathematical model selected and the related analysis rules. Any factor analysis defines the mathematical levels of the relationships among tests and a level of relationship is the loading of a test to a particular direction or vector in space. By grouping tests with high loadings on a particular vector, we can find those tests that best represent the vector and, because these tests have something in common, we now can think of them as representing a factor. If the loadings are high, the factor will be more robust than when the loadings are low. Additionally, factor A will be more distinct if tests loading high on factor A do not load high on other factors.

The next step is to name or label the factor by looking at the high test loadings on the factor and using the nature of the tasks to formulate a description. It is important to note that the factors are labelled by the viewer. The viewer should thus not accept the factor labels as fixed. Anyone can and should help name factors. Factor analyses of movement performance have been performed primarily to study the movement abilities of adult males, often in regard to military job requirements, such as predicting who will be successful in different phases of pilot training.

CHILDREN'S MOVEMENT ABILITIES

A comprehensive study of children's movement abilities was directed by Rarick and described in a book by Rarick et al (1976).

The Rarick project

The Rarick project was conducted, first, to describe a factor structure and, second, to describe person clusters or typologies. The factor structure was derived by the process used in the Fleishman (1964) study to find out how tests group or cluster. A second set of analyses was made to discover the grouping or clustering of persons who have similar performances across the factors and, thus, represent a type of mover. The two types of analyses identify test clusters and person clusters, and we can infer from them what the types of abilities and persons might be.

Test clusters

The Rarick project began by formulating an ability list and selecting tests for each. Forty-six tests were used to represent 12 abilities. The tests include seven measures of physical size and body composition (abilities 11 and 12), 17 measures of strength, endurance, and flexibility (abilities 1, 2, 3, 5, and 10), eight measures of manual control (abilities 6 and 7), and 14 measures of body control (abilities 4, 8, and 9). Five tests involving running, jumping, and throwing are listed in abilities 2 and 5 as strength and endurance, whereas others might consider these tests as measures of body control. The Rarick project included a variety of tests that were carefully pretested and well administered and many that were used by Fleishman (1964) examining the relationships among measures of physical size, body composition, strength, endurance, flexibility, manual control, and body control.

The Rarick project's main concern was to compare the movement factor structure of typically developing children and children with intellectual disabilities. The 46 tests were administered to 145 typically developing children, ages 6 to 9, and 261 children with intellectual disabilities divided into younger (ages 6–9) and older (ages 10–13) age groups. Our summary will focus on the typically developing children. The test data were correlated separately for males and females, with age partialled to remove the possible confounding effect of the 4-year age span within each of the age groups. Six factor analyses then were calculated separately for males and females, which made it possible to find factors that consistently appear, regardless of the analysis being employed.

Six comparable common factors (CCFs) were identified for the males and females in the Rarick project: (1) strength, power, and body size; (2) gross limb coordination; (3) fine visual–motor coordination; (4) fat or dead weight; (5) balance; and (6) leg power and coordination. These factors had three or more tests with loadings of 0.40 or higher and were found in at least four of the six factor analyses. A general inspection of the factors for males and females indicates a distinct similarity. The similarity of each factor was tested by calculating the cosines between factor axes to provide the agreement cosines listed for each factor in Table 6.5. Although not a correlation coefficient, an agreement cosine indicates the similarity of a factor for males and females in much the same way. There are strong similarities for all but comparable common factor 2 (cosine=0.73) and comparable common factor 6 (cosine=0.69), and the overall similarity is quite impressive. The level of performance may be

TABLE 6.5
Comparable common factors (CCF)[a]

Factor (agreement cosine)	Average loadings[b]	
	Boys	**Girls**
CCF 1: strength–power–body size (0.95)		
Bicycle with resistance	87	68
Height	85	47
Knee flexion	84	61
Grip strength right	80	64
Bi-acromial breadth	78	57
Weight	75	
Grip strength left	73	62
Knee extension	73	58
Elbow flexion	68	69
Bicycle without resistance	70	50
Elbow extension	66	65
Bicycle ergometer total		66
Physical working capacity (170)		53
CCF 2: gross limb–eye coordination (0.73)		
Target throw horizontal	80	60
Target throw vertical	79	42
Softball throw	72	68
Mat crawl	60	
Tyre run	52	60
CCF 3: fine visual–motor coordination (0.97)		
Purdue pegboard	78	68
Minnesota manipulative	72	75
Ring stacking	70	73
Golf ball placement	65	58
Two-plate tapping	65	54
Tyre run	62	
Pursuit rotor (40rpm)	57	
CCF 4: fat or dead weight (0.95)		
Abdominal skinfold	94	88
Subscapular skinfold	92	91
Triceps skinfold	82	86
Weight	49	77
Bi-iliac breadth		66
Bi-acromial breadth		57
Scramble		51
CCF 5: balance (0.89)		
Railwalk sideways	c	67
Stork test	57	55
Railwalk backwards	c	58
Railwalk forwards		58
Target throw vertical		50

TABLE 6.5

(Continued)

Factor (agreement cosine)	Average loadings[b]	
	Boys	**Girls**
CCF 6: leg power and coordination (0.69)		
Scramble	53	47
32m dash	c	81
137m dash	c	74
Vertical jump		70
Standing broad jump		58
Mat crawl		c

[a]Keogh and Sugden (1985) based on data from Rarick et al (1976). [b]Average of three orthogonal solutions with decimal point omitted. Blank cells indicate that two or more of the three loadings were less than 0.40. [c]Only two of three loadings were 0.40 or above. rpm, rotations per minute.

quite different, with males generally having higher mean performance scores, but the factors for males and females are very much the same. The factors for children with intellectual disabilities, analysed separately for younger and older males and females, were similar, although not to the extent for typically developing males and females. A major finding in the Rarick project is the similarity of factors identified for children, regardless of sex and intellectual level of functioning.

According to the factors in Table 6.5, comparable common factor 1 had many test loadings above 0.40 for what appears to be strength and body size, as listed for hypothesized abilities 1, 2, 3, and 12. Notice that strength did not divide into several factors, and endurance did not appear as a separate factor. Comparable common factor 6 included some of the tests proposed as explosive muscular strength, and the distinction seems to be that comparable common factor 6 is body control or coordination to run and jump, whereas comparable common factor 1 is limited to force production with few coordination problems to solve. This may be strength as a more direct output (comparable common factor 1) compared with strength as an indirect part of maximal performance in more skilful movements (comparable common factor 6).

Manual control was identified in CCF 3 in essentially the way listed in hypothesized ability 7. We use manual control to label this factor because it includes manipulate dexterity and some visual–spatial control, as discussed in Chapter 3. Throwing skills of accuracy and distance were the primary definers in comparable common factor 2, which the Rarick project called gross limb–eye coordination.

The overall power of the Rarick project can be seen in the six analyses accounting for an estimated 72% of the total variance for males and 68% for females. The reverse of this is that approximately 30% of the total variance was not attached or not related in describing factors for these tests and participants. Nevertheless, this is quite good when considering the difficulty of accounting for all of anything. The tests in the Rarick project were varied and were analysed in a rigorous, multiple fashion with a most important finding being the similarity in factors identified for males and females.

Person clusters

A second type of analysis was made in the Rarick project to identify person clusters, to make a graphic profile of relatively homogeneous groups of subjects. Using the factors identified for a group, the children's scores in that group were converted to standard scores for the tests used to define comparable common factors 1 to 6, except that comparable common factor 4 (fat or dead weight) was omitted. The level of performance in the form of a standard score was used to place a score of one child on one test in relation to those of all other children in the group. A profile was constructed for each child to describe the relative level of performance on each factor. A series of analyses was made to cluster or group individuals with similar profiles for the five factors shown in Table 6.5. Nine person clusters emerged and all but 10 of the 145 males and females were placed in one of the nine person clusters.

Typologies give a different view of factors or abilities because they refer to individuals rather than tests. One warning is that a different set of person clusters or profiles should be expected if this type of analysis is carried out separately for males and females. Combining males and females into one analysis will alter the standard scores if their means and distributions are not similar. This is illustrated in type 8, in which eight males and only one female are found to have quite high strength–power and gross limb–eye coordination (throwing accuracy and distance), with average performance in the other factors. The reverse is true in type 7, in which nine females and only one male are identified. It would be useful to place individuals in a typology within their sex group.

SUMMARY

The use of factor analysis was reviewed as a procedure for identifying factors and inferring the existence of abilities. Researchers began with a hypothesized set of abilities to be tested and adjusted in a sequence of studies, including a demonstration that factors (abilities) can predict achievement in a variety of situations.

Adult males' movement abilities have been reliably identified, although with rather limited applications. The Rarick project (Rarick et al 1976) is a starting point with a good preliminary structure and results, with an important finding being the similarity of factors for males and females, even though their mean performance levels generally are quite different. Another important contribution is the recognition of person clusters in addition to test clusters. The clustering of profiles should remind us that factors identify only abilities, whereas it is also appropriate to study how levels of abilities are combined in individuals to represent different types of movers.

The search for children's movement abilities has been limited primarily by the lack of systematic and continuing efforts. Part of this is the enormity and complexity of this line of research. Also, most studies to date have focused on other issues, such as test validations and perceptual-motor learning problems, which provide information about children's movement abilities only as a secondary and not as a continuing concern. In general, abilities usually become more complicated with age, which requires examining movement factors at different ages. Many movement factors have been found for adults, which means that the movement factors for children also must be numerous or must increase in number with age. A recent example of this is to be found in the validation of the Movement Assessment Battery for Children (Henderson et al 2007). Data from 1172 children across three age bands (3–6y, 7–10y, and 11–16y) were used with confirmatory factor analysis and structural equation modelling to explore the relationships between the tasks. In the younger group, a complex factor structure emerged, providing evidence for an independent general factor as well as specific factors representing the three components of the Movement Assessment Battery for Children, version 2 (MABC2): manual dexterity, aiming and catching,

and balance. In the middle age band, four correlated factors emerged with the additional one being the distinction between static and dynamic balance. In addition, a second-order general factor emerged explaining much of the variance in each primary factor. By age group 11 to 16 years the three-factor structure of the sections of the MABC2 was confirmed with little evidence of a general factor (Schulz et al 2011). The authors interpreted this as confirmation of the differentiation of abilities as the child develops; this finding needs to be confirmed and extended.

Summary

At 7 years of age, typically developing children will have acquired a total range of fundamental motor skills that naturally occur throughout development. They will have the basic units from which to build the skills that are required in daily life in response to increasingly complex environmental demands. From this age they are exposed to a wider variety of contexts that make increasing demands upon their abilities. In this chapter we have covered two major aspects of their abilities that will influence their participation and performance.

First, in the skills that require more of control and coordination, such as the development of spatial and temporal accuracy in coincidence timing, whether this is interception or continuous matching, the major increases in performance appear to occur between the ages of 6 and 7 years and 12 and 13 years. By the latter age, the performance either approaches that of adults, or the curve of improvement is shallower after age 12 or 13. From 7 years of age until their teenage years they become more proficient in their predication of moving objects and persons, allowing them to intercept or avoid, depending on the situation. In short, they are much better at establishing an accurate perception–action match. One can speculate whether this is due to the development of individual abilities such as visual perception or the more likely scenario that this development is more holistic in that the child, through experience, becomes more adept at solving the contextual movement problem in relation to his or her developing resources. These developing resources are functionally linked to the environmental situation as one process rather than as individual units.

Second, this profile of development also seems to be similar in some maximum performance tasks involving the manual skills of manipulation or tapping, and tasks involving reaction and movement time. There are large improvements on these tasks from age 7 to the teenage years, with less of a gain from then on. Improvement on these tasks enables the mover to have more time in which to anticipate and make predictions, thus contributing to an overall increase in tasks that require these qualities.

However, in tasks that involve maximum comparisons on tasks for which whole body actions are involved, development carries on after age 12 to 13, particularly in males. This is very much because of the changes that take place during puberty, which allow the movers to use their increased strength, speed, and endurance to increase their performance on tasks for which such qualities are at a premium. Thus, with the onset of puberty, both males and females are able to make good perception–action matches, but there is still much to come in terms of maximum total body performance. In Chapter 2, we note many of these changes and show how the child changes during puberty on maximum performance tasks. From this time on, because the functional tasks in which we engage are often a mixture of demands ranging from coordination to strength, flexibility, and endurance, the final product is often a combination of these factors with their relative contributions varying according to task demands.

REFERENCES

Adolph KE, Vereijken B, Shrout PE (2003) What changes in infant walking and why. *Child Dev* 74: 475–497. http://dx.doi.org/10.1111/1467-8624.7402011

Ammons RB, Alprin SI, Ammons CH (1955) Rotary pursuit performance as related to sex and age of pre-adult subject. *J Exp Psychol* 49: 127–133. http://dx.doi.org/10.1037/h0044345

Annett M (1970) The growth of manual performance and speed. *Br J Psychol* 61: 587–592. http://dx.doi.org/10.1111/j.2044-8295.1970.tb01274.x

Annett M (1996) In defence of the right shift theory. *Percept Mot Skills* 82: 115–137. http://dx.doi.org/10.2466/pms.1996.82.1.115

Anooshian GP (1975) Component analysis of stabilometer performance for elementary school boys. Master's thesis, University of California at Los Angeles.

Assaiante C (1998) Development of locomotor balance control in healthy children. *Neurosci Biobehav Rev* 22: 527–532. http://dx.doi.org/10.1016/S0149-7634(97)00040-7

Bachman JC (1961) Motor learning and performance as related to age and sex in two measures of balance coordination. *Res Q* 32: 123–137.

Bailey DC (1968) Longitudinal analyses of strength and motor development of boys ages twelve through seventeen years. PhD dissertation, University of Oregon.

Bard C, Fleury L, Carriere J, Belloc J (1981) Components of the coincidence anticipation behaviour of children aged from 6 to 16 years. *Percept Motor Skill* 52: 547–556. http://dx.doi.org/10.2466/pms.1981.52.2.547

Burton AW, Rodgerson RW (2003) The development of throwing behaviour. In: Savelsbergh G, David K, Van der Kamp J, Bennett S, editors. *Development of Movement Coordination in Children*. London: Routledge, pp. 225–239.

Chohan A, Savelsbergh GJ, van Kampen P, Wind M, Verheul MH (2006) Postural adjustments and bearing angle use in interceptive actions. *Exp Brain Res* 17: 47–55. http://dx.doi.org/10.1007/s00221-005-0239-z

Chohan A, Verheul MH, van Lampen PM, Wind M, Savelsbergh GJ (2008) Children's use of the bearing angle in interceptive actions. *J Motor Behav* 40: 18–28. http://dx.doi.org/10.3200/JMBR.40.1.18-28

Clarke HH (1971) *Physical and Motor Tests in the Medford Growth Boys' Growth Study*. Englewood Cliffs, NJ: Prentice Hall.

Connolly KJ (1968) Some mechanisms involved in the development of motor skills. *Aspects Educ* 7: 8–100.

Connolly KJ (1970) Response speed, temporal sequencing, and information processing in children. In: Connolly KJ, editor. *Mechanisms of Motor Skill Development*. New York: Academic Press, pp. 161–188.

Connolly KJ, Brown K, Bassett E (1968) Developmental changes in some components of a motor skill. *Br J Psychol* 59: 305–314. http://dx.doi.org/10.1111/j.2044-8295.1968.tb01145.x

Davol SH, Hasting ML, Klein DA (1965) Effect of age, sex, and speed of rotation on rotary pursuit performance by young children. *Percept Motor Skill* 21: 351–357. http://dx.doi.org/10.2466/pms.1965.21.2.351

Davol SH, Breakell SL (1968) Sex differences in rotary pursuit performance of young children: a follow up. *Percept Motor Skill* 26: 1199–1202. http://dx.doi.org/10.2466/pms.1968.26.3c.1199

Denckla MB (1973) Development of speed in repetitive and successive finger movements in normal children. *Dev Med Child Neurol* 15: 635–645. http://dx.doi.org/10.1111/j.1469-8749.1973.tb05174.x

Dorfman PW (1977) Timing and anticipation: a developmental perspective. *J Motor Behav* 9: 67–79.

Eckert HM, Rarick GL (1976) Stabilometer performance of educable mentally retarded and normal children. *Res Q* 47: 619–623.

Elliott JM, Connolly KJ (1974) Hierarchical structure in skill development. In: Connolly KJ, Bruner JS, editors. *The Growth of Competence*. London: Academic Press, pp. 135–168.

Espenschade AS (1940) Motor performance in adolescence. *Monographs of the Society for Research in Child Development* 5 (1, serial, no 24).

Fitts PM (1954) The information capacity of the human motor system in controlling the amplitude of movement. *J Exp Psychol* 47: 381–391. http://dx.doi.org/10.1037/h0055392

Fitts PM, Peterson JR (1964) Information capacity of discrete motor responses. *J Exp Psychol* 67: 103–112. http://dx.doi.org/10.1037/h0045689

Fleishman EA (1964) *The Structure and Measurement of Physical Fitness*. Englewood Cliffs, NJ: Prentice Hall.

Fulton CD, Hubbard AW (1975) Effect of puberty on reaction and movement time. *Res Q* 46: 335–344.

Gardner RA (1979) Throwing balls in a basket as a test of motor coordination: normative data on 1350 school children. *J Clin Child Psychol* 8: 152–155. http://dx.doi.org/10.1080/15374417909532911

Gentile AM, Higgins P, Miller EA, Rosen BM (1975) The structure of motor tasks. *Movement* 7: 11–28.

Glassow RB, Kruse P (1960) Motor performance of girls age 6 to 14 years. *Res Q* 31: 426–433.

Goetzinger CP (1961) A re-evaluation of the Heath rail walking test. *J Educ Res* 54: 187–191.

Halverson HM, Roberton MA, Langendorfer S (1982) Development of the overarm throw: movement and ball velocity changes by seventh grade. *Res Q Exercise Sport* 53: 198–205.

Hay L (1981) The effect of amplitude and accuracy requirements on movement time in children. *J Motor Behav* 13: 177–186.

Heath SR (1949) The rail walking test: preliminary maturational norms for boys and girls. *Motor Skill Res Exchange* 1: 34–36.

Henderson SE, Sugden DA, Barnett A (2007) *Movement Assessment Battery for Children*, 2nd edition. London: Harcourt Assessment.

Hodgkins J (1962) Influence of age on the speed of reaction and movement time in females. *J Gerontol* 17: 385–389.

Hodgkins J (1963) Reaction time and speed of movement in males and females of various ages. *Res Q* 34: 335–343.

Horn PW (1975) Pursuit rotor speed, sex differences, and reminiscence in young children. *J Psychol* 91: 81–85. http://dx.doi.org/10.1080/00223980.1975.9915801

Jacklin CN, Snow ME, Maccoby EE (1981) Tactile sensitivity and muscle strength in newborn boys and girls. *Infant Behav Dev* 4: 261–268. http://dx.doi.org/10.1016/S0163-6383(81)80028-8

Jordan DB (1966) Longitudinal analysis of strength and motor ages development of boys seven through twelve years. PhD dissertation, University of Oregon.

Kail R, Salthouse TA (1994) Processing speed as a mental capacity. *Acta Psychol (Amst)* 86: 199–225. http://dx.doi.org/10.1016/0001-6918(94)90003-5

Keogh JF (1965) Motor performance of elementary school children. (USPHS grants MH 08319-01 and HD 01059) Department of Physical Education, University of California at Los Angeles.

Keogh JF (1969) Change in motor performance during early school years. Technical report 2-69 (USPHS grant HD 1059). Department of Physical Education, University of California at Los Angeles.

Keogh JF, Sugden DA (1985) *Movement Skill Development*. New York: Macmillan.

Kerr B, Blanchard C, Miller K (1980) Children's use of sequence information in partially predictable reaction time sequences. *Journal of Experimental Child Psychology* 29: 529–549.

Kerr R (1975) Movement control and maturation in elementary-grade children. *Percept Motor Skill* 41: 151–154. http://dx.doi.org/10.2466/pms.1975.41.1.151

Konzack J, Borutta M, Topka H, Dichgans J (1995) The development of goal directed reaching in infants: hand trajectory formation and joint torque control. *Exp Brain Res* 106: 156–168.

Konczak J, Dichgans J (1997) The development toward stereotypic arm kinematics during reaching in the first three years of life. *Exp Brain Res* 117: 346–354.

Kuhtz-Buschbeck JP, Stolze H, Boczek-Funcke A, John K, Illert M (1998) Development of prehension movements in children: a kinematic study. *Exp Brain Res* 122: 424–432. http://dx.doi.org/10.1007/s002210050530

Leavitt JL (1979) Cognitive demands of skating and stick handling in ice hockey. *Can J Applied Sport Sci* 4: 46–55.

Lenoir M, Musch E, Janssens M, Theiry E, Uyttenhove J (1999) Intercepting moving objects during self motion. *J Motor Behav* 31: 55–67. http://dx.doi.org/10.1080/00222899909601891

Lenoir M, Musch E, Janssens M, Savelsbergh GJP (2002) Rate of change of angular bearing as the relevant property in a horizontal interception task during locomotion. *J Motor Behav* 34: 385–401. http://dx.doi.org/10.1080/00222890209601955

Montoye HJ, Lamphiear DE (1977) Grip and arm strength in males and females age 10–69. *Res Q* 48: 108–120.

Newell KM, Scully DM, Tenenbaum F, Hardiman S (1989) Body scale and the development of prehension. *Dev Psychobiol* 22: 11–13. http://dx.doi.org/10.1002/dev.420220102

Peacock WH (1960) *Achievement Scales in Physical Education for Boys and Girls Ages Seven Through Fifteen.* Chapel Hill: University of North Carolina Press.

Rarick GL, Smoll FL (1967) Stability of growth in strength and motor performance from childhood to adolescence. *Hum Biol* 39: 260–268.

Rarick GL, Dobbins DA, Broadhead GD (1976) *The Motor Domain and its Correlates in Educationally Handicapped Children.* Englewood Cliffs, NJ: Prentice Hall.

Rippee NE, Pangrazi RP, Corbin CB, Borsdorf L, Peterson G, Pangrazi D (1990) Throwing profiles of first and fourth grade boys and girls. *Phys Educ* 47: 180–185.

Salmoni AW, Pascoe C (1978) Fitts' reciprocal tapping task: a developmental study. In: Roberts CG, Newell KM, editors. *Psychology of Motor Behavior and Sport*. Champaign, IL: Human Kinetics, pp. 355–386.

Schulz J, Henderson SE, Sugden DA, Barnett A (2011) Structural validity of the Movement ABC-2 test: factor structure comparisons across three age groups. *Res Dev Disabil* 32: 1361–1369. http://dx.doi.org/10.1016/j.ridd.2011.01.032

Shea CH, Krampitz JB, Northam CC, Ashby AA (1982) Information processing in coincident timing tasks: a developmental perspective. *J Hum Movement Studies* 8: 73–83.

Shirley MM (1931) *The First Two Years: A Study of Twenty Five Babies. Postural and Locomotor Development.* Minneapolis: University of Minnesota Press.

Smits-Engelsman BCM, Sugden DA, Duysens J (2006) Developmental rends in speed accuracy trade off in 6–10 year old children performing rapid reciprocal and discrete aiming movements. *Hum Movement Sci* 25: 37–49. http://dx.doi.org/10.1016/j.humov.2005.12.002

Smoll FL (1974) Development of spatial and temporal elements of rhythmic ability. *J Motor Behav* 6: 53–58.

Smoll FL (1975) Variability in development of spatial and temporal elements of rhythmic ability. *Percept Motor Skill* 40: 140. http://dx.doi.org/10.2466/pms.1975.40.1.140

Spencer RMC, Zelaznick HN, Diedrichsen J, Ivry RB (2003) Disrupted timing of discontinuous but continuous movements by cerebellar lesions. *Science* 300: 1437–1439. http://dx.doi.org/10.1126/science.1083661

Sugden DA (1980) Movement speed in children. *J Motor Behav* 12: 125–132.

Surwillo WW (1977) Developmetal changes in speed of information processing. *J Psychol* 97: 97–102.

Thomas JR, Gallagher JD, Purvis GJ (1981) Reaction time and anticipation time: effects of development. *Res Q Exercise Sport Sci* 52: 359–367.

Vallis LA, McFadyen BJ (2005) Children use different anticipatory control strategies than adults to circumvent an obstacle in the travel path. *Exp Brain Res* 167: 119–127. http://dx.doi.org/10.1007/s00221-005-0054-6

Van Roon D, Caeyenberghs K, Smits-Englesman B, Swinnen SP (2008) Development of feedforward control in a dynamic manual tracking task. *Child Dev* 79: 852–865. http://dx.doi.org/10.1111/j.1467-8624.2008.01163.x

Wade MG (1980) Coincidence anticipation of young normal and handicapped children. *J Motor Behav* 12: 103–112.

Wade MG, Newell KM (1972) Performance criteria for stabilometer learning. *J Motor Behav* 4: 231–239.

Wann JP, Poulter DR, Purcell C (2011) Reduced sensitivity to visual looming inflates the risk posed by speeding vehicles when children try to cross the road. *Psychological Science Online*. http://dx.doi.org/10.1177/0956797611400917

Welford AT, Norris AH, Shock NW (1969) Speed and accuracy of hand movement and their changes with age. *Acta Psychol (Amst)* 30: 3–15. http://dx.doi.org/10.1016/0001-6918(69)90034-1

Williams HG (1973) Perceptual motor development in children. In: Corbin CB, editor. *A Textbook of Motor Development*. Dubuque, IA: William C. Brown, pp. 111–148.

Wolff PH, Hurwitz I (1976) Sex differences in finger tapping: a developmental study. *Neuropsychologia* 14: 35–41.

Zanone PG (1990) Tracking with and without target in 6 to 15 year old boys. *J Mot Behav* 22: 225–249.

Zanone PG, Kelso JAS (1994) The coordination dynamics of learning. In: Swinnen S, Heuer H, Massion J, Caeser P, editors. *Interlimb Coordination: Neural Dynamical and Cognitive Constraints*. San Diego, CA: Academic Press, pp. 462–490.

7
CEREBRAL PALSY

Cerebral palsy: the condition

In most countries worldwide, cerebral palsy is recognized as a condition that is defined primarily as a movement disorder. It has been noted throughout the ages, and in the 19th century it was formally recognized by the British orthopaedic surgeon William Little. In a lecture to the London Obstetrics Society in 1862, he described a disorder that was characterized by difficulties in reaching and grasping, and crawling, together with spasticity in the lower limbs. In this lecture many of the causes were outlined together with descriptions of features of diplegia and quadriplegia, as well as athetosis. It became known as Little's disease and since that time it has gained much attention, with early authors such as Freud in 1897 devoting a complete text to it (*Infantile Cerebral Paralysis*, 1968). In the early part of the 20th century much effort was devoted to treatment with universally accepted classification remaining unresolved. An early attempt at classification was provided by Minear (1956), who also provided guidelines for clinicians and researchers, and a number of studies began to examine aetiological factors and causal pathways (Minear 1956, Gage 1991).

Since the Minear (1956) guidelines, cerebral palsy has been described, analysed and defined in a number of different ways. In all cases of cerebral palsy there is evidence of brain damage, leading to difficulties with the coordination of movement, but the exact location of the damage does differ. The condition varies according to severity, location of the difficulties, and types of movements that are present, with some children having very little movement or control of their movements often in all four limbs, whereas others have fewer problems with the involvement of only one or two limbs. In addition, children with cerebral palsy often have associated difficulties such as sensory and cognitive problems, behavioural difficulties, and additional medical problems such as epilepsy (Pharoah et al 1998). Thus, the concern for parents

and professionals is the total development of the child, not simply a motor coordination difficulty.

Although this chapter concerns the development of children, it is pertinent to note that individuals with cerebral palsy survive well into adulthood, thus making quality of life an overwhelming issue. For individuals with cerebral palsy born between 1940 and 1950, 85% of the cohort survived to 50 years of age compared with the general population of 96% (Hemming et al 2006). Strauss et al (2008) produced a detailed analysis of life expectancy in cerebral palsy clarifying how it is measured, revised estimates, current age of the individual comparisons across countries and issues regarding quality of care. These estimates become important when examining individual profiles in the developing child and making provision for long-term individual support and intervention.

DEFINITION AND CLASSIFICATION

Definition

As with many conditions, the definition of cerebral palsy is not straightforward as it is a condition characterized by a wide range of symptoms that range in severity, type, and limb location. Bax (1964: 297) gave a classic definition of cerebral palsy as 'a non-progressive disorder of movement and posture due to a lesion of the immature brain'.

Additional comments were added by Bax et al (2005) to exclude disorders that were of short-term duration, due to progressive conditions or solely intellectual disability. The debate surrounding definition continues and as criteria for diagnosis do vary, in some cases considerably, comparisons across countries are often difficult. The definition alludes to cerebral palsy describing a number of disorders and this has been taken further by those who describe it as an 'umbrella term' that is used to cover a wide range of complex conditions, indicating that there is heterogeneity in the condition (Mutch et al 1992, Hagberg and Hagberg 1993). However, all the children will show the characteristics of a non-progressive disorder of motor function occurring as a result of brain damage. Mutch et al (1992) use it as an umbrella term for motor disorders, noting that it is non-progressive but adding that it can change, arising early in development as a result of lesions or anomalies in the brain. This raises several issues about what is meant by non-progressive and leads to identification of other conditions that are only tangentially related, leading some to ask whether or not the term is still useful (Stanley et al 2000). Kragelöb-Mann (2005) notes that, with the advance of magnetic resonance imaging (MRI), cerebral palsy may be described on functional/behavioural, neurological, and brain morphology levels, leading to the condition being studied within a range of neuroscience specialties. This would involve descriptions of the total child including the effect of various constitutional substrates on function that would necessitate common definitions and classification.

Despite the difficulties in defining the condition, ultimately most researchers and clinicians have come down in favour of its continuing usage because it is familiar to people and promotes understanding, it is short and unique, it gives considerable flexibility to our descriptions and understanding, and it appears to be more appropriate than any alternative. Baxter and Rosenbloom (2005: 507) in their editorial describe it as 'an old friend, and through familiarity still has a role…unlocking facilities for an affected child and obtaining research funding'.

This thinking was exemplified by a recent and comprehensive review of the term and its definition and classification in Bethesda, Maryland, at the International Workshop on the Definition and Classification of Cerebral Palsy (Bax et al 2005). The recommendation was that the concept should be retained as it is useful for management, epidemiology, and resources in public health and research purposes, but that it was a clinical descriptive term and not an aetiological diagnosis.

International workshop recommendations (Bethesda, Maryland, 2005)
The first part of the recommendations concerns definition and Bax et al (2005) developed the original definition, which was slightly modified in 2007 by many of the same group of authors. The latest version is as follows:

> Cerebral palsy (CP) describes a group of disorders of the development of movement and posture, causing activity limitations that are attributed to non-progressive disturbances that occurred in the developing fetal or infant brain. The motor disorders of cerebral palsy are

often accompanied by disturbance of sensation, cognition, communication, perception, and/or behaviour, by epilepsy and by musculoskeletal problems.

> Rosenbaum et al (2007, p. 9)

This is the most concise optimum definition, but the paper also recognizes that within each part there is a debate surrounding the appropriate wording. For example, terms such as 'activity limitations' are discussed within the International Classification of Functioning framework (WHO, 2001); 'fetal or infant brain' raises the issue of an upper age limit and, although it does not give an exact age, the authors do note that the symptoms will be apparent in the first 2 or 3 years of life and probably have occurred in the first year. Baxter and Rosenbloom (2005) note that substituting 'non-progressive disturbances that occurred in the developing of fetal or infant brain' for 'defect or lesion in the immature brain' possibly widens the condition to include developmental coordination disorder (DCD). While this is a possibility, there is a later chapter (Chapter 8) on DCD as it has a different history and separate body of literature. Blair and Love (2005), in their commentary on the new definition, query four areas:

- What is meant by non-progressive?
- What are the exact age limits for 'disturbance to occur' and the minimum age for it to be recognized in children who die early?
- What is the lower limit of severity required to be given the label of cerebral palsy?
- Are there other syndromes not mentioned that could meet the criteria?

It is clear that establishing a definition and subsequent classification to which all can sign up is a difficult task. However, the commentaries on the definition have stressed the crucial need for consistency such that accurate comparisons can be made for clinical and research work and the effective allocation of resources, and the most recent definition takes us some way to achieving these aims.

Classification

By type
The second part of the recommendations from the Bethesda Workshop involves classification, which is shown in Table 7.1 to include motor abnormalities, associated impairments, anatomical and radiological findings, and causation and timing (Bax et al 2005).

Bax et al (2005) divide these into nature and typology and functional motor abilities. In the former they list

TABLE 7.1
Components of cerebral palsy classification

Motor abnormalities

Nature and typology of the motor disorder: the observed tonal abnormalities assessed on examination (e.g. hypertonia or hypotonia) as well as the diagnosed movement disorders present, such as spasticity, ataxia, dystonia, or athetosis

Functional motor abilities: the extent to which the individual is limited in his or her motor function in all body areas, including oromotor and speech function

Associated impairments

The presence or absence of associated non-motor neurodevelopmental or sensory problems, such as seizures, hearing, or vision impairments, or attentional, behavioural, communicative, and/or cognitive deficits, and the extent to which impairments interact in individuals with cerebral palsy

Anatomical and radiological findings

Anatomical distribution: the parts of the body (such as limbs, trunk, or bulbar region) affected by motor impairments or limitations

Radiological findings: the neuroanatomical findings on computed tomography or magnetic resonance imaging, such as ventricular enlargement, white matter loss, or brain anomaly

Causation and timing

Whether there is a clearly identified cause, as is usually the case with postnatal cerebral palsy (e.g. meningitis or head injury) or when brain malformations are present, and the presumed time frame during which the injury occurred, if known

Reproduced with permission of the publisher from Bax et al (2005).

types of movements that are seen in children with cerebral palsy; more than one type can be seen in an individual but there should be a predominant one to which the child is assigned. They report that the reference and training manual of the Surveillance of Cerebral Palsy in Europe (SCPE) recommends the three groupings of spastic, dyskinetic, and ataxic, with dyskinetic further divided into dystonia and choreoathetosis.

SPASTICITY

Spasticity is the result of cerebral damage and is the most common characteristic of cerebral palsy with about 80% of cases showing some symptoms (Stanley et al 2000). However, there have been many interpretations of the meaning of spasticity. Lin (2004) presents a list of characteristics of spasticity, noting that they are so numerous it would be difficult to measure as the term includes many different aspects of motor dysfunction. It is accepted that these symptoms are diverse and present difficulties in measurement, but they would typically include abnormal control of voluntary movement with excessive co-activation of antagonistic muscles, hypertonia, hyperactive stretch reflexes, associated movements, and stereotypical movement synergies (Shumway-Cook and Woollacott 1995). The increased stretch reflex is often determined by passively stretching and extending muscle groups as they cross a joint (Gage 1991). There is an increased muscle tone (hypertonus) with a build-up of resistance followed by rapid release of tension accompanied by a positive

stretch reflex. This resembles a clasp-knife type of reaction and may occur at the beginning, middle, or end of the movement (Stanley et al 2000). Sugden and Keogh (1990) note that hypertonicity is not evenly distributed throughout the body, nor is it fixed and occurring all the time. A child may have a hypotonic trunk but show hypertonicity in the upper limbs, which may change as a result of changes in body position or actions and environmental context, illustrating the emphasis in this text on a dynamical system. In some severe cases, the spastic condition will limit the child to a small repertoire of movements, whereas in other cases hypertonicity can fluctuate, either increasing or decreasing during the course of a movement (Sugden and Keogh 1990).

Within a general framework emphasizing dynamic systems, Steenbergen and colleagues (2000) propose additional explanations to the stretch reflex for the presence of hypertonicity observed in spasticity noting that there are both neural and non-neural components that come into play. He accepts that the neural basis is reflected through the stretch reflex-generated muscle activity and motor unit activity which act as resistance to muscle lengthening, and passive stretch of relaxed muscle does generate reflex activity leading to hypertonia. But, in line with a dynamical explanation of motor behaviour, he proposes that non-neural components also can lead to an increased resistance to muscle lengthening thus increasing hypertonicity and spasticity. These non-neural components would include temperament of the individual, stress and fatigue, a reduced number of sacromeres with increased resistance to passive stretch and reduced flexibility of the muscle, both leading to a reduction in the range of joint motion. Steenbergen and colleagues (2000) conclude their summary of spasticity by noting that although the characteristics of spasticity tend to be constant across individuals, the variable symptoms that are present all interact to produce an individual disorder.

Spasticity is also categorized by the location of the impairment with three groups of quadriplegia, diplegia, and hemiplegia dominating.

- *Quadriplegia* involves all limbs equally or sometimes with arms affected more than the legs.
- *Diplegia* involves the legs being more affected than the arms.
- *Hemiplegia* involves either the right or left side of the body being solely affected or significantly more affected than the other side.

There are other categories such as monoplegia (one limb) or triplegia (three limbs), but these are rare and usually are included under the category of hemiplegia. A common type of spasticity is hemiplegia involving the location of the condition in one side of the body more than the other or totally in one side. It is generally not noted at birth unless it is very severe and becomes apparent when the child starts to favour one side more than the other in such activities as reaching and grasping. A strong hand preference is seen together with a primitive grasp, some hand fisting and asymmetry of hand use and the lack of hands joining at the midline. There is a general delay in the achievement of various motor milestones with a movement towards a strong preference to undertake activities with the less affected side, in activities such as crawling, creeping, and standing (Sugden and Keogh 1990). Children with spastic hemiplegia, however, often walk as overall balance is not the major problem and it is the hands that are usually more involved than the lower limbs. The onset of walking is sometimes delayed and if non-walking is present, it is usually correlated with either epilepsy or more serious general developmental problems (Bax and Brown 2004). The child walks with the shoulder on the involved side internally rotated, flexed at the elbow and ulnar deviated at the wrist. Often the hand is clenched with the thumb in the palm of the hand. Clinical reports note that restrictions to upper limbs are the more functionally limiting elements, but more surgery and botulinum toxin is often carried out on the lower limbs because of future implications for poor limb alignment and the risk of persistent pain (D Green, personal communication, March 2009).

DYSKINESIA

Dyskinesia is divided into the two areas of dystonia and athetosis with the former having few signs early in life except some possible variations in muscle tone, with abnormal postures and movements beginning around 6 months of life (Bax and Brown 2004). These characteristics involve involuntary movements around the mouth and arms and legs with difficulties in fine and gross motor control. These involuntary muscle contractions force certain parts of the body into abnormal, sometimes painful, movements or postures (Dystonia Medical Research Foundation, www.dystonia-foundation.org). Primary and secondary dystonias of childhood often generalize early in life, leading to deformity and pain as well as reduced participation and independence in children and young adults. Typical problems associated with dystonia include difficulties with mobility, physical function, speech and communication, swallowing, nutrition, bowel and bladder care, seating, limb positioning, sleep patterns, and emotional and social needs.

Athetosis, like spasticity, shows variability in expression across individuals, but the common feature is unsteady and fluctuating tone with often purposeless and bizarre movements that appear to be uncontrollable. The best estimate is that 10% to 20% of children with cerebral palsy can be classified in this group. These movements are assumed to be involuntary and include swiping, hitting, writhing, and rotary movements and are often due to continually changing muscle tone. The fluctuating tone makes it difficult for the child to remain in a stable fixed position; often children are unable to maintain stability of weight on their feet and constantly draw their feet up, taking the weight on one foot while the other 'paws' the ground. All of this action makes it difficult for the child to achieve a good postural stability. Spasms of flexion or extension heighten the problem and the grading of antagonist action is especially poor with muscle contraction of one group not counterbalanced by reciprocal inhibition of the antagonists (Sugden and Keogh 1990). Children with athetosis are generally hypotonic and show a delay in the achievement of movement milestones such as sitting, rolling over, and crawling, together with slow, abnormal involuntary movements often of a writhing variety and a constant motion.

ATAXIA

Like dyskinesis, ataxia is a less common form of cerebral palsy, comprising around 5% to 10% of the cerebral palsy population. Children with ataxia tend to have low muscle tone and demonstrate evidence of difficulties in balance and coordination, leading to difficulties in standing and walking. At birth the infant is floppy with reduced

TABLE 7.2
Classification of cerebral palsy subtypes by respondents

Cerebral palsy subtype	Case number									
	1	2	3	4	5	6	7	8	9	10
Spastic bilateral	12	26	24	29	21	4	16	3		5
Spastic unilateral	16		3			19				
Dyskinetic dystonic		2	1			1	10	9		
Dyskinetic choreoathetotic							1	14		
Dyskinetic non-classifiable					2		1	3	1	
Ataxic					1					
Non-classifiable							1		2	1
Total number of respondents	**28**	**28**	**28**	**29**	**24**	**24**	**29**	**29**	**3**	**5**

Reproduced with permission from the publisher from Gainsborough et al (2008).

muscle tone, being virtually the opposite of spasticity, and this hypotonicity produces an increased range of movements in all joints. Typically, children with ataxic cerebral palsy will walk with a wide-based gait utilized as a compensatory mechanism and they occasionally have a mild intentional tremor (Bax and Brown 2004). It is often associated with damage to the cerebellum and voluntary movements are present but they appear to be clumsy with over- or under-responding to movement challenges, and poor fixation of the head, shoulder, trunk, and pelvis. This inadequate response is often accompanied by wild arm movements, apparently compensating for the inadequacies of other parts of the motor control system. Like other forms of cerebral palsy, there is often delay in reaching motor milestones, and these are particularly detectable if they involve balance mechanisms. In addition, there are also abnormal movements, such as undesirable reflexes, not seen in typically developing children.

CONSISTENCY IN DIAGNOSIS

The diagnosis of cerebral palsy demands skilled expertise and because of the multiple symptoms within each category, the fluctuating nature of the condition, and the occasional mixed forms, it is not always possible to obtain 100% agreement between professionals. Gainsborough et al (2008) report on the validity and reliability of a surveillance of cerebral palsy in Europe, which outlined the collaboration between cerebral palsy surveys and registers in 14 centres in eight countries. Through the use of 10 text-based cases based on patient records, each 300 to 400 words in length, 30 professionals, including 26 doctors, gave a view as to the nature of each case. There was moderate to good level of agreement whether to include a child as a cerebral palsy case with 89% agreement.

However, when it came to examining subtypes, there was some disagreement between bilateral and unilateral spasticity, as shown by case 1 in Table 7.2, and there was also disagreement between spastic and dyskinetic (dystonic) types, such as case 7.

Two other important recommendations, concerning anatomical areas, come from the Bethesda workshop group. First, in addition to the usual method of classifying by severity in the arms and legs, they recommend that trunk and bulbar assessments are also made. Second, they recommend that it is important to distinguish between unilateral and bilateral involvement as this distinction has reasonably good reliability. However, despite the terms being in common usage, they recommend the abandonment of 'diplegia' and 'quadriplegia' in the diagnosis. They advise using a distinction between unilateral and bilateral together with a description of motor capabilities in both upper and lower extremities. They recognize the advances made in imaging technology and recommend that these be used wherever possible (Bax et al 2005).

The classification of cerebral palsy by type has a long history with the usual divisions being made on the nature of the motor disorder, concerning what the movements look and feel like, and the location of the disorder, that is where in the body the disordered movement occurs. Clinicians are skilled at diagnosing the condition and good agreement is often obtained. However, because of the complexity of the condition and the numerous symptoms, it is not always possible to obtain total agreement.

ASSOCIATED CHARACTERISTICS

Of particular interest in recent years has been the recognition that although motor impairment lies at the heart of cerebral palsy, it has become increasingly clear that in

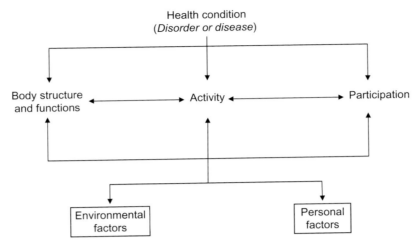

Fig. 7.1 The International Classification Model of Functioning, Disability, and Health. World Health Organization (2001).

many cases other functions are also impaired with corresponding effects on communication, behaviour, cognition, and sensory facilities all having a profound effect on the overall functioning of the child. Any intervention for a child should take account of these when collecting information to plan an intervention programme. Himmelman et al (2006) noted that in their study of 4- to 8-year-old children born between 1991 and 1998 with cerebral palsy in western Sweden, 61% were independent walkers, 31% were unable to walk, and 40% had intellectual disability, indicating that more children had learning problems in this population defined by motor impairment than those who could not walk. Other associated characteristics include epilepsy, sleep disorders, and self-reported quality of life difficulties (Varni et al 2005, Newman et al 2006, Carlsson et al 2008).

The Bethesda workshop (Bax et al 2005) on definition and classification has become a current benchmark by which cerebral palsy is defined and classified. It has been criticized as lacking clarity in some parts, such as what is meant by non-progressive or more definitive age limits (Blair and Love 2005), but overall it has moved the field on to a more comprehensive, collective definition and classification that benefits clinicians, researchers, parents, and, ultimately, the children. These approaches to classification overlap and complement the information presented in Chapter 12.

By ability and function
The International Classification of Functioning, Disability and Health (ICF 2001), developed by the World Health Organization (WHO), focuses on the 'components of health' and is intended for all people, not just those with disabilities. It is a classification system and can be used

with functional motor abilities providing and reflecting current views on the inter-relationship between health factors and context. It follows similar principles to the model used throughout this text emphasizing child resources, task, and environment. It is a useful tool to guide both research and clinical thinking in the field of childhood disability. The model is shown in Figure 7.1.

The ICF model clearly separates functioning and disability with key areas being the interactive relationships between health conditions such as disorder or disease and the environmental context in which the activity takes place. In addition, there is an emphasis on participation, a point that is taken up in Chapter 12 with a description of ecological intervention (Sugden and Henderson 2007) proposing that functioning is a combination of participation and learning with different factors affecting each one. Personal factors, or what in this text are referred to as child resources, are just one part of the story of appropriate functioning, albeit an important part.

One key change in the ICF model is the shift in language from negative terms such as impairment, disability, and handicap to the more neutral terms of body function, activity, and participation. A second change is that the term 'disability' is often viewed as a social construction and refers to a dynamic interaction between the person and his or her environment. In this text this idea has been taken further with a triad of influences, namely person–task–environment. WHO (2001: 28) chose a biopsychosocial model of health, functioning, and disability in order to provide 'a coherent view of different perspectives of health from a biological, individual and social perspective'.

In professional practice this type of thinking has a number of implications. One such example would be in the assessment of cerebral palsy that should be conducted in an environment conducive to the child's best performance. WHO (2001) introduces the terms 'capacity' and 'performance' with the former representing the child's best level of functioning after being provided with the most appropriate support and the latter referring to the child's current performance. It is the difference between potential and current performance and is similar to Vygotsky's (1978) concept of zone of proximal development, whereby the zone represents the difference between the child's current level of performance and the support from a more capable other. WHO (2001) notes some of the factors that may be influential in the child reaching this full 'capacity'.

There are models and classification systems that are being used as scales for gross motor and manual activities such as that advocated by ICF. A summary of two approaches in this vein follows, examining functional abilities using the Gross Motor Functional Classification System (GMFCS) and the Manual Ability Classification System (MACS).

GROSS MOTOR FUNCTION CLASSIFICATION SYSTEM

The recent trends in examining functions of children are in line with the ICF (WHO 2001) recommendations and this is addressed by the Gross Motor Function Classification System (GMFCS) devised by the team at McMaster University within the *CanChild* Centre for Disability Research. The GMFCS notes a child's current abilities and strengths in gross motor functioning concentrating on initiated movements in sitting and walking, shown in Box 7.1 (Palisano et al 1997, 2007).

Box 7.1 A closer examination

Gross Motor Function Classification System (GMFCS): Palisano et al (2007)
The classification system has five levels, with distinctions between the levels being made on functional criteria with an emphasis on the usual performance in home, school, and community settings. The classification system is closely related to the Gross Motor Function Measure by the same team, which measures function over time. The five levels of the classification system are shown below with a descriptor of function.

- I: walks without limitations;
- II: walks with limitations;
- III: walks using a hand-held mobility device;
- IV: self-mobility with limitations, may use powered mobility; and
- V: transported in a manual wheelchair.

These five levels are broken down in to the detail of what are the functional criteria for each one for five age groups: less than 2 years, 2 to 4 years, 4 to 6 years, 6 to 12 years and 12 to 18 years. For example, between ages 4 and 6 years, level II notes:

Children sit in a chair with both hands free to manipulate objects. Children move from the floor to standing and from chair sitting to standing but often require a stable surface to push or pull upon with their arms. Children walk without the need for a hand-held mobility device indoors and for short distances on level surfaces outdoors. Children climb stairs holding onto a railing but are unable to run or jump.

This type of description is laid down for each of the five levels in the five age groupings. The important point about this classification system is that it is functionally based. It is more firmly located in the ideals of the WHO's ICF and emphasizes daily functioning and what children can or cannot do, not quality of movement or potential for improvement. It is a different form of classification altogether from the more traditional ones. It provides a common language and standardized system to classify children with cerebral palsy, and with accompanying growth curves can help predict future gross motor development of children with cerebral palsy.

Agreement over GMFCS levels varied from 48% to 95% with a mean of 78%, but mostly there was clustering around two levels. Overall, the study found encouraging levels of agreement for deciding cerebral palsy cases for epidemiological registers but more variability for subtypes and GMFCS level. This variability was explained by differences both between and within individuals in interpreting guidelines, differences between centres and practices (with local guidelines often taking precedence), and the limitations in interpreting text-based cases. A final recommendation for the study was that regular training ought to be incorporated into individual registrars' standard practice.

Box 7.2 A closer examination

Manual Ability Classification System for Children with Cerebral Palsy (MACS): Eliasson et al (2006)
The aim of MACS is to provide a system to classify children's ability to use the hands for functional purpose in daily activities. It aimed to examine typical manual performance rather than maximum capacity and was devised as a manual equivalent of the GMFCS described in Box 7.1.

It measures the child's ability to handle objects in daily life and like the GMFCS it has five levels of success:

- I: Handles objects easily and successfully – may be slower and less accurate but there is no restriction of manual activities in everyday life.
- II: Handles most objects but with somewhat reduced quality and/or speed of achievement; alternative ways of performance might be used – no real restriction of independence but some activities may be avoided or achieved with limited success.
- III: Handles objects with difficulty; needs help to prepare and/or modify activities – performance is slow with only activities that have been adapted or set up performed independently.
- IV: Handles a limited selection of easily managed objects in adapted situations – requires effort and has limited success and requires constant support and/or adapted equipment for even partial achievement.
- V: Does not handle objects and has severely limited ability to perform even simple actions – requires total assistance.

The level is determined by someone who knows the child and not through a formal specific assessment, and typical performance is being sought. Validation is strong, using expert groups for construct validity followed by observations and discussion concerning video recordings with an expert group. Discussion posters at conferences and parental input contributed to the validation. Reliability was established through ongoing studies in Sweden and Australia giving inter-rater reliability between parents and therapists of 0.96 and a similar figure among therapists.

MANUAL ABILITY CLASSIFICATION SYSTEM FOR CHILDREN WITH CEREBRAL PALSY

A second functional classification system that has recently become very popular is the Manual Ability Classification System (Eliasson et al 2006). Again, this follows the principles laid down in the ICF model emphasizing functional ability. A closer examination of this is shown in Box 7.2.

These two classification systems illustrate how the functional movements of the child with cerebral palsy can be described and analysed and can also be used as one type of assessment to indicate any change in the child's performance. The move towards functional assessment rather than assessing impairment has practical implications and indicates a different way to view children, with their needs now being the central focus supporting them to achieve everyday functional skills, rather than chronicling what they cannot do.

CAUSATION AND CAUSAL PATHWAYS

The term 'causal pathways' is taken from Stanley et al (2000) and relates to the sequence of events, activities or conditions that precedes a particular condition. In the section on definition, the international workshop recommendations included causation but also recommended caution in interpretation. However, causation does remain a problem for all concerned with cerebral palsy. Baxter (2006) noted that in Swedish studies half of the children born with cerebral palsy are preterm, but that the causal pathways are poorly understood and attempts to intervene not terrible successful. This led him to note that 'most causal factors do not operate in isolation but synergise to make a disturbance more likely' (p. 3).

Multiple interacting variables
In the above quote, Baxter is stating that causation is not usually one factor producing a specific end result, but is noting that variables group together and evolve to create a dynamic system leading to an unknown impairment. This synergism starts in utero and extends to include antenatal factors creating casual pathways and eventually causal networks. To successfully prevent occurrence, it would be appropriate to direct attention to all of these. Improved antenatal care, such as replacement surfactant to aid respiration, has led to a greater chance of survival and diminished risk of cerebral palsy. However, paradoxically, improved survival rates in very young and small infants

(below 1000g) runs the risk of an increase in the condition (Stanley et al 2000).

Specific causal sources

Stanley et al (2000) proceed to analyse these causal pathways over a series of chapters involving the following categories.

Preconception and early pregnancy factors

These factors include family history and known and unknown genetic influences; infections and deficiencies such as iodine and thyroid hormone, reproductive disorders, toxic influences such as alcohol and carbon monoxide poisoning, hypoxia and ischaemia, and congenital infections.

Very preterm birth

Age at delivery and birthweight make separate contributions to causation even though they are often conflated. Very preterm birth, usually below 32 completed weeks of gestation, is the strongest predictor of later cerebral palsy and as gestational age decreases the risk increases with the incidence of cerebral palsy for neonates below that figure being 30 times greater than those born at term. Three possible pathways are suggested by Stanley et al (2000). First, some antenatal factor could lead to both preterm birth and cerebral palsy, for example a bacterial infection; second, preterm infants may be more susceptible to physiological disturbances such hypoxia or acidosis; third, early damage to the cerebral cortex, particularly white matter, can lead to preterm delivery and cerebral palsy.

Intrauterine growth restriction

Cerebral palsy risk increases with decreasing birthweight and this measure is also combined with gestational age at the time of birth, but because birthweight can be more accurately defined, it is often the marker that is used. It becomes more complicated because survival rates of children with very low birthweights are increasing, but this increases the risk of the survivors having some kind of difficulty such as cerebral palsy. Survival rates of infants born below 1500g have increased steadily from the 1970s, with Stanley et al (2000) reporting a change in western Australia from 300 survivors per 1000 live births in 1970 to over 800 per 1000 in 1994. With this increase comes the higher risk of cerebral palsy, with Escobar et al (1991) in their meta-analysis study showing a figure of 8% with cerebral palsy in children with a birthweight below 1500g.

Infants born small for gestational age are at risk for cerebral palsy and the reasons for this are multiple, with Stanley et al (2000) offering possibilities as to how this comes about. First, there may be factors that cause both

poor growth and cerebral palsy; second, that growth restriction, no matter what the aetiology, is causally linked to cerebral palsy; third, that growth restrictions cause conditions such as hypoglycaemia that may be responsible for cerebral damage; fourth, that fetuses with growth restrictions are more vulnerable to brain damages from other factors such as birth asphyxia; and finally, that already damaged fetuses cause poor growth, that is cerebral palsy produces poor growth.

Birth asphyxia

Birth asphyxia or lack of oxygen to the fetus during the process of labour has been a longstanding candidate for increased risk of cerebral palsy. However, Stanley et al (2000) note that birth asphyxia may not be as important as previously thought and that signs such as initiating and maintaining respiration are early indicators of cerebral palsy, not causal pathways. In addition, it is possible that many infants with birth asphyxia possibly had some antenatal event or condition that made them vulnerable to birth events.

Multiple pregnancies

Multiple pregnancies are associated with cerebral palsy with the rate of cerebral palsy being higher among births following multiple pregnancies. This explanation fits with many of the variables associated with cerebral palsy, with multiple pregnancies being linked to, for example, poor intrauterine growth, preterm delivery, and birth defects. Stanley et al (2000) suggest that this may increase as medical care improves and more multiple-born infants survive. The fact that there is a greater incidence of cerebral palsy in multiple than single pregnancies is an example of how, when the detail is examined, a singular statistic such as this is affected by multiple variables. For example, do low birthweight and prematurity have a covarying effect on the presence of cerebral palsy in multiple births? Bonellie et al (2005) showed that, for both singletons and twins, there was a higher rate among infants born preterm, and that the higher observed rates of cerebral palsy in twins was not simply due to the obvious differences between twins and singletons in birthweight and gestational age. Being a twin in itself was a factor but it was difficult to determine what it was about being a twin that has made it so.

Postnatally acquired cerebral palsy

A recognized factor in aetiology is that many children with cerebral palsy are the result of brain damage after birth, although the exact proportion is difficult to ascertain. Many children with postnatally acquired cerebral palsy have had risks beforehand such as low birthweight or short gestation, making both definition and prevalence figures difficult. Although it is clear that a significant proportion of all cerebral palsy is acquired postnatally, the pathway to this may start before the postnatal period begins. There is considerable variation as to what is the definition in the age range. Earlier limits were birth to 2 months but Stanley et al (2000) suggest that now the upper age limit ranges from 2 to 10 years, which is approaching the age of young adult brain damage, but most damage occurs during the first year postnatally. There is also the distinction between those who are within the diagnosis of cerebral palsy and those who are perfectly normal yet acquire brain injury through an incident such as a car accident. Causes of postnatally acquired cerebral palsy include both infection and trauma and the proportion of postnatally acquired cerebral palsy of all cerebral palsy cases varies between 1.4% and 60% with the huge difference usually being accounted for by differing age limits (Stanley et al 2000).

However, despite possible association of such causal factors, prevention remains difficult. For example, the question arises whether prescribing anticoagulants to large numbers of pregnant women is feasible. In addition, the large numbers of variables that make up the network of causal pathways conspire to make a complex system leading to a causal network. The evidence is not yet comprehensive enough for these factors to be accurately predictive or for them to be used as specific preventative methods. As Baxter (2006) notes, these causal factors do not usually operate on their own but come together and interact to provide the causal pathway.

An important study carried out in a number of European centres in England, Scotland, Ireland, Portugal, Sweden, Germany, and Finland was reported by Bax et al (2006). The study examined correlates of cerebral palsy and compared clinical findings with MRI brain studies. The major findings of the study are presented in Box 7.3.

In Box 7.3, Bax et al (2006) provide invaluable information that will go some way to reducing the prevalence of cerebral palsy. In addition to genetic and metabolic disorders, other factors are multiple and complex with variables such as infections, multiple pregnancies, and nutrition all prime candidates for increased awareness and monitoring.

PREVALENCE AND INCIDENCE

In examining the frequency of individuals who have a particular condition, the terms *prevalence* and *incidence* are both used and it is important to distinguish between the two. These differences are succinctly illustrated in Table 7.3 from Stanley et al (2000).

Prevalence

This term is used to determine the percentage of individuals with the condition in a whole population at any given time, and is measured by surveys identifying cases as a proportion of a population. Prevalence can be obtained by simply taking the number of cases in a suitable representative population or by looking at various incidence rates minus mortality, that is the proportion of live births that do not survive or change status, such as developing cerebral palsy postnatally. Changes in prevalence occur slowly over a protracted period of time as the whole age range of the population is involved. An important point to note is that prevalence rate is of great interest and use to those who are involved in planning service provision, with agencies such as health authorities using this information to allocate resources.

Stanley et al (2000) summarize the prevalence rates between 1959 and 1992 across regions in the four countries of Australia, Northern Ireland, England, and Sweden, giving an overall prevalence of 2 to 2.5 per live 1000 births. There was some variation with Sweden, England, and Australia dipping to around 1.5 in the early 1970s and then rising again to around 2 in the 1980s. In all cases of cerebral palsy there is a slight over-representation of males to females of roughly 1.1 to 1. More recently, prevalence of cerebral palsy in western Ireland from a population-based study set up through a register in 2002 found an overall prevalence of 1.8 per 1000 (Mongan et al 2006). The male to female prevalence was 68% to 32% and the rate of cerebral palsy in infants weighing less than 1500g at birth was 39 per 1000 compared with 1.3 per 1000 for those weighing more than 2500g. Bilateral spastic cerebral palsy was the most common subtype with 51% followed by spastic hemiplegia; 56% had intellectual impairments and 46% had experienced seizures. These figures are illustrative of the kinds of rates found in developed nations with comprehensive medical cover, but in other nations where pre- and postnatal care are not universal, higher rates will be present.

Incidence

This term is used to describe the number of new cases arising in a population and measured by following up a birth cohort and calculating the number of cases of cerebral palsy relative to the birth cohort. Thus, when looking at incidence, changes can take place quickly if some form of intervention or other influencing factor has occurred. Over time the changes in incidence, if continued, will lead to major changes in the prevalence rate. Incidence is a major focus of those involved in aetiology and prevention (Stanley et al 2000).

Box 7.3 A closer examination

Clinical and MRI correlates of cerebral palsy (Bax et al 2006)

A total of 432 children with cerebral palsy born between 1996 and 1999 in Europe were clinically assessed and 351 had brain scans. Data were obtained from parents, with obstetric, genetic, and metabolic information from medical records. (Percentages may not total 100 because of rounding.)

Prenatal findings

- A total of 39.5% reported an infection during pregnancy and, following interviews, an agreement was that 29.6% had a 'significant' infection. Colds, coughs, etc. were excluded. By 'significant', it was assumed that the infection could have contributed to the condition.
- 12% were from multiple pregnancies with four pairs both having cerebral palsy and seven others with a twin that did not survive.

Perinatal findings

- Over half of the children were born at term (54.5%).
- 10.9% were below 28 weeks; 16% between 28 and 31 weeks; and 18.3% between 32 and 36 weeks.
- 19.2% were below the 10th centile in birthweight.
- 70% of children were admitted to the special care infant unit after birth.

Clinical findings

The clinician was asked to record the topographical nature of the cerebral palsy in terms of the limbs involved and the type according to movement quality.

- A total of 34.4% were classified as diplegia; 26.2% as hemiplegia; 18.6% as spastic quadriplegia; 14.4% as dyskinesia; 3.9% as ataxia; and other accounting for 2.6%.

- Other characteristics included 28% with epilepsy; 31% of hemiplegia, 38% of diplegia, and 64% of quadriplegia with some kind of visual abnormality; and 7% with a hearing problem.

MRI findings

A total of 351 children had brain scans that were taken from 1 to 87 months with a mean age of 38 months.

- White matter damage of immaturity was the most common finding with 42.5% of the children showing this. It was found in 71.3% of those with diplegia, 34.1% of those with hemiplegia and 35.1% of those with quadriplegia.
- Basal ganglia and thalamic damage was found in 75.6% of the dystonic group and only occasionally seen in spastic quadriplegia and diplegia and not at all in the hemiplegic group.
- Focal cortical infarcts were almost exclusively found in hemiplegia (27.5%).
- 1.7% of the children had normal MRI results and these were distributed across all clinical cerebral palsy subgroups but making up half of the ataxic type.

Comment

The authors recommended that, on the basis of the study, all children with cerebral palsy should have a brain scan which can be related to the other findings. They also note that in the growing occurrence of malpractice suits, these kinds of data may have some relevance. Most children born before 34 weeks' gestation had white matter damage, but, unlike previous suggestions, the authors assert that there is little evidence for obstetric malpractice. It is more likely to be predisposing factors such as genetic and nutritional, and toxic factors, and infections during pregnancy that lead the child to be predisposed to an increased risk of hypoxic–ischaemic episodes. Those born after 34 weeks would not have been affected by perinatal processes. After excluding other possibilities of obstetric events, the authors were left with 70 children with either cortical/subcortical or basal ganglia damage born after 34 weeks, concluding that, from MRI information, only 19.9% of a population with cerebral palsy could be the result of obstetric mishap and many of these would not be malpractice, indicating that the overall incidence of malpractice would have been low.

TABLE 7.3
Cerebral palsy – measures of occurrence

Prevalence	Incidence
Existing/current cases in a population	New cases arising in a population
Planning of services	Aetiological studies
Prevalence is incidence minus mortality and migration	
Surveys to identify cases as a proportion of a specific population	Follow up a birth cohort
	Register cases of cerebral palsy and relate these to their birth cohorts
Very large surveys required to establish precise estimates	True incidence of brain defect/damage causing (likely to cause) cerebral palsy is not measurable
	Delay in ascertainment (months or years from cerebral defect)
	Cases lost due to deaths, out migration, and other losses from birth cohorts

Reproduced with permission of the publisher from Stanley et al (2000).

Incidence is a complex figure as it relies upon the definition of cerebral palsy including both motor impairment and a brain lesion, and therefore it depends on which one is taken as the defining characteristics as they usually do not express themselves at the same time. Stanley et al (2000) summarize the difficulties involved in this and how a true incidence is sometimes problematic because the numerator (number of individuals in a population) and denominator (number of cases) often cannot be obtained at the same time as motor impairment, such as at birth. A further complication arises in documenting evidence in that in some children with cerebral palsy movement disorganization (especially if accompanied by epilepsy) is noted earlier, whereas in others with less obvious motor signs (e.g. hypotonia) it is not identified until later. They note that it is important when examining rates for cerebral palsy to note definitions of denominators as it could be a rate per 1000 neonatal survivors, per 1000 live births or per 1000 total births, the last most common previously. Various other variables will have impact upon *incidence* and *prevalence*, such as age for inclusion, cause and age at acquisition, and exclusionary conditions (i.e. other than spasticity).

Although calculating rates of cerebral palsy is difficult because of the differing methodologies, with variation according to how it is calculated and who is included or excluded, the studies are relevant and are clear in that they state how the study was conducted. A simple distinction between prevalence and incidence is that the former is the proportion of the population experiencing the condition at a given moment in time, whereas the latter is the proportion of the population in which the condition arises. By studying prevalence and incidence rates conclusions can be drawn about the epidemiology that lead to better ways of prevention and allocation of resources. The potentially

rapid changes in incidence will lead to slower, but still clear changes in prevalence and together they provide evidence for the effects of intervention and lead to better methods for care and provision.

GROWTH AND DEVELOPMENT IN CHILDREN

A set of data on gross motor items of children with cerebral palsy was compiled by Hanna et al (2008) using the Gross Motor Function Measure (GMFM). They provided centiles for GMFM scores derived from 1940 assessments on a longitudinal sample of 650 children with cerebral palsy between the ages of 2 and 12 years who were receiving services and support at children's rehabilitation centres between 1996 and 2001. These centiles and graphs allow any child with cerebral palsy to be referenced to them, with the authors noting that one must consider whether this normative sample is appropriate for the child, and recognizing that it is typical for centile scores to vary widely on reassessment and not necessarily reflect a change in ability. The measures are only for showing who has cerebral palsy and the progression of the children through the various levels of the GMFM.

Our information on the progression of children with cerebral palsy during puberty is limited, particularly the effect of increasing skeletal growth on motor functioning. Van Eck et al (2008) examined this issue in a cohort of 100 children with cerebral palsy (37 females and 63 males, 73 ambulant and 27 non-ambulant) ranging in age from 9 to 13 years. The skeletal age was determined over a 3-year period through the use of radiographs, motor functioning was assessed using the GMFM and the severity of cerebral palsy was classified on the five-point scale of the Gross Motor Function Classification System (GMFCS).

There was a high prevalence of children with a deviation of more than 1 year of skeletal age in relation to chronological age, 42% to 55% in males and 38% to 57% in females, but in females only a small percentage had delayed skeletal age with most being advanced, whereas in males both delayed and advanced were equally divided. Other studies have found higher prevalence of both advanced and delayed skeletal age (Kong et al 1999). With respect to motor functioning, they found that there was little evidence to show that children with cerebral palsy were at risk for deterioration of motor skills as a function of skeletal maturity during puberty. One of the important features of this study is that it was a prospective longitudinal study and did not rely on retrospective or cross-sectional data. The authors did acknowledge that some children may have entered puberty before their lower age of 9 years and recommended using lower ages in any future work.

The research work on growth, particularly skeletal growth, has produced some variable results with differing percentages for both delayed and advanced skeletal age. A number of factors may account for this in addition to the known heterogeneity in children with cerebral palsy. These include different measures that are used to assess skeletal maturity, sex differences, severity of the condition, and whether or not the children were ambulatory. The skeletal maturity of the child is important and it is a vital intrinsic constraint in the production of movement; it is particularly important during growth spurts (such as during puberty) when the skeleton is growing quickly and has a larger interactional effect with the central nervous system.

Cerebral palsy and movement control
Cerebral palsy is a major condition defined with a movement problem at the core posing a number of questions about how control is achieved and what the major differences are between children with cerebral palsy and typically developing children. It is not unusual to find associated characteristics in children with cerebral palsy such as sensory difficulties and learning difficulties, but the defining characteristics involve problems in movement skill production and this hinders the children in their encounters in everyday life. This section turns to address these issues, using as a guide some of the variables that have been studied in typically developing populations. It is worth emphasizing that because of the heterogeneity of the condition, the variables described occur and influence movement to varying degrees in individual children with cerebral palsy.

CONSTRAINTS ON COORDINATION AND CONTROL

Constraints
The term 'constraints' is being used in many places throughout the book following the manner in which it is described by Newell (1986). He states that it can be used to mean to facilitate, encourage, or channel and not simply in its usual meaning of restricting, although this is included. Constraints thus become the influences on the children's movements and the development of these movements. In line with our model of motor outcomes being a function of the transaction between the mover's resources, the environmental context and tasks, constraints are involved in each part of the model.

As the resources of the child with cerebral palsy are atypical, it is not surprising that atypical movement responses are produced and that they show different movements to those that are seen in typically developing children. They are often the result of difficulties in muscle activation as shown by irregularities in reflexes, muscle tone, and tension and muscle synergies. There are examples of timing delays and of reversal of proximal–distal order of muscle activation. There is also a disruption of dynamic relationships among joint actions involving flexion–extension exchanges and related rates of change. Posture is often modified to aid movements, as seen in changes in trunk and head positions during reaching and grasping, which is a form of synergistic relationship on a larger scale. Problems become accumulative; poor use of sensory information is a limiting factor in postural control of ataxic children, which limits some of their movements. These in turn lead to difficulties with the movement outcome, which is often poor in quality. It may be that some of these responses are the best that can be accommodated within the resources of the child with cerebral palsy. Within a dynamical systems framework, the transacting variables all work together to discover the optimum solution to a movement problem that is present.

Any constraint can be *intrinsic* to the child in the form of his or her personal resources or *extrinsic* in the form of the task and the environmental array. Within a dynamical framework, the influence of intrinsic constraints works in a transactional manner with those that are outside the individual's resources. This transaction process, which has been a common feature throughout this book, is illustrated in the model shown below in Figure 7.2.

Intrinsic constraints
The intrinsic constraints are often defined as within the motor control systems such as managing and constraining the degrees of freedom through what has been called 'softly assembled' controllable units such as coordinative

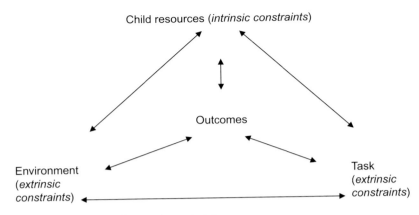

Fig. 7.2 Transactional process of intrinsic and extrinsic constraints.

structures. But it is not only direct motor control variables that are included as intrinsic variables. In addition, it is likely that the sensory system in children is not operating in a typical manner in that sensory feedback from a movement, for example, may not be accurate. Thus, the end result often is an impaired motor system working on impoverished and flawed sensory feedback information. Thus, this will heighten any movement problem by not only making movements difficult but also preventing, or at least weakening, any attempts at learning.

Other personal variables such as motivation, arousal, and anxiety are all intrinsic constraints with possible effects on a child's movement outcomes. As an example, I-Chun et al (2008) found that usage of assistive devices by children with cerebral palsy was influenced as much by cognitive and emotional variables such as self-concept and peer perception than by how much the device aided motor control. These emotional and cognitive variables are intrinsic constraints and within the resources of the child. When the children with cerebral palsy were asked about the usefulness of assistive devices and whether they used them, they accepted that the devices had a positive effect in terms of helping them but this was different across settings. At school, the devices helped them be independent and they were motivated to use them. At home, there was a different picture and the children did not worry about movements that were socially inappropriate, and thus the devices were seen as less necessary. Other factors that influenced usage were the physical environment and how facilitatory it was; their desired level of independence, whether they wanted help with pushing a wheelchair, for example; and finally their mothers' attitudes. These all changed as the context moved from school to home (I-Chun et al 2008). This type of study again shows how movement outcomes do not involve simple one-to-one relationships between variables and outcomes but are the result of a number of ever-changing dynamic circumstances. In addition, there is much information on the concept of resilience and how this affects outcomes in children with special educational needs and disabilities in general, and there is no reason to suspect that resilience and other personal variables are not strong factors in determining outcomes in children with cerebral palsy.

The list below proposes those variables that would typically be included in a list of intrinsic constraints:

- central nervous system properties;
- biomechanical properties;
- organization of motor control;
- degrees of freedom, coordinative structures;
- motivational influences;
- self-concept;
- resilience factors;
- morphological variables;
- cognitive variables; and
- emotional variables.

Despite the non-motor variables affecting movement outcomes, because of the nature of cerebral palsy, it is obvious that motor control intrinsic variables play a crucial role. As an example, the concept of coordinative structures, noted in earlier chapters, has regularly been proposed as fundamental to motor control. These are described as groups of muscles, often spanning several joints, that are constrained to act as a single unit that enables the muscle to act not singly, but as part of a self-regulatory unit. It would not be surprising, considering the degree of brain damage in children with cerebral palsy, that coordinative structures operate in an atypical manner. In typically developing children movement skill development is often facilitated through the formation of more elegant coordinative structures, enabling increased adaptability. Coordinative structures are concepts that aid in the understanding of how movement is controlled, and early developments show constraints limiting actions to isolated movements and not showing the smoothness and adaptability of later movements. For example, the young walker has a wide stance, with arms held high and taking single flat-footed steps, in contrast to later actions of the legs in a continuous motion with heel contact and arms swinging in the opposite direction to the legs. Older children can coordinate larger structures such as linking body rotation with arm and leg movements, thereby reducing the number of degrees of freedom by forming larger movement units rather than having a number of separate action units. The skilled performer's movements usually look smooth and typically have a holistic quality to them, rather than a series of individual parts. It would be expected that a child with cerebral palsy will show different development of these structures.

In addition, and linked to the concept of coordinative structures, are degrees of freedom, also noted in earlier chapters and described as the number of variables in a movement that are free to vary. Again, how they are utilized in children with cerebral palsy may show distinct differences to typical development. In running, a typically developing individual will be relatively stiff when developing the skill but later will be much looser in the arms and legs. This has been labelled as a progression from *freezing the degrees of freedom to freeing and utilizing them*. This progression, so often seen in typical skill development across a variety of movements, may take a totally different form in children with cerebral palsy. For example, the freezing of the degrees of freedom may remain longer or even become permanent because of the hypertonia noted in a condition with spasticity. Another difference may be in trying to successfully achieve an initial freezing of the degrees of freedom, so often a necessary characteristic to enable early control to be effective. This may prove to be impossible, causing a serious difficulty in a child with dystonia/athetosis who has problems with hypotonicity in the form of continuous and involuntary movement.

All children face the same challenges in trying to control the degrees of freedom, and it can be speculated that they do this in the first instance by limiting the range of movement until effective coordinative structures can be developed. Often these are never developed typically in children with cerebral palsy because of the intrinsic constraints that restrict what can be achieved. Thus, this leads to the production of unusual and atypical movements, in turn leading to inadequate coordination. However, it is unclear whether the coordination is constrained by problems in muscle activation or by the dynamic relationships needed to achieve higher levels of organization in muscle synergies. The various types of cerebral palsy will show different adaptations, with what is typically seen in children with spasticity showing different adaptations to those with dyskinesis.

The freezing to freeing of the degrees of freedom occurs as a natural consequence of the individual acquiring more motor control, and this progression facilitates control by releasing them, thus providing more adaptable skilled performance. In children with cerebral palsy it is speculated that this progression from freezing to freeing of the degrees of freedom may take a different form or not happen at all.

If the everyday action of reaching and grasping is taken as an example, differences are quite striking. A typically developing child of 8 years of age reaches with a smooth arm movement towards a target and as the hand approaches the target the fingers are progressively shaped to grasp the object. The child with spasticity will often show a jerky, clasp-knife action with rigid posture of the arm, indicating that the degrees of freedom have been frozen because of the neural damage. This makes the action sharp, often fast but uncontrolled, leading to a jerky movement, sometimes missing the target or finding the coordination of the reach and grasp being out of time. In addition, there is little natural progression from this to a state where degrees of freedom are released, thus aiding more flexible control and adaptable movements. The child with dyskinesis may have the opposite problem in finding difficulty in freezing the degrees of freedom and has freed them from the outset. Unfortunately, this freeing of the degrees of freedom is not always accompanied by the effective control of them. This is because of the hypotonus of the child, which produces a fluctuating wavering movement, again leading to a reaching and grasping performance that is not typical.

Models have been proposed about how muscles are organized and often have been likened to a mechanical system and acting like a mass spring. The forearm can act as a lever, the elbow a pivot resting in a flexed position and the flexors and extensors around the elbow joint viewed as two mass springs. With elbow extension, the flexor tendons are increased in tension because they are stretched with decreased tension in the extensor tendons. An equilibrium point is reached when the increased tension in the flexor tendons is equal to the decreased tension in the extensor tendons. If a limb is deflected from holding this equilibrium point and then is released, the limb will return to the equilibrium point, regardless of the amount of deflection. This model uses tendon tension as a primary means of control of muscle activity (Crossman and Goodeve 1963, Asatryan and Feldman 1965). Muscle activity is influenced by such variables as biomechanical properties of the limb such as the equilibrium point leading to different and often inadequate muscle synergies or coordinative structures (Sugden and Keogh 1990). This is particularly interesting for children with cerebral palsy as they are likely to have different and often unstable equilibrium points, thus changing the whole mechanical properties of the action.

It is pertinent to remember that a dynamical systems approach incorporates multiple subcomponents as agents of control, and change in one, such as flawed sensory input, will have an interactive effect across the motor control system. The corollary to this is that when intervening, by changing one aspect of this dynamic such as altering the task or manipulating the environment to the advantage of the child, there will be the same dynamic interactive effect but in a positive direction.

Extrinsic constraints

Extrinsic constraints are those that are outside of the personal resources of the child and yet they are ones that have an effect on the movement outcome, particularly in terms of support and intervention. The model of Bronfenbrenner (1979) outlines his way of looking at environmental influences on the child in his ecological account of child development. These environmental influences start with a micro system where the child is at the centre alongside close significant others and finishes with a macro system including such items as political influence and government policy. Thus, the extrinsic influences on a child will vary from those that directly influence his or her life to those that are more indirect and have to go through a number of stages in order for the effect to be seen in the child. It is accepted that national politics and local policies will influence the child's outcomes, but here the line is taken that only the more direct extrinsic variables are listed as it is possible to see the more immediate impact they have on the child's life. These extrinsic constraints include the environmental context in which the learning takes place and the task variables such as how practice is organized for the learning process.

A possible list of extrinsic constraints might include those listed below.

- Environmental constraints
  - Support from health and educational agencies
  - Support at home
  - Support and organization at school
  - Peer perception and support
  - Socio-economic status and culture
  - Community opportunities

  - Assistive devices
  - Expectations (of parents and school)
- Task constraints
  - Task process or function
  - Task variables – choice, difficulty
  - Manner of teaching and therapy-practice variables

The first six of the above list are environmental constraints and the last two involve task variables and how they are presented. Extrinsic constraints can be under the control of the parent, teacher, or therapist or are naturally occurring in the environment. In a text on intervention for children with developmental coordination disorder, and described in more detail in Chapter 12, Sugden and Henderson (2007) illustrate how movement outcomes are a function of multiple influences. They note the child's resources or intrinsic constraints but also examine the environmental and task influences or extrinsic constraints. They label their approach 'ecological intervention' to emphasize the multiple interacting variables.

In their ecological intervention, Sugden and Henderson (2007) subdivide the environmental constraints into home, school, health, and community, noting that these all have a direct or indirect effect on movement outcomes. Thus, in the home, the amount of time available is an important factor as are the routines of family life. In school, the amount of expertise that is available and the allocation of resources will also have a differential effect on outcomes. Similarly, in the health service, how often the child is seen, and how much advice is given, to whom and when is often variable and so will have a variable effect on outcomes. Participation is a crucial factor for a child with cerebral palsy, and thus community support and availability of such activities involving leisure is again a factor in determining outcomes. These factors of home, school, health, and community are not simply involved in direct intervention studies per se but are crucial variables in the everyday life of the child with cerebral palsy. Two children with exactly the same child resources and with the same condition (such as moderate hemiplegic cerebral palsy) may have the same personality factors such as resilience or motivation. However, because they are placed in different environmental settings, the outcomes for their movements and their lives in general are different. These differences all go to composing the dynamic, interactive, ecological system that we propose.

A crucial third part of our ecological and dynamical analysis of influences on outcomes for children with cerebral palsy is the constraint of the task and how it is presented (see Fig. 7.2). This is concerned with how children, when placed in the learning situation, learn the task. The issues of child resources have been taken into consideration, the environmental context is noted and used, and now the child has to learn a particular task whether at home, in school, or out in the community. For this we turn to the literature on how we acquire motor skills and the variables that affect the learning. These are described in detail by Schmidt and Lee (2005) and Sugden and Henderson (2007) and note such variables as task selection, task analysis, generalization of tasks, and practice variables. Many of these are covered in more detail in Chapter 12.

The two variables of environment and task and their subcomponents make up the external constraints in any analysis of outcomes for children with cerebral palsy. With such an array of influences it is not surprising that we see heterogeneity in not only the condition itself but also the developmental progression of the disorder as the individual moves through childhood to adolescence towards emerging adulthood. This is magnified when the full model of child resources, environmental, and task constraints all interact to produce the final movement outcome.

PROBLEMS IN COORDINATION AND CONTROL

Generic fundamental issues
The child with cerebral palsy has a number of interacting constraints that combine to make movements difficult. The constraints in the neural system start at fundamental levels leading through to, and interacting with, other intrinsic and extrinsic factors. Thus, problems with the whole motor coordination and control system including muscle tone and reflexes are factors that underlie the different movement skill development of children with cerebral palsy. The immediate and most direct impact is on muscle control, ranging from difficulties in controlling single motor units to problems in the organization of muscle synergies and recruiting appropriate coordinative structures. Poor muscle control provides great challenges to achieving typical development of posture, locomotion, and manual skills.

In addition to the difficulties in motor output is the poor quality of sensory information generated by aberrant muscle activity. Muscle and movement feedback of children with cerebral palsy provide sensory information about atypical and variable motor performance that make it difficult to modify movements in an appropriate manner. In addition, the neural system in children with cerebral palsy is 'noisy', making it difficult to separate a typical neural signal from noise in the system. Thus, the child is doubly disadvantaged with a limited motor output and the results not being fed back accurately. This culminates

in making the whole cycle of the integration of efferent output and afferent input both unstable and potentially inaccurate.

An examination of the proprioceptive functioning illustrates how this integration works and how, when one part of the system is providing inappropriate information, there is a cascading effect eventually resulting in poor coordination and control. For example, the functioning of the muscle spindle and detection of neural signals are important factors that affect many aspects of muscle control. The muscle spindle has both a motor and a sensory function that together regulate muscle stiffness. It is located in the muscle parallel with extrafusal fibres and is surrounded by a connective tissue capsule and plays a central role in alpha–gamma coactivation. Muscular contractions are regulated and controlled by independent but cooperative signals to alpha and gamma motoneurons in target muscles. The muscle spindle responds to changes in muscle length and/or it can be set to expect a specified amount of muscle stretch. If the muscle stretch is greater than expected, as when stepping into a hole while walking, the muscle spindle senses the discrepancy and adjusts muscle activity accordingly.

It would be expected that sensory information feedback from muscle spindle receptors of children with cerebral palsy describes aberrant, often misleading, muscle activity. For example, this occurs in children showing spasticity because of muscle hypertonicity and the positive stretch reflex accompanying the rapid muscle release that follows a build-up of resistance. In children with athetosis, this usually occurs because of hypotonicity in the muscle, as well as fluctuations in tone.

Another example of how sensory information can be misleading is in signal detection, which is a necessary feature of all sensory receptors in terms of differentiation between a real signal and any random noise in the system. A certain amount of noise always accompanies neural signals that are transmitted in the nervous system. Signal detection involves separating a signal that is 'real' from muscular activity and noise and using this as information for the forthcoming movement. It is likely that noise in the nervous system of children with cerebral palsy is often so high that signal detection is difficult, indicating that proprioceptive feedback in children with cerebral palsy is often not as accurate as in other children and thus may be difficult to analyse and use (Sugden and Keogh 1990). Within a dynamical systems approach the whole perception–action link as a holistic process is being degraded by the subcomponents or constraints and the process is seen as a single entity, constantly being moderated and tweaked by the constraints.

Basic muscle control involving motor and sensory processes

Typically, when a muscle group is activated there is corresponding synergistic coactivation of nearby muscles which can occur before, during, or after the primary muscle group depending on the task at hand. This coactivation helps produce the smooth, skilled, and accurate movement that we observe. Tedroff et al (2006) examined groups of children with cerebral palsy and compared them with typically developing peers on muscle recruitment patterns. Their results showed that children with cerebral palsy exhibited greater variability in patterns of muscle activation and more frequently failed to activate the primary muscle group first. This was often accompanied by atypical sequencing innervating another muscle before the one that was primarily responsible for the action. It appears that, in children with cerebral palsy, the synergistic relationship between primary muscle groups and those supporting the action are not as clearly defined, giving rise to the impaired movements that are observed. As this relationship depends on the nature of the task, that is whether the supporting groups act before, during, or after the primary muscle group activation, it would be interesting to vary the task to draw out these timing differences by using different tasks and compare children with cerebral palsy with those who are typically developing. One hypothesis would be that children with cerebral palsy are more fixed in their mode of responding than children who are typically developing. It would be interesting to see whether this projected 'fixed' responding manner is amenable to learning and to changes in the environmental and task constraints. Again, this type of thinking supports the notion that intrinsic constraints, in this case muscle sequence activation, are subject to moderation by extrinsic constraints in typically developing children. This may have value in intervention programmes for children with cerebral palsy.

A factor in muscle control is the need to be aware of muscle activity so that adjustments can be made. Awareness of muscle stretch has been studied by using vibration-induced illusions to give the impression that a muscle was being stretched (Tardieu et al 1984). The illusion was induced during isometric contraction by the application of vibration to the skin covering the muscle tendon as a means of stimulating the muscle spindle. Responses of children with cerebral palsy (ages 8–15 years) were compared with the responses of normal children (ages 8–14 years). The illusion of muscle stretch was experienced by all of the typically developing children but only half of the children with cerebral palsy.

In contrast to simple muscle activity, a more complicated but functionally important ability is awareness of total limb movement. Opila-Lehman et al (1985) note that both spastic and athetoid individuals generally have difficulties with proprioceptive awareness, with deficiencies usually being greater in children showing spasticity than in children more characterized by athetosis. Children with spasticity were less accurate than children with athetosis, who in turn were less accurate than typically developing children in reproducing arm movements. Jones (1976) proposed that a lack of awareness of forces operating on a joint may contribute to the movement skill problems of children with cerebral palsy. Using a passive movement task, the children were asked after each trial if the arm had been moved. Jones reported that children with spasticity and typically developing children made fewer errors in detecting movements and non-movements, whereas children with athetosis usually reported that movement activity had occurred, even when there was no movement. Jones (1976) noted that the children with athetosis displayed typical involuntary 'restlessness' in the arm held by the experimenter. This may have added neural noise that made it more difficult to detect movement and non-movement.

Control of muscle tension related to types of sensory awareness was analysed in a classic series of experiments by Harrison (1975a,b,c) as a means of studying overall muscle activity rather than isolated motor unit activity. She placed great emphasis on the role of proprioception in the muscle control problems of children with cerebral palsy and notes that hyperactivity of spinal motoneurons is a basic feature of spasticity. If the alpha motoneurons that supply spastic muscles have a lower activation threshold, then innocuous stimuli may elicit an abnormally strong contraction in spastic muscles. If muscle activity is aberrant, then muscle spindle afferent signals may be difficult to decipher and the child may be unable to use this sensory information properly when evaluating the appropriateness of a contraction, particularly when there are numerous simultaneous contractions. A closer examination of these studies is shown in Box 7.4.

Harrison also examined the responses that take place when a movement is disrupted (Harrison and Kruze 1987), looking at perturbations and any delay before adjustments are made that require the recapturing position, velocity, and timing of the original, intended movement. Both typically developing individuals and those with cerebral palsy were asked to produce rhythmical arm swings with random perturbations occurring by varying the force of resistance against elbow extension. Compared with typically developing individuals, individuals with cerebral palsy were less able to 'ride' both low- and medium-level perturbations and control and recognize different levels of muscle tension than were typically developing individuals. Improvement was possible when augmented

Box 7.4 A closer examination

Feedback and motor control: Harrison (1975b,c)

First series

Harrison (1975b) examined the ability to control and recognize different levels of muscle tension. The first task was to reproduce levels of muscle contraction (tension) that had previously been individually scaled. Individuals began by contracting forearm flexors as forcefully as possible.

Although the mean error of the group with spasticity was twice as large as the normal group, with greater inaccuracy at all tension levels, mean differences were not significant due to high within-group variability in the spastic group and this was shown when individual profiles were taken. Two of the six individuals with spasticity produced constant tension levels, regardless of the required tension level, indicating that they could not adjust to different tension levels. The other individuals increased and decreased tension levels appropriately, but they were particularly poor at producing low levels of tension. Harrison explains this in terms of signal detection, suggesting that gamma activity, as well as the contraction of other muscle groups, may produce a high level of noise, against which activity of forearm flexors is difficult to detect. The individuals with spasticity could not hold tension levels constant and took longer to reduce muscle tension, suggesting that they may need more time to decode and encode information about muscle activity and tension levels.

Second series

Harrison (1975c) tried to teach individuals with spasticity how to better control muscle tension, using augmented feedback from a visual display of electromyographic activity on a meter. The task involved contracting and relaxing as quickly as possible following a contraction. The result showed that relaxation was more rapid when subjects were provided with augmented visual feedback, but still did not reach the level of typically developing individuals without the feedback. She also examined the ability to maintain target levels of muscle tension. Individuals tensed forearm flexors to a target level and had to hold that tension level for 10 seconds. Tension levels of the individuals with spasticity without augmented feedback slowly drifted away from the target tension level. When provided with augmented feedback, they were better able to produce and hold the target tension level, but they drifted away near the end of the 10 seconds. Figure 7.3 shows the effect of visual feedback.

Training studies

Training studies involved teaching sequential and simultaneous control of both biceps and forearm flexors, to approximate a typical movement involving coordination of multiple muscle groups. Instruction began with

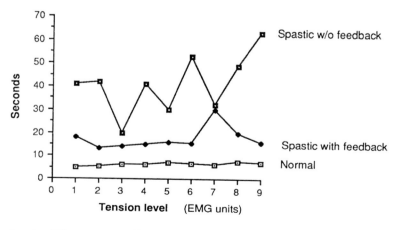

Fig. 7.3 Relaxation time by different groups with and without visual display. Reproduced with permission of the publisher from Harrison (1975).

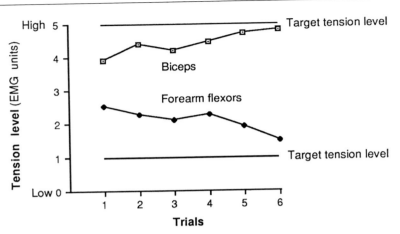

Fig. 7.4 Mean tension levels reproduced during simultaneous contractions. Reproduced with permission of the publisher from Harrison (1975).

individuals practising the production of a specified muscle tension in one specific muscle group followed by sequentially or simultaneously produced different combinations of tension levels in the biceps and forearm flexors. Knowledge of results was given at the end of each contraction as opposed to the continuous feedback provided in the tension-maintenance experiments. Results indicated that individuals with spasticity could learn sequential and simultaneous activity in two muscle groups in a manner similar to typically developing children. Figure 7.4 shows the improvement during six instructional trials for one combination of simultaneous muscle contractions. Accuracy of tension levels improved steadily so that the subjects were near the two target levels on the sixth trial.

Comment
An interesting observation was that some individual muscle contractions during combination contractions were more accurate than when the contraction was produced in isolation. This supports our general view that movements are greatly influenced by context, *even* when context is limited to the relationship of one muscle action to another. If the context is meaningful, with contractions producing a more functional movement, this may have a beneficial effect compared with a so-called nonsense movement taken out of context. There is also the possibility that mechanical factors may constrain tension levels when two or more muscles are active. Context and mechanical factors are here acting as positive constraints influencing the final production of coordination and control.

feedback was provided and control of individual muscle contractions also improved when made during combination contractions, which presumably provided context relationships to aid adjustment of muscle tension. In the child resources–environment–task model that has been consistently presented throughout the text, this indicates that by altering the constraint of the task and the instructions and manner of practice, improvement is possible.

A final observation on this series of studies is the variability of individuals with cerebral palsy. This is clearly the case when performance is taken across the group, thus supporting Mutch et al's (1992) observation that cerebral palsy is an umbrella term for a variety of characteristics. It is also the case that there is much intraparticipant variability in the performance of individuals with cerebral

palsy, thus suggesting that they are not able to regularly produce their best performance.

Postural control
As with all actions, postural control emerges from the transaction among the child, the task, and the environment, and thus all are understood in order to obtain a full understanding of postural control. Shumway-Cook and Woollacott (2007) define postural control as 'controlling the body's position in space for the dual purposes of stability and orientation' (p. 158).

Stability, often called balance, involves controlling the centre of mass in relation to the base of support whereas orientation involves controlling the body segments and the whole body in relation to the environment for a given task. Controlling the posture of the body in space is crucial to all of our movements, whether sitting on a chair or on the floor, moving around and/or using our hands to manipulate objects. All require postures, albeit of different kinds, with Shumway-Cook and Woollacott (2007) referring to them as 'systems'. These involve musculoskeletal components including joint range of motion, muscle properties, and biomechanical relationships between body segments. Neural components comprise motor processes, sensory and perceptual processes, and higher level cognitive processes for adaptation and such activities as anticipation.

When examining some of the processes required in postural control it is not surprising that a child with cerebral problems may show difficulties, and often the fundamental resources are lacking or maladaptive. For example, muscle tone is a component of posture and it has been noted that in children with cerebral palsy it is often impaired by being either too much or too little for the requirements of a given task. Tasks that are usually thought of as simple, such as static balance involving either sitting or standing upright, are dependent on a number of control processes. Even static balance involves small amounts of postural sway with body alignment, muscle tone, and postural tone all contributing to keeping the body upright. Body alignment allows the body to be in equilibrium with the least amount of energy expenditure. Muscle tone is the stiffness of the muscle and how much it resists being lengthened. Postural tone is the activity in antigravity postural muscles to counteract the forces of gravity (Shumway-Cook and Woollacott 2007).

In order that the body is tuned to the environment such that maintenance and alteration to postural control are appropriate, the perceptual systems play an important role. The person needs to know when and how to use the postural mechanisms, and for this an accurate picture of where the body is in space in relation to the environmental context is essential. Our visual, somatosensory (proprioceptors, cutaneous, and joint receptors), and vestibular senses provide us with this information. In children with cerebral palsy, for a variety of reasons, this sensory information is often inaccurate, and thus leads to inappropriate information being fed into a motor system that is not fully intact and accurate.

Shumway-Cook and Woollacott (2007) describe how coordination of muscle synergies (what have earlier been described as coordinative structures) influence postural control and divide the problems seen into the three parts of (a) sequencing problems, (b) timing problems, and (c) adapting postural activity to changing contextual demands. Some of their earlier work is shown as a closer examination in Box 7.5.

The overall results indicated that postural control problems in spasticity and ataxia are different. In the former, there was more difficulty with coordination of muscular activity, particularly in temporal ordering of muscle contractions; in the latter, the difficulties were found with related disorders in the sensory feedback mechanisms that monitor body position and motion with respect to vertical forces and surrounding objects. In spasticity, postural instability could be due to inappropriate muscle sequencing rather than weakness or inactivity in proximal muscles. Hypertonus usually is viewed as a primary cause of movement abnormalities, but it could be a compensatory means of stabilizing proximal limb segments during inappropriate ordering of muscle contractions. Also, ataxic tremor usually is attributed to aberrant muscle activity, but it appears to be more due to poor or inadequate use of sensory feedback information.

This work by Woollacott, Shumway-Cook and Nashner in numerous publications suggests that the normal sequencing of muscular activity patterns in children with, for example, spastic diplegia may be disrupted, reduced in amplitude, and slow with anticipatory postural control problems all affecting postural stability. This type of work confirms that the personal resources that a child with cerebral palsy possesses and brings to any movement situation have profound effects on posture, and the children are required to find individual and idiosyncratic solutions to these challenges. A first reaction to these challenges may be to think that they are so great that little can be done. But we do know that by changing the environment, by modifying the visual array, altering the task or varying other task variables such as instructions and different types of augmented feedback, the responses of the children are different and in many cases can be improved. This line of thought is developed further in Chapter 12.

Control of walking

In Chapter 4 there is a description of the progression in the development of walking in typically developing children. Development not only involves improvement in what can be described as normal walking, but also it can be varied to walk backwards, sideways, on tiptoes, and other ways. Normal walking involves a well-defined sequence of joint actions in the leg that are controlled by muscle activity and inertial momentum of the moving limb segments. The foot and ankle, because they are the junction between the floor and the leg, act as a pivot during walking and have a major influence on gait quality. These in turn depend upon actions occurring at the hip and knee joints. Muscle problems can limit and alter foot and ankle functioning in ways that lead to abnormal gait, and a comprehensive analysis of gait patterns is employed to examine how this occurs.

Box 7.5 A closer examination

Stance and posture control in selected groups of children with cerebral palsy: deficits in sensory organization and muscular coordination: Nashner et al (1983)

Aims and participants
Nashner et al (1983) compared muscle synergy responses of children with cerebral palsy with those of typically developing children when trying to maintain postural control in relation to changes in sensory information. Ten children with cerebral palsy who were only mildly impaired, could stand and walk, and were not currently in therapy were matched with 10 typically developing children.

Methods
Children were tested on an instrumented platform that allowed several permutations of physical and sensory perturbations. The platform was moved forwards or backwards in condition A to cause body sway opposite to the direction of platform movement, and was rotated down to the front or rear in condition B to cause ankle dorsiflexion or plantarflexion. Velocity of platform displacement was scaled to the height of each child and the platform in condition C was rotated in direct proportion to body sway. Kinaesthetic information indicating a vertical posture (relative to the platform) was in conflict with vestibular and visual information indicating forward or rearward leaning posture. An enclosure that was rotated in direct proportion to body sway maintained a constant visual surround in condition D and, in addition, visual information in condition D indicated a vertical posture in relation to the visual surround that was in conflict with kinaesthetic and vestibular information.
There were different combinations of platform movements and sensory perturbations, for example trying to stand still while reaching to grasp and push or pull a handle. Muscle synergy responses were measured by electromyographic recordings of gastrocnemius, tibialis anterior, hamstring, and quadriceps muscles for the standing task and in biceps and triceps muscles in the reaching task.

Results
There were different postural responses within the group of children with cerebral palsy. The three children with hemiplegic spasticity showed muscle synergy problems but maintained their upright posture during sensory conflict conditions C and D. The children with ataxia had nearly the opposite responses by showing appropriate muscle synergy characteristics but experiencing problems in maintaining upright posture, occasionally falling over.
   In both groups with cerebral palsy, onset latencies of muscle synergies were slow in response to forward and backward sway. Children with ataxia displayed the typical order of onset of muscle activation in which distal muscles were activated prior to proximal muscles. However, in the hemiplegic children with spasticity, the order of onset of muscle activation was reversed, becoming proximal to distal during movements that involved the affected leg and arm. The results from the three children with spastic diplegia and one child with athetosis were variable and not as clear; some had the order reversed (very much like the children with hemiplegia) whereas others had problems in both synergy order and response to sensory conflict (like the children with ataxia).

Discussion
Nashner et al propose that these findings concerning the mechanisms that governed the temporal order of action, as seen in the reversal of distal to proximal activation of muscle activity, contradict the assumptions about the role of reflex activity in postural control. For example, stretch reflexes (deep tendon reflex) in the gastrocnemius were clinically assessed as elevated in the hemiplegic children, a symptom that should have made them more responsive to platform perturbations. But responses to stretch of the gastrocnemius during forward and backward sway were delayed (150ms) compared with the response in typically developing children (95–110ms). This delay may have allowed the hamstrings to contract first, thereby reversing the normal distal to proximal ordering of muscle contractions. They proposed that this could not be attributed to elevated hamstring stretch responses because these, too, were slightly delayed when compared with normal children. The authors concluded that during stance, changes in stretch reflex mechanisms are not the cause of poor control of the spastic leg.

Typical walking

A number of techniques are available for analysing gait. A comprehensive gait analysis requires multiple measures, including EMG recordings, kinematic analysis, and force platform data, along with related computer analyses. Researchers and clinicians choose techniques that are appropriate and available for their particular purposes. Even then it is subject to the interpretation of researchers and clinicians trying to extrapolate specific information from a huge number of data (Ledebt 2003).

Comprehensive analyses of normal gait begin with the division of a single stride cycle into a swing phase and a stance phase for each leg (Inman et al 1981). The stance phase for the right leg begins at heel contact and continues through the time of double support, when the left leg also has contact with the floor. The swing phase is initiated as the leg swings to the rear and then forwards to heel contact. The stance phases of each leg overlap during the time of double support. Joint angles of the ankle, knee, and hip change throughout the stance and swing phases. Unnecessary muscle activity is kept to a minimum while maintaining balance, but muscle activity must provide sufficient force for forward progression. Muscles must hold as well as yield. Inertial momentum is also important because a moving leg provides some of the impetus for leg movement and allows muscles to be quiet at certain times in a well coordinated gait. Elaboration of this is found in Chapter 3.

Variables in walking in cerebral palsy

Gage (1991, p. 101) notes that children with cerebral palsy show some or all of the following characteristics:

- loss of selective muscle control;
- dependence on primitive reflex patterns for ambulation;
- abnormal muscle tone;
- relative imbalance between muscle agonists and antagonists across joints; and
- deficient equilibrium reactions.

These in turn produce the often idiosyncratic walking patterns we see in cerebral palsy.

Using a different set of criteria and taking a more constraints-led approach, Ledebt (2003) proposes the following three main characteristics of walking in children with cerebral palsy:

- limited range of motion;
- rotational deformities of bone; and
- weak joint power.

All of these in turn lead to problems of stability in stance, sufficient foot clearance during the swing, adequate step length, energy conservation, and appropriate swing-phase positioning of the foot. She continues to note that the above abnormalities rarely occur in isolation but are multiple and consist of both primary and secondary characteristics; it is important to separate the primary causes of any gait difficulties from the secondary ones that are compensations that a child will make to overcome the primary problem. A good example of this is toe-walking. One explanation posits that the cause is overactivity and strong contractions and shortening in the plantar flexors (Winters et al 1987), whereas an opposing view claims that toe-walking is compensation for weak plantar flexors and weak calf muscles (Kerrigan et al 2000). These two opposing explanations would lead to differing intervention strategies, with the former concentrating on lengthening or shortening the plantar flexors and the latter looking to strengthen them. In a summary of these, Ledebt (2003) provides evidence to come down in favour of the latter, believing that toe-walking is a compensatory activity for weak plantar flexors and weak calf muscles. Gage (1991) provides another example of the stiff knee gait leading to problems, with foot clearance in swing being produced by cospasticity of the rectus femoris and hamstrings. A compensation that is often made is hip abduction, allowing the leg to swing more freely. The cospasticity of the rectus femoris and the hamstrings thus become the primary cause and the hip abduction is the secondary or coping strategy.

Analysing walking in cerebral palsy

General gait differences between children with cerebral palsy and typically developing children have been reported by numerous other authors. For example, Skrotzky (1983) used computerized high-speed cinematography to compare the walking gaits of six children with cerebral palsy and 39 typically developing children. Children with cerebral palsy had decreased movement amplitude, shorter stride length, and slower gait velocity. Their movement patterns also were different including a lack of normal flexion–extension relationships in the lower limb and hip and differences in dorsiflexion and plantarflexion relationships at the ankle. In many children with cerebral palsy, pathological foot problems impose serious constraints on posture and walking. These conditions include equinus, which is related to prolonged or preterm activity of the soleus or gastrocnemius, caused by, among other things, continuous contractions of the posterior or anterior tibialis and the intensity of medial muscle contractions when the foot is in contact with the floor. Surgical and pharmaceutical interventions are often made to relieve these constraints.

The last 20 years has witnessed new techniques in examining and assessing actions such as walking. For example, motion analysis has allowed us to analyse the dynamic relationships of kinetic and kinematic features of locomotion by plotting measures of these features or higher order derivatives of the measures against each other, rather than plotting them separately against time. As an example, trajectories of joint angles are recorded during gait and are then plotted against each other to form a cyclic pattern for each stride. This provides a graphic display of the manner and extent to which two measures or a measure and its derivative are coordinated with each other.

DeBruin et al (1982) examined changes in hip angle plotted against changes in knee angle to provide a more objective analysis of gait development for use in assessing change following therapy. Walking of six normal and 15 children with cerebral palsy was filmed, and angle–angle plots for knee and hip joint movements of the right leg were detailed for one stride cycle of three children with cerebral palsy and one typically developing child. The first plot, for a typically developing female (age 11), was almost square with round corners and the coordination of knee and hip joint movements in this angle–angle plot shows a reasonably mature gait pattern. The angle–angle plots for the three children with cerebral palsy are quite different from this plot and from each other. A second plot is of a 9-year-old female with spastic diplegia, who in a clinical assessment had the most typical movements of the children with cerebral palsy. Her overall pattern of a rounded square is much smaller in size, indicating a reduced range of knee motion as well as increased flexion at heel strike. A third plot, of a 13-year-old female with spastic quadriplegia, shows that during the stance phase the hip starts to extend, as does her knee, rather than move towards flexion. In the swing phase, the pattern reverses, with both joints moving towards flexion. Concurrent flexion or concurrent extension, as represented in the diagonal plotting lines, is not indicative of a proficient gait and can be counterproductive. The fourth plot is of a 12-year-old female, also with quite severe spastic quadriplegia, and the location of her square-like but very small plot in the upper right indicates strong flexion contractures in both joints with a limited range of motion in both joints. Initial stance contact with her right foot was with the forefoot, whereas contact with her left foot was with the foot flat. The descriptions show not only the differences between plots of typically developing children and those of children with cerebral palsy, but also the variability and heterogeneous nature of the plots shown by children with cerebral palsy.

Beuter and Garfinkel (1985) used a different analysis, employing phase plane plots to describe knee and hip movements of three individuals with spasticity, three individuals with athetosis, and three typically developing individuals (ages 4–34) stepping over an object. The phase plane trajectories of typically developing individuals were orbital in shape with no intersections, whereas those of the individuals with cerebral palsy were quite different in size and shape with all but one having loops that intersected the trajectory line. These loops, which tended to occur in the extension phase, indicate retrograde motion and tended to occur earlier in the hip movement than in the knee. The authors saw the absence of loops as suggesting that the joint motion is a self-organizing system that is central to a dynamical explanation of motor behaviour. These dynamics involve decreasing flexion associated with flexion velocity that increases to a maximum, then decreases to zero at maximum flexion with the hip and knee then extending. In children with cerebral palsy, the intersecting loops in the phase plane trajectories indicate a fundamental change in the system dynamics with at least one more variable entering the system, thus making it more complex and changing the relationship between joint flexion and extension.

Walking prognosis in cerebral palsy

Of obvious interest to parents, clinicians, and researchers is whether there are any early signs that can give accurate predictions of later walking. There are some data that suggest that type of cerebral palsy can give an indication of later walking with general conclusions that those with hemiplegia and ataxia have greater potential for walking than children with hypotonia, whereas with other types the outcome is more variable (Watt et al 1989).

Ledebt (2003) analysed eight studies to determine if there were any common factors that are predictors of locomotion in children with cerebral palsy. First, she notes that those with hemiplegia and ataxia have a better outcome than those with dystonia, noting that a major predictor is the absence or persistence of primary reflexes. From her review of studies, those who showed persistence of reflexes such as the asymmetrical and symmetrical tonic neck reflexes, tonic labyrinthine reflexes, and supporting reflexes at 18 months rarely became ambulatory. She also notes that the rate of attainment of other milestones, such as sitting without support, is related to later walking status, but they are not predictors of the age at which walking will be achieved. Ledebt (2003) notes that, although there is great variability, the most reliable predictor for both aided and independent walking is the ability to sit unaided by the age of 2 years. On the other hand, negative predictors, that is the presence of those variables that are a hindrance to walking, include abnormal and postural primary reactions after 1 year of age and the inability to sit before 36 months. Other predictors include the probability that if a child with quadriplegic cerebral palsy is non-ambulatory aided or unaided by the age of 4, the chances of walking afterwards are very much diminished. In addition, it appears that the co-occurrence of other difficulties such as severe learning difficulties and epilepsy are also contributing factors with the explanation being that these are simply symptomatic of a more impaired neurological system.

The control of walking in children with cerebral palsy is a classic example of a dynamic system. The resources of the child, that is the type and extent of central nervous system (CNS) damage, bring with them changes in the intrinsic constraints, thereby affecting outcome. In addition, the extrinsic constraints, such as visual information flow, interact with these internal constraints to provide variability of outcome. With respect to this, Ledebt (2003) notes that kinematic and kinetic gait analyses have moved us forward in the description and prognosis of ambulation in children with cerebral palsy. However, she also adds caution in the interpretation of the data before they are used as the basis for treatment such as surgery, noting that there are often different explanations for the movement variations that are being observed. For example, in toe-walking she notes that often treatments improve the local characteristics without improving general gait efficiency and recommends that such variables as global levels of balance and the risk of falling also be considered. The development of walking in children with cerebral palsy depends upon a number of factors such as location and severity of the condition, the amount of support and practice the child receives, and any medical procedures that are engaged. With atypical neural substrates it is not surprising that we find different profiles from typical development in behavioural and kinematic measures. However, in the light of the ICF model, the important factor appears to be function, with a measure of the child's functional ability being the important variable as measured by the GMFM. As we have noted many times, outcomes are affected by multidimensional variables with the amount of appropriate experience being important, and one over which we have some measure of control.

Manual control

General functions
The arm and hand movements control objects often working together in multiple and sometimes different ways, and some of these have been described in Chapter 4. For example, using scissors to cut paper involves controlling the digits to open and close the scissor blades: the arm linkage system provides the support necessary to use the digits and also positions the scissors in relation to the paper. Manual control can be *unimanual* or *bimanual*, using one arm to control an object or using both arms, whether making the same or different movements.

One function of the *arm* is *support*, in which the arm linkage system is kept reasonably immobile in order to support the hand movements manipulating an object, such as with scissors. A second function of the arm is to *position the hand*, as when reaching to touch or grasp an object or transporting an object held in the hand. A third function of the arm is to *generate and modulate force*. When an object, such as a doorknob or screwdriver, is held firmly in the hand, the arm linkage system moves it by rotating the wrist to turn or twist it (Keogh and Sugden 1985).

One function of the *hand* is *grasp*, which includes picking up and holding an object, which can be performed either with the fingers scooping it up or the fingers opposing the thumb to pinch it, or with many variations thereof. When an object is held in the hand, we can describe the grip in two ways – either a power grip or a precision grip – indicating the type of functional control of the object. A second function of the hand is *manipulation*, in which fingers and thumb are used to change an object's position, as in tying shoelaces or turning a coin. Most manual movements combine these body units and their related functions. A spoon is transported and turned by arm movements while digital movements are used to control the position of the spoon to pick up food and place the spoon in the mouth.

Bimanual control is a matter of coordinating the two arm linkage systems, often while each system is making a movement different from the other. The two arm linkages can be used *separately*, such as one hand holding a jar while the other twists the top. Equally important are the *simultaneous* and *coordinated* use of the two arms in symmetrical and asymmetrical movements such as the two hands working together to roll pastry (Keogh and Sugden 1985).

Grips
Manual skills have also been classified with respect to anatomical and complexity criteria. For example, grips have been analysed as they are utilized in series of actions including those of transverse digital, adult digital, ventral clenched, adult clenched, oblique palmar, and transverse palmar (Fig. 7.5, which is the same as Fig. 5.8; Connolly and Elliott 1972).

Another example of value in the area of a classification system of manipulation is one by Connolly and Elliott (1984) and used by Sugden and Utley (1995) in

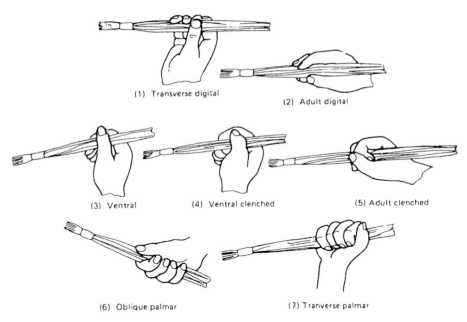

(1) Transverse digital   (2) Adult digital

(3) Ventral   (4) Ventral clenched   (5) Adult clenched

(6) Oblique palmar   (7) Tranverse palmar

Fig. 7.5 Grip variations of 3- and 4-year-old children when painting on an upright easel. Reproduced with permission of the publisher from Connolly and Elliott (1972).

children with cerebral palsy. In this classification, Elliott and Connolly present three categories of movement that encompass most manipulative movements and are called simple synergies, reciprocal synergies, and sequential patterns. Simple and reciprocal synergies involve movements that are simultaneous, with all the digits moving together in a single movement pattern.

- *Simple synergies* involve the thumb and digits working together as convergent flexors or extensors, such as squeezing a rubber ball. All the digits work in the same way.
- *Reciprocal synergies* involve movements in which the thumb and digits perform different activities, often with one flexing and the other extending, such as rolling a piece of plasticine between the thumb and first two digits.
- *Sequential patterns* involve the independent coordination of the digits in a sequence of movements, with some digits supporting an object while others move it. Turning a pencil end over end in one hand would be an example.

These tasks were used together with a selection of tasks from Brown (1987) by Sugden and Utley (1995) in their examination of functional manual skills in children with cerebral palsy. They organized tasks into Elliott and Connolly's (1984) groupings of simple synergies, reciprocal synergies, and sequential patterns, as well as

some additional bimanual tasks. The performance of the tasks was judged on a four-point scale with high being good performance. The mean for the non-hemiplegic hand scoring was 3.13 with the hemiplegic hand scoring 1.9, a difference that was significant. Of more importance was that the performance of the children revealed a change in strategy as the difficulty of the tasks increased. The simple strategies were usually performed with relative smoothness, but as the children performed the reciprocal tasks they became much more variable and less efficient. This was also true of the sequential patterns. Of interest was the finding that the bimanual tasks seemed to increase the fluency with which the children could use their hemiplegic hand, and this point is taken up in the section on bimanual skills. The authors looked at both fluency and efficiency of movement and by doing this they were able to examine how stability and change in one was accompanied by stability and change in the other and the complex interactions of the two noting the dynamic relationship between them.

Unimanual skills

Early classic works by Twitchell (1958, 1959) describe reaching and grasping problems of children with cerebral palsy. In the 1959 study, Twitchell reported that children with athetosis very often showed increased flexion of the arm, rather than the extension needed for a more efficient reaching movement. As reaching began, the arm was abducted at the shoulder, flexed at the elbow, and pronated at the wrist, so that the hand moved towards the head with fingers and thumb extended and remained like this with alternating flexion and extension of both the elbow and fingers. The hand showed wavering movements when approaching and touching the object and when withdrawing the hand it was often accompanied by a turning of head and eyes, and sometimes the trunk, indicating the dynamic interaction of postural control adjustments in control of manual movements. Often, when the object was grasped, it was dropped or held with an abnormally tight grip, a feature later analysed in detail by Forssberg and colleagues.

Film analyses of the grasping of 25 children with hemiplegia (ages 11mo to 15y) were reported by Twitchell (1958). First, there was a general slowness in speed of movement of the hemiplegic limb, starting with a delay of 1 to 3 seconds longer than the less involved limb in the initiation of reaching. A second general problem was overextension of fingers and occasionally of the wrist, which is different to normal preparation for grasping where fingers remain in a semiflexed position. The thumb, which was adducted at rest, remained in the adducted position. Grasp was weak, with an undulating change in grip power rather than a gradual reduction of power after grip was established again, a feature later taken up by Forssberg and colleagues (Forssberg et al 1991, 1992, 1999, Eliasson et al 1991, 1992, 1998, 2006). This was observed in everyday activities with children dropping objects normally expected to be carried. He also reported a difference in control of fixating muscles of the wrist during the process of grasping. When an object is grasped and the fingers flex around the object, wrist extensors normally fix the wrist and act synergistically with the flexors of the fingers to provide efficiency and power. Cerebral palsied children flexed the wrist towards the object, disrupting the fixation of the wrist, and lessened the leverage advantage of the fingers. When the wrist was artificially fixed in position by a splint, there was a doubling of grip strength. Twitchell suggests that wrist flexion is part of a flexor synergy of the upper extremity. Although the normal synergy is replaced by one ill suited to the effective and efficient performance of grasping, it may be the best adaptation that can be made by children with cerebral palsy within their intrinsic constraints. This provides a good example of how coordinative structures or synergies are recruited in a different manner to typically developing children, and yet with a relatively simple procedure the nature of the task can be change that changes the dynamics of the context, assisting the child to accomplish the movement.

There are two main functional requirements involved in the formation of finger grip during grasping: (i) the grip needs to adapt to the size, shape, and use of the objects to be grasped and (ii) the relative timing of finger movements for grasping must be coordinated with the reaching movement. Jeannerod (1986) filmed patients with pathological conditions, including two children with hemiplegia, as they reached to grasp an object. Grip formation of the normal and affected hands of the two children with hemiplegia are shown in Figure 7.6.

The non-hemiplegic hand of Child A who is typically developing (age 23mo) did not shape completely, but the desired pattern of extension followed by flexion was clearly present. On contact there was immediate flexion of the fingers for correct grip formation. However, the affected hand remained overextended throughout the movement. Child B (age 5y) had better use of the normal limb in a pincer grasp of a small object. The index finger in the affected hand remained extended with incomplete flexion of the extended finger. Finger grip formation was not observed during reaching.

In a series of articles, Eliasson and Forssberg and colleagues in Sweden have conducted extensive work on hand function in typically developing children and those with cerebral palsy (Forssberg et al 1991, 1992, 1999, Eliasson et al 1991, 1992, 1998, 2006). Much of their work has been directed to prehensile force control when the children are manipulating objects, with the basic finding that children with cerebral palsy have difficulties with fingertip force control and amplitude control when they are manipulating objects with the additional problem of slower movements and prolonged delays during movement phases. They report that typically developing children have the ability to simultaneously initiate the grip and load forces by the use of what they call a 'grip-lift synergy' and are able to accomplish this by 4 years of age. This is very much in line with the description of what we have called coordinative structures, which are softly assembled according to the contextual need and the suggestion that the assembly of these could be impaired in children with cerebral palsy. Eliasson and Forssberg (Forssberg et al 1991, 1992, 1999, Eliasson et al 1991, 1992, 1998, 2006) have confirmed that children with cerebral palsy have difficulties in anticipatory control without extensive practice even though they can adjust their grip according to the object's weight. However, this is a sequential process, not the simultaneous one that is seen in typically developing children. The children with cerebral palsy have what Eliasson et al (2006) call an 'impaired grip-lift synergy' with the hand first pressing the object down onto the tabletop and exhibiting variable grip forces before the lifting takes place. Thus, the action becomes laboured and sequential in contrast to the smoother anticipatory simultaneous actions of the typically developing child.

The question Eliasson et al (2006) asked was whether this impairment, which produced large differences

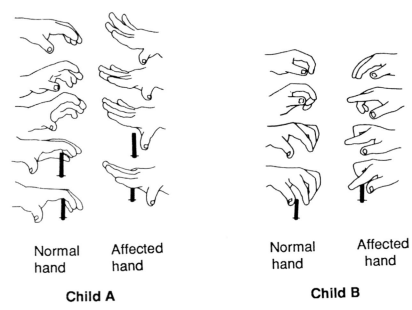

| Normal hand | Affected hand | | Normal hand | Affected hand |

Child A **Child B**

Fig. 7.6 Formation of finger grip of normal and affected hands of two patients with hemiplegic cerebral palsy. Reproduced from Jeannerod (1986).

between the two groups from 6 to 10 years of age, changed as the children with cerebral palsy developed. A closer examination of this question is shown in Box 7.6.

Unimanual skills in children with cerebral palsy differ in several ways to those of children who are typically developing. In terms of grips, they are often either fixed in stereotypical positions or fluctuating in hand posture, both of which result in atypical movements and inefficient and/or ineffective actions. In addition, lifting and grasping strategies appear to consist of two sequential actions rather than the simultaneous grip–lift strategy that is usually observed in typically developing children.

Bimanual skills

In everyday life there is constant use of the hands both separately and together, unimanually or bimanually, which can be both symmetrical, doing the same thing with both hands, or more usually asymmetrical, doing one thing with one hand and another action with the other. Thus, actions such as tying a knot, unscrewing the top of a jar, or stabilizing a piece of paper while writing often figure in our daily routines. Both hands have to come together to complement each other by working in time and space in a coordinated manner.

The research on bimanual movements points to a recognition that often the movements of one limb may affect the movements of the other. That is why performing different movements with each limb is often difficult – the rubbing tummy–tapping head type movements – showing

that there is a tendency to link or couple the limbs in time and space. Most of the literature has confirmed this tendency in the timing of the hands and with rather less attention being paid to the spatial influence between the hands (Steenbergen et al 2003). This tendency to 'couple', as this linking phenomena is called, could be seen as of interest and of benefit to those individuals who have impairment in one limb but are relatively unaffected in the other. Thus, in the condition of hemiplegic cerebral palsy whereby one side of the body is more affected than the other, this tendency for the two hands to work together may have both theoretical and practical implications. Both of these are addressed here as it is difficult to separate them, but more work on the practical and intervention side is presented in Chapter 12.

Work with healthy adult populations has confirmed that timing is very often coupled. Kelso et al (1983) found that when individuals reached for a target unimanually, Fitts' law was confirmed. Fitts' law (Fitts 1954) specifies a linear relationship between the distance of the object to be reached and the width of the object with the following formula: movement time=a+b $\log_2(2A/W)$.

This relationship has been confirmed often in adults and under varying conditions. When Kelso et al (1983) used bimanual tasks with both hands working to aim for different targets of different lengths, the normal relationship specified by Fitts' law broke down and when the hands were reaching for different targets they still arrived at the target at the same time. This tendency of

Box 7.6 A closer examination

Development of hand function and precision grip control in individuals with cerebral palsy: a 13-year follow-up study: Eliasson et al (2006)

This study took the rarely examined development of hand functions in children, with the authors noting that, despite the lack of studies, there is some evidence to suggest that improvements can be made. They note that the effects of occupational therapy, particularly when combined with botulinum toxin and constraint-induced therapy, have shown results and that although the long-term development is unclear, hand function is dynamic and susceptible to change.

Methods

Twelve children with cerebral palsy took part in the study, six with hemiplegia and six with diplegia, and all participated in the first data collections in 1989–90 when they were 6 to 8 years of age. Of the 12, 10 returned in 2002–03 to participate and were then 19 to 20 years of age. All had been in mainstream schools and all had access to paediatric rehabilitation programmes. The Jebsen–Taylor test of hand functioning was used to test speed and dexterity and the Manual Ability Classification System (see page 185) was used to describe hand function competence in daily life. The Jebsen–Taylor test consists of seven subtasks including grasping differently weighted objects between the thumb and index finger, stacking checkers, simulated eating, and turning over cards. The writing task is excluded. Each subtest is quantified in terms of the length of time taken to complete the task.

Results and comments

The times for the Jebson–Taylor test decreased on average by 45% between the first trial at 6 to 8 years and the second trial at 19 to 20 years of age. All subtests, except for card turning, decreased, but only the reduction for the simulated eating was significant. The time to complete the grip–lift task decreased by 22%, which was mainly due to a faster preload phase, indicating that the movement was becoming less sequential. In addition, the participants pushed down the object before lifting, suggesting a less sequential force generation. There was also some improvement in anticipatory force control to the weight of the object.

At 6 to 8 years of age the children with cerebral palsy had not developed force coordination patterns typical for their age but had a rather immature pattern. Even as adults, although there was clearly some development, they still retained a sequential initiation of grasping and reaching with a press downwards on to the tabletop. Anticipation of force according to an object's weight and texture was absent at 6 to 8 years as the children could not scale grip and load during grasping on the basis of previous experience. This partially improved by the second session at 19 to 20 years of age. Overall, there was improvement in hand functions despite variability within the sample group, suggesting that development had taken place and increased hand function is not simply an early years phenomenon and is not static. The authors conclude that hand function capability is amenable to intervention, suggesting that functional and structural plasticity in the brain is possible.

the limbs to couple has been explored many times since the Kelso study, with researchers varying the difficulty of the movements and also moving into the realm of spatial coupling (Swinnen et al 1998, Bogaerts and Swinnen 2001). In children, too, the phenomenon of coupling has often been reported, with authors such as Fagard et al (2001) and Jeeves et al (1988) noting that maturation in interhemispheric communication and the corpus callosum was related to the coordination of bimanual movements.

In individuals with cerebral palsy, and in particular those with hemiplegic cerebral palsy, there are obvious problems with everyday tasks that require the use

of both limbs, and, in spite of this, as Steenbergen et al (2003) have noted, there is a scarcity of work examining bimanual actions in children with hemiplegic cerebral palsy. In studies that have examined the differences between the more and less involved sides in individuals with hemiplegic cerebral palsy, the evidence points to a proximal to distal increase in movement asymmetry. Steenbergen et al (2003) propose that this is because distal tasks, such as grasping, pose severe problems possibly because the hand and fingers are controlled totally by the damaged hemisphere, whereas movements of the trunk (proximal movements) are controlled on a bilateral basis, with some from the more intact hemisphere. This is why, when moving with the involved side, many individuals show a preference for trunk movement as well as arm movements when reaching and grasping.

Two studies examined reaching and aiming or pointing in both unimanual and bimanual conditions and analysed the differences between them (Sugden and Utley 1995, Utley and Sugden 1998). These studies also looked at spatial variables and hand postures, as well as the usual temporal variables, and are outlined in Box 7.7.

Work by Steenbergen et al (2000) and Rice and Newell (2001) showed that coupling also occurred at the interjoint level, as in elbow and shoulder movements, with often the unimpaired side adapting to the impaired side. Overall, the results on coupling in hemiplegic cerebral palsy show coupling at the level of the kinematics of end effector and at interjoint level with the unimpaired side able to respond flexibly between unimanual and bimanual movements. This tendency to couple has been taken forward with interesting possibilities for rehabilitation with what has become known as Hand–Arm Bimanual Intensive Training (HABIT; Charles and Gordon 2006). This is described in more detail in Chapter 12, but is based on some of the principles of coupling, that is using both hands in cooperation with each other during activities of daily living.

In summary, several general observations can be made of the limited information about manual movements of children with cerebral palsy:

- Movements generally are slow, variable, and often weak.
- Natural movement patterns are disrupted by differences in muscle synergies (e.g. producing flexion instead of extension) and poor timing.
- Grip formation during reaching often is poor or absent.
- The forces that are exerted during the grasping of an object are variable and often not directly related to the efficient accomplishment of the task, and, finally, more corrections are needed during reaching, which indicates poor programming of movements.
- Children with cerebral palsy do couple their limbs in bimanual movements and this could lead to more specific and targeted intervention. Using bimanual movements and the natural tendency to couple may be a way towards exploiting different task presentations.

In addition to the above, we know that proprioceptive information is often poor in children with cerebral palsy, and thus again there is the situation with an impaired motor system working on less efficient sensory information.

Although this presents a picture of the resources of the child being less effective, it does also present challenges to researchers and clinicians about how the contextual environment and the selection and presentation of tasks can be modified to maximise the potential of the children.

Visuomotor skills

The emphasis in this section has been on movement skill problems related to inadequate muscle activation. It is important also to consider problems in adapting movements to environmental conditions and task requirements, particularly in terms of perception and use of visual input. Is visuoperceptual development inadequate, as a result of brain damage or impoverished movement experiences, in ways that constrain the adaptation of movements beyond the limitations imposed by poor neuromotor coordination?

The everyday task of handwriting and drawing provides us with some clues in this complex area. Both handwriting and drawing demand that the child not only provides purposeful goal-directed movement but also does so with great accuracy and the process is constantly monitored and/or directed by vision. This applies in many skills, but in these it is emphasized because of the continuous nature of the task, in that it involves a sequence of actions over a continuous period of time and there is ongoing feedback. In some classic studies, Abercrombie (1970) views normal visuoperceptual development as progressing from more global perceptions that provide general approximations of the visual world to more analytical perceptions that provide more detail and better information about relationships among figure features. She believes the more global level of visuoperceptual development can be limited by inadequate experience, particularly the lack of skilled movement experiences, and children with cerebral palsy are often slower in developing adequate eye movement control and have more impoverished movement experiences. These may lead to delays in visuoperceptual development that limit movement skill development.

A second possibility is that, although visuoperceptual development is adequate, a child cannot use visual information to organize a movement response. Abercrombie reported that some children made many changes of patterns, constructed with sticks or blocks, that they knew were not correct, but they made matters worse by altering the generally adequate global shape in an effort to improve relationships and details. She saw this as a conflict in which they viewed the general approximation as no longer sufficient, but they were not able to improve on what they had done initially. In general, children with neurological disorders generally take more time to write legibly, and the ability of those with hemiplegic cerebral

Box 7.7 A closer examination

Bimanual coupling in children with hemiplegic cerebral palsy: Sugden and Utley (1995) and Utley and Sugden (1998)

In these two studies the authors noted the tendency in typically developing children and adults to couple and conducted two studies to analyse the phenomenon in children with hemiplegic cerebral palsy. In both studies the experimental paradigm was the same: children with hemiplegic cerebral palsy reached and pointed or grasped with one hand, then the other, followed by a reach and grasp with both hands together. The analysis involved an examination of unimanual impaired hand reaching compared with reaching in a bimanual condition. In the first study (Sugden and Utley 1995) the children reached in their own preferred time whereas in the second study (Utley and Sugden 1998) the reaching and grasping was done at speed, as fast as possible. In both experiments, the movements were captured on real-time video plus kinematic analysis with points on shoulder, elbow, wrist and thumb, and first finger.

All of the children in the two studies were classified as hemiplegic, with cerebral palsy, and aged between 6 and 10 years. They were all moderately impaired and could make an effort to reach and grasp with the involved limb. In both studies three measures of coupling were used. The first was one of overall timing: did the timing of the two hands change in the unimanual and bimanual conditions? Second, trajectory: did this alter in the two conditions? Third, finger and hand shaping: was there any difference between the two conditions?

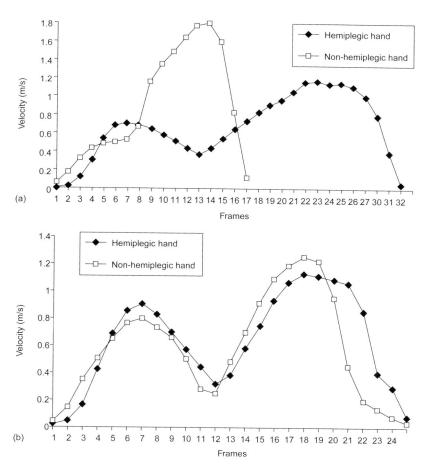

Fig. 7.7 Unimanual (a) and bimanual (b) reaching and grasping at preferred speed. Experiment 1. Reproduced with permission of the publishers from Utley and Sugden (1998).

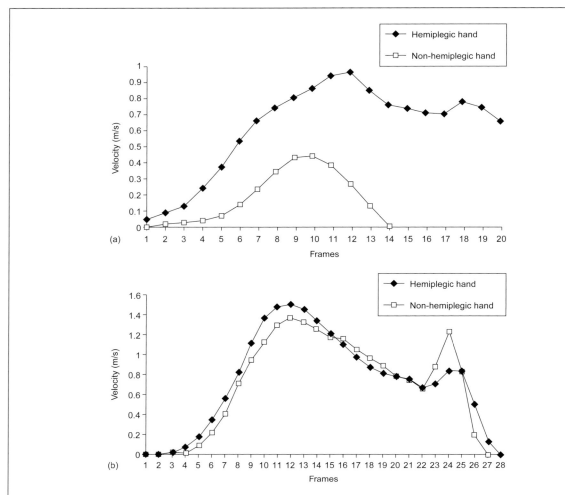

Fig. 7.8 Unimanual (a) and bimanual (b) reaching and grasping as fast as possible. Experiment 1. Reproduced with permission of the publishers from Utley and Sugden (1998).

The results were consistent across the two studies. In the first instance, nearly every child showed evidence of coupling, that is in the bimanual condition there was a movement of the two hands to work together. However, the manner in which this occurred varied. First, it was in the area of timing that most coupling took place. In the bimanual condition, there were several instances of the impaired limb 'moving' to the speed of the unaffected limb when compared with the unimanual condition. In many cases this involved a speeding up of the impaired limb, while occasionally the unaffected limb slowed down. On other occasions, in the unimanual condition, the hemiplegic limb occasionally never reached the target. Examples of these are shown in Figures 7.7 and 7.8.

In Figure 7.7b, in the bimanual condition, the hemiplegic hand speeds up and the non-hemiplegic hand slows down so they both work in time together. In Figure 7.8a, in the unimanual condition, the hemiplegic hand never hits the target, but does so when coupled with the non-hemiplegic hand (7.8b). In the area of trajectory, there were instances of the impaired limb taking a lower trajectory in the bimanual condition rather than the high 'slapping' movements during the unimanual condition. In only a few instances did hand shaping change as a result of the two hands working together, and when it did with a better shaping from the impaired hand, no other changes took place. It was as though changing this aspect of reaching and grasping was all the system could deal with at one particular time.

The two studies have implications for both theoretical explanations of movement behaviour and clinical work for children with hemiplegic cerebral palsy.

palsy depends on several factors including severity, extent of sensory loss, degree of spasticity, and the presence of dystonia (Berninger and Rutberg 1992, Bumin and Kavak 2008).

Howard and Henderson (1989) provide an example that takes us beyond eye–hand coordination to involve mobility within the environment. Children aged 7 to 14 years were asked to judge their body size in relation to a door opening. Two groups of cerebral palsied children, with either spasticity or athetosis, and a third group of nonhandicapped children were matched on mental age. Children with cerebral palsy included some who were ambulatory and some who were in wheelchairs. The children were shown a door opening in which height and width could be adjusted by moving blinds from the top or the sides. They were tested first on changes in door height and were asked to indicate when the space was just big enough for them to walk through without bending and without knocking off their hat. A similar procedure was used for door width.

Spatial-body judgements of physically normal children were more accurate than those of cerebral palsied children. The magnitude of the group difference is illustrated by some children with cerebral palsy estimating that a wheelchair could get through a 2.4m gap while others saying it could not. There was no relationship between severity of handicap and visuoperceptual accuracy. We do not know if this difference in visuoperception was a result more of brain damage or limitations in movement skill experiences.

Judgements of children with athetosis were more accurate than those of children with spasticity, whereas Nashner et al (1983) found that spastic children were able to resolve visual, kinaesthetic, and vestibular sensory conflicts while trying to maintain postural control. Although judgements of spatial accuracy and resolution of sensory conflicts are quite different aspects of visuomotor functioning, the differences in results among spastic children indicate the difficulty in determining causal relationships.

PARTICIPATION: RECREATIONAL AND LEISURE ACTIVITIES

The World Health Organization's adoption of the ICF (WHO 2001) has moved the focus from a concentration on disability to the functioning of the child with cerebral palsy in everyday life. This is exemplified by the DMCFS and MACS, described earlier. The emphasis on participation in the ICF (2001) model moves the debate from one that is concentrated on personal resources, where limitations are seen as the determining factor, towards how the environmental circumstances and context can be modified such that individuals with cerebral palsy can participate.

It moves us from a concentration on the consequences of any disorder to an emphasis on components of health and how they can be modified so that support is given to all.

When out-of-school recreation and leisure activities are examined in samples of children with disabilities (including cerebral palsy) and typically developing children, there are differences according to sex, age, and disability (King et al 2010). Children without disabilities enjoyed a widening and more intense social participation and greater levels of enjoyment as they became older, across all age groups of 6 to 8 years, 9 to 11 years and 12 to 14 years. This did not occur in the children with disabilities, with 12- to 14-year-olds reporting less satisfaction than those aged 6 to 8 years of age. The authors make a plea for the creation of community-based recreational centres and improved information for parents.

The King et al (2010) study shows us the consequences of not optimally providing information and support for children with disabilities, and yet there is good evidence that children with cerebral palsy can be involved in a wide range of recreational and leisure activities and that they experience a high level of enjoyment irrespective of their personal resource limitations (Majnemer et al 2008). They note that information collected about a child should include not only their physical ability but also how much the child enjoys or would enjoy leisure and recreational activities and whether and how this increased participation leads to any improvement in quality of life. Parush and Rihtman (2008) ask the question as to what constitutes leisure activities in children with cerebral palsy and whether the same instruments as those used in typically developing children can be used to assess participation and enjoyment. They conclude by asking whether leisure activities requires a new definition for a population of children with cerebral palsy, which is traditionally defined as those activities that are freely chosen and are enjoyable. Imms (2008) presents a description of leisure which seems to better fit a population such as children with cerebral palsy. She notes:

> Leisure is defined in terms of activity, time and meaning. It includes activities performed for pleasure or to restore ourselves, and which provide an opportunity for expressing or forming our identity.
>
> (p. 1878)

As the ICF model has moved the thinking away from simply the child's resources, it is pertinent to examine how the resources of the child interact with his or her activities and level of participation. Morris et al (2006) used a postal survey to obtain details of cerebral palsied children's impairments and factors affecting their activities and participation. Their findings showed that disability does affect activities and participation but does not prevent participation, and they use the term 'participation intensity' to take the debate a little further. They argue that from an equity perspective there should be a systematic assessment of whether the participation of a child with cerebral palsy is consistent with his or her potential and then measure how much this can be improved/ameliorated by technology or the removal of barriers interacting with the child's personal preference.

Coster and Khetani (2008) recommend that the measurement of participation should reflect three key issues:

1 Activity and participation should be differentiated, with activities being simply the execution of a particular task, whereas participation indicates an involvement in what WHO calls life situations that Coster and Khetani (2008) characterize as organized sequences of activities directed to a personally or socially meaningful goal.

2 Whether it is objective or subjective aspects of participation that are being measured, with the former being the observation of whether a child is participating and the latter indicating the extent to which this has meaning to the child.

3 Who is the appropriate person to respond when children are being assessed often depends on whether it is objective or subjective aspects that are being measured. In the former, parents and others close to the child may provide valuable information, but when it is subjective information that is required the child is the most appropriate respondent. The belief is that it is preferable to assess participation through self-report or direct observation with proxy measures being utilized by teachers and parents.

In order to look at the effect of changing children's resources on participation, Wright et al (2008) assessed children's participation before and after botulinum toxin treatment. Thirty-five children with cerebral palsy aged 3 to 12 years were assessed at baseline and at 2 months and 6 months following botulinum toxin treatment. Following a dose of BoNT-A there was a significant reduction in dynamic spasticity as a measure of body structure and function, and activity and participation measures increased. However, the strength of the relationship between the changes in body structures and functions and activity and participation was no more than fair, with correlations around 0.3 to 0.4. The authors conclude that the various levels of the ICF (WHO, 2008) are complex, and activity gains after interventions, such as through

BoNT-A, are likely to be influenced by a combination of a variety of child and environmental factors.

A significant review of the literature on participation in children with cerebral palsy was conducted by Imms (2008), with the studies reported on using cross-sectional, population-based or qualitative methodologies using a person–environment–occupation framework (similar to the task–child resources–environment model used throughout this text). The first part of the review examined general participation factors, noting that children with disabilities experienced greater participation restriction than their peers and that children with cerebral palsy had poorer participation than other disability groups, with large individual variations reported. Most of these studies examined personal child factors as the determining cause of participation restriction. A second part of her review examined environmental factors that influenced participation. She notes that, within a dynamic systems framework and socio-political understanding of disability, there is an increased focus on changing the environment to enable and facilitate participation. These studies highlighted the effect of the community, social and attitudinal barriers, and time-consuming bureaucracy, as well as the eminently practical factors such as the availability of transport help from family and friends. Participation with peers has usually been considered from the perspective of play, with Imms (2008) reporting on both positive and negative experiences. The positive ones were a sense of solidarity with other children and enjoying the challenges of play, with the negative ones being bullied, being exploited and sometimes being included only to make a game work. School participation showed varied results according to differing educational systems, but Imms (2008) concluded that not enough is being done to reduce bullying and to ensure that schools are physically accessible. Participation in leisure activities also showed both positive and negative experiences being present with such variables as family gatherings, reciprocity in friendships, equal treatment, and avoidance tactics from other participants and mocking actions all working in a dynamic way to produce participation outcomes.

Children with cerebral palsy have consistently been found to have lower levels of participation and those with greater functional impairment are the most restricted. They do participate, but at a reduced level, and they are rarely fulfilled in this important area of daily functioning. However, there is insufficient research evidence to make definitive statements about what happens as children get older, and the changing nature of participation such that alterations to the environmental context would bring substantial changes for the better.

This evidence from theory, empirical work, and practical experience is that there is cause for optimism. A dynamical theoretical model of task–child–environment leaves us in control of two of these three components of participation outcomes. From empirical work there is strong evidence that participation varies by location of home, type of school, provision of facilities, attitudes of significant players including peers, and health and community involvement. For professional evidence, one has only to visit a selection of regional or local health centres or talk with parents and the children themselves to recognize that these variables are not only crucial in children's participation, but also under our control, and, if there is a will, can be modified.

Summary

The term cerebral palsy is an umbrella term for a group of individuals who have a motor disorder as their primary and defining characteristic, but who are a heterogeneous group with respect to severity and type and the variety of co-occurring characteristics they evidence. The definitions, aetiology, classifications, and characteristics of children with cerebral palsy are important as they make up part of the dynamical system that eventually produces a movement outcome. The biological basis for the disorder, which is some form of neurological impairment, means that movements are atypical, with a variety shown depending on the type of cerebral palsy. This atypicality often starts with fundamental neural transmission and goes all the way through to functional actions of walking and other gross motor skills and manual activities, such as reaching and grasping, and is particularly influential in restricting the flexibility and adaptability in their

responses to novel movement problems that they encounter in everyday life. These in turn lead to differences both in the performance of and ultimately participation in everyday activities.

The chapter has concentrated on the resources of the child, and in the model that has been presented throughout the text, the child's resources are only part of the story when examining movement outcomes. Yet, they are an important part of the story and without them it is not possible to examine how the children's movement qualities can be improved through modification of the other two parts, namely the task and the environment. These are both examined in Chapter 12 when analysing assessment and intervention.

An examination of the movement capabilities of children with cerebral palsy has ranged from simple control of motor units to global participation in recreational activities, and we have shown that at all levels the modification of the task or the environment has effects on the movement outcomes. From feedback on simple movements (e.g. Harrison 1975c) through changing visual arrays (Nashner et al 1983), to bimanual coordination (Sugden and Utley 1995), changing the nature of the task or the context has influenced the final movement. It is appropriate that the final part of this chapter has addressed the issues of participation in leisure and recreation activities as this has implications for the issues that are raised when the wider environmental context is examined. The resources of the child are crucial and powerful variables when examining their movement competence, but they do not operate in isolation from the task and environment, which together provide the total dynamic system that is the fundamental unit of any comprehensive analysis.

REFERENCES

Abercrombie MLJ (1970) Learning to draw. In: Connolly K, editor. *Mechanisms of Motor Skill Development*. New York: Academic Press, pp. 307–335.

Asatryan DG, Feldman AG (1965) Functional tuning of nervous system with control of movement or maintenance of steady posture: 1. Mechanographic analysis of the work of the joint on execution of a postural task. *Biophysics* 10: 925–935.

Bax MDM (1964) Terminology and classification of cerebral palsy. *Dev Med Child Neurol* 6: 295–297. http://dx.doi.org/10.1111/j.1469-8749.1964.tb10791.x

Bax MDM, Brown K (2004) The spectrum of disorders known as cerebral palsy. In: Scrutton D, Damiano D, Mayston M, editors. *Management of the Motor Disorders of Children with Cerebral Palsy*. London: Mac Keith Press, 9–21.

Bax MDM, Goldstein M, Rosenbaum P, Leviton A, Paneth N, Dan B, Jacobsson B, Damiano D (2005) Proposed definition and classification of cerebral palsy, April 2005. *Dev Med Child Neurol* 47: 571–576. http://dx.doi.org/10.1017/S001216220500112X

Bax MDM, Tydeman C, Flodmark O (2006) Clinical and MRI correlates of cerebral palsy. *JAMA* 296: 1602–1608. http://dx.doi.org/10.1001/jama.296.13.1602

Baxter P (2006) Cerebral palsy: synergism, pathways, and prevention. *Dev Med Child Neurol* 48: 3. http://dx.doi.org/10.1017/S0012162206000016

Baxter P, Rosenbloom L (2005) CP or not CP? *Dev Med Child Neurol* 47: 407. http://dx.doi.org/10.1017/S001216220500099X

Berninger V, Rutberg J (1992) Relationship of beginning writing: application to diagnosis of writing disabilities. *Dev Med Child Neurol* 34: 198–215. http://dx.doi.org/10.1111/j.1469-8749.1992.tb14993.x

Beuter A, Garfinkel A (1985) Phase plane analysis of limb trajectories in nonhandicapped and cerebral palsied subjects. *Adapted Physical Activity Quarterly* 2: 214–227.

Blair E, Love S (2005) Definition and classification of cerebral palsy: commentary. *Dev Med Child Neurol* 47: 510. http://dx.doi.org/10.1017/S0012162205241002

Bogaerts H, Swinnen SP (2001) Spatial interactions during bimanual coordination patterns: the effect of directional compatibility. *Motor Control* 2: 183–199.

Bonellie SR, Currie D, Chalmers J (2005) Comparison of risk factors for cerebral palsy in twins and singletons. *Dev Med Child Neurol* 47: 587–591.

Bronfenbrenner U (1979) *The Ecology of Human Development: Experiments by Nature and Design*. Cambridge, MA: Harvard University Press.

Brown JK (1987) A neurological study of hand function of hemiplegic cerebral palsy. *Dev Med Child Neurol* 3: 287–304.

Bumin G, Kavak ST (2008) An investigation into factors affecting handwriting performance in children with hemiplegic cerebral palsy. *Disabil Rehabil* 30: 1374–1385. http://dx.doi.org/10.1080/09638280701673609

Carlsson M, Olsson I, Hagberg G, Beckung E (2008) Behaviour in children with cerebral palsy and without cerebral palsy. *Dev Med Child Neurol* 50: 784–789. http://dx.doi.org/10.1111/j.1469-8749.2008.03090.x

Charles J, Gordon AM (2006) Development of hand–arm bimanual intensive training (HABIT) for improving bimanual coordination in children with hemiplegic cerebral palsy. *Dev Med Child Neurol* 48: 931–936. http://dx.doi.org/10.1017/S0012162206002039

Connolly KJ, Elliott J (1972) Evolution and ontogeny of hand function. In: Blurton-Jones N, editor. *Ethological Studies of Child Behaviour*. Cambridge: Cambridge University Press, pp. 329–383.

Coster M, Khetani MA (2008) Measuring participation in children with disabilities: issues and challenges. *Disabil Rehabil* 30: 639–648. http://dx.doi.org/10.1080/09638280701400375

Crossman ERFW, Goodeve PJ (1963) Feedback control of hand movements and Fitts' law. Paper presented at the meeting of the Experimental Psychological Society, Oxford, July 1963. Published in *Quarterly Journal of Experimental Psychology* 1983; 35A: 251–278.

DeBruin H, Eng P, Russell DJ, Latter JE, Sadler JTS (1982) Angle–angle diagrams in monitoring and quantification of gait patterns for children with cerebral palsy. *Am J Phys Med* 61: 176–192.

Eliasson AC, Gordon AM, Forssberg H (1991) Basic coordination of manipulative forces of children with cerebral palsy. *Dev Med Child Neurol* 33: 661–670. http://dx.doi.org/10.1111/j.1469-8749.1991.tb14943.x

Eliasson AC, Gordon AM, Forssberg H (1992) Impaired anticipatory control of isometric forces during grasping by children with cerebral palsy. *Dev Med Child Neurol* 34: 216–225. http://dx.doi.org/10.1111/j.1469-8749.1992.tb14994.x

Eliasson EC, Ekholm C, Carltedt T (1998) Hand function in children with cerebral palsy after upper-limb tendon transfer and muscle release. *Dev Med Child Neurol* 40: 612–621.

Eliasson AC, Forssberg H, Hund Y-C, Gordon AM (2006) Development of hand function and precision grip control in individuals with cerebral palsy: a 13 year follow-up study. *Pediatrics* 118: 1226–1236. http://dx.doi.org/10.1542/peds.2005-2768

Elliott J, Connolly K (1984) A classification of manipulative hand movements. *Dev Med Child Neurol* 26: 283–296. http://dx.doi.org/10.1111/j.1469-8749.1984.tb04445.x

Escobar GJ, Littenberg B, Petiitti DB (1991) Outcome among surviving very low birthweight infants: a meta-analysis. *Arch Dis Childhood* 66: 204–211. http://dx.doi.org/10.1136/adc.66.2.204

Fagard J, Hardy-Leger I, Kervella C, Marks A (2001) Changes in inter-hemispheric transfer rate and the development of bimanual; coordination during childhood. *J Exp Child Psychol* 80: 1–22. http://dx.doi.org/10.1006/jecp.2000.2623

Fitts PM (1954) The information capacity of the human motor system in controlling the amplitude of movement. *J Exp Psychol* 47: 381–391. http://dx.doi.org/10.1037/h0055392

Forssberg H, Eliasson AC, Kinoshita H, Johanson RS, Wrestleing G (1991) Development of human precision grip. I: Basic coordination of force. *Exp Brain Res* 85: 451–457. http://dx.doi.org/10.1007/BF00229422

Forssberg H, Kinoshita H, Eliasson AC, Johanson RS, Wrestleing G (1992) Development of human precision grip. II: Anticipatory control of isometric forces targeted for object's weight. *Exp Brain Res* 90: 393–398.

Forssberg H, Eliasson AC, Redon-Zouiteni C, Mecuri E, Dubowitz L (1999) Determinate forces in grasping in children with unilateral brain lesions. *Brain* 122: 1157–1175. http://dx.doi.org/10.1093/brain/122.6.1157

Freud S (1897) Die infantile Cerebrallahmung. In: H. Nothnaget, editor. *Specielle Pathologie und Therapie*, Volume 9, Part 3. Vienna: Holder, pp. 1–327.

Freud S (1968) *Infantile Cerebral Paralysis*. Russin LA, translator. Miami: University of Miami Press.

Gage JR (1991) *Gait Analysis in Cerebral Palsy*. Oxford: Mac Keith Press.

Gainsborough M, Surman G, Maestri G, Colver A, Cans C (2008) Validity and reliability of the guidelines of the surveillance of cerebral palsy in Europe for the classification of cerebral palsy. *Dev Med Child Neurol* 50: 828–831. http://dx.doi.org/10.1111/j.1469-8749.2008.03141.x

Hagberg B, Hagberg G (1993) The origins of cerebral palsy. In: David TS, editor. *Recent Advances in Paediatrics*. Edinburgh: Churchill Livingstone, pp. 67–83.

Hanna SE, Barlett DJ, Rivard LM, Russell DJ (2008) Reference curves for the Gross Motor Function Measure: reference curves for clinical description and tracking over time for children with cerebral palsy. *Phys Ther* 88: 506–607. http://dx.doi.org/10.2522/ptj.20070314

Harrison A (1975a) Components of neuromuscular control. In: Holt KS, editor. *Movement and Child Development*. London: Mac Keith Press, pp. 34–50.

Harrison A (1975b) Studies of neuromuscular control in normal and spastic individuals. In: Holt KS, editor. *Movement and Child Development*. London: Mac Keith Press, pp. 51–74.

Harrison A (1975c) Training spastic individuals to achieve better neuromuscular control using electromyographic feedback. In: Holt KS, editor. *Movement and Child Development*. London: Mac Keith Press, pp. 75–101.

Harrison A, Kruze R (1987) Peryrbation of a skilled action: 1. The responses of normal and cerebral palsied individuals. *Hum Movement Sci* 6: 37–65. http://dx.doi.org/10.1016/0167-9457(87)90021-2

Hemming K, Hutton JL, Pharoah POD (2006) Long-term survival for a cohort of adults with cerebral palsy. *Dev Med Child Neurol* 48: 90–95. http://dx.doi.org/10.1017/S0012162206000211

Himmelman K, Beckung E, Hagberg G, Uvebrandt P (2006) Gross and fine motor function and accompanying impairments in cerebral palsy. *Dev Med Child Neurol* 48: 417–423. http://dx.doi.org/10.1017/S0012162206000922

Howard EM, Henderson SE (1989) Perceptual problems in cerebral palsied children: a real world example. *Hum Movement Sci* 2: 141–160. http://dx.doi.org/10.1016/0167-9457(89)90014-6

I-Chun Huang, Beveridge SE, Sugden DA (2008) Children's perceptions of their use of assistive devices in home and school settings. *Disabil Rehabil* 42: 95–105.

Imms C (2008) Children with cerebral palsy participate: a review of the literature. *Disabil Rehabil* 30: 1867–1884. http://dx.doi.org/10.1080/09638280701673542

Inman VT, Ralston HJ, Todd F (1981) *Human Walking*. Baltimore, MD: Williams and Wilkins.

Jeannerod M (1986) The formation of the finger grip during prehension: a cortically-mediated visuomotor patter. In: Whiting HTA, Wade MG, editors. *Themes in Motor Development*. Dordrecht: Martinus Nijhoff, pp. 183–205.

Jeeves MA, Silver PH, Milne AB (1988) Role of the corpus callosum in the development of a bimanual motor skill. *Dev Neuropsychol* 4: 305–325. http://dx.doi.org/10.1080/87565648809540415

Jones B (1976) The perception of passive joint movements by cerebral palsied children. *Dev Med Child Neurol* 18: 25–30. http://dx.doi.org/10.1111/j.1469-8749.1976.tb03601.x

Kelso JAS, Putnam CA, Goodman D (1983) On the space–time structure of human inter limb coordination. *Q J Exp Psychol* 35A: 347–375.

Keogh JF, Sugden DA (1985) *Movement Skill Development*. New York Macmillan.

Kerrigan DC, Riley PO, Rogan S, Burke DT (2000) Compensatory advantages of toe walking. *Arch Phys Med Rehab* 81: 38–44.

King G, Law M, Hurley Y, Petrenchik T, Schwellnus H (2010) A developmental comparison of the out-of-school recreation and leisure activity participation of boys and girls with and without physical disabilities. *Int J Disabil Dev Educ* 57: 77–107. http://dx.doi.org/10.1080/10349120903537988

Kong CK, Tse PW, Lee WY (1999) Bone age and linear skeletal growth of children. *Dev Med Child Neurol* 41: 758–765. http://dx.doi.org/10.1017/S0012162299001528

Kragelöb-Mann I (2005) Cerebral palsy: towards developmental neuroscience. *Dev Med Child Neurol* 47: 435. http://dx.doi.org/10.1017/S0012162205000836

Ledebt A (2003) Locomotion in children with cerebral palsy: early predictive factors for ambulation and gait analysis. In: Savelsbergh G, Davids K, van der Kamp J, Bennett S, editors. *Development of Movement Coordination in Children*. London: Routledge, pp. 177–187.

Lin JP (2004) *The Assessment and Management of Hypertonus in Cerebral Palsy: A Physiological Atlas*. London: Mac Keith Press.

Majnemer A, Shevell M, Law M, Birnbaum R, Chillingaryan G, Rosenbaum P, Poulin G (2008) Participation and enjoyment of leisure activities in school-aged children with cerebral palsy. *Dev Med Child Neurol* 50: 751–758. http://dx.doi.org/10.1111/j.1469-8749.2008.03068.x

Minear WL (1956) A classification of cerebral palsies. *Pediatrics* 18: 841–852.

Mongan D, Dunne K, O'Nuallain S, Gaffney G (2006) Prevalence of cerebral palsy in the West of Ireland 1990–1999. *Dev Med Child Neurol* 48: 892–895. http://dx.doi.org/10.1017/S0012162206001952

Morris C, Kurinczuk JJ, Fitzpatrick R, Rosenbaum PL (2006) Do the abilities of children with cerebral palsy explain their activities and participation? *Dev Med Child Neurol* 48: 954–961. http://dx.doi.org/10.1017/S0012162206002106

Mutch L, Alberman E, Hagberg B, Kodma K, Perat MV (1992) Cerebral palsy epidemiology: where are we now and where are we going? *Dev Med Child Neurol* 34: 547–551. http://dx.doi.org/10.1111/j.1469-8749.1992.tb11479.x

Nashner LM, Shumway-Cook A, Marin O (1983) Stance posture control in select groups of children with cerebral palsy: deficits in sensory organization and muscular coordination. *Exp Brain Res* 49: 393–409. http://dx.doi.org/10.1007/BF00238781

Newell KM (1986) Constraints on the development of coordination. In: Wade MG, Whiting HTA, editors. *Motor Development in Children: Aspects of Coordination and Control*. Amsterdam: Martinus Nijhoff, pp. 341–361. http://dx.doi.org/10.1007/978-94-009-4460-2_19

Newman CJ, O'Regan M, Hensey O (2006) Sleep disorders in children with cerebral palsy. *Dev Med Child Neurol* 48: 564–568. http://dx.doi.org/10.1017/S0012162206001198

Opila-Lehman J, Short MA, Trombly CA (1985) Kinaesthetic recall of children with athetoid and spastic cerebral palsy and of non-handicapped children. *Dev Med Child Neurol* 27: 223–230.

Palisano R, Rosenbaum P, Bartlett D, Livingstone M (2007) *Gross Motor Function Classification System Expanded and Revised*. Hamilton, Ont.: CanChild Centre for Childhood Disability research, McMaster University.

Palisano R, Rosenbaum P, Walter S, Russell D, Wood E, Galuppi B (2007) Development and reliability of a system to classify gross motor function in children with cerebral palsy. *Dev Med Child Neurol* 39: 214–223. http://dx.doi.org/10.1111/j.1469-8749.1997.tb07414.x

Parush LLS, Rihtman T (2008) Participation of children with cerebral palsy in leisure activities supports the current ICF health paradigm. *Dev Med Child Neurol* 50: 726–726. http://dx.doi.org/10.1111/j.1469-8749.2008.03072.x

Pharoah POD, Cooke T, Johnson MA, King R, Mutch L (1998) Epidemiology of cerebral palsy in England and Scotland, 1984–89. *Arch Dis Child Fetal Neonatal* 71: 21–25. http://dx.doi.org/10.1136/fn.79.1.F21

Rice MS, Newell KM (2001) Interlimb coupling and hemiplegia because of right cerebral vascular accident. *Occup Ther J Res* 21: 12–28.

Rosenbaum P, Paneth N, Leviton A, Goldstein M, Bax M (2007) The definition and classification of cerebral palsy. *Dev Med Child Neurol* 49: 1–44. http://dx.doi.org/10.1111/j.1469-8749.2007.00001.x

Schmidt RA, Lee TD (2005) *Motor Control and Learning: A Behavioural Emphasis*. Champaign, IL: Human Kinetics.

Shumway-Cook A, Woollacott MH (2007) *Motor Control: Theory and Practical Applications*. Baltimore, MD: Williams & Wilkins.

Skrotzky K (1983) Gait analysis in cerebral palsied and non handicapped children. *Arch Phys Med Rehabil* 64: 291–295.

Stanley F, Blair E, Alberman E (2000) *Cerebral Palsies: Epidemiology and Causal Pathways*. London: Mac Keith Press.

Steenbergen B, Van Thiel E, Hulstijn W, Meulkenbroek RGJ (2000) The coordination of reaching and grasping in spastic hemiparesis. *Hum Movement Sci* 19: 75–105. http://dx.doi.org/10.1016/S0167-9457(00)00006-3

Steenbergen B, Utley A, Sugden DA, Thieman PS (2003) Discrete bimanual movement co-ordination in children with hemiparetic cerebral palsy. In: Savelsbergh G, Davids K, van der Kamp J, Bennett S, editors. *Development of Movement Coordination in Children*. London: Routledge, pp. 156–176.

Strauss D, Brooks J, Rosenbloom L, Shavelle R (2008) Life expectancy in cerebral palsy: an update. *Dev Med Child Neurol* 50: 487–493. http://dx.doi.org/10.1111/j.1469-8749.2008.03000.x

Sugden DA, Keogh JF (1990) *Problems in Movement Skill Development*. Columbia, SC: University of South Carolina Press.

Sugden DA, Utley A (1995) Interlimb coupling in children with hemiplegic cerebral palsy. *Dev Med Child Neurol* 37: 293–310. http://dx.doi.org/10.1111/j.1469-8749.1995.tb12008.x

Sugden DA, Utley A (1995) A vocabulary of grips in children with hemiplegic cerebral palsy. *Physiotherapy – Theory and Practice* 11: 17–30. http://dx.doi.org/10.3109/09593989509022403

Sugden DA, Henderson SE (2007) *Ecological Intervention for Children with Movement Difficulties.* London: Harcourt Assessment.

Swinnen SP, Jardin K, Verschueren S, Meulenbroek RGJ, Franz EA, Dounskaia N, Walter CB (1998) Exploring interlimb constraints during bimanual graphic performance: effects of muscle grouping and direction. *Behav Brain Res* 90: 79–87. http://dx.doi.org/10.1016/S0166-4328(97)00083-1

Tardieu G, Tardieu C, Lespargot A, Roby A, Bret MD (1984) Can vibration-induced illusions be used as a muscle perception test for normal and cerebral palsied children? *Dev Med Child Neurol* 26: 449–456. http://dx.doi.org/10.1111/j.1469-8749.1984.tb04470.x

Tedroff K, Knutson LM, Soderberg GL (2006) Synergistic muscle activity during maximum voluntary contractions in children with and without cerebral palsy. *Dev Med Child Neurol* 48: 789–796. http://dx.doi.org/10.1017/S0012162206001721

Twitchell TE (1958) The grasping deficit in infantile spastic hemiparesis. *Neurology* 8: 13–21. http://dx.doi.org/10.1212/WNL.8.1.13

Twitchell TE (1959) On the motor deficit in congenital bilateral athetosis. *J Nerv Ment Dis* 129: 105–132. http://dx.doi.org/10.1097/00005053-195908000-00001

Utley A, Sugden DA (1998) Interlimb coupling in children with hemiplegic cerebral palsy during reaching and grasping at speed. *Dev Med Child Neurol* 40: 396–404.

Van Eck M, Dallmeijer AJ, Voorman JM, Becher JG (2008) Skeletal maturation in children with cerebral palsy and its relationship with motor functioning. *Dev Med Child Neurol* 50: 515–519. http://dx.doi.org/10.1111/j.1469-8749.2008.03010.x

Varni JW, Burwinkle TM, Sherman SA, Hanna K, Berrin SJ, Malcarne VL, Chambers HG (2005) Health-related quality of life of children and adolescents with cerebral palsy: hearing the voices of children. *Dev Med Child Neurol* 47: 592–597.

Vygotsky L (1978) *Mind in Society: The Development of Higher Psychological Processes.* Cambridge, MA: Harvard University Press.

Watt JM, Robertson CM, Grace MG (1989) Early prognosis for ambulation of neonatal intensive care survivors with cerebral palsy. *Dev Med Child Neurol* 42: 292–296.

WHO (2001) *International Classification of Functioning, Disability and Health.* Geneva: World Health Organization.

WHO (2008) *International Statistical Classification of Diseases and Related Health Problems 10th Revision.* Geneva: World Health Organization.

Winters TF, Gage JR, Hicks R (1987) Gait patterns in spastic hemiplegia in children and young adults. *J Bone Joint Surg* 69A: 437–441.

Wright FV, Rosenbaum PL, Goldsmith CH, Law M, Fehlings L (2008) How do changes in body functions and structures, activity and participation relate to children with cerebral palsy? *Dev Med Child Neurol* 50: 283–289.

8
DEVELOPMENTAL COORDINATION DISORDER

Development of movement skill competence

As they reach school age, most children have developed a range of movement competencies that equip them for the requirements of the home, school, and community environment. They have been exposed to the normal motoric demands at home and in play situations, and they have developed a range of agility and manual skills that serve them well in the classroom, out on the playground, playing with friends, and participating in other activities of daily life. Thus, most children show competence for their age in skills such as agility, running, jumping, hopping, and climbing; in more fine motor activities such as writing, drawing, copying, and manipulating small objects; in self-care skills such as eating, dressing, and using the toilet; and in activities requiring competence with objects such as balls and bean bags thrown and received. The acquisition of such skills and abilities has been well documented in texts of motor development (Keogh and Sugden 1985, Haywood and Getchell 2001, Piek 2006, Gabbard 2011).

There are other children, however, who do not develop fully in this way. Often they have been late to achieve developmental motor milestones outside of typical limits with, for example, large delays in walking or difficulty with a pincer grip or they are simply poor at many of the skills noted above. Very often these children show no outward signs of physical disability and rarely show movements that are pathological such as the jerkiness or the continuous motion often seen in cerebral palsy. However, their motor skills are poor and appear to lag behind those of their peers, placing them at a disadvantage in a number of areas of the school curriculum, in the home environment, or in daily interaction with their peers in social and recreational contexts. The children are often first noticed by parents who identify differences between their children and others or in the early years of schooling by educational professionals. Over the years, a number of

terms have been used to describe these children, but more recently the term *developmental coordination disorder* (DCD) is the one that has attracted wide support (APA 1987, 1994, 2000; and confirmed by consensus statements, Polatajko et al 1995, Sugden 2006).

The history of the study of children whose motor coordination is poor takes many forms, in part because of the involvement of differing professionals ranging from medical and health personnel to physical educationists, general educators, and psychologists. The interest of many of these professionals has been stimulated by questions concerning the motor development and learning of children and the effect any impairment in this area has on the functional motor activities of daily living. Others have taken a slightly different tack by concentrating on the remediation of poor motor performance and the relationship of this to a wider range of skills such as school readiness and academic success (for a review see Kavale and Forness 1995). The effects of impaired motor skill on both activities of daily living and academic performance are part of the criteria set by the *Diagnostic and Statistical Manual of Mental Disorders 4th Revision* (DSM-IV) (APA 2000), and later in the chapter the debate surrounding this effect is discussed.

Historical context

As with many disorders that have interested a variety of professionals, children with DCD emerge from a complex, diverse history with multiple strands. Jack Cratty, in numerous publications (e.g. 1969, 1975a,b, 1994) and with a history of providing support in motor development clinics, helped to bring attention to children with awkward movements, so-called 'clumsy children', and proposed various means of identification and intervention schedules. In addition, he also chronicled the history of research into the area, identifying a number of specific time periods (Cratty 1994).

Cratty (1994) notes that up to the beginning of the 1900s there were explorations by neurologists examining obvious brain damage and the relationship between location and severity of brain damage and consequent motor behaviour. This was all part of an attempt to identify any direct links between brain and behaviour. Following this came a period from around 1910 up to the mid-1960s when, particularly in the USA, motor incoordination was inextricably linked with other disorders in children such as general and specific learning disability and inattention and hyperactivity (Kephart 1956, Getman 1963, Delacato 1966, Barsch 1965). It was during the latter part of this period that the concentration on the link between motor performance and other disabilities became prominent, and this association was often reflected in the terminology that was used, such as minimal brain damage or minimal cerebral dysfunction and occasionally minimal cerebral palsy. Around this time, minimal brain damage or minimal neurological disorder and other similar terms were diagnostic terms used for children of average intelligence who exhibited a variety of learning disabilities. Consequently, motor assessment became important because deficits in motor control were thought to be more reliable measures of the integrity of the central nervous system than others that are more indirect such as attentional and social difficulties. This line of thought has continued to the present with many children with DCD showing co-occurring characteristics such as attentional, social, and cognitive difficulties (Kaplan et al 1998, Kadesjo and C Gillberg 1999, Rasmussen and C Gillberg 2000, Green and Baird 2005). Furthermore, it is interesting to note that this association, and the subsequent proposal that improvements in motor competence can improve other learning disabilities, is one that has had a more recent resurrection with both clinical practices and commercial concerns promoting this link, a topic to which attention is directed later in this chapter and in Chapter 12.

Cratty notes a third historical period from the mid-1960s to his writing (Cratty 1994) when 'clumsy children' were studied in a more sophisticated manner, with an examination of the sensory and motor aspects of the condition together with accompanying social and emotional difficulties. Continuing this theme of periods it could be argued that since the late 1980s and early 1990s there has been an explosion of interest in the topic with more research and clinical work being reported and, additionally, other manifestations which, in Cratty's chronology, indicate a fourth period. This final/latest period has a number of characteristics and is shown in Box 8.1.

The above points are addressed throughout the chapter together with a description of the condition, an examination of diagnostic criteria and an elaboration of the characteristics of the child, both motor and non-motor items, and the developmental progression of the condition. At times, because of necessity, assessment and intervention are mentioned, but the detail of these topics is left to Chapter 12. Recent texts on the topic of problems in motor development that are recommended for consultation include Cermak and Larkin (2002), Dewey and Tupper (2004), Sugden and Chambers (2004), and Geuze (2007).

Terminology

Over the years many terms have been used to describe children who are awkward in their movements, with labels such as the *clumsy child* (Dare and Gordon 1970, Keogh et al 1979, Lord and Hulme 1987, Losse et al 1991, Geuze and Kalverboer 1994). Until relatively recently, the *clumsy child* or the *clumsy child syndrome* was the most common label attached to these children, presumably because the label actually defined the types of movements the children exhibited. It is rarely used now as a label, mainly because it is seen as such a pejorative term, although it is occasionally seen as a description of the movement, as is the term physical awkwardness. Other terms that have been employed include *perceptual motor dysfunction* or *perceptual motor difficulties* (Laszlo et al 1988), which emphasize the part that sensory processes play in the performance of motor skills. In contrast to this, the terms *movement* or *motor difficulties* and *movement skill problems* (Sugden and Keogh 1990, Sugden and Sugden 1991, Wright et al 1995) have been used to illustrate that movement difficulties are the core component of the condition. This term does not explain why these difficulties may occur, but it does identify the defining characteristic. The term *dyspraxia* has been and still is a popular label to apply to these children by parents, the occupational and physical therapy professions, and the media. The label has been widely used, although it is not without its severe critics who note that it has been borrowed from the adult clinical literature, has concentrated on the planning of movements rather than the movement itself, and has had a number of different definitions with very little final consensus. In addition, it often incorporates a number of co-occurring characteristics in the definition itself rather than as secondary or associated characteristics. These would make consistent and reliable diagnosis very difficult (Henderson and Henderson 2002; see Box 8.2).

The history of terminology has also produced more general terms, which have been used to describe coordination difficulties alongside other types of disorders. Thus earlier terms such as *minimal brain damage* (MBD), *minimal cerebral dysfunction*, and *minimal neurological damage/dysfunction* (MNDE; for a review see Kavale and

---

Box 8.1 A closer examination

Recent developments in DCD

- A condition involving significant impairment of motor control affecting activities of daily living has had formal recognition by both the World Health Organization (WHO 1992) and the American Psychiatric Association (APA 1994, 2000).
- The terminology has changed from 'clumsy children' to DCD or dyspraxia. DCD is becoming the most widely used term internationally, and, although there are advocates of dyspraxia, DCD is the preferred term of the DSM (APA 1994, 2000) and the term is used worldwide by both researchers and practitioners.
- Two consensus statements have examined both APA and WHO coverage of the condition and proposed modifications. These have made it easier for researchers and clinicians to ensure that accurate comparisons across samples can be made (Polatajko et al 1995, Sugden 2006). In addition, a recent publication, an interdisciplinary clinical practice guideline, was proposed by Germany and Switzerland reflecting current practice (Blank et al 2012).
- The increase in visibility of the topic is exemplified by nine world DCD conferences, starting in London in 1993, with Lausanne, Switzerland, the most recent venue for the world conference, in 2011, with over 25 countries represented.
- The issues of comorbidity and co-occurring associated characteristics are now common themes, with an acceptance that these are probably the rules in children with DCD rather than the exceptions (Kaplan et al 1998, Kadesjo and C Gillberg 1999, Rasmussen and C Gillberg 2000, Green and Baird 2005). There is an interesting paradox emerging from the seemingly disparate views that DCD is firmly established as a separate disorder yet it is recognized that in most cases it has co-occurring characteristics with a range of associated difficulties.
- Subgroups of children with DCD have been suggested with recognition that a distinctive characteristic of the group is heterogeneity yet the core characteristic of movement difficulty remains (Dewey and Kaplan 1994, Hoare 1994, Miyahara 1994, Wright and Sugden 1996, Macnab et al 2001; for a review see Visser 2007).
- Previously, research had concentrated on the period 6 to 11 years, but now it is beginning to include other phases of development that previously received scant attention. Studies of both children in their early years and emerging adults are now being conducted, and we are beginning to see an approach to the topic that concentrates more on the entire lifespan and the differences that each phase portrays (Cousins and Smyth 2003, 2005, Piek 2003, Chambers and Sugden 2006, Kirby et al 2008a,b, Piek et al 2008).
- Studies are beginning to be conducted on the underlying neurological substrates using techniques such as functional magnetic resonance imaging (fMRI) (Querne et al 2008, Zwicker et al 2009).
- Issues of assessment and intervention are now regularly addressed with examinations of differing perspectives from theoretical, empirical, and experiential viewpoints (Pless et al 2001, Wilson 2005, Polatajko and Cantin 2006, Sugden and Dunford 2007, Barnett 2008, Sugden 2007).

Forness 1995) have all been used to include children who show a variety of difficulties such as inattention, hyperactivity, and incoordination with the inference that some form of neurological disorder is present. More recently the term *atypical brain development* (ABD) has been used in a similar manner to indicate that coordination difficulties probably do not occur in isolation but in conjunction with other characteristics with an underlying atypicality in brain development (Kaplan et al 1998). A related but slightly different approach is taken by Gillberg and colleagues (RH Gillberg and Rasmussen 1982, IC Gillberg et al 1983, 1989) who use the term DAMP, which is an abbreviation for disorder of attention motor control and perception. This indicates again that the condition is not simply one of motor control but involves other characteristics as well. DAMP differs from ABD and MBD in that it usually takes behavioural characteristics of DCD and attention-deficit–hyperactivity disorder (ADHD) but does not in the label refer directly to any underlying brain malfunction. These terms have been used to describe separate conditions that deal not only with motor disorders but also overlapping developmental disorders and often differ according to the different professional disciplines of those involved. A selection of terms is shown in Table 8.1.

TABLE 8.1

A selection of terms used to describe children now labelled as having developmental coordination disorder

Term	Reference
Clumsy child	Numerous authors including Dare and Gordon (1970)
Clumsy child syndrome	Gubbay (1975), Keogh et al (1979), Lord and Hulme (1987), Losse et al (1991), Cratty (1994)
Perceptual motor difficulties	Laszlo et al (1988)
Movement/motor difficulties	Keogh and Sugden (1985), Henderson et al (1989)
DAMP	RH Gillberg and Rasmussen (1982), C Gillberg et al (1983), IC Gillberg et al (1989)
Atypical brain development	Numerous including Kaplan et al (1998, 2001) and Lunsing et al (1992)
Minimal brain dysfunction	C Gillberg et al (1983), IC Gillberg et al (1989)
Dyspraxia	Numerous including Dewey (1995), Portwood (1996)

DAMP, disorder of attention motor control and perception.

All of the above terms have been generally super-seded by the current term – *DCD* – which is now the one that is most widely used throughout the world. Henderson and Henderson (2002) note that terminology has both theoretical and practical implications. Consistent termi-nology would help comparisons across research samples and in clinical situations a condition defined and labelled is more likely to receive help and support. Henderson and Henderson (2002) debate the merits of the three labels DCD (APA 2000), specific disorder of motor function (WHO 1992), and developmental dyspraxia, and the dis-cussion is outlined with A closer examination in Box 8.2.

Recently, Sinani et al (2011) examined gesture pro-duction, often called dyspraxia, in two groups of children with DCD and typically developing age-matched and younger children and showed that both groups with DCD performed poorer than their age-matched peers, and the clinical sample of children with DCD performed poorer than a school sample and were more like the younger groups. From the various profiles of the different groups of children, the authors proposed that the term 'dyspraxia' should be used to indicate a particular component of DCD rather than as an alternative diagnostic term.

Although all labels bring with them various negative connotations and simplistic descriptions, the term DCD is a logical progression in that the condition is developmen-tal and it is concerned with a lack of or impaired motor coordination as the core characteristic. This is not to say that the debate about terminology has ended; it still goes on, but currently DCD is widely accepted as the most appropriate.

Who are the children?

A common and often quoted characteristic of children with DCD is 'heterogeneity' (e.g. Hoare 1994, Hadders-Algra 1999, Macnab et al 2001, Green and Baird 2005),

which reflects the broad range of characteristics found in children with DCD with both strengths and difficulties. It is true that each individual child will show a different profile and may have more or fewer characteristics than a child with the similar label of DCD, but this is not unusual in any disorder. For example, a child with learning dis-ability may have a unique profile but at the core there will be some quality such as a cognitive limitation that is fundamental to their learning difficulty. The same is true of children with DCD who exhibit different motor profiles and with characteristics outside of the motor domain but often associated with DCD. However, at the core of the condition is a fundamental difficulty with coordination, leading to problems with movement in everyday func-tional activities.

Three profiles of children are illustrated in Box 8.3. They are taken at different stages of their lives to illustrate how difficulties are often present throughout life but may change in how they are manifested. An analogy can be made with the condition of dyslexia in which early in life word attack skills are often impaired or even lacking, but with age, although the individual may become relatively competent in reading, often a residual spelling problem remains.

These are three different individuals at different stages of childhood and emerging adulthood showing profiles that overlap in some areas and are independent of each other in others. Yet all three start with the same fundamental characteristic, namely that of impairment in some area of motor functioning. All three are relatively awkward in movements requiring agility and balance; two have difficulties with handwriting, whether it is slow or illegible; two have some associated characteristics such as attentional difficulties or lack of social skills; all are concerned about the effect their impaired motor functions have on their daily lives; and all are of at least average

---

Box 8.2 A closer examination

Terminology: Henderson and Henderson (2002)
As part of an article that reviewed the then current state of our understanding of DCD, the authors first addressed the question of terminology and specifically examined the most common terms in usage:

- DCD (APA 1994, 2000)
- specific developmental disorder of motor function (WHO 1992)
- developmental dyspraxia.

They first summarized the *usage* by noting that different countries employ different terminology. For example, at the time of writing Italy used dyspraxia; the Netherlands used DCD; and in the UK it varied, as it did in the USA, although DCD was recognized for parents seeking private help through health insurance companies.

Second, they examined the term *specific developmental disorder of motor function* (WHO 1992) and, although they found merit in the term, they preferred the term 'coordination' in DSM-IV to the term 'function' in the *International Classification of Diseases, 10th Revision* (ICD-10), noting that it went to the core of the difficulty, whereas function could be impaired with a number of causes not all attributable to motor control. Coordination is preferred as it implies intentionality; it involves spatial and temporal aspects of any action; most actions involve a sequence of movements; and, finally, a coordinated action should be directed to environmental contexts.

They regarded the term *dyspraxia* as unhelpful primarily because of the confusion of the meaning of the term, which to their knowledge has never had a consistent set of criteria. They used the term 'apraxia' to construct their arguments and extended this reasoning to the term 'dyspraxia', with the authors relegating the term in the same manner. Henderson and Henderson noted that apraxia is used in the literature of acquired disorders and they questioned the relevance of this literature to developmental disorders. They noted that apraxic patients do not often show motor problems but that their problems are more of a planning nature and, although children with motor problems do exhibit planning difficulties, they are rarely of the extreme type, as exemplified by the apraxic patient who can only wave goodbye in the context of leaving and not to a verbal command.

The article concludes with the following statement:

Given our implacable hostility to the association of the developmental disorder with those of acquired disorders referred to as apraxia, our approval of the term coordination…we have no alternative but to endorse the label 'DCD'.

(p. 18)

---

intelligence. Not all of them have had recent assessments, yet, if they had, it is likely that two of them would have received a diagnosis of DCD (Jack and Peter) and the third (Linda), although not with an overall low performance, has serious problems in specific areas that cause concern. So what are the diagnostic criteria for DCD?

Diagnostic criteria for developmental coordination disorder

DIAGNOSTIC AND CLASSIFICATION MANUALS
Diagnosis, descriptions, and assessment are often inextricably linked, with description being a more general term outlining the condition and assessment used as a tool to determine whether diagnostic criteria have been reached.

It is possible to conduct assessments without a diagnosis being made, but the converse is not true, with some form of assessment or collection of information being a necessity for a diagnosis. The details of assessment are shown in Chapter 12, but some specific to children with DCD are included here as they relate to the diagnostic criteria.

Until relatively recently the diagnostic criteria for DCD have been variable or localized and even idiosyncratic. However, since 1987, when the DSM-III first included DCD as a condition (APA 1987), the diagnostic criteria have become tighter, with the result that researchers and clinical workers around the world are now better able to compare like with like when discussing the children with whom they are involved. DSM-IV (APA 1994) picked up after DSM-III, and this was consolidated

Box 8.3 A closer examination

Examples of children with movement difficulties

Example 1: Jack

Jack is 7 years of age and both his parents and his teachers have noted that he has problems with a variety of movement activities. He is an only child and his parents report that, after a typical birth and early few months of development, he was late to walk (16mo) and always had difficulties with manipulating fine objects. However, it was not until he started school at 4 years old that they noticed just how much difficulty he was having in comparison with the other children.

At school, in the classroom, his drawing and letter formation was always poor. This has continued and he is now receiving special instruction in handwriting. In physical education and out in the playground his agility skills are such that he is starting to be excluded from playground games by his peers. His running is slow and cumbersome and in activities such as jumping and hopping he often falls over, much to the amusement of his friends in class. His throwing is awkward and he can rarely throw overhand accurately enough for one of his friends to catch it, but remarkably he is a good catcher and this often helps him compensate for his other difficulties, making it possible for him to participate in some ball games. He also has difficulty with putting on his coat as he seems unable to plan the action, often being confused with how to approach this seemingly simple everyday task. This poor planning does occur in other areas with his inability to organize himself in the short term, such as order in washing and dressing, and in the long term, in terms of what he needs during the day and where he needs to be, conspiring to make his day confusing and frustrating.

At the moment, in school, he appears to be coping with his movement difficulties and is showing no adverse signs of becoming emotionally upset or socially isolated. He is of average ability, can read at an age-appropriate level, and is eager to answer questions in class. However, because of his slow and often illegible handwriting he is starting to fall behind his classmates in some work and his handwriting-specific tutoring is beginning to mark him out from the rest of the class, even though the teacher is keen on making her extra work as inclusive as possible in the course of normal lessons.

At home his main difficulty is that he is slow in most areas of self-care at times when speed is of an essence. Thus without help he is slow to wash and dress himself and eat, and he often forgets what is required for his day at school. His parents are very supportive and do not wish to place him under too much pressure, but also they would like to give as much help as possible so that the difficulties do not become worse. He attends a local child development centre where he is seen by an occupational therapist who has formally assessed him on both normative- and criterion-referenced test with parental input. On all of these measures Jack falls in the lowest 5% of children for his age group, showing particular difficulties in balance and agility and manual skills, but with average catching ability. Jack is an easy-going child with competent social skills and friends both at school and at home.

Example 2: Linda

Linda is 14 years of age, attends secondary school, and is well above average in all of her academic subjects, being particularly proficient in the maths and science areas. She tells everyone that she wants to go to university to become an engineer. Linda is a very tall and gangly child who, when moving, looks as though her four limbs are controlled by four different motors – in short she appears very awkward and ungainly and she is easily picked out in a crowd of similar-aged girls. One particular problem that she has is with dancing; she is part of a group of children who go to the local youth centre around two or three times a week for their social activities and dancing is a major part of this. She is very reluctant to take part as she knows how awkward she looks and she cannot perform movements quickly enough to keep time with the rhythm. She also has difficulty styling her hair like the other girls.

In school she has difficulties with all aspects of physical education, with the result that she takes no part in extracurricular school activities of a physical nature, and therefore her skills do not improve. In the classroom with her academic subjects she achieves highly and is in the top 10% of a good school year. Her handwriting is very neat but painfully slow, which is starting to cause difficulties as national testing comes around. In practical subjects such as design and food technology she is careful, meticulous, and well organized but again very slow. She pays attention in class and is well structured and organized in her approach to her work. At home, apart from the youth centre, she spends much of her time in her bedroom slowly completing school work. A further complication is that she, like the other girls, has a mobile phone but she is very slow to text and when the girls are in a group she phones instead so as not to stand out. She has not been formally tested for well over 3 years, but when she was she scored at the 20th centile overall on a standardized test of motor proficiency. This did not seem too bad but on closer examination it showed that she was quite typical in ball skills; in the lowest 1% in balance and agility; and around the 10th centile on manual skills. Furthermore, when a speed test of handwriting was conducted she scored in the lowest 1%, albeit with very neat writing (Barnett et al 2007).

Socially she appears quite gauche and immature, which does not help when she is trying to make friends with her peer group. Currently she has some good friends, but she is shy and this, coupled with her physical awkwardness, both generally and when trying to dance, is making her anxious and her parents worried about her immediate adolescent future. Finally, she cannot ride a bicycle; she tried for a while but found it so difficult she gave up.

Example 3: Peter

Peter is 20 years of age and is in his second year at an institute of further education following a social science course. Throughout his school career his grades in most subjects were around the median and he progressed from school to his local further-education institute. Although he achieved generally quite satisfactory marks at school, his progression was not without a number of hitches and pitfalls. First, many of his motor skills have always been very poor indeed; an exception to this is his handwriting, which has always been neat and an acceptable speed. However, most of his other motor skills have given him great trouble both in and out of school.

From an early age Peter has been very awkward in his movements, bumping into people in the street and corridors at school. He has a history of accidents such as dropping objects, knocking over vases, and falling off his bicycle. He only learned to ride a bike after years of trying, but now that he can just about control it he is reluctant to do so as he feels he may be a danger to both himself and other road users. He has always had difficulty with physical education as the school he attended had a concentration on team sports, which put a great strain on his agility and ball skills, which have always been poor. This led him to being excluded from out-of-class and out-of-school physical activities for a number of his formative adolescent years. The problems all seem to be with his agility and skills, which are more gross than fine in nature. His manipulation skills have always been relatively good: he writes quite well and at speed and his keyboard and phone skills are also well within a normal range.

Peter has a number of associated characteristics that heighten his poor motor skills and often leave him socially isolated. All of these associated characteristics surround the general area of attention. First, he appears to be a long time coming to attention – he gives the impression of being miles away. Second, when he starts to pay attention, the time span is quite short even for a topic in which he has shown interest in the past. Third, and connected to the second, he is highly distractible and moves off topic very quickly when he sees something else which may not even have an apparent interest. Finally, he is impulsive and often moves, talks, or generally reacts before the full information has been presented.

The consequence of this is that Peter is becoming socially isolated at college, and it has recently become worse because of his failure to either drive or ride a bike. He gave up riding a bike because of his fear of causing danger, and, although he is taking driving lessons, he is reliant on public transport and others' good will for lifts to social events, etc., and it will be a long time before he is competent enough to be on the road on his own.

with the text revision version (DSM-IV-TR; APA 2000). In addition, a similar set of criteria was developed for *International Classification of Diseases-10* (ICD-10) by the World Health Organization (1992). There are some differences, with aspects that are present in one and not in the other, and slightly different terminology. For example, the labels are different: in DSM-IV it is the title of this chapter – developmental coordination disorder – whereas ICD-10 notes that specific developmental disorder of motor function is one of three terms to describe the disorder, the others being clumsy child syndrome and developmental dyspraxia (see Box 8.2). There are other small differences such as ICD-10 excluding children with IQs below 70 and DSM-IV simply saying that any motor impairment should be over and above that associated with learning disability.

However, the two classifications are largely in agreement with each other, and, as Henderson (1994) notes, the very fact that DCD has a specific entry in both important volumes and is now recognized as a separate developmental disorder places it in the same category as other developmental disorders requiring separate aetiological investigation, diagnostic criteria, assessment schedules, and intervention protocols.

In a detailed and comprehensive review of clinical and research diagnostic criteria, Geuze et al (2001) analysed 176 publications for the manner in which they diagnosed children and 41 publications that had used the term DCD to classify children. They found that inclusion criteria for the condition were largely adhered to, but instruments, cut-off points, exclusionary criteria, and additional criteria all varied. Much of what they reported on is currently still valid, with additional work complementing and occasionally modifying their conclusions. More recently, Albaret and de Castelnau (2007) produced a review of the issues surrounding diagnosis and, in addition, gave a summary of some of the assessment instruments that are employed.

DESCRIBING THE CONDITION
When describing the condition of DCD in DSM-IV (APA 2000) the following is stated:

> A marked impairment in the development of motor coordination...The manifestations of this disorder vary with age and development. For example, younger children may display clumsiness and delays in achieving developmental milestones (e.g. walking, crawling, sitting, tying shoe laces, buttoning shirts, zipping pants). Older children may display difficulties with the motor aspects of assembling puzzles, building models, playing ball and printing or handwriting.
>
> (pp. 56–57)

WHO (1992) uses the term 'specific developmental disorder of motor function' and describes it as

> A disorder in which the main feature is a serious impairment in the development of motor coordination that is not solely explicable in terms of general intellectual retardation or any specific congenital or acquired neurological disorder. Nevertheless, in most cases a careful examination shows marked neurodevelopmental immaturities such as choreiform movements of

unsupported limbs or mirror movements and other associated motor features, as well as signs of impaired fine and gross motor coordination.
>
> (F82)

Both of these manuals have been used by clinicians and researchers as a starting point for their work, although of late DSM-IV (APA 2000) has become more of a standard reference point. The diagnostic criteria for DSM-IV are discussed in the following pages while, as noted earlier, recognizing that ICD-10 does provide complementary, additional, and occasionally slightly different views.

The London, Ontario, Consensus Statement 1994
In 1994 in London, Ontario, Canada, a meeting of researchers and clinicians provided a first consensus statement highlighting the condition and providing a more detailed statement than was provided in DSM-III/IV (APA 1987, 1994). The London Consensus (Polatajko et al 1995) was a landmark document and proposed a standardization of published research in the field of DCD. This consensus confirmed DSM-III/IV in the use of the term DCD and noted that the condition was chronic, usually lifelong, and associated with an impairment of both functional performance and quality of movement and could not be explained by factors such as age or intelligence or by other recognizable disorders. The statement also confirmed the high incidence of associated features such as low self-esteem and, at the time of writing, poorly understood causal factors. In addition, the statement noted that causation was multifactorial, thus leading to a variety of symptoms and subtypes. Multiple modes of assessment and intervention were proposed with settings of home, school, and play areas all recognized together, with various individuals – parents, teacher, and health professionals – all participating in intervention. This meeting was the pioneer in critically analysing the condition using both formal criteria and the experience of researchers and clinicians.

The Leeds Consensus Statement 2006
The London Statement brought a new order to the study of DCD, such that researchers and clinicians now had some guidance for common ground for the identification of the children with movement difficulties. A further look at the field took place 10 years on from this meeting. Between 2004 and 2006 a series of seminars were held at the University of Leeds, UK, sponsored by the Economic and Social Research Council of the United Kingdom with worldwide attendees coming together to try and achieve consensus on the condition with respect to definition, characteristics, diagnosis, assessment, and intervention.

The Leeds meetings provided the opportunity to revisit, revise, and produce a new consensus statement incorporating both the London Statement and some modifications, which had emerged from more recent clinical and research work.

The conclusions from Leeds began with a statement that DSM-IV-TR (APA 2000) provides a useful basis on which to form a diagnosis of DCD, although a number of clarifications and amendments were proposed. The Leeds Consensus Statement (Sugden 2006) accepted these and made the following comments with respect to modifications or extensions.

- It noted that the long-term prognosis of individuals with DCD is variable: a small proportion do appear to improve, but more often adolescence and adulthood are characterized by continuing motor difficulties in addition to social and educational problems and medical and psychiatric consequences.

- The problems experienced are severe and persistent and exist despite appropriate movement learning experience. As a consequence of these difficulties, and without adequate support and/or specific intervention within the family, school, and work environments, an individual with DCD will be placed at a significant disadvantage. DCD is an idiopathic condition.

- Its onset is apparent in the early years but would not typically be diagnosed before 5 years of age. It has a varying, but significant, impact throughout the lifespan.

- The difficulties described as DCD are recognized across culture, race, socio-economic status, and sex, although most studies find a higher prevalence in males than females.

- Descriptions of children with DCD change as the children develop. In the younger years there are parent reports of the children having great problems dressing in the morning, being disorganized, and having difficulties with their clothes and bathroom activities.

- At school they are often poor and slow at handwriting and in the playground are reluctant to engage in normal playground activities, even if they are invited, which they are often not.

- As they enter middle childhood, such social activities as bike riding present difficulties, while very often the writing problem continues. This latter trait is a particular hindrance to the pupil as they enter secondary school where the ability to write legibly and fast is usually seen as a prerequisite for success.

- There is recent evidence to show that difficulties continue into emerging adulthood, with the social consequences of motor problems being at the forefront and the specific case of driving being a challenging issue. In this period of emerging adulthood, co-occurring characteristics take on a particularly important role, often leading to social and/or emotional difficulties (Geuze 2007, Kirby et al 2008a,b).

DSM-IV CRITERIA

The London, Ontario (1995) and Leeds (2006) Consensus Statements aimed to achieve consistency in terminology, definitions, and diagnosis such that researchers and clinicians are clear about the population under investigation. They are seen as confirming DSM-IV criteria with suggested modifications and comments on the four diagnostic criteria, two of which are inclusive and two exclusive (APA 2000, p. 58):

- *Criterion A*: 'Performance in daily activities that require motor coordination is substantially below that expected given the person's chronological age and measured intelligence.'
- *Criterion B*: 'The disturbance in criterion A significantly interferes with academic achievement or activities of daily living.'
- *Criterion C*: 'The disturbance is not due to a general medical condition (e.g., cerebral palsy, hemiplegia or muscular dystrophy) and does not meet criteria for a Pervasive Developmental Disorder.'
- *Criterion D*: 'If mental retardation is present, the motor difficulties are in excess of those usually associated with it.'

An examination of each criterion in turn results in elaborations, commentaries, and in some cases suggested alterations from the Leeds Consensus (Sugden 2006). Currently, two pieces of work are being developed that will influence these criteria. First, a draft of DSM-V is out and comments are being requested. Second, Rainer Blank and a group of international colleagues have recently developed a comprehensive document detailing diagnosis and intervention for the German and Swiss systems (Blank et al 2012).

Criterion A and commentary

> Performance in daily activities that require motor coordination is substantially below that expected given the person's chronological age and measured intelligence. This may be manifested by marked delays in achieving motor

milestones (e.g., walking, crawling, sitting), dropping things, 'clumsiness', poor performance in sports, or poor handwriting.

(APA 2000, p. 58)

It is now generally recommended that an individually administered and culturally appropriate norm-referenced test of general motor competence be employed to apply Criterion A. DSM-IV does not provide guidance on how to interpret 'substantially below', but a usual cut-off point for Criterion A is applied to performance at or below the fifth centile. (Observational checklists are often used as an initial screening tool.) It is recognized that the fifth centile is arbitrary and can be seen as both too high and too low. For example, if the usual statistics are employed, two standard deviations (approximately 2.5%) is the common marker and ICD-10 recommends this. Conversely, 15% is a figure that is often used and, although it is often recommended to monitor children within this figure, it is not really practical to use this as a defining percentage for the condition. Thus, 5% has been thought to be both reasonable and part of custom and practice in both clinical and research settings (Sugden 2006). In a slightly different vein Geuze et al (2001) propose the 15th centile for clinical purposes and the 5th centile for research purposes, leading Albaret and de Castelnau (2007) to state that different cut-offs should be used depending on whether clinical (15th centile) or research (5th centile) evaluation is the objective. It is worth noting that in tests of motor impairment the figures of 5% and 15% are often used, thus leading us to report these percentages.

In a recent, large, UK birth cohort study, a prevalence/incidence figure of between 1.7% and 4.9% was proposed (Lingam et al 2009). They examined the prevalence of DCD in children aged 7 years as part of the Avon Longitudinal Study of Parents and Children (ALSPAC) with data on approximately 7000 children. All four criteria on DSM-IV-TR (APA 2000) were addressed:

- using subtests of the Movement ABC (MABC) for Criterion A
- using handwriting and parent questionnaire for Criterion B
- using neurological information available from the ALSPAC database for Criterion C
- excluding any child with a Wechsler Intelligence Scale for Children (WISC) score of less than 70 for Criterion D.

Combining the four criteria, 149 children met the DSM criteria for DCD. This group of children comprised the lowest 5% on Criterion A and 10% on Criterion B.

Of these, 30 were excluded with a known neurological diagnosis or an IQ less than 70, leaving 119 who met the full DSM-IV criteria for DCD. This gave a prevalence of 1.7% of children with a mean age of 7 years and 6 months and a sex ratio of 1.8:1 males to females. If children scored between the 5th and 15th centile on the MABC and between the 10th and 15th centile on the activities of daily living or failed the handwriting test, a further 22 children were identified. This gave a prevalence of 4.9% with a sex ratio of 1.7:1 males to females. The authors conclude that, using the strict DSM-IV criteria, 17 children per 1000 are identified as having DCD and 49 per 1000 have probable DCD.

The Lingam et al (2009) study with its large numbers may require us to re-examine the prevalence figures, as it shows figures lower than those usually presented. In all studies of prevalence it is prudent to examine the criteria and cut-off points that lead to the figures.

When making a diagnosis, caution is recommended to clinicians and researchers when applying and interpreting tests, noting that the tests themselves do not indicate diagnosis. This only comes about when a full range of information is collected from a variety of sources, with the professional making a diagnosis or not as a result of the total amount of information presented (Barnett 2008).

Criterion B and commentary

'The disturbance in criterion A significantly interferes with academic achievement or activities of daily living.' There is a negative impact on activities of daily living – such as dressing, feeding, riding a bicycle – and/or on academic achievement such as through poor handwriting skills. Core aspects of the disorder include difficulties with gross and/or fine motor skills, which may be apparent in locomotion, agility, manual dexterity, complex skills (e.g. ball games) and/or balance.

(APA 2000, p. 58)

Establishing a direct link between poor motor coordination and academic achievement is complex, but an obvious area is the specific skill of handwriting, which is often affected in children with DCD and is known to adversely affect academic achievement. For school-age children handwriting is also an activity of daily living and it is an important part of learning and assessment across the school curriculum, with much time being spent writing during the school day. Knowledge and skills are assessed through the medium of handwriting and it continues to be a needed skill in adulthood, as at university most examinations are still handwritten and lecture notes are usually taken by hand. It has been well established that poor fluency in writing is related to reduced quantity and quality of written content and poor handwriting can lead to academic underachievement (Briggs 1970, Simner et al 1996).

Handwriting may be assessed for a variety of reasons including identification, description, quantification, monitoring, and intervention. For any of these applications it is usual to consider measurement issues for this particular skill, with attention being given to two different aspects in the assessment of handwriting:

- the final product (in terms of quality and speed of production)
- the writing process (how writing evolves and the posture of the writer).

It is also usual to consider the skill in a wider context in terms of how the skill has been taught and what other literacy and language skills the child possesses. In addition, in other areas of the curriculum such as physical education, design technology, food technology, and science practicals, it is easy to see how a child with movement difficulties would have problems.

Other areas of academic achievement are less easy to substantiate and have a history of controversy. For example, proposals have been made that academic areas such as reading are strongly and directly linked to motor incoordination (Fawcett and Nicolson 1995, 1999, Nicolson and Fawcett 1999). This is not a new phenomenon: researchers and clinicians have proposed this link for a number of years (Kephart 1956, Getman 1963, Barsch 1965, Delacato 1966). These older theoretical and clinical constructs have had challenges over the years, with writers such as Cratty (1975a,b) and Kavale and Forness (1995) making strong criticisms. More recently, these links have been made theoretically through a biological substrate such as the cerebellum, an impairment in which has often led to it being proposed as the underlying cause of difficulties experienced by children with dyslexia and those with DCD. The logical progression is that some intervention protocols for children with dyslexia have at their core motor activities. In Chapter 12 these protocols are examined in more detail, but suffice here to note that again they have come under substantial criticism (Bishop 2007).

Activities of daily living typically would include consideration of self-care, play, leisure, and schoolwork. There is evidence to show that the views of the child, parents, teachers, and relevant others do differ with respect to what they believe are activities of daily living. Thus,

from a clinical point of view, with the aim of a successful intervention, it is now recommended that the child's views should be at least as important as the others' views and in many cases take precedence (Dunford et al 2005). In the clinical environment, when designing intervention programmes, skilful work by the clinician and/or teacher is required to handle the situations in which views differ widely. A slightly different approach to Criterion B is taken by Watkinson et al (2001) who, through a self-assessment instrument, used playground participation as a means of assessing 'interference', as specified in Criterion B. Summers et al (2008) used qualitative interviews of parents to examine the impact of DCD on their children's daily routines in Australia and Canada, illustrating not only differences between children with DCD and controls but also the more fundamental importance of collecting information from a variety of sources to build an accurate and total profile of the child. Thus one would recommend that, when assessing activities of daily living, the views of all interested parties, particularly the child, are taken and used together with an analysis of different environmental contexts.

An example of differences between children with DCD and their typically developing counterparts on activities of daily living is illustrated in a parent report study by Geuze (2005), who looked at motor milestones, activities of daily living, and school activities, with some of the results shown in Table 8.2.

Whereas it may seem that some children who are typically developing experience difficulties, it is clear that, as a group, children with DCD are experiencing many more problems across a wide range of tasks.

A final comment on Criterion B is that it often appears as a criterion for a number of developmental disorders (APA 2000). In other words, it is a general criterion that covers and applies to a number of conditions, but it is particularly relevant to DCD. Appropriate movement skills are critical to activities of daily living; indeed it is hard to think of those daily activities that do not involve movement and thus it is an essential part of the identification criteria. The effect on academic activities through handwriting has similar strong evidence, whereas the direct effect of movement activities on other academic areas such as reading is less well supported.

Criterion C and commentary

The disturbance is not due to a general medical condition (e.g., cerebral palsy, hemiplegia or muscular dystrophy) and does not meet criteria for a Pervasive Developmental Disorder.

(APA 2000, p. 58)

TABLE 8.2
Differences between children with DCD
and TDC as reported by parents

Activity	TDC % slow or late	DCD % slow or late
Walking	5	33
Bicycle riding	11	54
Feeding	35	60
Dressing	0	47
Handwriting	30 poor	57 poor; 20 bad
Gym	5	20

Based on data from Geuze (2005). DCD, developmental coordination disorder; TDC, typically developing children.

A conventional neurological examination is often conducted to rule out major neurological conditions (e.g. definite disorders of posture, tone, reflexes). However, this is not always the case and it may be unrealistic to expect on all occasions. Criterion C notes that the disturbance is not due to a general medical condition (e.g. cerebral palsy, hemiplegia, or muscular dystrophy) and does not meet criteria for a 'pervasive developmental disorder' (p. 58). DCD does not imply aetiology but is a symptom-based diagnosis. One difficulty with the DSM-IV criteria for diagnosing DCD has been the lack of clarity surrounding Criterion C, as there are many medical conditions that have a lack of motor control as one 'symptom' among others and a known condition such as cerebral palsy, hemiplegia, or muscular dystrophy should exclude a diagnosis of DCD. With more recent advances in various areas of medicine and genetics it may be that this criteria is revisited. At the moment there is the possibility, in borderline cases of mild cerebral palsy, of the two conditions being confused and even overlapping.

The Leeds Consensus recommended the acknowledgement that overall the evidence suggests that DCD is a unique and separate neurodevelopmental disorder, which can and often does co-occur with one or more other neurodevelopmental disorders. Commonly, these include ADHD, autistic spectrum disorder (ASD), specific language impairment (SLI), and developmental dyslexia. It would appear to be inappropriate to exclude the possibility of a dual diagnosis of DCD and a pervasive developmental disorder, and both could be given if the situation arose. This would help in giving a clearer profile of the child's capabilities (see later section on co-occurring characteristics).

Criterion D and commentary
Currently in the new DSM-V criteria, which has been sent out for review, this criterion is missing and thus the concept of discrepancy is not employed. However, until DSM-V is published we are reviewing DSM-IV, with a commentary at the end of this section on the implications of the anticipated changes in DSM-V.

Under DSM-IV Criterion D, if an intellectual disability is present, the motor difficulties are in excess of those usually associated with it.

Ideally, a measure of IQ should be made to establish the general level of intellectual ability. Where this is not feasible a teacher's opinion or other relevant data such as national tests may be acceptable. Learning disability is defined in DSM-IV as an IQ score below 70. The Leeds Consensus Statement recommended that children with a measured, or presumed, IQ below 70 should not be given a diagnosis of DCD, as these children are known to have a higher risk of motor difficulties. Within a typical range of intelligence, above 70, the relationship between IQ and motor competence is low, but as soon as the IQ drops below 70 the relationship begins to rise and continues to do so as the IQ falls, reaching a stage in which most children with severe to profound learning disability show some sign of motor impairment. For this reason it is appropriate to exclude those with presumed IQs below 70, as the primary diagnostic category would be different to DCD, with motor impairment shown as a co-occurring characteristic (see Chapter 9 on intellectual disabilities). For example, Sugden and Wann (1987) when working with children with moderate learning disability (IQs 50–75) found 30% of 8-year-olds and 50% of 12-year-olds scored below the fifth centile on the Test of Motor Impairment (Stott et al 1984).

By employing IQ or some other measure of ability, the concept of discrepancy is being introduced; this is the notion that motor ability is out of line with other abilities. In other developmental disorders such as dyslexia this has been a very hotly debated concept and this is addressed in Chapter 10 on other developmental disorders. Suffice to note here that it has not figured quite as strongly in the DCD literature, being an exclusionary clause, noting that any impairment should be over and above any generic intellectual disability that is present.

If Criterion D is excluded from the new DSM-V, IQ is not part of the criteria and takes away the discrepancy concept. This is a laudable step forward as any discrepancy concept is very difficult to invoke in a practical manner. However, it does not mean that a child with an intellectual disability will automatically be diagnosed as DCD, as this is unlikely to be a primary identifying characteristic. It is more likely that an intellectual disability is diagnosed with a co-occurring characteristic of motor difficulties, which paves the way for intervention which might have been previously absent. However, unless a lower cut-off

IQ is proposed, below which one should not diagnose DCD, there is always the possibility that a dual diagnosis is given such as intellectual disability and DCD, with a subsequent rise in the prevalence of DCD.

Criteria C and D are both exclusionary criteria and the Leeds Consensus reiterates DCD as a 'specific and separate' disorder which may (frequently) co-occur with other developmental disorders. There was agreement that the terms minimal brain dysfunction and ABD were not helpful to diagnosis.

The issue of diagnosis of DCD is complex with numerous variables playing a significant role. The DSM-IV criteria with modifications from the two consensus statements have provided us with a significant step forward and more and more researchers and clinicians worldwide are addressing this with the result that comparisons across contexts are more easily made. However, consistent diagnosis is never easy and strictly adhering to DSM-IV is often difficult when one includes the cost of ruling out differential diagnosis.

In the last few years, more attention has begun to be paid to those individuals who are outside of the usual range of study of 6 to 11 years, with the result that the current situation can be accurately called one in which a lifespan approach to motor coordination difficulties is coming to the fore.

Early and later identification of children with DCD

The majority of studies on children with movement difficulties involve children between 6 and 11 years of age. DSM-IV, when quoting prevalence rates, uses these two ages as their range. However, it is clear that for most individuals movement problems do not simply start when they are 6 years of age nor do they usually finish when they are 11.

EARLY YEARS

The lower age limit of children with DCD usually included in descriptive or experimental studies (including intervention studies) is around 5 or 6 years of age (Geuze et al 2001). However, when interviewing parents of children with DCD about the natural history of their child's motor coordination problems most report these to have been present before the child entered school (Pless et al 2001). Indeed, it is probably illogical to assume that motor coordination problems only 'emerge' at (pre)school entry. It is usually clear that there are already many task and environmental demands placed on preschool children allowing those with non-optimal motor behaviour to be noticed (Chambers and Sugden 2002, Jongmans 2005). It is also true that, in the home, parents and carers have often noticed that the child is somehow different.

Inter- and intra-individual variability in motor performance are major challenges in identifying children with poor motor coordination at a young age. Longitudinal research among infants between 9 and 21 months has shown intra-individual fluctuations in infants' scores over time within the gross and fine motor domain. Both show periods of 'leaps and bounds' and periods in which children gain motor skills in steady increments can be observed (Thelen and Ulrich 1991, Ulrich 1997). In addition, different children show different pathways to master motor skills, although preferred patterns can be detected (Darrah et al 2003). Both phenomena carry with them the risk of either wrongly identifying a child as being delayed in acquiring motor skills or underestimating the consequences of deviant motor behaviour at an early age. Similarly, in the ages between 2 and 5 years, this variability both within the child and within a group of children is often due to lack of experience.

As a result, population screening methods to identify young children with motor coordination difficulties have so far not been widely introduced, although infant and young children's development charts do provide a global evaluation of children's motor development (Peabody Developmental Motor Scales, Folio and Fewell 1983; Denver Developmental Screening Test II, Frankenburg et al 1992; Bayley 1993). Screening methods could be beneficial, as they allow for identification of 'true-positive' cases, which, in turn, would facilitate early intervention. Recently attempts to remedy this have been made by researchers such as Chambers and Sugden (2002, 2006) who devised a checklist aimed at identifying children with movement problems between the ages of 3 and 5 years and followed this up with intervention schedules, with early results providing cautious optimism. One firm stance that was taken by the groups producing the Leeds Consensus and by Chambers and Sugden (2006) was that a diagnosis of DCD should not be given below the age of 5, primarily because of both the variability of experience before formal schooling and the instability of development between the ages of 2 and 5 years. This does not mean that the difficulties are not addressed; indeed, if a child is having obvious difficulties between these ages, these difficulties can be addressed using a three-tier approach that is analogous to the three-tier approach in reading problems, in which each tier is followed by one of increasing intensity, with reference to the child's response to intervention. This approach is described further in Chapter 12.

Most vital information concerning the early years comes from retrospective descriptions by parents of children later identified as DCD (Pless et al 2001). These signs represent more functional activities of daily living such as a child's quality of performance during play, sport, locomotion, meals, and dressing at preschool age. Which (combination of) signs when present at preschool age will lead to DCD is currently not known, and the ways of assessing these signs reliably in early childhood, leading to a later diagnosis of DCD, is still a major challenge.

LATER YEARS AND EMERGING ADULTHOOD

Just as there is a paucity of studies examining movement difficulties in the early years, a similar situation exists with older children. In many ways this is not surprising. By 11 or 12 years of age, many of the tasks that were challenging to children with movement difficulties early in life have been overcome or compensations have been made. For example, by this age self-care skills such as washing, dressing, and using cutlery have been learned, although often in a rather mechanical manner. Those skills that posed problems are simply omitted from the repertoire of the children. Prime candidates for these are skills such as sports and athletic endeavours. However, this does not mean that no problems remain for, as is illustrated in the case studies above, new problems arise. In addition, it is also known that the problems noted early in life very often stay through to emerging adulthood. Longitudinal studies such as those conducted by Gillberg and colleagues (e.g. RH Gillberg and Rasmussen 1982, C Gillberg et al 1983, IC Gillberg et al 1989), Cantell et al (1994), and Losse et al (1991) give good illustrations of this (see later section on progressions).

There has been some recent work examining difficulties that appear in adulthood, not as part of any progression studies. Cousins and Smyth (2003, 2005) selected adults aged between 18 and 65 with a history of motor disorders in childhood and engaged them in motor tasks. The results showed that coordination difficulties were common across the lifespan and, although there was a continuum of impairments with some participants approaching normal performance on some tasks, many were clearly impaired on a variety of tasks, and the group as a whole performed more poorly than controls on the entire range of tasks. A summary of the findings is shown in Table 8.3.

Many showed the same difficulties that they had reported as children, yet there were some tasks that were obviously specific to adults such as car driving, as reported in our case study of Peter. About half of the group had a higher-education qualification, illustrating that motor problems were not necessarily a barrier to education, but there were also reports of being unable to maintain employment commensurate with their academic qualifications. Cousins and Smyth (2005) in a review article note that '... they felt they could not perform tasks quickly enough, and could not learn new systems that

TABLE 8.3

A list of tasks performed significantly worse by adults with self reports of development coordination disorder (index group) than by matched controls

Self ratings

Bumping into objects

Balance

Manual dexterity

Catching and hitting objects

Handwriting

Construction

Actual motor tests

Manual dexterity

Handwriting speed (not errors)

Some measure of construction

Obstacle avoidance speed (not errors)

Static and dynamic balance

Aiming and catching

Clap and catch

Reaction and movement time

Based on data from Cousins and Smyth (2003).

were introduced to the workplace after they were taken on as employees' (p. 131).

Recent work by a number of individuals is starting to make an impact on how we view emerging adults and adults with motor coordination difficulties. Kirby, in a series of publications with colleagues (Kirby et al 2008a,b, 2010, 2011), has promoted the status of this group of individuals, noting that not only do coordination difficulties remain but also that they are different to the ones seen in childhood and bring with them associated social and other difficulties. For example, driving has already been noted, but Kirby showed that adults with motor coordination difficulties do drive and pass their test, but they drive fewer miles than average adults of the same age, engage in fewer social interactions, and tend not to have serious accidents, although they do have less serious ones such as hitting gate posts. This does tend to suggest that they are aware of their limitations and adjust their lives accordingly. Kirby et al (2008a) note that an increasing number of students in the UK are arriving at university and college with a diagnosis of DCD and requesting Disabled Students' Allowances to gain support. In comparison to students with dyslexia those with DCD receive less support in terms of the amount, but the type of support they receive is very similar to those students with dyslexia. The authors also note the changing difficulties of the students with DCD, with the problem not residing solely within the motor domain but being seen in their social and organizational skills and what the authors label as weaknesses in executive functioning (Kirby et al 2011).

In Box 8.4 these points made by Kirby et al (2008b) are elaborated.

For different reasons, the phases of early years and emerging adulthood will begin to attract more research and clinical emphasis. In the early years, there are the known benefits of early intervention, although this is not without its pitfalls, with self-fulfilling prophecy and incorrect identification being two. Both of these can be moderated by the judicious manner in which intervention is provided (see Chapter 12). For the phase of emerging adulthood, it is now clear that without intervention motor skill difficulties are unlikely to go away and in adulthood they not only continue but change in nature and are accompanied by numerous co-occurring characteristics.

Co-occurring characteristics

There have always been children who have a motor difficulty not only as their main characteristic but also their only one, with the work by Peters and Henderson (2008) clearly showing this. However, at the beginning of the chapter, relating to the history of DCD, it was noted that one of the defining features of current day work in the area is the acceptance that co-occurring characteristics are the norm rather than the exception in this population of children. Indeed, the topic is so important that a whole chapter (Chapter 11) is devoted to other developmental disorders that have motor difficulties as additional characteristic features. The difference between this section and that chapter is that here children are identified with a motor disorder as the core characteristic and defining feature, whereas in Chapter 12 it is the other developmental disorders, such as SLI, that are the focus of attention, with motor disorders seen as a co-occurring characteristic. This is a subtle distinction and probably not one that can always stand a rigorous analysis because of the continuous, rather than discrete, nature of the disorders. However, this distinction is useful for an overall picture of how co-occurring characteristics play an important role in the total picture of the child. Certainly, as is shown in Chapter 12 on assessment and intervention, co-occurring characteristics play a crucial role in constructing a profile and selecting priorities, which lead to appropriate intervention.

In noticing that children with DCD do not usually display a single discrete disorder, Kaplan et al (2006) discuss the merits of the terms comorbidity, co-occurrence, and continuum. They come down in favour of discarding comorbidity because it is misleading, as it specifies that the underlying constitutional substrates are independent and not causally related. They therefore favour co-occurring and continuum to describe associations among developmental disorders, with the former employed when there are common aetiologies present or absent, and a continuum used to indicate the range of abilities across a number of domains.

DCD is a developmental disorder with children showing profiles that differ according to their motor characteristics, as shown in Box 8.3. However, this heterogeneity is not only shown in the motor domain but also in associated characteristics and overlaps with other developmental disorders (Henderson and Hall 1982, Henderson et al 1994). Green and Baird (2005) point out that the issues raised by the extent of associated characteristics and/or overlapping conditions are not simply academic ones, because they directly affect intervention, support, and provision. Owing to the overlap or co-occurring characteristics there is a long history of giving children more generic labels than DCD. Early ones such as minimal brain damage or dysfunction (Pasamanick and Knobloch 1966) have largely disappeared, primarily because there was seldom any evidence of brain damage. More recently, this has been revived by Kaplan et al (1997) who came up with the term *ABD* and has shown the overlap of DCD with other developmental disorders such as ADHD, dyslexia, and pervasive developmental disorders such as the ASD. Later in this chapter, there is a section on 'Underlying biological substrates' (page 242), which examines possible organic problems in children with DCD, and in Chapter 10, on other developmental disorders, there is a discussion as to why there are co-occurring characteristics across developmental disorders. A model from Morton (2004) is presented to examine this from biological, cognitive, and behavioural viewpoints. Suffice to note that terms such as atypical brain damage are attempts to explain co-occurring characteristics by reference to some underlying biological substrates not specifically identified.

The literature on associated characteristics focuses on two methodologies. First, there is a group of studies that examine DCD and follow this by analysing associated characteristics. The second method is to look at other developmental disorders such as ADHD and determine whether or not the individuals could also have a diagnosis of DCD or have movement difficulties that are not diagnosed as such. Much of the literature dealing with the latter is summarized in Chapter 10. Attentional difficulties in children have been widely studied with respect to associated coordination difficulties, with the Swedish studies of the Gillberg groups being the most prominent in this area (C Gillberg et al 1983, IC Gillberg and C Gillberg 1989, IC Gillberg et al 1989, Hellgren et al 1994, Rasmussen and C Gillberg 2000). This group of studies found that

Box 8.4 A closer examination

Adults and DCD: Kirby et al (2008b)

Aim

The study aimed to examine the characteristics of students aged 16 to 25 who had reported coordination difficulties since childhood and who were in further or higher education at the time.

Methodology

A total of 109 individuals originally took part with 93 in the final sample, recruited from colleges and universities across the UK. The 93 participants completed a web-based or paper-based questionnaire. The aim was to mirror DSM-IV criteria but by using a self-reporting methodology. Criterion A could not be addressed in this way unless they had had previous formal assessment. Criterion B was met by the items surrounding activities of daily living. Criterion C was met by excluding those who had responded positively to questions about general medical conditions. It was assumed that Criterion D was met as all were attending higher or further education, thus potentially eliminating anyone with a full scale IQ below 70. A total of 93 individuals were identified and placed in groups:

1   DCD only (23)
2   DCD and dyslexia, ADHD, ASD (36)
3   Dyslexia only (23)
4   No formal diagnosis (11)

Results

In comparison with the dyslexia group, the DCD-only group reported significantly more difficulties in childhood relating to seven questions about motor activities. For example, more than twice the number reported difficulties in playing team games and in riding a bicycle, whereas both groups reported high levels of writing difficulties, which appeared to be a persistent problem. Persons with DCD, whether on its own or in combination, were more likely to be living at home than the dyslexia group (DCD only 71%, dyslexia 17%). Students with dyslexia were more likely to receive Disabled Students' Allowances or Disability Living Allowance than students with DCD (dyslexia 74%, DCD 29%). No differences were found between the type of support offered by colleges and universities to students with different disability conditions (Table 8.4).

The students also reported on their strengths and weaknesses, with those with DCD reporting greater difficulties with executive functioning-type tasks and the surprising finding of strengths in social and communication skills among the DCD-only group.

Conclusion

Most of the differences were found between the DCD-only group and the dyslexia-only group with the DCD-plus group being somewhere in between. The issue of handwriting remained a problem and the question of whether, after a reasonable amount of practice time throughout schooling, handwriting should be discarded in favour of teaching proficient keyboard skills was raised by the authors. They also noted that in further and higher education few professionals can actually assess the students, and recommended professional training emphasizing a multidisciplinary approach to advice, assessment, and support.

TABLE 8.4
Type of support received by condition

Type of support	DCD (n=23) (%)	DCD plus (n=36) (%)	Dyslexia only (n=23) (%)	No diagnosis (n=11) (%)
Extra examination time	76	74	78	18
Laptop	48	34	52	9
Note taker	14	18	4	27
Mentor/coach	24	26	26	27
Student support	62	76	74	9
Other	19	16	17	27

children with coordination difficulties overlapped with, and were at high risk for, attentional disorders. To emphasize this they used the term DAMP to indicate the overlap between perceptual and attentional disorders. In a similar vein, Kaplan et al (1997) in Canada identified ADHD in 41% of children with DCD, and 17% of children with ADHD met the criteria for DCD. This overlap of DCD with attentional and social and emotional difficulties is also reported by Green and Baird (2005), who showed that 53% of children with DCD were reported by their parents to have activity and attentional problems. These co-occurring problems have been reported to have long-term effects and more pervasive influence than simply DCD or ADHD on their own.

Other co-occurring conditions and characteristics that have been reported include SLI (Powell and Bishop 1992, Hill 1998), and Hill et al (1998) found a 60% incidence of DCD in a sample of children with SLI. Literacy skills have long been associated with poor coordination, particularly in reading, with studies showing a consistent linking of DCD and ADHD (Green and Baird 2005). Again this is covered in more detail in Chapter 10.

C Gillberg and Kadesjo (2003) report on a series of studies showing strong relationships among ADHD, autism, and movement difficulties. Kadesjo and C Gillberg (1999) showed almost half of children with ADHD to also have DCD in a total population study in Karlstad, Sweden. Similar rates of comorbidity were obtained in other populations studies (RH Gillberg and Rasmussen 1982, Landgren et al 1996). An interesting reason for this is proposed by Denkla (1974) who, using tests of rapid alternating coordination, concluded that 'overflow movements' or 'associated movements' were signs of both impaired motor coordination and hyperactivity.

Social and emotional problems often occur in tandem with the motor difficulties in children of school age, and, although there is uncertainty about any causal effect and indeed in which direction this would be, there is good evidence for a relationship. This relationship is taken further in Chapter 12, in which there are many programmes that target the movement capabilities of the child, often using the phrase '*learning to move*', as well as those that use movement for other purposes, with '*moving to learn*' being the primary aim. In the former there is an emphasis on the acquisition of movement skills per se and in the latter on how movement skills can be used to enhance learning in other domains.

There is a strong body of literature pointing to the relationship between movement difficulties and social and emotional problems such as low self-esteem, poor self-concept, and emotional difficulties (Henderson et al 1989, Losse et al 1991, Maeland 1992, Cratty 1994, Schoemaker

and Kalverboer 1994). Skinner and Piek (2001) worked with children aged 8 to 10 and 12 to 14 with and without DCD using Harter's theory of motivation to examine perceived competence and social support, and their influences on self-worth and anxiety. The major findings showed that children with DCD had lower self-perceptions and global self-worth than their typically developing peers, and this was evident across a number of domains. Their perceptions were clearly lower in the athletic and physical appearance areas but also in other areas. As Skinner and Piek (2001) succinctly note, 'Children and adolescents with DCD are less happy with their lives, and place less value on themselves than their coordinated counter parts' (p. 91).

It is not a foregone conclusion that there is a direct cause and effect from poor coordination to social and emotional difficulties, but the evidence is building up and the possibility of this directional effect cannot be ignored. An interesting additional finding by Skinner and Piek was that those with DCD perceived themselves as having lower social support and acceptance in their social group than their peers. Adolescents appeared to be more affected than younger children, being more unhappy with their lives, having greater anxiety, and more social and emotional problems and receiving less support than younger children. A natural progression was to examine the relationship between social and emotional and motor variables in younger children (Piek et al 2008) with the aim of determining whether this relationship had early precedents. There were moderate relationships between motor ability and anxiety/depression that were significant enough for the authors to recommend further investigation. Table 8.5 shows examples of some co-occurring characteristics.

Developmental progression

There was a time when it was thought that children would 'grow out' of the movement problems simply through a passage of time and maturation. However, there has not been enough evidence to substantiate this proposal and what evidence we do have points to an equivocal picture. As the condition began to be better defined in the 1990s, researchers began to look at both the short- and long-term consequences and effects of the condition, with the result that some longitudinal studies were undertaken with school-age children (Losse et al 1991, Cantell et al 1994, 2003, Piek 2003). In addition, other commentators noted that progression does not always include school-age children, and progressions from birth through to entering school have also been examined (for a summary see Sugden and Wright 1998). More recently, what happens in adulthood after DCD in childhood has

TABLE 8.5
Co-occurring characteristics with DCD

Co-occurring characteristic	Percentage overlap	Reference
ADHD	60	Rasmussen and C Gillberg (2000)
Specific language impairment	60	Hill (1998)
Reading difficulties	55	Kaplan et al (1998)
Social, emotional, and behaviour difficulties	82	Losse et al (1991), Skinner and Piek (2001)

Rasmussen and C Gillberg (2000) reported that 80% of children with a combined diagnosis of DCD and ADHD had poorer outcomes, compared with only 13% in a control group, leading them to say that it was a combination of problems that gave the most pessimistic outcomes. DCD, developmental coordination disorder; ADHD, attention-deficit–hyperactivity disorder. From data reported by Rasmussen and Gillberg (2000).

become a significant point of interest (Cousins and Smyth 2005, Kirby et al 2008a,b).

A developmental perspective was taken by Missiuna et al (2007) who, in an article they called 'A trajectory of troubles', examined parents' perspectives of their children with DCD between the ages of 6 and 14 years. They found that there was an evolution in parents' concerns as the child developed, with earlier concerns focusing on the pure motor and play activities. This would seem logical as these activities are central to a child's life at this time. As the child developed these concerns changed to self-care, academic, and peer relationship problems in middle childhood, and because of frustration they evolved through to self-esteem and emotional issues later. Missiuna et al (2007) called for more parent awareness and professional training in order for the children to receive appropriate help to try to prevent this progression of difficulties.

The examination of developmental progressions can be undertaken in different ways. One way is to look retrospectively at children and involves taking children at a specific moment in time and then following them as they develop. This can be done over a short or long period of time, with other variations involving the number of times the children are examined. Another method is to look retrospectively. Here an examination of a group of individuals is performed from the present time by looking back at reports from the individual concerned or from others involved in their lives. Prospective studies have great advantages in that ongoing reports and observations can be accurately made, but they are rare and expensive. Retrospective studies have the advantage of being relatively economical but are plagued by distortions of memory and recall. Other differences in studies of developmental progressions surround the populations under study. Some studies focus on whole populations and thus are strong on prevalence and showing how individuals move in and out of the conditions. Others focus on risk

groups, often using smaller numbers, giving detailed pictures of the nature of any condition.

BIRTH TO SCHOOL AGE
Although the condition is not usually diagnosed until children are of school age, there are some conclusions that can be drawn from studies that look at the stability or otherwise of motor characteristics of children between birth and school age. Large cohort studies such as the Collaborative Perinatal Project (Nichols and Chen 1981), which looked at a cohort of 30 000 children, showed, through re-examination of the data (Sugden and Keogh 1990), that children with low Bayley scores at 8 months were nearly twice as likely to have neurological soft signs at 7 years of age, but this risk did not continue to the same degree, and the further away from each other the measures were taken, the less predictive they were. The low neuromotor performance of low birthweight children was well documented by Mutch et al (1993), who reported results from the 1992 Scottish Low Birth Weight Study Group. Sugden and Keogh (1990) make the obvious comment that, in the early years, movement behaviours are the most common response, so they may not be quite as discriminative as they are in later years. This was partially true in a Scottish developmental screening programme, in which there was a high proportion of children with minor neurological disorders in the first year, and this made movement problems too common to be a predictor of other problems. Another way to examine this is to take a group of children identified for at-risk factors and compare them to a control group. Children with very low birthweights (below 1000g) were examined and compared to those in a control group (Hall et al 1995). By 8 years of age, 50% in the low birthweight group scored below the fifth centile on the MABC compared with 8% in the control group.

A common method of identifying preschool-age children who are at risk is to perform population screening, but as Jongmans (2005) points out, screening is not suitable for diagnosis. She notes the advantages of early screening such as finding true-positive cases at an early age, which is an aid to providing support and resources to parents and may also prevent secondary problems. However, she also notes the downsides of many screening instruments lacking validity and the problem of identifying 'false' positives, that is those children who are identified as at risk through screening but subsequently show no problems. She concludes by recommending the assessment of children with appropriate instruments throughout their lifespan because a single test at one point in time does not give the full dynamic picture of what motor development entails. An example of multiple assessments examining stability over time is described by Darrah et al (1998, 2003) who examined 45 typically developing infants monthly from 2 weeks of age until they were walking. Over the year, 31% of children at some time received a score in the lowest 10%, suggesting instability in the emergence of gross motor skills in typically developing infants.

An example of work in this area is shown in Box 8.5. These and other results show that difficulties at birth in some and often many children persist, with problems up to and beyond school age, but individual prediction about future performance is difficult as these figures relate to group statistics. What we do know is that some children with very low birthweights, born preterm, and/or with neurological signs at birth will not survive; others will develop recognizable disorders such as cerebral palsy; and for the remainder there will be a higher incidence of persistent coordination difficulties. However, some children in this group do develop typically and one challenge to professionals working with these children is to isolate those variables that contribute to more successful outcomes.

PROGRESSION DURING THE SCHOOL YEARS

There have been relatively few studies pointing to definitive outcomes of children showing problems with motor coordination. Early studies such as Knuckey and Gubbay (1983) gave cause for some optimism. They tested the same children at 10 and 18 years of age and found that only the most severe had not overcome their difficulties, and the outcomes were reasonably optimistic, but they lost 50% of the original children in the study. Cantell et al (1994, 2003) originally assessed children at school-entry age, again at 11 and 15 years of age, and finally at 17. Of the children who evidenced movement difficulties at 6, labelled 'clumsy' in their study, 65% of them continued to have motor problems up to 11 years of age and just under 50% at 15, with the remainder in an 'intermediate' group not clearly distinguishable from either the movement

problem group or the control group. By 17 all groups had improved, but Cousins and Smyth (2005) still arrive at the conclusion that as many as one-half of children with movement difficulties continue to show them well into adolescence, with those exhibiting severe difficulties most at risk.

It is not only the motor problems that appear to persist, with a number of studies showing associated difficulties. In the Cantell et al (1994) study the children with motor difficulties rated themselves lower on scholastic competence and had fewer hobbies. Lower academic prowess has also been reported by Geuze and Borger (1994), and, although this seems to be a feature, Cousins and Smyth (2005) alert us to the confounding variable of lower academic status and are cautious about making a direct link between movement problems and academic performance. This body of literature has implications for the definition of DCD, as having an effect on academic performance is part of the Criterion B for diagnosis in DSM-IV-TR (APA 2000).

A 10-year follow-up study by Losse et al (1991) examined the children on a number of variables including motor, social, and academic areas and is described in Box 8.6.

One factor that is impossible to control in these longitudinal studies is the type of experiences the children have had during these years. In particular, the evidence for the effect of intervention over long periods of time is only starting to trickle through. Sugden and Chambers (2003) examined the effect of intervention using teachers and parents over a 4-year monitoring study of children with DCD using standardized tests and interview data. The children were part of an intervention protocol, three to five times a week, that lasted 16 weeks (8wks each with parents and teachers), with periods of no intervention beforehand and none afterwards, attempting to control for both maturational growth and temporary gains. Over a 4-year period 26 children were followed and the results split into three subgroups. First there was a group, constituting approximately one-half of the children who, after intervention, moved out of the category of DCD as defined by DSM-IV (APA 1994) and never moved back in. A second group of five children moved out of the DCD category immediately after intervention, but over the next 2 years steadily moved back in. A third group was quite variable with most moving in and out of the category but with two children seemingly unaffected by the intervention. Single participant analysis showed that individual progressions differed quite substantially and that this type of analysis involving full-group, subgroup, and individual analysis might be useful in unlocking the way to predictions about progressions. Thus, when examining developmental

Box 8.5 A closer examination

Prematurity and Movement Difficulties: Jongmans et al (1998)

Aim

The investigation examined the differences between children born preterm and those in a typical referral group on a number of perceptual motor measures at 6 years of age; whether any difficulties are accompanied by other problems; how these problems relate to other outcomes; and the relationship between perceptual measures at 6 years and measures taken during the neonatal period relating to weight, gestational age, and the presence or absence of brain lesion.

Methods

A final total of 156 (78 boys and 78 girls) at-risk children participated in the study with a mean birthweight of 1306g and gestational ages ranging from 25 to 34 weeks with a mean of 30 weeks. Three different reference groups ($n=88$, $n=60$, $n=64$) were selected for the perceptual motor and neurological tests. In addition, a sample of 215 term children was available for cognitive and reading tests.

Tests used included

- MABC (Henderson and Sugden 1992)
- Developmental Test of Visual–Motor Integration (VMI) (Beery 1967)
- Examination of the Child with Minor Brain Damage (Touwen 1979)
- British Ability Scales (Elliott 1979)
- Rutter Scales – parent and teacher scales (Rutter 1967).

Results

- On MABC prematurely born children scored significantly lower than the reference groups, but the VMI scores did not reach significance.
- On the Examination of the Child with Minor Brain Damage the preterm group showed significantly more neurological signs as they also did on the British Ability Scales and on reading ability.
- Overall 48% of the premature group had perceptual motor difficulties, 15 as their sole difficulty.
- Of the preterm-born children 81 passed both MABC and VMI; 54 failed one; and 21 failed both. Those who failed both read fewer words than the other children, and both groups who failed at least one showed more neurological problems than those who passed.

Conclusion

At 6 years of age there was a high presence of perceptual motor difficulties in the preterm group (48%), with 44% falling between the 5th and 15th centile on MABC and 19% below the 5th centile. This was very much in line with other studies such as that of Mutch et al (1993), who reported that at 4 years of age 20% of preterm children scored below the 10th centile. It was also clear that some children have perceptual motor problems as their sole difficulty, and 15 (20%) out of the 75 who failed the perceptual motor tests were in this category. The extent of the perceptual motor difficulties also seemed to be positively related to the number of other problems encountered by the preterm children. The authors make the case for the problems not to be underestimated and state that they deserve the attention of professionals: 'Although the origins of their difficulties may be different, we believe our data on prematurely born children to be generalisable to the larger population of children with coordination difficulties' (p. 650).

progression of a group of children with DCD, a more complete analysis would include the events that happened in the children's lives between the measurement periods.

A number of individuals have worked with groups of children within a wider definition than just DCD and have conducted classic longitudinal research on the progression

Box 8.6 A closer examination

A 10-year follow-up of 'clumsy' children: Losse et al (1991)

Aim

'Clumsy' children were originally assessed to ascertain the condition more clearly when compared with a typically developing control group, and 10 years later the researchers returned and assessed the children again together with life stories to signal any changing situation.

Children

A sample of 32 children, 16 of whom were designated as 'clumsy' and 16 controls, was assessed on a number of variables including neurodevelopmental status (The Neurodevelopmental Test Battery), general motor competence (The Henderson Revision of the Test of Motor Impairment), intelligence (WISC), self-concept (The Harter Perceived Competence Scale for Children), and leisure interests (interview questionnaire and interview). School records were also consulted to determine progress in school.

Results

- In terms of motor performance, the 'clumsy' children were significantly poorer then typically developing children in their motor skills on a standardized test 10 years on and the records from physical education teachers confirmed this difference.
- Originally the children had been matched on intelligence, academic achievement, and social and emotional status. Differences in verbal IQ, academic achievement, parts of the Harter scale, and incidences in social and behavioural problems were present 10 years on.
- In terms of academic achievement, 14 of the 16 participants in the control group were about to sit public examinations, compared with only six of the 'clumsy' group.
- The 'clumsy' group had more involvement with the police, more experience of being bullied, and poor concentration and a lack of organization in class.

Overall the 'clumsy' group continued to show more pervasive problems than the control group and all had some difficulties at school, not always in physical education lessons and sports, with many showing handwriting difficulties. However, there were one or two who originally had poor scores but no longer had difficulties in school. Comments of the children often revealed a deep sense of failure with comments such as 'I don't like sport because I'm no good at it…Teachers don't help people like me who are not very good' or 'I dreaded hockey. I don't like the teacher's attitude, she shouted at me' (Losse et al 1991, Table VII, p. 61).

Discussion

The authors discuss two questions surrounding the progression of motor difficulties through childhood.

- The first surrounds the natural history of motor difficulties and they cautiously suggest that 'clumsiness' is not confined to childhood but does continue well beyond those years.
- The second is the wider implications that motor difficulties in the early years have for the development of other abilities and achievements, concluding that there are co-occurring difficulties, but whether these are caused by the motor difficulties has yet to be resolved.

of children with difficulties including movement problems. Some of these studies have started at birth and followed the children into adolescence. The Groningen Perinatal Project looked at the incidence of MND in term populations of infants born in the University Hospital in Groningen between 1975 and 1978. From just over 3000 children, 21% were considered 'suspect' neurologically and 5% 'abnormal' neurologically. These were followed up with assessments at 6 years of age (Hadders-Algra et al 1985, 1986); at 9 years of age (Hadders-Algra et al

1988a,b); and at 12 years of age (Lunsing et al 1992). Many of the children rated as neurologically impaired developed movement difficulties; some had recovered before the first follow-up study at 6 years of age but often with speech and language problems. By 12, many of the children originally with MND appeared to be typically developing, whereas during puberty some children who were typical at birth seemed to develop neurological problems with more males than females showing problems (Lunsing et al 1992). In many males this development did reverse back to typical development, suggesting some kind of recalibration during the pubertal period. In females at this time there appeared to be a steadier, more linear developmental profile. This type of change adds weight to the argument that greater change and variability are evident during periods of maximum development.

The other important set of longitudinal studies that have taken motor skills as one of a number of characteristics is the series conducted by Gillberg and colleagues (RH Gillberg and Rasmussen 1982, IC Gillberg and C Gillberg 1989, Rasmussen and C Gillberg 2000). They chronicled the progression of children with attention, motor, and perceptual dysfunctions and referred to them as DAMP. Over 3000 children were followed over a period of more than 10 years from 6 years of age. They noted as one of their findings that motor and perceptual problems declined over the years but that this should not be taken to mean there were no more problems. The hard signs of perceptual motor dysfunction had reduced but underlying problems such as behaviour, health, and school achievement remained. The authors pointed to DAMP being a neurodevelopmental disorder with changing clinical landmarks that still continued to cause difficulties throughout childhood and adolescence. These studies, which look at behaviours other than motor, are important as they show that the motor problems may disappear but re-emerge in other areas.

The age period from 16 until the early 20s is often referred to as 'emerging adulthood', and there has been a paucity of information about what happens to children with DCD as they move into this period. One reason for this has been a lack of suitable test instruments to assess the adult population but these are now starting to emerge. Kirby et al (2010) have developed a checklist by using two groups, one in England and one in Israel, providing an English and Hebrew version. The checklist contains 40 items in three subscales:

- movement difficulties in childhood
- current movement difficulties
- current other difficulties.

The overall checklist and the three subscales of the Adult Developmental Coordination Disorders/Dyspraxia Checklist (ADC) were able to distinguish clearly between a DCD group and controls. More research is recommended to obtain clear cut-off points, but it was noted that the tool remained sensitive to groups across two countries of differing cultures.

Until the last few years, most of the work examining characteristics of children with DCD has concentrated on the age range between 5 and 6 and 11 and 12. This is not surprising as during the primary schooling years many demands are made in the movement domain and it is an important period for the development, acquisition, and consolidation of those skills that respond to these demands. However, both logic and research would suggest that children in the main neither suddenly start to have difficulties at 5 years of age nor do they grow out of them by 12. The age of 5 is one that children often start to come into contact with other children such that comparisons can be made, but often the difficulties have been noted earlier by parents. Similarly, it can be assumed that some children will withdraw from some movement experiences, having consistently failed in them, some will compensate through the use of other activities, and many will have acquired some of the routine activities such as those in the self-care area. However, in the majority of cases difficulties still persist, often with a change of emphasis; different tasks become important according to environmental demands and problems arise in other areas such as in the social and lifestyle domains. The work of Piek, Jongmans and others in the early years (Jongmans 2005, Piek et al 2008) and that of Cousins and Smyth and Kirby in the emerging adult phases (Cousins and Smyth 2003, 2005, Kirby et al 2008a,b, 2010, 2011) are bringing a new understanding and shedding new light on this complex field.

Core motor characteristics of children with DCD

The diagnosis of children with DCD in itself presents some characteristics but does so only within tight diagnostic procedures. In order to show more detail, depth, and insight into the difficulties of these children, different ways of examining the condition are presented and each part is explored in detail. The core of the difficulties of children with DCD by definition is a motor condition, and this section describes the characteristics using the motor component as the starting point. However, motor difficulties can be described in various ways, and in this section they are examined from differing angles all contributing to the core characteristic.

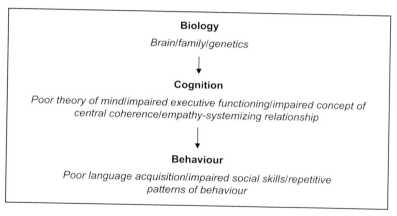

Fig. 8.1 Morton's (2004) causal model of developmental disorders (e.g. autism).

MORTON MODEL

The Morton model is used again in Chapter 10 on developmental disorders, and here it is used with some modification. Morton (2004), extending earlier work with Frith (Morton and Frith 1995), has provided us with a useful way of examining developmental disorders in general, and his model is shown here to illustrate some of the key features of DCD. Morton (2004) takes conditions such as dyslexia and attention-deficit disorder and examines them from biological, cognitive, and behavioural perspectives. He calls it 'causal modelling' that links the biological aspects of a developmental disorder such as dyslexia to the observable behavioural symptoms through the intermediary variable of cognition. Thus, in the case of dyslexia, he links familial traits, genetic studies, and possible cerebellum difficulties to poor, unexpected reading difficulties through such cognitive constructs as phonological difficulties, impaired short-term memory, and visual-processing deficits. In the case of autism, he links the biological information we have on autistic individuals with the behavioural symptoms of delay or absence of language acquisition, social problems, and restrictive or repetitive stereotypical patterns of behaviour through various cognitive constructs. These include undeveloped theory of mind, poor executive functioning, a lack of central cohesion, and the empathy-systematising debate from Baron-Cohen (2007). It is not the accuracy of Morton's explanations that are influential, as the component parts of behaviour, cognition, and biology will change, but it is the model itself that provides a useful tool for us to examine and analyse these disorders. Figure 8.1 is a simple model adapted from Morton using a causal modelling explanation to examine the condition of autism.

MORTON MODEL AND DCD

The model can be applied to the condition of DCD, albeit with some modifications which involve a slight change in one of the headings. Morton's (2004) examples all apply to developmental disorders that are predominantly cognitive in nature such as autism, dyslexia, and ADHD, and thus the intervening, linking variable is logically named 'cognition'. Such cognitive concepts as theory of mind or executive control can be added to others such as memory and attention, all of which play a major role in the interplay between biology and behaviour.

Although cognition plays a significant part in the performance of motor skills, it is not the only intervening variable and many would argue that it is not even the most important. In the motor skills domain such cognitive concepts as memory and attention have been utilized, but there are also others that are distinctly not cognitive in nature such as controlling degrees of freedom, morphological constraints, and coordinative structures. For those reasons, we are proposing that the central part of the model be modified and labelled 'constraints' using Newell's description of the role and examining the possibilities of these as multiple, explanatory variables linking biology to behaviour. This label more accurately describes the many variables that act in this way.

In order to explain this modified model (Fig. 8.2), it is presented in a different order to the Morton original, enabling a final concentration on the intervening constraints.

- First, behavioural symptoms are described, which is a follow-on from the diagnostic criteria and the types of information that have been collected from a variety of sources. These are the symptoms that first give rise to concern and initial identification.

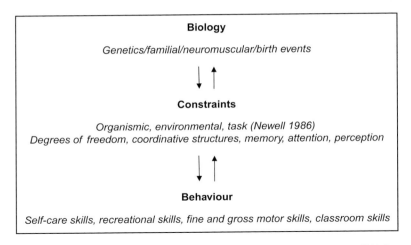

Fig. 8.2 Proposed causal modelling of developmental coordination disorder. Adapted from Morton (2004).

This level is no different to the Morton model from which it is taken.

- A second label is biology, and, although there are few studies that have made definitive contributions, there is a beginning of interesting work in this area with the advent of more sophisticated methods of examining both neurological processes (fMRI) and more genetic material being made available. Again this is no different to the Morton model.

- The third heading is labelled constraints and as noted above this is a change from the original model, which is labelled cognition. Constraints, like cognition in the Morton model, are the possible intervening variables between biology and behaviours.

- In the model in Figure 8.2 there is also a transactional effect of the variables involved, with a two-way influence between experience and biological variables being mediated by constraints.

In the earlier sections of the book there are a number of discussions concerning explanations of both motor learning and motor development. These have been drawn upon from two camps. First there is the long history of cognitive explanations of motor behaviour, as exemplified through information processing systems. Thus such topics as attention, various forms of memory, reaction time, and the formation of motor schemas are all fundamental to this train of thought (for a review see Schmidt and Lee 2005). Indeed, if this was the only explanation of motor development, the use of this to examine DCD under the heading of 'cognition' would be entirely appropriate as in the other developmental disorders. However, as has been detailed earlier in the text, this is not the only explanation and a second approach, which has been labelled a dynamical systems approach, is currently prominent. In this the main features are not cognitive, although these are included; the main characteristics are the multiple subsystems that cooperate dynamically to produce the end result within an ecological framework. These subsystems can be child resources or in the context of the environment or in the task itself. Even in the child itself, the subsystems are not seen as totally cognitive; rather, the whole neuromuscular system is viewed as a self-organized unit using such concepts as softly assembled degrees of freedom and coordinative structures (see pages 190–193 for details).

The dilemma becomes what to call the intermediate level of causation that Morton labels 'cognitive'. We have selected the word 'constraints' as the one that most accurately describes the modification of Morton's model, and it is used in a different way from the normal definition, which usually involves a restriction. Newell (1986) notes that in his model, and the way it has subsequently been used in the dynamical systems literature, constraints can permit, channel, encourage, or limit and discourage motor behaviour, and these constraints can be *organismic*, which includes both structural and functional, *environmental*, or *task*. This model is almost identical to the one used throughout the book and based on the work of Keogh and Sugden (1985), although they use the term transactional influences.

In Newell's model, organismic constraints first involve *structural constraints* that are time dependent and 'hard-wired' into the perceptual motor system, including such processes as speed of neural transmission. *Functional constraints* are more easily changed over a shorter period and may depend on children's experiences and learning. *Environmental constraints* involve the culture and child-rearing practices set in an ecological

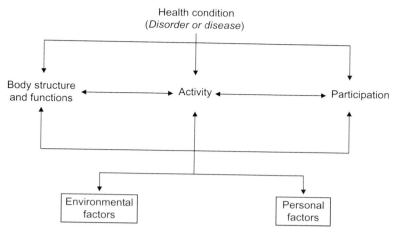

Fig. 8.3 The International Classification of Functioning, Disability and Health model. World Health Organization (2001).

context described earlier in the book (Bronfenbrenner 1979). *Task constraints* are due to the specific demands of the task and again are described in more detail earlier in the book (pages 193–194).This is included in our modification of Morton's model shown in Figure 8.2.

This manner of presenting the condition is very much in keeping with the International Classification of Functioning, Disability and Health (ICF) model of functioning, disability, and health reproduced from Chapter 7 (Fig. 7.1) and shown in Figure 8.3.

The ICF model clearly separates functioning and disability, with key areas being the interactive relationships between health conditions such as disorder or disease and the environmental context in which the activity takes place.

It could be argued correctly that the modified Morton model itself does not quite have distinct sections in that there is overlap between them. For example, the biological items could be seen as constraints and such concepts as memory are often seen as simply descriptions of behaviour at a different level. It is worth recognizing that the original Morton model could attract similar criticism. The fundamental issue is that this model offers a different and more structured manner in which to analyse the difficulties in a child with DCD and, probably more importantly, offers ways forward concerning priorities for not only assessment and intervention, but also avenues for theoretical explanations of the condition.

Motor behavioural characteristics of DCD

It is logical to start with the behavioural characteristics as these constitute the central core of any identification and diagnosis of children with DCD, and surround difficulties with motor skills that are evident when children with DCD

are compared with their peers on standardized tests, on criterion referenced checklists, and from observation in activities of daily living. These chronicle motor behaviours in the home, in the classroom, and in various forms of recreational activities. Very often our measurements are led by these tools with standardized tests examining abilities in such areas as balance, manual skills, agility, coordination, and ball skills.

Everyday descriptions attest to children with DCD having difficulties on a variety of motor tasks; these will include reports from parents reporting that the children were late in reaching the major motor milestones such as walking, jumping, and running, or in manipulation tasks such as picking up objects or pouring liquids without spilling. The difficulties occur in different contexts: in the classroom, on the playground, at home, and in recreational activities. The difficulties often stay with the children as they develop through childhood and through adolescence to emerging adulthood, and, although the symptoms change as they get older, the underlying difficulties with motor tasks present in everyday activities and expected of individuals at that stage of their development remain. In addition, a number of associated characteristics are often present (for reviews see Geuze 2007).

DIFFERENT PERSPECTIVES

Activities of daily living (Criterion B of DSM-IV; APA 2000) are seen as representative of behavioural characteristics in Morton's modified model, and there are differences not only in what activities different children have difficulties with but also, within the same child, what different individuals view as the difficulties. Children with DCD have difficulties with a wide range of activities of daily living, but children, parents, and teachers do not always select the same activities of daily living as representative of the difficulties the child is experiencing.

Dunford et al (2005) examined this and found that parent and teacher concerns were easily elicited by simply asking, 'What are your main concerns?'. However, children required something more concrete and structured such as the Perceived Efficacy and Goal Setting System (PEGS) (Missiuna et al 2004) in order to express their concerns. PEGS consists of 24 pictures organized in pairs, with one showing a competent child and the other showing one having difficulties. The child is asked to choose the picture they are most like. Using PEGS, children were much more likely to select difficulties in self-care such as dressing and leisure activities than parents and teachers. The children were motivated to be the same as their peers with comments such as 'because everyone else can'; they also perceived that their lack of competence in skills excluded them from playing with their peers with comments such as 'to join in with friends'. Some children wanted to be better at dressing so that they could get ready for school in the morning, whereas others were motivated by wanting to be quicker at changing for physical education. Parents often voiced quite general concerns about the children's motor skills or about the perceived impact this was having on schoolwork, specific activities, and/or school behaviour. In contrast to the children, they did not identify many self-care issues or leisure activities as concerns. Parents may not perceive leisure interests to be an appropriate focus for intervention, so the relationship between participation in physical activity and long-term health may need to be explained. Teachers seemed to raise general concerns about motor skills and, not surprisingly, focused on the impact that this was having on the child's school life. Handwriting issues were frequently raised and teachers often commented on discrepancies between the child's written work and other academic skills. Even when presented with numerous self-care and leisure interests to select, teachers focused consistently on printing, scissor use, and finishing schoolwork on time. From studies such as this it appears that gaining the views of children

is essential, as it ensures that self-care and leisure tasks are addressed as part of intervention.

DIFFERENT PROFILES

Not all children with DCD will show all of the characteristics and be impaired across all tasks. For example, some will show more problems with manual skills, whereas others will have more difficulties with agility and balance. Some attempts have been made, using standardized tests such as MABC (Henderson and Sugden 1992, Henderson et al 2007), to break down motor skills into component parts such as ball skills, manual skills, and balance. When tested on these, children with DCD do not always score low on each part, often showing uneven profiles. For example, Kirby et al (unpublished), in an analysis of over 150 children tested on MABC and all scoring in the lowest fifth centile, showed that varying profiles emerged: 56% of the children scored low in all three categories of balance, ball skills, and manual skills; 35% had problems in only two areas; and a minority group of 9% had scores in one category that were so low they tipped the overall score into the lowest fifth centile. This heterogeneity within the group of children with DCD is a finding that has strong all-round support, making the task of specifically locating the defining characteristics of the condition a difficult one. However, the central core is a motor difficulty and this motor difficulty shows a number of ways in which it can be expressed. One could make a simple analogy with a child exhibiting a language disorder that could be shown as one of expression, reception, or both. In Table 8.6 there are three examples of children all of whom would fit into Criterion A of DSM-IV (APA 2000), indicating significant impairment of movement, but with very different profiles.

In Example 1 the scores are evenly balanced and the child looks to be having difficulties in all areas. In Example 2 only two areas are of concern with balance being fine. In Example 3 the child again had two areas of concern with this time manual dexterity being fine. From the above examination of the profiles of children on any standardized test, there are clearly different profiles,

TABLE 8.6
Different profiles of children with DCD

	Movement ABC scores			
	Total	**Aiming and catching**	**Manual dexterity**	**Balance**
Example 1	45	12	18	15
Example 2	45	9	8	28
Example 3	45	6	28	11

Movement ABC, Movement Assessment Battery for Children.

which in turn will have implications for any intervention. The message is clear: it is not enough to diagnose DCD or even take an overall score from a standardized assessment instrument; the overall detailed profile of the child is required (see Chapter 12).

SUBGROUPS

A small number of studies have examined intragroup differences and similarities by looking for subgroups using factor and cluster analytic techniques and, as Visser (2007) notes, the results vary considerably. Much of the variance between these studies can be attributed to the measures used for selection of participants and the tests used in the analysis. Using cluster analysis on the results of six tests Hoare (1994) found five clusters of children:

- Cluster 1 with low scores in kinaesthetic acuity and running;
- Cluster 2 with poor scores of kinaesthetic acuity and balance;
- Cluster 3 with low scores overall but particularly on perceptual tasks;
- Cluster 4 with good kinaesthesis but poor visual scores, suggesting that there is not a generalized perceptual difficulty and it is much more specific; and
- Cluster 5 with good perceptual scores but poor motor execution.

Other researchers have continued in a similar manner with Macnab et al (2001) trying to replicate Hoare's study but with children who appeared to have more severe difficulties. There have been some minor differences between studies, but Macnab et al (2001) came close to replicating the clusters found by Hoare (1994). A slightly different approach was taken by Wright and Sugden (1996) who used the eight subcomponents of the MABC test within the balance, manual skills, and ball skills sections together with the four sections of the MABC checklist. In order to reduce the number of measures used in the cluster analysis, a factor analysis was first conducted, reducing these 12 measures to five factors which were fed into the cluster analysis. This revealed four clusters:

- Cluster 1 comprised children who were only moderately impaired and were so across all measures.
- Cluster 2 involved catching on its own.
- Cluster 3 consisted of children who were impaired overall with a specific deficit in those tasks that involved a moving environment.
- Cluster 4 contained those who were poor on the manual skill tests on the MABC test.

Other examples examining subtypes are from Miyahara (1994), Dewy and Kaplan (1994), and Lyytinen et al (1988), all providing slightly differing results. This should not be surprising for a number of reasons. First, compared with other domains, such as language disorders, the number of factor and cluster analytic studies in the motor domain on impaired children have been few. There has not been a consensus on what tests to feed into the factor and cluster studies with the result that a variety of tests have been employed. It is well known that the results of any factor analytic study are dependent on what variables are fed in with different tests providing different results. In addition, the selection of participants has differed across studies with a range of criteria employed and different percentage cut-off points. However, although these exercises have not brought a consensus on the specific subtypes, there have been some common findings (Visser 2007). There has been a factor of generalized impairment found in nearly all of the studies and, as Visser (2007) explains, this is logical as it can be a common feature no matter what tests are employed. This is an area where more definitive work can be obtained by adhering to the now internationally recognized criteria for participant selection and some commonly agreed tests.

'PURE' CASES OF DCD

A common feature of any group of children with DCD is heterogeneity and there have been examples in this chapter. This involves not simply the differences in the motor characteristics, as described earlier under Subgroups and Different profiles, but also refers to the co-occurrence of other characteristics, which was described earlier in this chapter and will appear later in Chapter 10. With respect to this latter point, it has already been stated that co-occurring characteristics are the rule rather than the exception. However, 'pure' cases of DCD do exist, with some children having a significant motor impairment that is their sole difficulty. Peters and Henderson (2008) employed a single-case study approach to examine the journey of children with DCD from identification through to assessment. Some of the results and cases are shown in Box 8.7.

Underlying biological substrates

A comment that is commonly made about DCD is that there are heterogeneous characteristics and this heterogeneity takes more than one form. Hadders-Algra (2003), when examining the evidence for a relationship between brain lesions at an early age and clumsiness, noted that heterogeneity in terminology has hampered research in this area, and it could be added that, even with the acceptance of the term DCD, there is still heterogeneity in

---

Box 8.7 A closer examination

The contribution of single-case studies: Peters and Henderson (2008)
The authors examined in detail six males and one female with DCD from a larger cohort of clinically referred children. One male is shown here as an example of a 'pure' case of DCD.

Participant A
This participant is a male aged 7 years who weighed 3.5kg at birth after a term Caesarean section. He achieved the major motor milestones but by 7 struggled with both fine and gross motor tasks. He looked awkward when running and jumping, could not ride a bicycle, and had problems with writing, drawing, scissors, and buttons and laces. He was fit and healthy but scored below the first centile on MABC. He was within the normal range on VMI (Beery 1967) and had no adverse signs in a clinical examination. He was also within the normal range on the British Picture Vocabulary Scale (Dunn et al 1997); on the Autistic Spectrum Screening Questionnaire (Ehlers et al 1999); and on the Strengths and Difficulties Questionnaire (Goodman 2001). He eventually did learn to ride a bike and enjoyed football despite not being skilled, but his handwriting was poor.

This child was fairly well adjusted, had friends, and played musical instruments. He did get upset at having poor motor skills but this was a consequence of a lack of coordination, not a co-occurring characteristic. The motor impairment did impact on his activities of daily living. The authors say of Participant A 'XX is one of the few children who could safely be described as a "pure" case of DCD' (p. 100).

---

behavioural characteristics, which make the link between lesions and motor difficulties problematic.

Our current knowledge about the direct relationship between brain and behaviour in DCD is not at an advanced stage. fMRI studies are beginning to be used for both clinical and research work and we have informal evidence for the continued presence of DCD in families, together with the start of more data-based gene studies (Piek 2006). This work also showed the possibility of a shared genetic structure with ADHD, and, when DCD and ADHD were comorbid, there was a joint heritability of 66%. Using a model that is based upon a gene–environment interaction, such as part of a dynamic system, gives a wider scope for at-risk factors. In ADHD studies, as in cerebral palsy studies (see Chapter 7), such variables as maternal smoking and lead exposure have been linked to the condition. In DCD there are few similar studies, but the AVON Longitudinal Study of Parents and Children (Hibberlin et al 2007) reports links between low seafood intake at 32 weeks' gestation and problems in motor coordination, pro-social behaviour, and communication.

It is pertinent to note that, when examining the possible underlying biological substrates, there is the tacit assumption that the influence is always one way. That is, any biological mechanism will have an effect through constraints to subsequent behaviour. However, as our modified Morton model on page 239 shows, this is not always the case. It is known that the neural system is relatively plastic and influence is not just one way, with environmental experiences having an effect on fundamental biological systems, as would be expected from any dynamic system.

MINIMAL BRAIN DAMAGE
The search for biological substrates in DCD has been one with a long history, and global terms such as MBD have been used as descriptors of children showing impaired movements as well as other difficulties. Relationships between actual brain damage in individuals with head injuries and clumsiness in movement have been reported for many years. In time this relationship was subtly reversed when children with clumsy movements showing no overt brain damage were labelled as MBD or MND. The label of MBD was very popular during the 1960s and 1970s and included children with a wide range of difficulties, some motor, others impaired attention, overactivity, and unexpected learning disabilities (Kavale and Forness 1995). It has not been commonly seen in recent years, but others such as ABD (Kaplan et al 1998) and MND (Hadders-Algra 2003) have become prominent.

The term MBD and others like it such as MND have long been associated with motor disorders and an interesting feature of this is that the search for neural damage is a paradoxical one because, if it is found, it would normally lead to a non-DCD diagnosis under the current DSM-IV criteria! Criterion C states that a diagnosis should not be given if the condition is due to a general medical condition. In the discussion earlier in the chapter on Criterion

C, it was noted that this was a difficult criterion to work with and, as imaging techniques improve, one that would probably need to be revised or at least modified.

If some form of MBD or MND was found it would be useful to determine whether the damage was prenatal, perinatal, or postnatal. Hadders-Algra (2003) proposes that there are two basic forms of MND: simple and complex. Simple MND is the most common in school-age children, has little clinical impact, involves a normal but 'non-optimally wired brain', and has its origins in genetics or a stressful early life (Hadders-Algra 2003, p. 46). Complex MND is more specific and perinatally acquired and shows more distinct and serious brain dysfunction, possibly due to lesions early in life. These are the children who Hadders-Algra (2003) proposes as having motor difficulties and possibly learning and attention problems.

Specific areas of the brain
A specific area of the brain that has been the subject of much discussion over the last few years is the cerebellum. Ivery (2003), when reviewing cerebellar involvement in developmental disorders including those in the motor domain, notes that evaluating causal brain–function relationships can be a tricky business, especially in developmental disorders, because neural abnormalities can be subtle. Through techniques such as magnetic resonance imaging (MRI) he concludes that there is some evidence to suggest that cerebellar abnormalities have been linked to autism, ADHD, and dyslexia but still suggests causal accounts are speculative for a number of reasons. First, it is not clear why a common neural abnormality should be related to very different developmental disorders. If it is, why, and what is the pathway? Second, a localized pathology would seem too simplistic, and, third, patients with cerebellar disorders do not often appear to develop symptoms similar to those seen in autism, ADHD, or dyslexia. However, he does caution against rejecting a cerebellar involvement, citing work on cerebellar influence in temporal tasks. When discussing children with DCD he recognizes that a relationship would seem reasonable as movement difficulties are symptoms of patients with cerebellar ataxia and also notes that there may be a subgroup of children with movement difficulties who have timing problems with a possible relationship to the cerebellum. There is an acceptance that this work is very much at an early stage, and, given the heterogeneous nature of the condition, there may be a multitude of neurological profiles.

Links between brain networks and cognitive functions associated with DCD have been reported with executive function, and its possible corresponding biological substrates were examined by Querne et al (2008). They list executive function to be those cognitive abilities that control and regulate behaviours such as planning and inhibiting actions and shifting from one action to another, with attentional functions and working memory also included. They use fMRI on a go–no-go task in which children are asked to perform rapid responses on frequent go trials and inhibit the response on infrequent no-go trials. Motor inhibition has been found to be associated with brain regions such as the anterior cingulated cortex (ACC), middle frontal cortex (MFC), orbitofrontal cortex, and inferior parietal cortex (IPC). Querne et al (2008) compared 8- to 13-year-old children with DCD with controls on this task and found that overall the children with DCD obtained similar inhibition scores to the typically developing children, but that the responses were slower and more variable and there were more errors of omission. The fMRI, using structural equation modelling, indicated that path coefficients from MFC and ACC to IPC increased in children with DCD, especially in the left hemisphere, and that some path coefficients in the right hemisphere decreased in children with DCD compared with typically developing children. The authors cautiously propose that children with DCD may be characterized by abnormal development of hemispheric specialization.

Very young children with neonatal encephalopathy have been examined to establish motor outcomes and the relation with patterns of lesions found from MRI scans. Mercuri and Barnett (2003) report on a number of infants examined by MRI between 1991 and 1996 who had neonatal encephalopathy and Apgar scores below 5 at 1 minute. All were prospectively followed up at 3, 6, 12, and 24 months and then yearly on a structured neurological examination. Between 5 years and 6 months and 6 years and 6 months they were examined on standardized tests of motor impairment. The results showed that the severity of the outcome depended to a large extent on the amount of basal ganglia lesions being associated with cerebral palsy, microcephaly, dystonic, or severe global delay. In addition, only one in seven children with basal ganglia lesions had completely normal motor outcomes. The overall percentage of children with minor motor abnormalities such as clumsiness was relatively low at around 15%, which is different to preterm-born children who had a very clear relationship between white matter lesions and clumsiness.

Overlapping biological substrates have been found in DCD and other disorders, showing that it is not just in the usual behavioural symptoms that co-occurring characteristics are present. Scabar et al (2006) note the frequent association between DCD and SLI and also the link between language impairment and epileptiform discharges during sleep, which resemble benign epilepsy with centrotemporal spikes (BECTS). They investigated this association in children with DCD, first by looking for the sleep discharges in the DCD children, and second by taking a group of children with BECTS and investigating the occurrence of DCD. Their investigations showed that over 70% of children with DCD also had nocturnal epileptiform discharges and, in a population of children with BECTS, 30% would have been identified as children with DCD. They use this information to promote another term denoting co-occurring characteristics – that of Hereditary Impairment of Brain Maturation – which is somewhat akin to ABD (Kaplan et al 1998) but different in that ABD does not refer to genetics.

The link between behaviours and biological underpinnings has a long history in many human facilities and it is not surprising that this relationship is being investigated in greater detail in DCD with the advance of sophisticated technology. fMRI studies such as the one by Querne et al (2008) are a possible route forward, but all of them are dependent on not simply the technology but also clarity in the definition and assessment of the condition, to ensure that both parts of the relationship are accurately delineated.

Constraints: perceptual, cognitive, and motor

The original model from Morton (2004) uses the term 'cognitive process' to explain how the biological substrates are mediated to produce the behavioural symptoms that are seen. This concept is extended here and labelled *constraints*, as the mediating influences from biology through to behaviours and vice versa, acknowledging that they involve more than simply cognitions. A study of these has both theoretical and practical implications. On a theoretical level, if the bidirectional level of these constraints can be understood, our knowledge of all forms of motor development, both typical and atypical, will be enhanced. From a practical viewpoint, identifying influential constraints will increase the chance of successful support and intervention.

The previous reviews of the behavioural signs of DCD, followed by what are speculative biological substrates underlying the condition, are enhanced through the intermediary constraints of perceptual, cognitive, and motor processes. Through the use of standardized tests, criterion-referenced measures, clinical reports, interviews with children, parents, and teachers, and observations, the motor skills of children showing difficulties have been well described. These constraints are described with an analysis of the differences in these components between children with DCD and typically developing children. The section has been divided into topic headings such that an understanding of the components can be easily accessed. However, it is pertinent to remember the holistic nature of motor tasks when performed in context.

A model of constraints that is used in Chapter 12 is extended and shown in Figure 8.4.

Sensory and Perceptual Factors

Among the subsystems that are proposed as making up motor performance, there is general agreement that

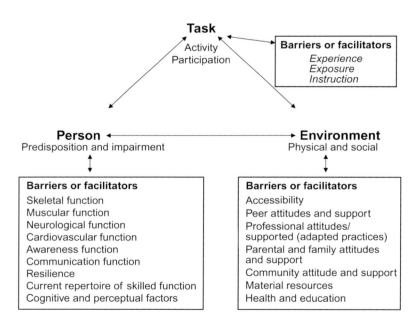

Fig. 8.4 Constraints interacting in movement skill production. Reproduced with permission of the publisher from Hultzer (2007).

perceptual processes would be a major one, with the obvious observation that information has to enter the system so that it can be used for motor output. It is another matter how the information enters, whether it is through indirect levels of processing or direct through a perception–action match. Most of the studies have invoked more a processing approach to perception rather than a direct perception–action linkage, but, as we have presented throughout the book, the situation has changed with respect to typical development, which has moved to an emphasis on direct perception and dynamic systems. This approach is now being seen in children who develop atypically. Among the perceptual processes that we possess, two stand out, with respect to motor performance, as being of primary importance: vision and kinaesthesis. We refer back to Chapter 6, which details some of the development of these two primary senses.

Vision

In the control of movement vision has many important roles and these are described in detail in Chapters 2 and 11. It specifies the environment in terms of space and time and thus has a huge effect on the final movement product. Visual information, in the form of the location of objects when stationary, is crucial to such skills as reaching and grasping; the location of moving objects, requiring prediction and anticipation, is also provided by vision and linked to the motor system so that actions can be made; ongoing visual information is used in the control of movements, allowing limbs to make ongoing corrections in response to information about the limbs and their positions given the environmental demands. Finally, vision is used to monitor and provide information about the end result of any movement, whether or not it has been successful, and how much correction, if any, is required for the next attempt at a particular task. It should be noted here that adequate vision on its own is not a sufficient condition for successful movement to occur; it has to be linked to action through perceptual–cognitive process such as anticipation, prediction, and memory.

Hulme and Lord showed that children with DCD had poorer visual perception than typically developing children in a series of studies involving line-length matching, size constancy judgements, and discrimination of shape, area, and slope. From these studies they proposed that poor visual perception was a contributory factor to the difficulties that children with DCD exhibited (Hulme et al 1982a,b, Lord and Hulme 1987, 1988). Although these results are persuasive, as Hill (2005) points out, it is difficult to give full support to them because of the complexity of processes occurring between sensory input and motor output, making exact location of any deficit problematic.

Schoemaker et al (2001) examined the relationship between visual perception and motor performance using the Developmental Test of Visual perception (Hammill et al 1993). In a population of children with DCD she found that less than 50% of the children had poor scores in visual motor skills and no significant correlations were found between visual perceptual ability and motor skills, as measured by the MABC test (Henderson and Sugden 1992).

The results from the individual studies on the role that vision plays in determining the exact nature of the problems faced by children with DCD is unclear. In some of the studies quoted above, vision has not been found to play a significant part. Yet, our knowledge of motor performance leads us to say that this has to be incorrect as vision is widely acknowledged to play a major role in the performing and learning of motor skills. In a meta-analysis of deficits associated with DCD, Wilson and McKenzie (1998) found the greatest deficiency was in visual–spatial processing.

More recent studies have begun to examine vision in a different way by analysing what it does for the mover in tasks in which such variables as prediction are involved. Wilmut and Wann (2008), working with children and young adults with DCD (6–23y of age) and age-matched controls, examined the ability to organize a movement in response to advance visual information. Participants were seated and required to make movements on a Plexiglas semi-opaque tabletop in response to types of pre-cue information. Both eye movements and hand latencies were measured. With no pre-cuing information the DCD group were as quick as the typically developing group in initial hand movements but were less efficient at modifying directional errors. However, when pre-cuing visual information was given, the typically developing group was better able to use this by refining their movements. This was only the case in the DCD group when there was no ambiguity in the cues, and this group had particular difficulties using predictive motion cues. They perseverated with a strategy of fixating the target before moving rather than employing the faster strategy of using the advanced information.

It may be that in individual studies the exact nature of sensory difficulties and the relationship to DCD has not been found. It also may be that in children with DCD who have different profiles the nature of the perceptual problems are different. Thus, it may point to the heterogeneity of DCD as a condition, with vision playing a minor role in some cases but a more major one in others. The studies of Wilmut and Wann (2008) and others (e.g. Mon-Williams et al 1999) that analyse the use of vision rather than simple variables such as acuity may move us in the right direction concerning any differences in children with DCD. Other studies using subgroup analysis and single-subject designs may also give us better insight into this.

Kinaesthesis
Earlier, in Chapter 2, we discussed some of the conundrums surrounding kinaesthesis and other sensory input. We are favouring a holistic approach to sensory input in which there is an integrated system with all senses working in collaboration. However, we also recognize that the majority of studies have not been conducted in this manner and thus we present here some traditional data on kinaesthesis followed by a more recent look at the area.

The sensory source that provides us with information about posture, location, force, speed of limbs in space, and the forces exerted by muscles is known as kinaesthesia. This information is provided by joint receptors, muscle spindles, tendon organs, and skin receptors and is used for the evaluation and planning of movements. Very often the term kinaesthesia is used interchangeably with the term proprioception, although the latter is often reserved as a wider term to include many sensory systems working together, such as vestibular mechanisms in the ear working in conjunction with vision to provide information about the position and movements of the body and its parts. In its purest form kinaesthesis is the ability to detect the movement of the body and its parts without the use of vision. However, very often kinaesthesis is used in conjunction with other senses, particularly vision, as part of an overall system that builds redundancy into our processing capacity (Hill 2005).

Again, like vision, it is accepted that kinaesthesis is a vital component in our ability to perform purposeful skilful movement, but, again like vision, the exact role it plays in distinguishing between skilful and unskilful performers is still unclear. Hill (2005) provides the example of ball catching to illustrate the part kinaesthesis has to play in an everyday recreational skill. She notes that the movement of the head and hands, often not in the field of vision, must be coordinated to the position of the ball in flight in order to make a successful catch. This is done via a link-up between vision, which specifies ball position, and kinaesthesis and effector processes, which are working together to place the hands in the correct position to catch the ball. Often this link-up will prove difficult for children with DCD and is a good reason why, when teaching ball skills, the skilful teacher will start by ensuring that the ball is thrown low enough to be in the same field of vision as the hands, so that vision and kinaesthesis are working together.

As kinaesthesis is accepted to be an integral part of skilled performance, efforts to isolate it in children

with problems seemed to be a promising start. Laszlo and Bairstow in the 1980s began a series of studies examining kinaesthesis first in typically developing children and then in children with difficulties (Laszlo and Bairstow 1985). They made the logical argument that, as kinaesthesis is known to be a factor in skilled performance, it may be deficient or impaired in children with DCD, and an improvement in this process may lead to an overall improvement in skilled performance. Using their Kinaesthetic Sensitivity Test, Laszlo and Bairstow (1985) tested two aspects of kinaesthesis, namely acuity and perception with memory. They provided normative data on typically developing children that showed steady improvement up to the age of 12 on these tasks, and they reported that children with DCD performed worse than typically developing children of the same age. Although a logical step, the study was not without its critics who pointed out that only a narrow band of kinaesthetic ability was being tested, which mainly consisted of passive movements, the scoring system may be inappropriate, and it did not always discriminate between skilled and unskilled performers (Lord and Hulme 1987, Sugden and Wann 1987, Elliott et al 1988).

Other methods of examining kinaesthetic processes in children with DCD were pursued in a series of studies by Smyth and Glencross using a reaction-time paradigm, which found that poor coordination was associated with impaired kinaesthetic skills but not visual ones (Smyth and Glencross 1986, Smyth 1994, 1996). Similarly, a number of cross-modal studies, matching vision and kinaesthesis, are pointing towards difficulties for children with DCD (Hulme et al 1982a, Lord and Hulme 1987, 1988).

There appears to be a paradox with kinaesthesis for, if we take a movement skill that we know involves kinaesthesis and try to examine its role, it is extremely difficult to isolate kinaesthesis from other processes that are ongoing and contributing to the final skilled product. When kinaesthesis is isolated for the purpose of study, it is at a stage where the skill is non-contextual and less meaningful, thus lessening its relationship to real life. This apparent paradox becomes solvable if kinaesthesis is viewed as just one part of the input process and is combined with vision, touch, and audition. This is the view we prefer and have described in Chapter 2.

Some lines of research have attempted to do this by examining how kinaesthesis and vision interact with each other and analysing how information taken in through one sense is transferred to another (Sigmundsson et al 1977, von Hofsten and Rösblad 1988, Smyth and Mason 1997, Sigmundsson 1999). The general conclusion is that when children with DCD are using kinaesthesis on its

Box 8.8 A closer examination

Visual–proprioceptive mapping in children with developmental coordination disorder: Mon-Williams et al (1999)

Aim

The aim of this study was to determine whether children with DCD have a specific difficulty with using vision in visual–proprioceptive mapping tasks and also to examine the effect that different conditions of task presentation have upon this facility.

Children

The study included 32 children selected by their teachers as having motor impairment. This was reduced to eight children after the administration of the MABC test and checklist. This experimental group was age-matched to three control groups of children with no movement skill problems, aged 5, 6 and 7 years, each group containing eight children.

Procedure

In the *first experiment*, the task involved the seated child matching the position of a point or their finger on a table placed in front of them. In the first condition, called visual proprioception to proprioception (VP:P), the child had to point with the unseen index finger of the dominant hand under the table to a position on the shield visible from above and also marked by the index finger of the child's non-dominant hand. In the second condition, known as vision to proprioception (V:P), the child had to point under the table to a visible target on top of the table without the assistance of the non-dominant hand, which was kept in the lap. In the third condition, called proprioception to proprioception (P:P), the child placed the non-dominant hand at a location above the table and pointed to the same location below the table with the dominant hand, but both hands had vision occluded by an opaque shield. Direct measurement of the child's ability to match limb position was taken through the use of electromagnetic position trackers, which were attached to the fingernail of the dominant hand and gave a three-dimensional positional location for the hand as it moved.

In *Experiment 2* trackers were placed on the wrist of each arm to track movement. Two conditions were employed. In the first the child could see the position of the dominant arm and had to match this with the unseen, non-dominant arm (VP2:P2); in the second both hands were unseen and the child had to match the limbs on the basis of only proprioceptive information (P2:P2).

Results of Experiment 1

The results showed no differences between the three age control groups, with children making errors between 8 and 15mm. The P:P condition produced more errors than the other two conditions, which showed no differences between them. When the typically developing children were compared with the children with DCD there was a significant difference between them and also showing an interaction effect for task. This interaction effect showed the children with DCD making equivalent errors in the VP:P and P:P conditions, but more errors on the V:P condition. The tracker showed the DCD group positioning the arm away from the body in the VP:P and V:P conditions, whereas the control groups had this bias in all three conditions. Both groups had a bias towards the contralateral side, with the DCD group showing high variability of position.

Results of Experiment 2

Again the results showed a clear effect of task, with the P2:P2 condition being consistently inferior to the VP2:P2 condition. Overall, again the children with DCD made significantly more errors than the typically developing children. Children with DCD tended to position the dominant arm above and further away from the body in the VP2:P2 condition but not in the P2:P2 condition, whereas for the control groups this occurred in both conditions.

Conclusion

In both experiments children with DCD produced more errors than their age-matched peers in both spatial- and limb-matching tasks, which was to be expected, but they specifically performed more poorly by not taking advantage of having sight of the spatial location of one arm in the V:P condition. This condition is unique in that it forces cross-modal matching, which is not necessary in either the VP:P or P:P conditions, leading to the conclusion that it may not simply be the case that a deficit in either visual perception or kinaesthesis is a possible contributory factor to poor motor performance in children with DCD. The likelihood is that it is more complex than this, with an interweaving of visual and kinaesthetic cross-modal matching, which is constantly being demanded in activities of daily living, being a possibility.

own without vision, there is a decrement in performance when compared with typically developing children. A closer examination into some of these factors is found in Box 8.8, which describes a study by Mon-Williams et al (1999).

From research evidence and clinical experience it is clear that perceptual variables in the form of visual and kinaesthetic processing are crucial to the skilled performance of motor skills with the logical progression that any deficit would be a contributing factor to the low skill seen in children with DCD. However, what is not clear is the exact nature of this contribution and there is a need for research that takes daily tasks in realistic, meaningful environments to more clearly identify the relative contributions of vision and kinaesthesis. This work would directly affect the types of interventions that we would be confident in providing.

COGNITIVE FACTORS

Cognitive factors is a loose term that is often used to describe the process of taking in information by the sensory system, through to the effector system, and producing the end movement. Variables that have been examined include attentional processes; use of prediction; speed of decision through reaction time; efficiency of memory; and response preparation and selection. Many of these are found to be overlapping and in some studies more than one variable is studied. Using motor behaviour as problem solving is also seen as a cognitive process.

The study of motor behaviour has a long and distinguished history in examining cognitive variables such as memory and attention (for reviews see Schmidt and Lee 2005, Magill 2007). Attention and memory processes are crucial for the planning of any movement. Attention involves the process of selecting out relevant information from both the environment and the child's intrinsic systems such as proprioception. Similarly, memory can involve memory of the environmental layout or context and motor memory of efferent action. This motor memory has had several candidates as the unit of analysis over the years, but the evidence points more to general and larger units such as synergies/coordinative structures than the micro ones of individual muscles or motor units. In typically developing children in memory for movements improves greatly in the 6- to 12-year-old age range, and various researchers have found differences between children with DCD and typically developing children on both attention and memory variables (Chapter 3; Keogh and Sugden 1985, Dwyer and McKenzie 1994, Skorji and McKenzie 1997).

Reaction time

If a simple ability is examined, such as the time taken to respond to various stimuli (often used as a cognitive factor), the general finding is that, as a group, children with DCD take longer to respond than typically developing children. Van Dellen and Geuze (1988) proposed that slowness in children with DCD was a consequence of cognitive decisions in response selection. The children in their study were slower to respond, but their movements were just as accurate as those of typically developing children. It does appear that, as the task becomes more complex or more demanding, children with DCD fall differentially behind their typically developing peers (van Dellen and Geuze 1988, Vaessen and Kalverboer 1990). The Vaessen and Kalverboer (1990) study is interesting as it used a dual-task paradigm, with children responding to reaction-time stimuli as they were walking on a balance beam. They varied the motor component, that is, the balance beam, and the cognitive loading by making the reaction task more difficult, and they found that it was the cognitive loading that caused the decrement in performance.

An examination of both reaction time and movement time in children with DCD was conducted by Henderson et al (1992), who found that children with DCD were slower to react to both simple and complex reaction-time tasks than their typically developing peers, and their movement times were also slower when the targets were small. The task involved a simple reaction time but also a second with an aiming component that effectively transformed the reaction-time task into a coincidence-timing task. Thus the children had to pay due attention to the timing of the task with respect to an external signal and not just the speed of their own reactions. The study comprised 12 children with DCD aged between 7 and 11 years who were matched with similar-aged peers. Overall the results show children with DCD to be slower in reacting and moving in a simple aiming task and to have higher absolute errors in a coincidence-timing task, with the most sensitive discrimination variable being the movement time to a small target.

These studies together with others, such as that on vision and proprioception by Mon-Williams et al (1999), illustrate some of the complexities in teasing out the underlying cognitive variables that may contribute to the motor problems those children with DCD show. Hill (2005) concludes her summary of speed issues in DCD by suggesting that they are a central deficit in the planning and control of action and may be an explanation as to why children with DCD are typically slower and have difficulties with everyday tasks such as drawing and handwriting.

Closely related to speed of processing is keeping time to some external driver, as it demonstrates the ability to align internal timing mechanisms to map on to the demands of a task that has temporal requirements. A tapping task, in which the child has to tap in time to some external audible tone, is often used as an indicator of timing ability. The length of time between consecutive taps is measured and the variability in this length of time is a measure often used in analysis. Williams et al (1992) used this type of task by requiring the children to tap to a tone and then continue after the tone was stopped. The results showed the children with DCD to be more variable than controls and the timing variability deficit was explained more by a central timing mechanism problem than by any delay in executing the motor response.

How information is used to aid movement preparation and execution is a crucial part of the action process. For example, movements are often made in response to environmental demands; occasionally these demands require fast actions and any information that can be obtained in advance is advantageous to the mover if it is utilized appropriately. Wilmut and Wann (2008) looked at the ability of children with DCD to organize movements in response to advance information. Working with typically developing individuals and individuals with DCD (both groups aged 6–23y), they presented pre-cuing information on a task involving fast hand movement. When no pre-cues were present the individuals with DCD were as fast on initial hand movements as the typically developing group even though they were less efficient in correcting directional errors. However, when pre-cuing was introduced, the group with DCD could only use the information if there was no ambiguity and they often continued to stay with strategies that were slower and less efficient. This study again illustrates the impaired flexibility of action responses and associated strategies in individuals with DCD, with such characteristics having an influence on their performance of skills in everyday life.

Internal modelling and imagery
More recent analysis of cognitive variables offers different and promising lines of investigation. In a number of articles, Wilson and colleagues' examination of imagery in children with DCD has resulted in an internal modelling deficit hypothesis, which proposes that children with DCD have an impaired ability to represent action (Wilson et al 2001, 2004, Williams et al 2006). The experimental paradigm that they use is one that involves mental rotation of an object such as a hand, numbers, or letters, or the whole body, and the child having to make a decision as quickly as possible about its orientation with different forms of instructions and support. These careful studies indicate

that children with DCD may have impaired ability in using imagery and an inability to utilize internal models of motor control accurately. Williams et al (2006) provided partial support for an internal modelling hypothesis but are cautious, noting that the heterogeneous nature of DCD makes it unlikely that this inability is the sole explanatory, psychological cause of the condition. However, the Wilson group is offering novel and interesting ways of looking at DCD, rather than staying with more traditional methods. It does appear to hold promise for an explanation of some of the difficulties that children with DCD evidence and it also may give lines to pursue for intervention.

It is clear that both perceptual and cognitive variables make a substantial contribution to the impaired coordination we see in children with DCD. This is logical because of the great bodies of literature that have shown cognitive variables to be a determining factor in motor performance of children and adults who exhibit typical performance.

MOTOR CONSTRAINTS
All definitions of DCD include motor ability as the core characteristic of the condition and the overt everyday behaviours have been identified and measured many times and in different ways. When these behaviours are broken down into their component parts, we can see more clearly some of the motor constraints that typify the condition.

Balance
Balance is an ability chosen as an example of a motor constraint because, first, it is such a fundamental ability upon which other actions are dependent and, second, it is a human activity that is not only highly dependent on the two perceptual factors of vision and kinaesthesis but is used in many tests of motor impairment such as MABC (Henderson et al 2007). Thus poor balance has become one of the defining features of children with DCD. A number of researchers have found that children with DCD tend to rely on vision more than their age-matched counterparts and this would fit well with findings from younger typically developing children who exhibit similar characteristics (Wann et al 1998, Geuze 2003). For example, in a simple task of walking in the light or dark to a light emitting device, children with DCD walked more slowly and swayed more during the dark condition than their typically developing peers (Deconick et al 2006).

Tsai et al (2008) studied balance in children with DCD and those who were typically developing by analysing data from large groups of children (64 DCD, 71 typically developing) and in a narrow age band (ages 9–10y) when balancing ability is reasonably stable. They noted the heterogeneity of children with DCD and tried to reduce this by including those children with DCD who had specific balance difficulties. They measured static balance on both legs with eyes open and shut using analysis of sway as the dependent measure. When standing on the dominant leg children with DCD showed greater total path length in all conditions and a greater sway area when they had their eyes closed. On the non-dominant leg the finding was that children with DCD had poorer performance than typically developing children in all conditions.

A comprehensive analysis was taken by Geuze (2005) who reviewed balance problems in children with DCD and concluded that under normal static circumstances balance in these children was not usually a problem. However, when novel balance activities were introduced or the children had to regain control after losing balance they showed poor corrective strategies.

The work on balance in children with DCD is quite extensive, mainly because it is used in most tests of motor impairment. However, the situation is complex because of a number of factors associated with both the child with DCD and the test that is being administered. For example, the well-reported heterogeneity in children with DCD means that a child could be diagnosed despite not having a difficulty with balance if the child displays poor fine motor and ball skills. The tasks that are used to measure balance also vary considerably from static to dynamic, through eyes open or shut, to measures that simply involve time in or out of balance, through to more sophisticated motion analysis measures. The Geuze (2005) conclusion that children with DCD in many circumstances have satisfactory balance is interesting. It may be that when children with DCD are presented with a straightforward balance task with which they are familiar, and with plenty of time to organize themselves they have few problems. However, when asked to perform novel balance activities, or respond quickly to out of balance situations, they cannot spontaneously recruit synergies or coordinative structures that enable them to deal with this novel situation. They may be poor at flexibly dealing with new situations.

Different paradigms that potentially lead to the concept of embodied cognition as described in Chapter 1 were utilized in two studies by Chen et al (2011a,b). Both studies involved a suprapostural task to be performed, visual and cognition, while being engaged in a postural balance task. In both cases the children with DCD swayed more than the typically developing children when they were performing the suprapostural cognitive task. In the 2011a study, the results from typically developing children mirrored previous results, with adults showing, during the performance of a suprapostural task such as tracking or detecting size variations in visual patterns, a reduction in postural activity. In children with DCD this was the

opposite, and the 2011b study using a digital memory task again showed that, when a difficult suprapostural task was involved, children with DCD swayed more than their typically developing counterparts.

Differences from a dynamical theory perspective
Explanations of the differences between children with DCD and typically developing children from both theoretical and practical perspectives have concentrated largely on the processing arena primarily because this has been the major experimental paradigm over the last 30 or 40 years or so. However, as we have noted in earlier chapters, dynamical systems theory and an ecological view of perception (that it is direct) have become relatively mainstream in their application to a better understanding of the motor development of both typically and atypically developing children. This work emphasizes the coupling of perception and action within the child and the coupling of the child to the context in which they perform these actions. We argue that studying perception independent of perception–action coupling in children with DCD may be a reason why some studies have not detected the differences that may exist in the motor abilities between children with DCD and typically developing children. This failure to detect the hypothesized differences may be due to testing such attributes in isolation, which lacks ecological validity. They note that information in the form of metric units, as typically employed in information processing studies, is not appropriate for determining sensitivity to the environmental array. They provide examples of how activities such as stair climbing and crossing the road are related not to absolute metrics but to performer- or body-scaled ratios.

A series of studies (Johnson and Wade 2009, Chen et al 2011a,b) examined first how children with DCD compared with typically developing children at adjusting judgements of their maximum capabilities in response to actual capabilities, and second, differences between the two groups of children when recording changes in postural motion while engaged in suprapostural tasks requiring perceptual and cognitive effort. These studies are shown in Box 8.9.

Taken together these studies challenge standard processing accounts of the performance differences, especially with respect to issues regarding hypothesized 'executive control' differences. The data from the studies described in the box suggest that the locus of the motor differences resides in the strength of the link between perception and action or cognition and action. Clearly the biomechanics of the postural system influence both perceptual and cognitive performance in an 'embodied' context. Wade et al (2005) note that studying visual

Box 8.9 A closer examination

Perception–action coupling in children with DCD: Johnson and Wade (2008) and Chen et al (2011a,b)
In the Johnson and Wade (2008) study the task required participants to judge a horizontal reach in which the children had to bend at the hip to reach out to a ball on a pedestal. Before they actually reached, they had to estimate the maximum distance that the ball could be away from them in order for it to be reached under a number of experimental conditions. There were three experimental conditions that were varied involving the hands (one or both); feet on blocks of varying length; and the support surface in being rigid or compliant (concrete or high-density foam). The standard condition was a one-handed reach with a standard foot-length block on a rigid floor, and the measures used were judged horizontal reach maximum versus actual horizontal reach maximum. Under all three experimental conditions children's actual horizontal reach maximum was reduced. In these altered conditions, children with DCD made smaller or incorrect alterations to the altered conditions in their estimations. The interactions of group by condition are shown in Figures 8.5, 8.6 and 8.7.

   The conclusions were that children with DCD appeared less adept at detecting when their action capabilities were altered, and they appeared to have learned more conservative strategies. They appeared to use fewer

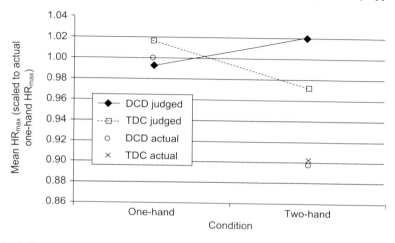

Fig. 8.5 Hand manipulation: group × condition interaction. Reproduced with permission of the publisher from Johnson and Wade (2009).

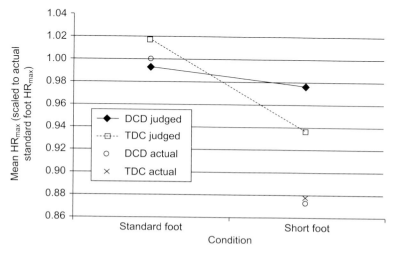

Fig. 8.6 Foot manipulation: group × condition interaction. Reproduced with permission of the publisher from Johnson and Wade (2009).

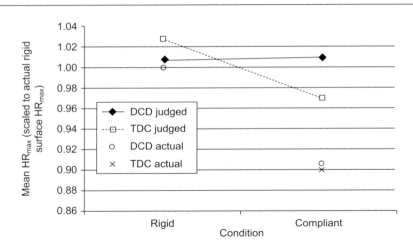

Fig. 8.7 Support surface manipulation: group × condition interaction. Reproduced with permission of the publisher from Johnson and Wade (2009).

exploratory movements, leading to difficulty in detecting their own capabilities. It is as though they did not appear to know their own capabilities.

The Chen et al (2011a,b) studies recorded postural motion during a suprapostural task protocol. In the 2011a study the task was a visual–perceptual one requiring participants to determine a difference in two vertical lines (same or different) present in sharp- and faded-image form.

The central hypothesis for this study was that changes in perceptual demand and subjective workload of the suprapostural visual task would differentiate the two groups of children (DCD vs typically developing). The results show that overall positional variability was greater in the DCD group than the typically developing group.

The typically developing children reduced their postural motion in the high-difficulty condition compared with the low-difficulty condition. The children with DCD did not record such a reduction.

This suggests that children diagnosed with DCD have a diminished perception–action coupling in situations where perceptual task demand is high, thus reducing functional integration of postural activity with suprapostural task demand.

In the second study (Chen et al 2011b) a similar protocol was employed but using a cognitive memory task as opposed to a visual–perceptual task. The task was a digit memory recall (maximum number of digits correctly retained over a 10s span). The maximum was the high-difficulty condition, and 50% of the maximum was the low-difficulty condition. Again the central finding was reduction in postural motion for both groups when compared across task difficulty. The reduction between low- and high-difficulty conditions was significant for the typically developing group but not for the DCD group.

The group by task difficulty was significant for both head and torso motion in the medial–lateral direction.

It would seem that the ability to modulate posture when engaged in a suprapostural task requiring an increase in either visual (Chen et al 2011a) or cognitive effort (Chen et al 2011b) produces a diminished response in children with DCD compared with their typically developing peers.

perception on its own in children with DCD may be a mistake and may explain why some studies have not found a difference between children with DCD and typically developing children. The reason could be that testing such attributes in isolation is far removed from an ecologically valid task set in context involving visual perception. They note that information in the form of metric units, the measure used in information processing studies, is not appropriate for measuring sensitivity to the environmental array. They provide examples of how activities such as stair climbing and crossing the road are related not to absolute metrics but performer- or body-scaled ratios.

In a related theoretical vein invoking a perception–action paradigm, but using a different experimental setup, Whitall et al (2006) looked at auditory motor coupling in children with DCD. They noted that research on perception–action coupling had mainly concentrated on vision as the sensory system with the conclusion that children with DCD are generally poorer in auditory motor coupling than typically developing children, being more variable and slower. However, little had been done with audition. Whitall et al (2006) used a task involving clapping while walking in place in response to an auditory signal. They chose to use this dual task as it involves 'interference' in a classic information processing paradigm, but in dynamical systems this is reconceptualized as 'self-organization'. This coupling had been confirmed in previous studies with adults and young children able to combine the two actions of clapping and walking with different patterns of coordination (Getchell and Whitall 2003). When examining this phenomenon in children with DCD, Whitall et al (2006) compared them with age-matched peers and an adult group and found both developmental differences and differences related to DCD.

In absolute deviation of relative phasing, that is how closely individuals timed their foot strike or clap to a metronome beat, there were differences between the adults and the two groups of children but not between children with DCD and those with typical development. When variability of relative phasing was examined, that is the tightness of the metronome and clap or step within trials, there was a difference between the DCD group and the other two groups with the DCD group coupling less stably. In addition, adults and the typically developing group adopted absolute four-limb coupling patterns, which in the DCD group were absent. Unstable auditory motor coupling mechanisms in children with DCD are an explanation that would fit nicely within a dynamical systems framework, and also there is the possibility that even without auditory cueing children with DCD may lack control of segmental interactions of the four limbs.

The work examining dynamical explanations of some of the difficulties that are experienced by children with DCD is in its infancy and yet does show promise. Its advantages over other explanations include the more complete and total picture that it promises. It does not simply concentrate on the sensory input or the difficulties that may lie therein, or on the cognitive explanations and such concepts as motor programmes or schemas to give insight into motor behaviour. Indeed, it takes all of these and treats them as constraints in a system that is self-organized, with multiple components that are integral parts in any action and with these constraints being at various levels within the child–task–environment transaction. These advantages are similar to the ones that are proposed for dynamical explanations of any individual whether adult or in childhood, including those children

diagnosed with DCD. The disadvantages are that to date we have very few studies utilizing paradigms that provide empirical support for this. However, we are minded by the fact that evidence for positions comes from three different arenas: theoretical, empirical, and experiential (Sugden and Dunford 2007). The theoretical position, we believe, is strong, and the empirical support is also becoming strong in adults and even in typically developing children. Our position is that, if it is strong in these two populations, it is not parsimonious or sensible to look for alternative explanations in children with DCD.

Participation and activities

In Chapter 9, on cerebral palsy, participation was examined from a number of different angles, and in children with DCD the same variables apply when looking at their participation in leisure and recreational activities. It is about choice, opportunity, satisfaction, ease of access, and suitability. Their poorer motor skills are a factor in these, but the environmental context is a much bigger factor than their personal resources.

Magalhaes et al (2011) note that most literature in this area focuses on motor skill functions not participation, with a concentration on handwriting, dressing and self-care, ball skills, and sport. Few deal with family lifestyles, neighbourhood support, and community involvement, with those that do showing increased participation. Even at a young age there is evidence to show that children with DCD participate less than their peers and they are less independent and have lower levels of enjoyment. However, when they do participate, the diversity of activities and intensity is similar in both groups (Bart et al 2011). Similar results were found in a longitudinal study by Green et al (2011) in which children with DCD had less frequent participation and were more isolated, but when they were engaged enjoyment levels were similar.

The message from these and other studies on participation is clear: the motor impairments that children with DCD show are not the cause of their diminished access to and participation in leisure and recreation activities. It has much more to do with the other two parts of our consistent theme throughout this text, namely the task and the environment. This is why, in our chapter on assessment and intervention (Chapter 12), we stress that to improve the lives and skills of children with DCD, increased participation has to be a factor in tandem with improved learning.

Summary

Over the last 30 years there has been a huge interest in children who are now given the label DCD. From relatively narrow beginnings there is now detailed literature on all aspects of the condition, from definitions and characteristics with explanatory variables through to assessment and diagnosis leading to intervention approaches.

With the advent of the DSM-III (APA 1987) and IV (APA 1994) and with the forthcoming DSM-V in 2013 there has been a much better definition and diagnosis of the condition. This work has been supplemented and aided by ICD 10 (1992). Work on prevalence of the condition has been helped by a tightening of the criteria such that 2% to 4% seems to be a reasonable figure to propose. It is hoped that this will result in research studies that enable us to make comparisons across countries. However, to do this effectively there is a need for increased rigour in the assessment process with suitable instruments that directly address the criteria.

Some strides have been made in the area of examining underlying causation with the work on biological underpinnings, but this is very much in its infancy. Work on perceptual and cognitive strategies is much more advanced and there is a reasonably consistent picture emerging, albeit with the qualifier that the population is heterogeneous in nature. Paradoxically, where the research appears to be lacking is in the underlying motor variables that affect performance. This is a developmental disorder that has at its core a motor deficit both in the definition and in the behavioural characteristics, yet cognitive variables have been studied far more often as explanatory variables. The work from the stable of dynamical systems provides us with great opportunities to remedy this and go to the heart of the difficulties.

At the core of DCD is a motor disorder and an impairment of everyday movement tasks, both of which are fundamental to the definition. There are co-occurring characteristics in most children with DCD, but they are not the primary defining characteristics (DSM-IV; ICD-10). At the recent World DCD Conference in Lausanne (IX), Newell, a leading figure in motor learning, control, and development but not DCD, pinpointed areas of research that appeared to need boosting within the area of DCD. The surprising one he noted was the area of 'coordination', which is in the title of the disorder. He then outlined areas of coordination that would appear to be ripe for study in this group of children. If the area of coordination is examined in more detail, then learning can be better facilitated, and couple this with modes of improving participation and the end result may be an improved overall lifestyle of children with DCD.

REFERENCES

Albaret J-M, de Castelnau P (2007) Diagnostic procedures for developmental coordination. In: Geuze RH, editor. *Developmental Coordination Disorder: A Review of Current Approaches*. Marseille: Solal, pp. 27–82.

APA (1987) *Diagnostic and Statistical Manual of Mental Disorders: DSM III*, 3rd edition. Washington, DC: American Psychiatric Association.

APA (1994) *Diagnostic and Statistical Manual of Mental Disorders: DSM IV*, 4th edition. Washington, DC: American Psychiatric Association.

APA (2000) *Diagnostic and Statistical Manual of Mental Disorders: DSM IV*, 4th edition text revision. Arlington, VA: American Psychiatric Association.

Barnett A (2008) Motor assessment in developmental coordination disorder: from identification to assessment. In: Sugden DA, Kirby A, Dunford C, editors. Special issue of *International Journal of Disability Development and Education: Children with Developmental Coordination Disorder* 55: 113–129.

Barnett A, Henderson SE, Scheib B, Schultz J (2007) *Detailed Assessment of Speed of Handwriting*. London: Pearson Assessment.

Baron-Cohen S (2007) Theories of the autistic mind. *The Psychologist* 21: 112–116.

Barsch RH (1965) *Achieving Perceptual Motor Efficiency*. Seattle, WA: Special Child Publications.

Bart O, Jarus T, Erez Y, Rosenbergh L (2011) How do young children with DCD participate and enjoy daily activities? *Res Dev Disabil* 32: 1317–1322. http://dx.doi.org/10.1016/j.ridd.2011.01.039

Bayley N (1993) *Bayley Scales of Infant Development*, 2nd edition. San Antonio, TX: Therapy Skill Builders.

Beery KE (1967) *The Developmental Test of Visual-Motor Integration*. Chicago, IL: Follett.

Bishop DVM (2007) Curing dyslexia and attention deficit hyperactivity disorder by training motor coordination: miracle or myth? *J Paediatr Child Health* 43: 653–655. http://dx.doi.org/10.1111/j.1440-1754.2007.01225.x

Blank R, Smits-Englesman B, Polatajko H, Wilson P (2012) European Academy for Childhood Disability (EACD): recommendations on the definition, diagnosis and intervention of Developmental Coordination Disorder (long version). *Dev Med Child Neurol* 54: 54–93. http://dx.doi.org/10.1111/j.1469-8749.2011.04171.x

Briggs D (1970) The influence of handwriting on assessment. *Educ Res* 13: 50–55. http://dx.doi.org/10.1080/0013188700130107

Bronfenbrenner U (1979) *The Ecology of Human Development*. Cambridge, MA: Harvard University Press.

Cantell MH, Smyth MM, Ahonen TP (1994) Clumsiness in adolescence: educational, motor and social outcomes of motor delay detected at 5 years. *Adapted Physical Activity Quarterly* 13: 61–73.

Cantell MH, Smyth MM, Ahonen TP (2003) Two distinct pathways for developmental coordination disorder: persistence and resolution. *Human Movement Sci* 22: 413–431. http://dx.doi.org/10.1016/j.humov.2003.09.002

Cermak SA, Larkin DA (2002) *Developmental Coordination Disorder*. Albany, NY: Delmar Thompson Learning.

Chambers ME, Sugden DA (2002) The identification and assessment of young children with movement difficulties. *Int J Early Years Educ* 10: 157–175. http://dx.doi.org/10.1080/0966976022000044717

Chambers ME, Sugden DA (2006) *Coordination Disorders in the Early Years*. London: Whurr.

Chen F-C, Tsai C-L, Stoffregen TA, Wade MG (2011a) Postural responses to a suprapostural visual task among children with and without developmental coordination disorder. *Res Dev Disabil* 32: 1948–1956. http://dx.doi.org/10.1016/j.ridd.2011.03.027

Chen F-C, Tsai C-L, Stoffregen TA, Chang C-H, Wade MG (2011b) Postural adaptations to a suprapostural memory task among children with and without developmental coordination disorder. *Dev Med Child Neurol* 54: 155–159.

Cousins M, Smyth MM (2003) Developmental coordination impairments in adulthood. *Human Movement Sci* 22: 433–459.

Cousins M, Smyth M (2005) Progression and development in developmental coordination disorder. In: Sugden DA, Chambers ME editors. *Children with Developmental Coordination Disorder*. London: Whurr, pp. 119–134.

Cratty BJ (1969) *Perceptual and Motor Development of Infants and Children*. New York: Macmillan.

Cratty BJ (1975a) *Remedial Motor Activity for Children*. Philadelphia, PA: Lea and Febiger.

Cratty BJ (1975b) *Physical Expressions of Intelligence*. Englewood Cliffs, NJ: Prentice Hall.

Cratty BJ (1994) *Clumsy Child Syndromes: Descriptions, Evaluation and Remediation*. Chur, Switzerland: Harwood Academic.

Dare MT, Gordon N (1970) Clumsy children: a disorder of perception and motor organisation. *Dev Med Child Neurol* 12: 178–185. http://dx.doi.org/101111/j1469-87491970tb01886x

Darrah J, Redfern L, Maguire TO, Beauln MJ, Watt J (1998) Intra-individual stability of rate of gross motor development in full term infants. *Early Human Dev* 52: 169–179. http://dx.doi.org/10.1016/S0378-3782(98)00028-0

Darrah J, Hodge M, Magill-Evans J, Kembhavi G (2003) Stability of serial assessments of motor and communication abilities in typically developing infants – implications for screening. *Early Human Dev* 72: 97–110. http://dx.doi.org/10.1016/S0378-3782(03)00027-6

Deconinck FJA, De Clercq D, Savelsbergh GJP, Van Coster R, Oostra A, Dewitte G, Lenoir M (2006) Visual contribution to walking in children with DCD. *Child Care Health Dev* 32: 711–722. http://dx.doi.org/10.1111/j.1365-2214.2006.00685.x

Delacato CH (1966) *Neurological Organization and Reading*. Springfield, IL: Charles C Thomas.

van Dellen T, Geuze RH (1988) Motor response processing in clumsy children. *J Child Psychol Psychiatry* 29: 489–500. http://dx.doi.org/10.1111/j.1469-76101988tb00739x

Denkla MB (1974) Development of motor coordination in normal children. *Dev Med Child Neurol* 16: 729–741. http://dx.doi.org/10.1111/j.1469-8749.1974.tb03393.x

Dewey D (1995) What is developmental dyspraxia? *Brain Cogn* 29: 254–274. http://dx.doi.org/10.1006/brcg.1995.1281

Dewey D, Kaplan BJ (1994) Subtyping and developmental motor deficits. *Dev Neuropsychol* 10: 265–285. http://dx.doi.org/10.1080/87565649409540583

Dewey D, Tupper D, editors (2004) *Developmental Motor Disorders: A Neuropsychological Perspective*. New York: Guilford.

Dunford C, Missiuna C, Street E, Sibert J (2005) Children's perceptions of the impact of developmental coordination disorder on activities of daily living. *Br J Occup Ther* 68: 207–214.

Dunn LIM, Dunn LMM, Whetton J, Burley J (1997) *British Picture Vocabulary Scales*, 2nd edition. Windsor: NFER-Nelson.

Dwyer C, McKenzie BE (1994) Impairment of visual memory in children who are clumsy. *Adapted Physical Activity Quarterly* 11: 179–189.

Ehlers S, Gillberg C, Wing L (1999) A screening questionnaire for Asperger Syndrome and other high functioning Autism Spectrum Disorders in school age children. *J Autism Dev Disord* 29: 129–141. http://dx.doi.org/10.1023/A:1023040610384

Elliot CD (1979) *British Ability Scales*. Windsor: NFER-Nelson.

Elliott JM, Connolly KJ, Doyle AJR (1988) Development of kinaesthetic sensitivity and motor performance in children. *Dev Med Child Neurol* 30: 80–92. http://dx.doi.org/10.1111/j1469-8749.1988.tb04728.x

Fawcett AJ, Nicolson RI (1995) Persistent deficits in motor skill acquisition of children with dyslexia. *J Motor Behav* 27: 235–240. http://dx.doi.org/10.1080/00222895.1995.9941713

Folio MR, Fewell RR (1983) *Peabody Developmental Motor Scales*. Allen, TX: DLM Teaching.

Frankenburg WF, Dodds J, Archer P, Shapiro H, Bresnick B (1992) The Denver II: a major revision and restandardization of the Denver Developmental Screening Test. *Pediatrics* 89: 91–97.

Gabbard C (2011) *Lifelong Motor Development*. San Francisco, CA: Benjamin Cummins.

Getchell N, Whitall J (2003) How do children coordinate simultaneous upper and lower extremity tasks? The development of dual motor task coordination. *J Exp Child Psychol* 85: 120–140. http://dx.doi.org/10.1016/S0022-0965(03)00059-6

Getman GN (1963) *The Physiology of Readiness Experiment*. Minneapolis, MN: PASS.

Geuze RH (2003) Static balance problems in children with developmental coordination disorder. *Human Movement Sci* 22: 527–548. http://dx.doi.org/10.1016/j.humov.2003.09.008

Geuze RH (2005) Motor impairment in DCD and activities of daily living. In: Sugden DA, Chambers ME, editors. *Children with Developmental Coordination Disorder*. London: Whurr, pp. 19–46.

Geuze RH, editor (2007) *La Maladress chez les Enfants Presentant un Trouble D'acquisition des Coordination Motrices: Revue des Approches Actuelles* [*Developmental Coordination Disorder: A Review of Current Approaches*]. Marseille: Solal, pp. 197–227.

Geuze RH, Borger H (1994) Response selection in clumsy children: five years later. *J Human Movement Stud* 27: 1–15.

Geuze RH, Kalverboer AF (1994) Tapping a rhythm: a problem of timing for children who are clumsy and dyslexic. *Adapted Physical Activity Quarterly* 11: 203–213.

Geuze RH, Jongmans MJ, Schoemaker MM, Smits-Englesman BCM (2001) Clinical and research diagnostic criteria for developmental coordination disorder: a review and discussion. *Human Movement Sci* 20: 7–47. http://dx.doi.org/10.1016/S0167-9457(01)00027-6

Gillberg C, Kadesjo B (2003) Why bother about clumsiness? The implications of having developmental coordination disorder (DCD). *Neural Plasticity* 10: 59–68. http://dx.doi.org/101155/NP200359

Gillberg C, Carlstrom G, Rasmussen P, Waldenstrom E (1983) Perceptual, motor and attentional deficits in seven-year-old children. Neurological screening aspects. *Acta Paediatrica Scandinavia* 72: 119–124. http://dx.doi.org/10.1111/j.1651-2227.1983.tb09675.x

Gillberg IC, Gillberg C (1989) Children with preschool minor neuro-developmental disorders. IV: Behaviour and school achievement at age 13. *Dev Med Child Neurol* 31: 3–13.

Gillberg IC, Gillberg C, Groth J (1989) Children with preschool minor neurodevelopmental disorders. V: Neurodevelopmental profiles at age 13. *Dev Med Child Neurol* 31: 14–24. http://dx.doi.org/10.1111/j.1469-8749.1989.tb08407.x

Gillberg RH, Rasmussen P (1982) Perceptual motor and attentional difficulties in six-year-old children: background factors. *Dev Med Child Neurol* 24: 752–770. http://dx.doi.org/10.1111/j.1469-8749.1982.tb13697.x

Goodman R (2001) Psychometric properties of the Strengths and Difficulties Questionnaire (SDQ). *J Am Acad Child Adolesc Psychiatry* 40: 1137–1345. http://dx.doi.org/10.1097/00004583-200111000-00015

Green D, Baird G (2005) DCD and overlapping conditions. In: Sugden DA, Chambers ME, editors. *Children with Developmental Coordination Disorder*. London: Whurr, pp. 93–118.

Green D, Lingham R, Mattocks C, Ridoch C, Ness A, Emond A (2011) The risk of reduced physical activity in children with probable developmental coordination disorder: a prospective longitudinal study. *Res Dev Disabil* 32: 1332–1342. http://dx.doi.org/10.1016/j.ridd.2011.01.040

Gubbay SS (1975) *The Clumsy Child*. London: Saunders.

Hadders-Algra M (1999) Differentiation of developmental coordination disorder with the help of a standardised neurological assessment. Paper presented at the Developmental Coordination Disorder 4th International Conference, Groningen, The Netherlands, July.

Hadders-Algra M (2003) Developmental coordination: is clumsy motor behaviour caused by a lesion of the brain at an early age? *Neural Plasticity* 10: 39–50. http://dx.doi.org/10.1155/NP.2003.39

Hadders-Algra M, Touwen BCL, Olinga AA, Huisjes HJ (1985) Minor neurological dysfunction and behavioural development: a report from the Groningen Perinatal Project. *Early Human Devt* 11: 221–229. http://dx.doi.org/10.1016/0378-3782(85)90076-3

Hadders-Algra M, Touwen BCL, Huisjes HJ (1986) Neurologically deviant newborns: neurological and behavioural development at the age of six years. *Dev Med Child Neurol* 28: 569–578.

Hadders-Algra M, Huisjes HJ, Touwen BCL (1988a) Perinatal correlates of major and minor neurological dysfunction at school age – a multivariate analysis. *Dev Med Child Neurol* 30: 472–481. http://dx.doi.org/10.1111/j.1469-8749.1988.tb04774.x

Hadders-Algra M, Huisjes HJ, Touwen BCL (1988b) Perinatal risk factors and minor neurological dysfunction: significance for behaviour and school achievement at nine years. *Dev Med Child Neurol* 30: 482–491. http://dx.doi.org/10.1111/j.1469-8749.1988.tb04775.x

Hall A, McLeod A, Counsell C, Thomson L, Mutch L (1995) School attainment, cognitive ability and motor function in a Scottish very- low-birthweight population at eight years: a controlled study. *Dev Med Child Neurol* 37: 1037–1050. http://dx.doi.org/10.1111/j.1469-8749.1995.tb11965.x

Hammill DD, Pearson NA, Voress JK (1993) *Developmental Test of Visual Perception*, 2nd edition. Austin, TX: Pro-Ed.

Haywood KM, Getchell N (2001) *Lifespan Motor Development*, 3rd edition. Champaign, IL: Human Kinetics.

Hellgren L, Gillberg IC, Bagenholm A, Gillberg C (1994) Children with deficits in attention motor control and perception (DAMP) almost grown up: psychiatric and personality disorders at age 16 years. *J Child Psychol Psychiatry* 35: 1255–1271. http://dx.doi.org/10.1111/j.1469-7610.1994.tb01233.x

Henderson L, Rose P, Henderson SE (1992) Reaction time and movement time in children with developmental coordination disorder. *J Child Psychol Psychiatry* 33: 895–905. http://dx.doi.org/10.1111/j.1469-7610.199.2tb01963.x

Henderson SE (1994) Editorial. *Adapted Phys Activity Q* 11: 111–114.

Henderson SE, Hall D (1982) Concomitants of clumsiness in young school children. *Dev Med Child Neurol* 24: 448–460. http://dx.doi.org/10.1111/j.1469-8749.1982.tb13649.x

Henderson SE, Henderson L (2002) Towards an understanding of developmental coordination disorder. The second G Lawrence Rarick Memorial Lecture. *Adaptive Phys Activity Q* 19: 11–31.

Henderson SE, Sugden DA (1992) *Movement Assessment Battery for Children: Manual*. Sidcup: Psychological Corporation.

Henderson SE, May DS, Umney M (1989) An exploratory study of goal setting behaviour, self concept and locus of control in children with movement difficulties. *Eur J Special Needs Educ* 4: 1–13. http://dx.doi.org/10.1080/0885625890040101

Henderson SE, Barnett AL, Henderson L (1994) Visuo-spatial difficulties and clumsiness: on the interpretation of conjoined deficits. *J Child Psychol Psychiatry* 35: 961–969. http://dx.doi.org/10.1111/j.1469-7610.1994.tb02305.x

Henderson SE, Sugden DA, Barnett A (2007) *Movement Assessment Battery for Children 2: Kit and Manual*. London: Harcourt Assessment.

Hibberlin JR, David JM, Steer C, et al (2007) Maternal seafood consumption in pregnancy and neurodevelopmental outcomes on childhood (ALSPAC study). An observational cohort study. *Lancet* 369: 578–585. http://dx.doi.org/10.1016/S0140-6736(07)60277-3

Hill EL (1998) A dyspraxic deficit in specific language impairment and developmental coordination disorder? Evidence from hand and arm movements. *Dev Med Child Neurol* 40: 388–395. http://dx.doi.org/10.1111/j.1469-8749.1998.tb08214.x

Hill EL (2005) Cognitive explanations of the planning and organization of movement. In: Sugden DA, Chambers ME, editors. *Children with Developmental Coordination Disorder*. London: Whurr, pp. 47–71.

Hill EL, Bishop DVM, Nimmo-Smith I (1998) Representational gestures in developmental coordination disorder and specific language impairment: error types and the reliability of ratings. *Human Movement Sci* 17: 655–663. http://dx.doi.org/10.1016/S0167-9457(98)00017-7

Hoare D (1994) Subtypes of developmental coordination disorder. *Adapted Phys Activity Q* 11: 158–169.

von Hofsten C, Rösblad B (1988) The integration of sensory information in the development of precise manual pointing. *Neuropsychologia* 26: 541–572.

Hulme C, Biggerstaff A, Morgan G, Mckinlay I (1982a) Visual kinaesthetic and cross modal judgements of length by normal and clusmy children. *Dev Med Child Neurol* 24: 461–471. http://dx.doi.org/10.1111/j.1469-8749.1982.tb13650.x

Hulme C, Smart A, Moran G (1982b) Visual perceptual deficits in clumsy children. *Neuropsychology* 30: 475–481.

Hultzer Y (2007) Systematic ecological modification approach to skill acquisition in adapted physical activity. In: David WE, Broadhead GD, editors. *Ecological Task Analysis and Movement*. Champaign, IL: Human Kinetics, pp. 170–195.

Ivery RB (2003) Cerebellar involvement in clumsiness and other developmental disorders. *Neural Plasticity* 10: 141–153.

Johnson DC, Wade MG (2009) Children at risk for developmental coordination disorder: judgement of changes in action capabilities. *Dev Med Child Neurol* 51: 397–403. http://dx.doi.org/10.1111/j.1469-8749.2008.03174.x

Jongmans M (2005) Early identifcation of children with developmental coordination disorder. In: Sugden DA, Chambers ME, editors. *Children with Developmental Coordination Disorder.* London: Whurr, pp. 155–167.

Jongmans MJ, Mercuri E, Dubowitz L, Henderson SE (1998) Perceptual motor difficulties and their concomitants in six-year-old children born prematurely. *Human Movement Sci* 17: 629–653. http://dx.doi.org/10.1016/S0167-9457(98)00016-5

Kadesjo B, Gillberg C (1999) Attention deficits and clumsiness in Swedish 7-year-old children. *Dev Med Child Neurol* 40: 796–804. http://dx.doi.org/10.1111/j.1469-8749.1998.tb12356.x

Kaplan BJ, Crawford SG, Wilson BN, Dewey DM (1997) Comorbidity of developmental coordination disorder and different types of reading disability. *J Int Neuropsychol Soc* 3: 54.

Kaplan BJ, Wilson BN, Dewey DM, Crawford SG (1998) DCD may not be a discrete disorder. *Human Movement Sci* 17: 471–490. http://dx.doi.org/10.1016/S0167-9457(98)00010-4

Kaplan BJ, Crawford S, Cantell M, Kooistra L, Dewey D (2006) Comorbidity, co-occurrence, continuum: what's in a name? *Child Care Health Dev* 32: 723–731. http://dx.doi.org/10.1111/j.1365-2214.2006.00689.x

Kavale KA, Forness SR (1995) *The Nature of Learning Disabilities.* Hillsdale, NJ: Lawrence Erlbaum Associates.

Keogh JF, Sugden DA (1985) *Movement Skill Development.* New York: Macmillan.

Keogh JF, Sugden DA, Reynard CL, Calkins J (1979) Identification of clumsy children: comparisons and comments. *J Human Movement Studies* 5: 32–51.

Kephart NC (1956) *The Slow Learner in the Classroom.* Columbus, Ohio: Charles Merrill.

Kirby A, Sugden DA, Beveridge SE, Edwards L, Edwards R (2008a) Dyslexia and developmental coordination disorder in further and higher education. *Dyslexia* 14: 197–213.

Kirby A, Sugden DA, Beveridge SE, Edwards L (2008b) Developmental coordination disorder in adolescents and adults in further and higher education. *J Res Special Educ Needs* 8: 120–131. http://dx.doi.org/10.1111/j.1471-3802.2008.00111.x

Kirby A, Edwards L, Sugden DA, Rosenbaum S (2010) The development and standardization of the Adult Developmental Co-ordination Disorders/Dyspraxia Checklist (ADC). *Res Dev Disabil* 31: 131–139. http://dx.doi.org/10.1016/j.ridd.2009.08.010

Kirby A, Edwards L, Sugden DA (2011) Emerging adulthood in developmental coordination disorder: parent and young adult perspectives. *Res Dev Disabil* 32: 1351–1360. http://dx.doi.org/10.1016/j.ridd.2011.01.041

Kirby A, Sugden DA, Edwards L (unpublished) Profiles of children with developmental coordination disorder on the Movement Assessment Battery for Children.

Knuckey NW, Gubbay SS (1983) Clumsy children: a prognostic study. *Aust Paediatr J* 19: 9–13.

Landgren M, Pettersson R, Kjellman B, Gillberg C (1996) ADHD, DAMP and other neurodevelopmental/psychiatric disorders in 6-year- old children: epidemiology and co-morbidity. *Dev Med Child Neurol* 38: 891–906. http://dx.doi.org/10.1111/j.1469-8749.1996.tb15046.x

Laszlo JI, Bairstow P (1985) *Test of Kinaesthetic Sensitivity.* London: Senkit PTY in association with Holt Rinehart & Winston.

Laszlo JI, Bairstow PJ, Bartrip J, et al (1988) Clumsiness or perceptuo-motor dysfunction? In: Colley A, Beech J, editors. *Cognition and Action in Skilled Behaviour.* Amsterdam: North Holland, pp. 293–316. http://dx.doi.org/10.1016/S0166-4115(08)60629-9

Lingam R, Hunt L, Golding J, Jongmans M, Emond A (2009) Prevalence of developmental coordination disorder using the DSM IV at 7 years of age: a popluation based study. *Pediatrics* 123: e693–e700. http://dx.doi.org/10.1542/peds.2008-1770

Lord R, Hulme C (1987) Perceptual judgements of normal and clumsy children. *Dev Med Child Neurol* 29: 250–257. http://dx.doi.org/10.1111/j.1469-8749.1987.tb02143.x

Lord R, Hulme C (1988) Visual perception and drawing ability in clumsy and normal children. *Br J Dev Psychol* 6: 1–9. http://dx.doi.org/10.1111/j.2044-835X.1988.tb01075.x

Losse AM, Henderson SE, Elliman D, Hall D, Knight E, Jongmans M (1991) Clumsiness in children: do they grow out of it? A ten year follow-up. *Dev Med Child Neurol* 33: 55–68. http://dx.doi.org/10.1111/j.1469-8749.1991.tb14785.x

Lunsing RJ, Hadders-Algra M, Huisjes HJ, Touwen BCL (1992) Minor neurological dysfunction from birth to 12 years. I: Increase during late school age. *Dev Med Child Neurol* 34: 399–404. http://dx.doi.org/10.1111/j.1469-8749.1992.tb11451.x

Lyytinen H, Ahonen T (1988) Developmental motor problems in children: a 6 year longitudinal study. *J Clin Exp Psychol* 10: 57.

Macnab JJ, Miller LT, Polatajko HJ (2001) The search for subtypes in DCD: is cluster analysis the answer? *Human Movement Sci* 20: 49–72. http://dx.doi.org/10.1016/S0167-9457(01)00028-8

Maeland AF (1992) Identification of children with motor coordination problems. *Adapted Phys Activity Q* 9: 330–342.

Magalhaes LC, Cardoso AA, Missiuna C (2011) Activities and participation in children with developmental coordination disorder: a systematic review. *Res Dev Disabil* 32: 1309–1316. http://dx.doi.org/10.1016/j.ridd.2011.01.029

Magill RA (2007) *Motor Learning and Control: Concepts and Applications,* 8th edition. New York: McGraw-Hill.

Mercuri E, Barnett A (2003) Neonatal brain MRI and motor outcomes at school age in children with neonatal encephalopathy: a review of personal experiences. *Neural Plasticity* 10: 51–57. http://dx.doi.org/10.1155/NP.2003.51

Missiuna C, Pollack N, Law M (2004) *Perceived Efficacy of Goal Setting in Young Children System (PEGS).* San Antonio, TX: Psychological Corporation.

Missiuna C, Moll S, King S, Law M (2007) A trajectory of troubles: parents' impressions of the impact of developmental cordination disorder. *Physical and Occupational Therapy in Pediatrics* 27: 81–101. http://dx.doi.org/10.1080/J006v27n01_06

Miyahara M (1994) Subtypes of students with learning disabilities based upon gross motor functions. *Adapted Phys Activity Q* 11: 368–383.

Mon-Williams MA, Wann JP, Pascal E (1999) Visual-proprioceptive mapping in children with developmental coordination disorder. *Dev Med Child Neurol* 41: 247–254. http://dx.doi.org/10.1017/S0012162299000523

Morton J (2004) *Understanding Developmental Disorders.* Oxford: Blackwell. http://dx.doi.org/10.1002/9780470773307

Morton J, Frith U (1995) Causal modelling: a structural approach to developmental psychopathology. In: Cicchetti D, Cohen DJ, editors. *Developmental Psychopathology, Volume 1: Theory and Methods.* New York: Wiley, pp. 357–390.

Mutch L, Leyland A, McGee A (1993) Patterns of neuropsychological function in a low-birthweight population. *Dev Med Child Neurol* 35: 943–956. http://dx.doi.org/10.1111/j.1469-8749.1993.tb11576.x

Newell KM (1986) Constraints on the development of coordination. In: Wade MG, Whiting HTA, editors. *Motor Development in Children: Aspects of Coordination and Control*. Dordrecht: Martinus Nijhoff, pp. 341–361.

Nichols PL, Chen TC (1981) *Minimal Brain Dysfunction: A Prospective Study*. Hillsdale, NJ: Lawrence Erlbaum.

Nicolson RI, Fawcett AJ (1999) Developmental dyslexia: the role of the cerebellum. *Dyslexia* 5: 155–177. http://dx.doi.org/10.1002/(SICI)1099-0909(199909)5:3<155::AID-DYS143>30CO;2-4

Pasamanick B, Knobloch H (1966) Terospective studies on epidemiology of reproductive casualty: old and new. *Q J Behav Dev* 12: 7–26.

Peters JM, Henderson SE (2008) Understanding developmental coordination disorder and its impact on families: the contribution of single case studies. In: Sugden DA, Kirby A, Dunford C, editors. Special issue of *Int J Disabil Dev Educ: Children with Developmental Coordination Disorder* 55: 97–112.

Piek JP (2003) The role of variability in early infant motor development. *Infant Behav Dev* 25: 452–465. http://dx.doi.org/10.1016/S0163-6383(02)00145-5

Piek JP (2006) *Infant Motor Development*. Champaign, IL: Human Kinetics.

Piek JP, Bradbury GS, Elsley SC, Tate T (2008) Motor coordination and social-emotional behaviour in preschool-aged children. In: Sugden DA, Kirby A, Dunford C, editors. Special issue of *Int J Disabil Dev Educ: Children with Developmental Coordination Disorder* 55: 143–152.

Pless M, Carlsson M, Sundelin C, Persson K (2001) Preschool children with developmental coordination disorder: self-perceived competence and group motor skill intervention. *Acta Pediatrica* 90: 532–538. http://dx.doi.org/10.1080/080352501750197674

Polatajko HJ, Cantin N (2006) Developmental coordination disorder (dyspraxia): an overview of the state of the art. *Semin Pediatr Neurol* 12: 250–258. http://dx.doi.org/10.1016/j.spen.2005.12.007

Polatajko HJ, Fox M, Missiuna C (1995) An international consensus on children with developmental coordination disorder. *Can J Occup Ther* 62: 3–6.

Portwood M (1996) *Developmental Dyspraxia: Identification and Intervention*. London: David Fulton.

Powell RP, Bishop DVM (1992) Clumsiness and perceptual problems in children with developmental coordination disorder. *Dev Med Child Neurol* 34: 755–765. http://dx.doi.org/10.1111/j.1469-8749.1992.tb11514.x

Querne L, Berquin P, Vernier-Hauvette MP, et al (2008) Dysfunction of the attentional brain network in children with developmental coordination disorder: an fMRI study. *Brain Res* 1244: 89–102. http://dx.doi.org/10.1016/j.brainres.2008.07.066

Rasmussen P, Gillberg C (2000) Natural outcome of ADHD with developmental coordination disorder at age 22 years: a controlled longitudinal community based study. *J Am Acad Child Adolesc Psychiatry* 39: 1424–1431. http://dx.doi.org/10.1097/00004583-200011000-00017

Rutter M (1967) A children's behaviour questionnaire for completion by teachers: preliminary findings. *J Child Psychol Psychiatry* 8: 1–11. http://dx.doi.org/10.1111/j.1469-7610.1967.tb02175.x

Scabar A, Devescovi R, Blason L, Bravar L, Carozzi M (2006) Comorbidity of DCD and SLI: significance of epileptiform activity during sleep. *Child Care Health Dev* 32: 733–739. http://dx.doi.org/10.1111/j.1365-2214.2006.00705.x

Schmidt RA, Lee TD (2005) *Motor Control and Learning: A Behavioral Analysis*. Champaign, IL: Human Kinetics.

Schoemaker MM, Kalverboer AF (1994) Social and affective problems of children who are clumsy: how early do they begin? *Adapted PhysActivity Q* 11: 130–140.

Schoemaker MM, van der Wees M, Flapper B, Verheji-Jamsen N, Scholten-Jegers S, Geuze R (2001) Perceptual skills of children with developmental coordination disorder. *Human Movement Sci* 20: 73–94. http://dx.doi.org/10.1016/S0167-9457(01)00031-8

Sigmundsson H (1999) Intermodal-matching and bimanual coordination in children with eye-hand coordination problems. *Nordisk Pysioterapi* 3: 55–64.

Simner ML, Leedham CG, Thomassen AJWM (1996) *Handwriting and Drawing Research: Basic and Applied Issues*. Amsterdam: IOS Press.

Sinani C, Sugden DA, Hill EL (2011) Gesture production in school versus clinical samples of children with Developmental Coordination Disorder and typically developing childen. *Res Dev Disord* 32: 1270–1282. http://dx.doi.org/101016/j.ridd.2011.01.030

Skinner A, Piek JP (2001) Psychosocial implications of poor motor coordination in children and adolescents. *Human Movement Sci* 20: 73–94. http://dx.doi.org/10.1016/S0167-9457(01)00029-X

Skorji V, McKenzie B (1997) How do children who are clumsy remember modelled movements? *Dev Med Child Neurol* 39: 404–408.

Smyth MM, Mason UC (1997) Planning and execution of action in children with and without developmental coordination disorder. *J Child Psychol Psychiatry* 38: 1023–1037. http://dx.doi.org/10.1111/j.1469-7610.1997.tb01619.x

Smyth TR (1994) Clumsiness in children: a defect of kinaesthetic perception? *Child Care Health Dev* 20: 27–36. http://dx.doi.org/10.1111/j.1365-2214.1994.tb00372.x

Smyth TR (1996) Clumsiness: kinaesthetic perception and translation. *Child Care Health Dev* 22: 1–9. http://dx.doi.org/10.1111/j.1365-2214.1996.tb00417.x

Smyth TR, Glencross DJ (1986) Informtion procesing deficits in clumsy children. *Aus J Psychol* 38: 13–22. http://dx.doi.org/10.1080/00049538608256413

Stott DH, Moyes FA, Henderson SE (1984) *The Test of Motor Impairment*. San Antonio, TX: The Psychological Corporation.

Sugden DA, editor (2006) *Developmental Coordination Disorder As A Specific Learning Difficulty: Economic Science Research Council Seminar*. Cardiff: Dyscovery Trust.

Sugden DA, Chambers ME (2003) Intervention in children with DCD: the role of parents and teachers. *Br J Educ Psychol* 73: 545–561. http://dx.doi.org/10.1348/000709903322591235

Sugden DA, Chambers ME, editors (2004) *Children with Developmental Coordination Disorder*. London:Whurr.

Sugden DA, Dunford CD (2007) The role of theory empiricism and experience in intervention for children with movement difficulties. *Disabil Rehabil* 29: 3–11. http://dx.doi.org/10.1080/09638280600947542

Sugden DA, Keogh JF (1990) *Problems in Movement and Skill Development*. Columbia, SC: University of South Carolina Press.

Sugden DA, Sugden L (1991) Assessment of movement skill problems in seven- and nine-year-old school children. *Br J Educ Psychol* 61: 329–345. http://dx.doi.org/10.1111/j.2044-8279.1991.tb00990.x

Sugden DA, Wann C (1987) The assessment of motor impairment in children with moderate learning difficulties. *Br J Educ Psychol* 57: 225–236. http://dx.doi.org/10.1111/j.2044-8279.1987.tb03156.x

Sugden DA, Wright H (1998) *Motor Coordination Disorders in Children.* Thousand Oaks, CA: Sage Publishers.

Sugden DA, Kirby A, Dunford C, editors (2008) Developmental coordination disorder. *Special issue of Int J Disabil Dev Educ* 55: 93–187.

Summers J, Larkin D, Dewey D (2008) What impact does developmental coordination disorder have on daily routines? In: Sugden DA, Kirby A, Dunford C, editors. Special issue of *Int J Disabil Dev Educ: Children with Developmental Coordination Disorder* 55: 131–142.

Thelen E, Ulrich BD (1991) Hidden skills: a dynamic systems analysis of treadmill stepping in the first year. *Society for Research in Child Development Monographs* 56: 1–98.

Touwen BCL (1979) *Examination of the Child with Minor Neurological Dysfunction,* 2nd edition. London: SIMP/Heinemann.

Tsai C-L, Wu S-K, Huang C-H (2008) Static balance in children with developmental coordination disorder. *Human Movement Sci* 27: 142–153. http://dx.doi.org/10.1016/j.humov.2007.08.002

Ulrich BD (1997) Dynamic systems theory and skill development in infants and children. In: Connolly KJ, Forssberg H, editors. *Neurophysiology and Neuropsychology of Motor Development.* London: Mac Keith Press, pp. 319–345.

Vaessen W, Kalverboer AF (1990) Clumsy children's performance on a double task. In: Kalverboer AF, editor. *Developmental Biopsychology: Experimental and Observational Studies on Children at Risk.* Ann Arbor, MI: University of Michigan Press, pp. 223–240.

Visser J (2007) Subtypes and comorbidity in developmental coordination disorder. In: Geuze RH, editor. *Developmental Coordination Disorder: A Review of Current Approaches.* Marseille: Solal, pp. 9–25.

Wann JP, Mon-Williams M, Rushton K (1998) Postural control and coordination disorders: the swinging room revisited. *Human Movement Sci* 17: 491–513. http://dx.doi.org/10.1016/S0167-9457(98)00011-6

Watkinson EJ, Dunn JC, Cavaliers N, Calzonetti K, Wilhelm L, Dwyer S (2001) Engagement in playground activities as a criterion for diagnosing developmental coordination disorder. *Adapt Phys Activ Q* 18: 18–34.

Whitall J, Getchell N, McMenamin S, Horn C, Wilms-Floet A, Clark JE (2006) Perception-action coupling in children with and without DCD: frequency locking between task-relevant auditory signals and motor responses in a dual motor task. *Child Care Health Dev* 32: 679–692. http://dx.doi.org/10.1111/j.1365-2214.2006.00676.x

WHO (1992) *International Statistical Classification of Diseases and Related Health Problems, Volume 1,* 10th edition. Geneva: World Health Organization.

Williams HG, Woollacott MH, Ivry R (1992) Timing and motor control in clumsy children. *J Motor Behav* 24: 165–172. http://dx.doi.org/10.1080/00222895199299941612

Williams J, Thomas PR, Maruff P, Butson M, Wilson PH (2006) Motor, visual and egocentric transformation in children with developmental coordination disorder. *Child Health Care Dev* 32: 633–647.

Wilmut K, Wann J (2008) The use of predictive information is impaired in the actions of children and young adults with developmental coordination disorder. *Exp Brain Res* 191: 403–418. http://dx.doi.org/10.1007/s00221-008-1532-4

Wilson PH (2005) Practitioner review: approaches to assessment and treatment of children with DCD: an evaluative review. *J Child Psychol Psychiatry* 46: 806–823. http://dx.doi.org/10.1111/j.1469-7610.2005.01409.x

Wilson PH, McKenzie BE (1998) Information processing deficits associated with developmental coordination disorder: a meta analysis of research findings. *J Child Psychol Psychiatry* 39: 829–840. http://dx.doi.org/10.1017/S0021963098002765

Wilson PH, Maruff P, Ives S, Currie J (2001) Abnormalities of motor and praxis imagery in children with developmental coordination disorder. *Human Movement Sci* 20: 135–139. http://dx.doi.org/10.1016/S0167-9457(01)00032-X

Wilson PH, Maruff P, Butson M, Williams J, Lum J, Thomas PR (2004) Impairments in the internal representation of movement in children with developmental coordination disorder (DCD): a mental rotation task. *Dev Med Child Neurol* 46: 754–759. http://dx.doi.org/10.1111/j.1469-8749.2004.tb00995.x

Wright HC, Sugden DA (1996) A two-step procedure for the identification of children with developmental coordination disorder in Singapore. *Dev Med Child Neurol* 38: 1099–1106. http://dx.doi.org/10.1111/j.1469-8749.1996.tb15073.x

Wright HC, Sugden DA, Walkuiski J, Tan J (1995) Identifying children with motor difficulties. *J Sports Sci* 13: 82.

Zwicker JG, Missiuna C, Maled LA (2009) Neural correlates of developmental coordination disorder. *J Child Neurol* 24: 1273–1281. http://dx.doi.org/10.1177/0883073809333537

9
CHILDREN WITH INTELLECTUAL DISABILITY

General descriptions

Intellectual disability is defined as significantly subaverage intellectual functioning present from birth or early infancy that causes limitations in the ability to conduct typical activities of daily living. Like many others (e.g. Odem et al 2007) we recognize that intellectual disability, along with other terms such as mental retardation, is a social construction, but we also recognize the value of such terms. Odem et al (2007) propose the following three purposes for this construct:

- To enable persons to receive specialist and often additional help from education, health, and/or social services.
- To allow a framework for research and clinical investigations that can be utilized across countries and cultures.
- To plan appropriate programmes that address the specific needs of such individuals.

Terminology and Definitions

Terminology is a huge issue with respect to this group of individuals; even though the *Diagnostic and Statistical Manual of Mental Disorders* (DSM) and *International Classification of Diseases* (ICD) use mental retardation, we choose to use the term intellectual disability.

Both ICD-10 (WHO 1992) and DSM-IV-TR (APA 2000) use the term 'mental retardation', but in many countries, such as the United Kingdom, this term is rarely used because of its negative connotations. The term mental retardation has acquired an undesirable social stigma, and, because of this stigma, doctors and health care practitioners have begun replacing it with the term 'intellectual disability'. As noted above we choose to use the term intellectual disability but using also the *definitions* provided by DSM-IV and draft DSM-V for mental retardation. If we take the current DSM-IV definition of

intellectual disability, it involves the following characteristics (APA 2000):

- Significantly subaverage intellectual functioning: an IQ approximately 70 or below on an individually administered IQ test.
- Concurrent deficits or impairments in present adaptive functioning in meeting expectations of culture and peer group in at least two of the areas of communication, self-care, home living, social/interpersonal skills, use of community resources, self-direction.
- Functional academic skills, work, leisure, health, and safety. The onset is before 18 years of age.

The code based on degree of intellectual functioning involves the following:

- Mild: IQ 50 to 75. Includes approximately 85% of the population with intellectual disability. Individuals in this group can live independently with some community support.
- Moderate: IQ 35 to 50. Includes approximately 10% of the population with intellectual disability. Individuals in this group can often lead relatively normal lives with oversight. Individuals in this group live typically in group homes with others.
- Severe: IQ 20 to 25. Includes 3% to 4% of the population with intellectual disability. Individuals in this group can usually master basic skills of daily living, such as cleaning and dressing. They typically live in a group-home setting.
- Profound: IQ less than 20. Individuals in this group make up 1% to 2% of the population with intellectual disability. They can achieve acceptable levels of basic communication and self-care skills. This group often has other associated cognitive disorders.

Draft proposals are now available for DSM-V, which is anticipated to go to press in 2013, and there are proposed changes to the criteria set by DSM-IV. On the DSM-V website the label 'mental retardation' is retained as the overall title, but immediately under it, and followed by the criteria, the term intellectual disability is used. The draft proposals note that the change in terminology is consistent with such variables as international opinion. There are also changes to the wording of cut-off points, with regard to cultural sensitivity, and adaptive functioning is based on factor analytic studies of adaptive behaviour. Of particular interest is that the code is no longer based on strict IQ measures and is more to do with functionality, including adaptive behaviours. The proposed draft changes are as follows:

- Current intellectual deficits of two or more standard deviations below the population mean, which generally translates into performance in the lowest 3% of a person's age and cultural group, or an IQ of 70 or below. This should be measured with an individualized standardized, culturally appropriate, psychometrically sound measure.
- And concurrent deficits in at least two domains of adaptive functioning of at least two or more standard deviations which generally translates into performances in the lowest 3% of a person's age and cultural group, or standard scores of 70 or below. This should be measured with an individualized standardized, culturally appropriate, psychometrically sound measure. Adaptive behavior domains typically include:
  - Conceptual skills (communication, language, time, money, academic)
  - Social skills (interpersonal skills, social responsibility, recreation, friendships)
  - Practical skills (daily living skills, work, travel)
- With onset during the developmental period.
                                    (www.apa.org)

The code of different levels of intellectual disability is no longer based on an IQ test.

As noted above, persons with intellectual disability have significantly below average intellectual functioning that limits their ability to cope with two or more activities of normal daily living (adaptive skills). These activities include the ability to communicate; live at home; take care of oneself, including making decisions; participate in leisure, social, school, and work activities; and be aware of personal health and safety.

Persons with intellectual disability also have varying degrees of impairment. While recognizing that each individual case is different, clinicians find it helpful to classify a person's level of functioning. Intellectual functioning levels are currently based on the results of developmental quotient tests and IQ tests, or on the level of support needed. In DSM-V these levels are not based on IQ tests but a wider range of functional adaptive measures. Support is categorized as intermittent, limited, extensive, or pervasive. Intermittent means occasional support; limited means support such as a day programme in a sheltered workshop; extensive means daily, ongoing support; and pervasive means a high level of support for all activities of daily living, possibly including full-time nursing care. Based only on IQ test scores, about 3% of the total population are considered to have intellectual disability. However, if classification is based on the need for support, only about 1% of people are classified as having significant cognitive limitation.

Causes

A wide variety of medical and environmental conditions can cause intellectual disability. Some are genetic; some are present before or at the time of conception; and others occur during pregnancy, during birth, or after birth. These would include transplacental infections, prenatal exposure to toxins and teratogens, prenatal malnutrition, birth injury, hypoxia, childhood infections (e.g. meningitis), and childhood exposure to environmental toxins. The common factor is that something typically impairs normal neurological development. Worldwide undernutrition has been regarded as a major determinant of cognitive development (Emerson and Hatton 2007), and the range is considerable, from zero per cent in the USA to 18% in India (United Nations Children's Fund 2006). However, identification of a specific cause is possible in only about one-third of people with mild intellectual disability and two-thirds of people with moderate to profound intellectual disability.

Some children with intellectual disability are immediately recognized because of some chromosomal atypicality, with Down syndrome being the most obvious one and the one to which knowledge and attitudes have changed substantially in recent years. The condition was first recognized in the mid-19th century, but it was 1959 before Lejeune and colleagues noted the now familiar 47 chromosomal abnormality instead of the usual 46. Around 90% of people with the syndrome will have an extra chromosome associated with chromosome number 21; the remainder have a translocation in which part of chromosome 21 attaches itself to another chromosome, or a mosaic condition in which the 47 chromosomes are not evenly distributed across all cells, with some having the regular 46 (Sugden and Keogh 1990).

Characteristics
Sugden and Keogh (1990) note four characteristics that are fundamental to children with intellectual disability.

- The first is a lower level and rate of learning, and this includes all forms of learning from formal instruction to incidental learning. This learning includes intellectual, social–behavioural, and language.
- Second is the impaired ability to use knowledge and skills in situations different from those in which they were first learned. Skills seem 'welded' to the context in which they were learned, with little or no transfer or generalization.
- Third, Sugden and Keogh (1990) note the heterogeneity of learning problems in children with intellectual disability, with some having general difficulties across all domains, and others having difficulties in only one or two areas. This may seem to overlap with Chapter 11, on other developmental disorders, but the major difference is that the children described in that chapter will be in a typical range of intelligence (IQ >70).
- Fourth, although some children with intellectual disability have abnormalities apparent at birth or shortly thereafter, in the majority of children with intellectual disability symptoms are more related to learning disabilities that are not noticeable until the preschool period.

Symptoms become apparent at a younger age in those more severely affected. Usually, the first problem parents notice is a delay in language development. Children with intellectual disability are slower to use words, put words together, and speak in complete sentences. Their social development is sometimes slow because of cognitive impairment and language deficiencies. Children with intellectual disability may be slow to learn activities of daily living including the ability to dress and feed themselves. Some parents may not consider the possibility of cognitive impairment until the child is in school or preschool and is unable to keep up with age-appropriate expectations.

Children with intellectual disability are somewhat more likely than other children to have behavioural problems, such as explosive outbursts, temper tantrums, and physically aggressive behaviour. These behaviours are often related to specific frustrating situations compounded by an impaired ability to communicate and control impulses. Older children may be gullible and easily taken advantage of or led into minor misbehaviour.

About 10% to 40% of people with intellectual disability also have a mental health disorder (dual diagnosis). In particular, anxiety and depression are common, especially in children who are aware that they are different from their peers or who are maligned and mistreated because of their disability.

Diagnosis
Many children are evaluated by teams of professionals, including a paediatric neurologist or developmental paediatrician, a psychologist, speech pathologist, occupational or physical therapist, special educator, social worker, or nurse. For children who would fall into the range of 'mild' intellectual disability this is often not identified until the school years, and, in countries such as the UK, they would not be labelled as a distinct category. They are much more likely to be distinguished by the level of educational need they show and the provision given as required. Children within this range are most likely to be educated in mainstream school with specialist help given within the regular classroom setting. This specialist help would be graded according to the child's need.

In many other countries, and with children who show a higher level of intellectual disability, a first step in the evaluation of a child suspected of having intellectual disability might be the testing of intellectual functioning and looking for a cause. Whereas the cause of the child's intellectual disability may be irreversible, identifying a causal disorder for the disability may allow a reliable prediction of the child's future course, which might prevent further loss of skills and permit interventions that can increase the child's level of functioning, and counselling may be given to parents on the risk of having another child with that disorder.

Newborn infants with physical abnormalities or other symptoms suggestive of a condition associated with intellectual disability often need tests to detect possible metabolic and genetic disorders. Imaging tests, such as computed tomography or magnetic resonance imaging, may reveal the presence of structural problems within the brain. An electroencephalogram records the brain's electrical activity to evaluate a child for possible seizures. A chromosome analysis, urine and blood tests, and bone radiographs can also help rule out suspected causes of intellectual disability.

Some children who show delays in learning language and mastering social skills may have conditions other than intellectual disability. As hearing problems interfere with language and social development, a hearing evaluation is typically performed. Emotional problems and learning disorders can also be mistaken for intellectual disability. Children deprived of normal love and attention for extended periods of time may seem to have intellectual disability. A child with delays in sitting or walking (gross motor skills) or in manipulating objects (fine motor skills) may have a neurological disorder not associated with intellectual disability.

As mild developmental problems are not always noticed by parents, developmental screening tests, during well-check visits to a doctor, can evaluate a child's cognitive, verbal, and motor skill development. Parents can help the doctor determine the child's level of functioning by completing a Parents' Evaluation of Developmental Status test (www.pedstest.com). Children who perform significantly below their age level on these screening tests are referred for formal testing.

Formal testing often comprises interviews with parents, observations of the child, and norm-referenced tests. Tests such as the Wechsler Intelligence Scale for Children –Fourth Edition Integrated (WISC® – IV) measure intellectual ability; other tests, such as the Vineland Adaptive Behavior Scales Second Edition (Vineland-II), assess communication, daily living skills, social abilities, and motor skills. Generally, these tests accurately compare a child's intellectual and social abilities with those of typically developing children (TDC) in the same age group. However, children of different cultural backgrounds, non-English-speaking families, and very low socio-economic status are more likely to perform poorly on these tests. For these reasons, a diagnosis of intellectual disability requires that all test data be integrated with information obtained from parents and direct observations of the child. A diagnosis of intellectual disability is appropriate only when both intellectual and adaptive skills are significantly below average.

There is a strong cautionary note with respect to IQ tests as there has been a history of misuse and inappropriate placement. This has involved employing them in cultures for which the tests were not suitable and persevering with strict cut-offs when not only is there a built-in error in IQ tests, but an administrative change in cut-offs changes substantially the status of individual children. A change in the definition in 1969 from one to two standard deviations below the mean meant that some children who were previously 'retarded' under the old definition were now 'cured'. This cautionary note is very much in line with the new proposals for DSM-V.

Prevention and prognosis

Prevention applies to environmental, genetic, and infectious disorders as well as to accidental injuries. Fetal alcohol syndrome is a common and totally preventable cause of intellectual disability. The March of Dimes and other groups concerned about the prevention of intellectual

disability focus much of their efforts on alerting women to the damaging effects of ingesting alcohol or smoking during pregnancy. The effect of these behaviours can cross the blood–brain barrier and as a consequence the damaging effects of both directly impact the developing fetus. Genetic testing may also be a recommendation for those who have a family member or other children with a known inherited disorder, particularly those related to intellectual disability, such as phenylketonuria, Tay–Sachs disease, or fragile X syndrome. Identification of a gene for an inherited disorder allows genetic counsellors to help parents evaluate the risk of having an affected child. Couples who plan to have children are often advised to receive necessary vaccinations, such as against rubella. Women at risk for infectious disorders that may be harmful to a fetus, such as rubella and human immunodeficiency virus, are often tested before becoming pregnant.

Proper prenatal care lowers the risk of having a child with intellectual disability. Folic acid and vitamin supplements taken before conception and early in pregnancy can help prevent certain kinds of brain abnormalities. Advances in the practices of labour and delivery and in the care of preterm infants have reduced the rate of intellectual disability in such cases.

Tests such as ultrasound, amniocentesis, chorionic villus sampling, and various blood tests administered during pregnancy can identify conditions that often result in intellectual disability. Amniocentesis or chorionic villus sampling is often used for women at high risk of having an infant with Down syndrome, especially those aged 35 years and older, and for those with family histories of metabolic disorders. The maternal serum alpha-feto-protein is a helpful screen for neural tube defects, Down syndrome, and other abnormalities. A few conditions, such as hydrocephalus and severe Rhesus incompatibility may be treated during pregnancy. Most conditions, however, cannot be treated, and early recognition can serve only to prepare the parents for the circumstances surrounding the birth of a child with atypical developmental issues.

As some forms of intellectual disability coexist with serious physical problems, the life expectancy of children with intellectual disability may be shortened, depending on the specific condition. In general, the more severe the cognitive disability and the more physical problems the child has, the shorter the life expectancy (Landesman and Ramey 1989). However, a child with mild intellectual disability has a relatively normal life expectancy, and advances in health care have improved the long-term health outcomes for people with all types of developmental disabilities. Many people with mild to moderate intellectual disability are able to support themselves, live independently, and can be successfully employed in jobs that require basic intellectual skills.

From the above narrative regarding both definition and diagnosis it is expected that delayed motor development is a characteristic of children who are diagnosed with an intellectual disability. With a wide range of diagnostic values, especially the IQ score, it is not surprising that the inherent variability is large in young children diagnosed with intellectual disability. Owing to this variability investigations into the motor abilities of the population are often compromised. Much of the research on the motor development of children with intellectual disability has focused on a specific group of children diagnosed with Down syndrome. The range of diagnostic and behavioural characteristics for this group is somewhat narrower than the population at large diagnosed as intellectual disability. Children born with Down syndrome have IQs typically in the range of 50 to 65 and are excellent candidates for research studies because they can understand instructions in experimental protocols. As a consequence, a good deal of the research and clinical description of the motor behaviour of this population discussed in this chapter reflects knowledge about individuals with Down syndrome.

Constraints on control and coordination

Any discussion about motor behaviour must reflect the ongoing interactions among the *task*, the *performer*, and the *environment* (see Fig. 1.5 in Chapter 1 and throughout this text). The ongoing dynamic interactions among these three factors always influence both the performance and the acquisition of a motor skill. In the case of a person diagnosed with intellectual disability, the performer in this 'trinity' has the added constraint of a set of known motor and cognitive challenges.

To better understand the motor impairments that seem to be a consequence of intellectual disability a distinction is drawn between the *phylogenetic* and the *ontogenetic* aspects of motor development.

- By *phylogenetic* we refer to the evolutionary characteristics that the developing child carries with him or her as part of the evolution of the human species: from a motor or control and coordination perspective we are talking about the development of posture, locomotion, reaching and grasping, and the skill set, or what are referred to in the motor development literature as 'fundamental motor skills'.
- *Ontogenetic* motor development relates more to the development of individual skill sets that form part of, and are necessary for, an individual's activity in their own societal or cultural context. With respect to individuals diagnosed with intellectual disability we are

referring to the necessary skill development of activities of daily living: skills needed for employment, and skills that enhance opportunities for successful social interaction and participation in recreational and sport-related activities, which themselves promote relationships and friendships.

PHYLOGENETIC ASPECTS OF MOTOR DEVELOPMENT

Fundamental motor skills

There is strong evidence from a variety of sources to show that children with intellectual disabilities have delays in the achievement of major motor milestones. The general picture is that the more severe the intellectual disability the greater the delay that particular group will have in achieving motor milestones, and they will also exhibit lower motor ability. For example, Sugden and Wann (1987) examined children with mild intellectual disability (ages 8 and 12 and with mean IQs of 63 and 65, respectively) on the Test of Motor Impairment (Stott et al 1984). The recommended cut-off for TDC is at the 5% level, and, when this was used with the children with intellectual disability, the percentages that fell below this point were 30 for the 8-year-olds and nearly 50 for the 12-year-olds. Thus not only were children with intellectual difficulties showing motor difficulties at least six times the prevalence of TDC, but, from this study, they appear to be worse as they get older.

Of those individuals who fall into the mild category (approximately 85% of the intellectual disability population), a good number are persons with Down syndrome. An added advantage of studying individuals with Down syndrome is that they represent a much less variable subset of those with mild intellectual disability (IQs between 50 and 75). This permits a more robust set of research conclusions because the participants share a more stable set of traits and behaviours. In such a recognized group as Down syndrome, we find that there are marked delays in achieving mastery of fundamental skills. For example, Carr (1970) calculated age and movement quotients of children with Down syndrome using the Bayley Scales. The test items included early posture and locomotion as well as manual skills and the two major characteristics of children with Down syndrome were delay and variability. Carr (1975) also suggested that the rate of achieving and learning skills was slower in children with Down syndrome, which in effect means that, as they get older, the gap between them and their typically developing peers becomes wider.

Individuals with Down syndrome have a more closely defined profile of physical characteristics: they are typically shorter in height, and have higher levels of hypotonia and ligamentous laxity (thought to contribute to reduced coordination and control), which in turn produces hypermobility and may account for delays in postural control and locomotion when compared with typically developing peers. What is surprising is that studies investigating hypotonia of muscle mass do not reveal striking differences in controlling muscle stiffness. One might reasonably expect reduced performance of activities requiring both kinematic (coordination) and kinetic (control) to be directly related to differences in monitoring such kinetic factors as muscle stiffness.

Studies by Davis and Kelso (1982) and Latash and Corcos (1991) report that the ability to generate a range of length–tension values in reproducing specific joint angles showed no differences between a group of participants with Down syndrome and age-matched typically developing controls. Participants with Down syndrome can regulate muscle stiffness equally as well as their typically developing peers; the only difference of note was that the participants with Down syndrome were less capable of such regulation over extreme values, suggesting a limitation in range only. Joint laxity can lead to a variety of orthopaedic problems, which can limit participation in sport and recreation activities. Obesity is also a problem that occurs with early termination of growth coupled with reduced levels of physical activity.

Development of these motor skills includes the fundamental motor 'milestones' noted by the early developmental theorists who we discussed in Chapter 1. The overall progress of the phylogenetic aspects of motor development when we compare children with Down syndrome to their typically developing peers is illustrated in Table 9.1 from data compiled by Henderson (1986).

Developmental milestones
As can be readily observed from Table 9.1 the developmental delays between children with Down syndrome and their typically developing peers on a range of both gross and fine motor skills can vary, on average, by as little as 2 months (e.g. holding the head steady) to as much as 19 months for the first time a child can walk independently (36mo for Down syndrome and 17mo for TDC). In addition the age range for attaining these 'milestones' is greater for children with Down syndrome than TDC. Recall that one of the key themes of this book is the important relationship between movement and cognitive development (what we refer to as '*embodied cognition*'); it should come as no surprise therefore that the

TABLE 9.1
Selected developmental milestones for children with Down syndrome

	Children with Down syndrome		Typically developing children	
	Average age (mo)	Range (mo)	Average age (mo)	Range (mo)
Gross motor activities				
Holds his or her head steady	5	3–9	3	1–4
Pulls to stand	8	4–12	5	2–10
Stands alone	18	12–38	11	9–16
Walks alone	19	13–48	12	9–17
Walks upstairs, assisted	30	20–48	17	12–24
Fine motor activities				
Grasps a hanging ring	6	4–11	4	2–6
Passes objects from hand to hand	8	6–12	5.5	4–8
Pulls the string of a toy	12	7–17	7	5–10
Builds a tower of cubes	20	14–32	14	10–19
Copies a circle	48	30–60+	30	24–40
Personal/social/self-help activities				
Smiles spontaneously	3	2–6	2	1–5
Feeds his- or herself a biscuit	10	6–14	5	4–10
Plays pat-a-cake and/or peek-a-boo	11	9–16	8	5–13
Drinks from a cup	20	12–30	12	9–17
Uses a spoon or fork	20	12–36	13	8–20

Adapted from Henderson (1986).

developmental lag in phylogenetic motor development between children with Down syndrome and TDC (i.e. sitting upright, postural control, independent walking) is mirrored by delays in cognitive development.

Hypotonia and reflexes

There has been a long-held view that the early motor development of children with Down syndrome is characterized by hypotonia and an abnormal timetable for the emergence and dissolution of reflexes. Hypotonia in later childhood can lead to limitations in motor skill, and it is possible that some of the unusual postures that children with Down syndrome exhibit when sitting, for example, could be the result of hypotonia. The development of reflexes in children with Down syndrome are often delayed (Cowie 1970) and often this is noted as being related to delays overall in motor development.

The usual assumption made for these developmental delays observed in children with intellectual disability has been that the underlying cause can be attributed to neurological deficits. Although this may well be logical as it is based on clinical observation and evaluation, it is only more recently that attempts have been made to seek data-based (empirical) confirmation of this assumption. The impetus for this line of investigation came initially from the work of the late Esther Thelen, on the origin of the step reflex (Thelen 1986). It should be noted here that the 'step reflex' is a phylogenetic characteristic present in the neurological system of all humans. Thelen and her research team at Indiana University reported that the seemingly 'random' supine kicking of newborn infants was an identifiable rhythmic (periodic) activity, closely resembling the frequency of the step reflex that is the coordinative mechanism that supports the emergence of locomotion in young infants at a point when TDC are physically mature enough to both stand upright independently and begin to walk. Thelen provided empirical support for this line of thinking by supporting young, prewalking infants over a small treadmill and demonstrating that the motion of the treadmill would elicit in the infant a step cycle that was the movement response that enables the young infants to walk. Employing the protocol developed by Thelen for TDC infants, Ulrich et al (1992) investigated the step reflex in children diagnosed with Down syndrome. In addition, they reported on a treadmill training programme for infants with Down syndrome (Ulrich et al 2001). The results of these two studies are summarized in Box 9.1.

In the first half of this text we referred to the work of Karen Adolph (Adolph and Berger 2006), who noted that in some instances the role of experience was just as important, and sometimes more important, than neural/maturational variables or biomechanical variables.

Studies such as the one by Ulrich in Box 9.1 would seem to bear this out.

Postural development

Again, with postural development there has always been an assumption that the main driver for any delay or limitation was the neural system. Sugden and Keogh (1990) reported on studies that looked at severity of disability and neurological functioning and concluded that 'cognitive ability is a less important determinant of the ability to walk than is neural integrity' (p. 77).

Although they were correct in noting that a minimum cognitive requirement is not necessary for walking, they did not take into consideration other factors that may determine early postural control and the onset of walking.

Other research comparing aspects of postural development (a precursor to independent walking) has shown similar results that call into question the assumption that these delays are due to a neurological deficit. Butterworth and Cicchetti (1978) reported that discrepant visual feedback appeared more disruptive to infants with Down syndrome than TDC when they were standing, compared with when they were sitting. They argued that postural control is dependent on congruence between the variables affecting postures, such as vestibular and vision, and that infants with Down syndrome have a higher threshold for detecting discrepancies. When they were seated in a more stable position the effects were minimal, but when standing only a minor change was necessary for the child with Down syndrome to become unstable. They did not detect the minor change and make the necessary adjustment, thus becoming unstable.

Several studies reviewed and reported by Newell (1997) lead to a general conclusion that the underlying *phylogenetic* mechanisms, in most cases, do not reliably distinguish between TDC and children with intellectual disability, and this leads to the conclusion that the developmental range of progression suggests more of an overlap of the two groups, rather than a clear division between the two. This makes the study of children with intellectual disability more challenging than merely concluding that the differences are embedded in a theory that argues for deficit in neurological substrates. Note also that no single theory or aetiology can explain what clinical observation has confirmed many times over: namely that children with a diagnosis of intellectual disability show a substantial lag in both motor and general cognitive development.

Reaching and grasping

Early research on reaching and grasping from the Hester Adrian Centre at the University of Manchester in England invariably came to the conclusion that children with Down

Box 9.1 A closer examination

Infant walking: Ulrich et al (1992)

In their 1992 study Ulrich et al replicated the Thelen and Ulrich (1991) study using infants with Down syndrome as participants. Testing the infants with Down syndrome once a month they demonstrated that much like their typically developing peers they responded to the treadmill by producing steps without the benefit of practice. Overall the participants with Down syndrome demonstrated treadmill stepping consistently at 14 months, albeit later than their typically developing peers, but clearly the infants with Down syndrome were eliciting a pattern of behaviour similar to functional locomotion. Ulrich et al (1992) demonstrated that six out of a group of seven infants with Down syndrome, 11 months old, showed a similar step reflex response to the typically developing infants tested earlier by Thelen and Ulrich (1991). This was later confirmed in a second study by Ulrich and Ulrich (1995). The conclusion was that, from a neurological perspective, the substrate necessary to permit walking was present in both infants with Down syndrome and TDC probably very early in development (in utero), and this challenged the long-held assumption that the onset of locomotion was predicated on a certain level of neurological development. In a follow-up study, Ulrich et al (2001) employed a treadmill training paradigm, whereby cooperating parents trained their children on a customized treadmill, having been trained by the research team to both position their child on the treadmill and carry out the training protocol. Participants with Down syndrome were randomly assigned to two groups (training and control), with both groups receiving paediatric physical therapy, but the training group practiced on the treadmill for 8 minutes per day, 5 days per week until the infants could walk independently as defined by item number 62 on the Bayley Scale of Infant Development (Bayley 1993). The main results are illustrated in Figure 9.1. The three measures recorded were 'raises self to stand', 'walks with help', and 'walks independently'.

As can be observed, the experimental training group completed all three of the criterion measures well ahead of the control group. The differences all favoured the training group with two of the three criterion measures (walk with help and walk unaided) showing a significant difference. The first criterion, 'raises self to stand', showed an advantage for the training group but the difference was not significant.

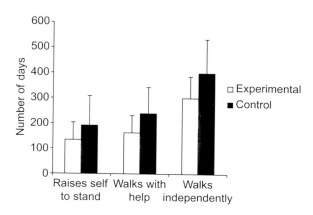

Fig. 9.1 Progression to upright locomotion in typically developing children and children with Down Syndrome. Redrawn from data from Ulrich (2001).

syndrome are more variable and delayed in their manipulation skills than their typically developing peers. There was some evidence that infants with Down syndrome were not only slower in achieving reaching and grasping milestones (Cunningham 1979) but they were also more variable in age of achievement. For example the 12 infants with Down syndrome could reach and make contact with an object at almost 24 months and reach and grasp at 3 years and 6 months. The respective milestones in their 12 typically developing peers were 16 months and 24 months. In addition, the standard deviations of the children with Down syndrome were three times those of TDC and the range was four times the size.

Grips were also examined by the same Hester Adrian group; Moss and Hogg (1981) compared grips of children with Down syndrome with those of a group of TDC up to 4 years of age. Their overall finding was that children with Down syndrome increased their number of grips with age, but they used fewer precision grips than the TDC group. Four of the grips are illustrated in Figure 9.2, with two palmar and two digital grips shown. Older TDC used the two digital grips over 30% of the time, whereas the children with Down syndrome only used them half as often even though they were on average 6 months older.

Sugden and Keogh (1990) concluded that children with Down syndrome were both delayed and more variable in the performance of their manual skills; they showed less visual anticipation; and, as they became older, they used fewer precision grips and continued to use grips that appeared to be immature and less effective. In conclusion they note that 'it appears that there are qualitative differences in reaching and grasping rather than just a general slowness in rate of development' (p. 85).

This statement is supported by Charlton et al (2000), who were interested in whether children with Down syndrome were qualitatively different to TDC in their reaching and grasping. Their reach was more jerky and variable and there was a greatly reduced use of precision grips compared with age-matched TDC. However, they found that the overall timing of the reach was influenced by task goals and object properties, the same as TDC such that, when different sizes of objects were presented, both TDC and children with Down syndrome were able to use the intrinsic properties of the object size. Children with Down syndrome are delayed in their reaching and grasping and are more variable in both temporal and spatial aspects of reaching and grasping. However, the finding that they are susceptible to similar body-scaled ratios and object properties as TDC may provide cues for intervention. Neural explanations do not seem to offer the final say in the matter.

This work by Charlton et al (2000) is in line with research that has addressed questions focusing on the link between perception and action – research that investigates skilled actions in a manner different from earlier research. In a similar vein Newell (1997) reviewed the results of several studies on adults and children with intellectual disability that strongly suggested that the underlying phylogenetic mechanisms *do not*, in most cases, always reliably distinguish between TDC and children with intellectual disability. There is more overlap between the two groups than separate categorization, and as noted this presents a severe challenge to theoretical explanations of the observed differences in children with intellectual disability who show a substantial lag in both motor and general cognitive development. It would appear that opportunities for action perceived by the actor diagnosed with intellectual disability are essentially similar to those observed in their typically developing peers. This observation from Newell's (1997) review focuses less on measures that report performance errors (e.g. changes in RT or MT) and more on the ability of the individual to detect, or be sensitive to, the perceptual information that permits accurate execution of the demands of the task in question, and the scaled relationship between the action required and the demands of the task.

Two examples of studies that have investigated the perceptual motor behaviour in children with Down

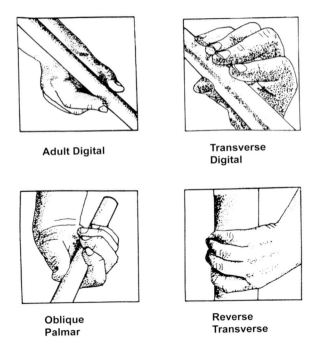

Fig. 9.2 Four grips observed by Moss and Hogg. Reproduced with permission of the publisher from Moss and Hogg (1981).

syndrome are by Savelsbergh et al (2000) and Wade et al (2000). These are reviewed more closely in Box 9.2.

The role of posture and the influence of optical flow in individuals with intellectual disability have not been widely studied in the research literature. Butterworth and Cicchetti (1978) suggested a relationship in the strength of coupling between optical flow and its impact on postural motion as a direct function of developmental age in the months when infants transition from sitting to standing. Infants with Down syndrome might possibly need to rely more on visual information longer than typically developing infants as they begin to develop independent walking. Alternatively, the recorded differences may be due more to general aspects of postural control, that is a consequence of general muscle strength and coordination. Clearly, more research on these problems needs to be directed at this population. Similarities and differences between individuals diagnosed with intellectual disability and their typically developing peers, and the underlying causes, remain equivocal. There is substantial evidence that functional perceptual–motor coupling is consistent, irrespective of diagnosis; errors in performance focus more on the inherent slow responsiveness of children and adults diagnosed with intellectual disability. This is borne out by the studies reported in the two Boxes 9.1 and 9.2 discussed above. It is clear that children with intellectual disability do have differences and some performance

Box 9.2 A closer examination

Coupling of information and movement: Savelsbergh et al (2000) and Wade et al (2000)

The Savelsbergh et al (2000) paper reviewed a series of studies that examined functional coupling of information and movement. The authors reviewed studies that focused on the reaching and grasping of objects (prehension), catching, and postural control, as it relates to the role of vision and optical flow. With respect to reaching and grasping, participants were asked to reach for and grasp a series of small cups of varying size – scaled to both above and below the hand size of each participant. The question asked in this study was: does a body-scaled relationship exist between the width of the cup to be grasped and the hand width of the participant? The study recorded the point at which the reaching child switched from a one-hand to a two-hand reach and grasp. This study was essentially the same as the study by Newell et al (1989) reviewed earlier in Chapter 4. They demonstrated a strong body-scaled relationship between the grasping ability of young, typically developing infants and the size of the object being grasped. The results of Savelsbergh et al (2000) concerning children with Down syndrome are illustrated in Figure 9.3. The data demonstrate that the 'dimensionless' variable (the ratio of cup width to hand size) was essentially the same for both the participants with Down syndrome and TDC, suggesting some level of phylogenetic invariance.

With respect to catching (Fig. 9.4), participants with Down syndrome recorded more errors than their typically developing peers – due in all likelihood to timing errors such as completing the catch too late. When the focus was on the use of the temporal information available to complete the catch, the differences were not apparent between the two groups. Errors by the Down syndrome group were more likely to be a result of slowness of movement. No differences were seen in anticipatory timing.

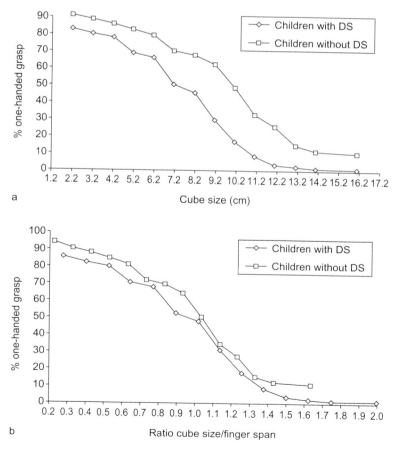

Fig. 9.3 Cup width to hand size. DS, Down syndrome. Reproduced with permission of the publisher from Savelsbergh et al (2000).

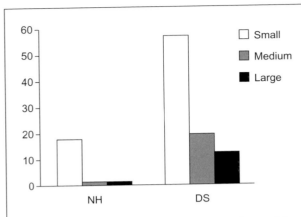

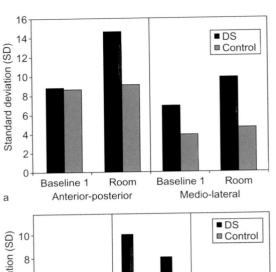

Fig. 9.4 Catching errors. Reproduced with permission of the publisher from Savelsbergh et al (2000).

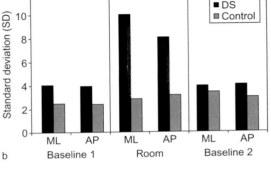

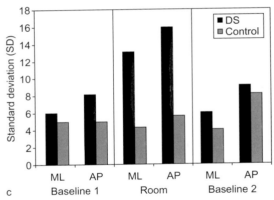

A study on the role of optical flow and its influence on postural control was reported by Wade et al (2000). This study recorded the postural motion of two groups of young participants (Down syndrome and age-matched TDC) in a moving room protocol originally developed by Lee and Lishman (1975). Postural motion was recorded as changes in optical flow were generated from three separate room motion conditions: *radial flow* (front wall only), *lamellar flow* (side wall only), and *global flow* (whole-room movement). The results (Fig. 9.5) of the Wade et al study showed that the Down syndrome group recorded significantly higher levels of postural motion than the matched TDC group. These data supported the Butterworth and Cicchetti (1978) data for postural response to optical flow when standing.

The three graphs in Figure 9.5 depict motion recorded as ground reaction force (a); standard deviation of acceleration at the hip (b); and standard deviation of acceleration at the head (c). In all three graphs it is clear that the participants with Down syndrome record higher postural motion than their matched typically developing peers, and Wade et al (2000) concluded that the reason for these large differences may be attention-related issues rather than a direct response to imposed optical flow.

Fig. 9.5 Ground reaction force (a), standard deviation of acceleration at the hip (b), and standard deviation and acceleration at the head (c). Reproduced with permission of the publisher from Wade et al (2000).

deficits in their motor skills. However, through work looking at how children with intellectual disabilities detect information and pick up relevant information by actively exploring the environment, we can provide them with guidelines about their own movement capabilities in order to improve their skills.

Burton (1990) designed a study to quantify the perceptual sensitivity of children with intellectual disability and TDC. The movement constraints were in the form of a barrier, scaled to the height of each individual participant. The scaled relationship was between the height of the participant and the height of the barrier, in much the same way as cup width and hand width in the grasping studies reported by Savelsbergh et al (2000). The results of this study are presented in Box 9.3.

We are left with a puzzle. In the language of science we say the results are 'equivocal'. Some research suggests that the differences among groups of intellectual disability may be anchored primarily in the general slowness of the participants with intellectual disability ('knowing how') and not in their ability to couple perceptual information to their movements; other data suggest just the opposite – namely perceptual difficulties ('knowing what') account for the discrepancies in motor performance! Accurately perceiving the movement constraints in the environment may explain more about the observed movement deficits than the actual ability to perform the required activity or skill. As Newell (1997) has noted

> There are many factors, however, that can delay the development of the fundamental posture, locomotion prehension, and communication skills. The theoretical implications of the relationship between cognitive deficits and motor delays is not, however, as straightforward as it might first appear.
>
> (p. 222)

ONTOGENETIC ASPECTS OF MOTOR DEVELOPMENT
This area of study is concerned more with how individuals diagnosed with intellectual disability learn the motor skill activities that can support self-sufficiency such as activities of daily living: washing, dressing, shopping, eating, and the many activities necessary to live independently. In addition, the motor activities necessary for work and recreation all require learning the necessary motor skills to be employed or to participate in a sport or recreational activity. The central question here is: 'What can be trained or learned?' As with phylogenetic motor abilities, lower average performance and greater variability are characteristics of individuals with intellectual disability when performing and learning ontogenetic activities.

Box 9.3 A closer examination

Assessing the perceptual–motor interaction in children with intellectual disability and TDC: Burton (1990)
The purpose of this experiment was to design a gross motor task that would quantify the perceptual sensitivity of children with intellectual disability and TDC to the relationship between their personal constraints and the constraints in the environment in a movement context.

Participants
Three groups of young children were volunteer participants in this experiment: 17 preschool children with intellectual disability (mean age 6y), 25 typically developing kindergarteners (mean age 6y 3mo), and 27 typically developing fourth graders (mean age 10y 6mo). The participants with intellectual disability included two children with Down syndrome and all qualified for early-childhood special education by demonstrating either developmental delay or a sensory, physical, social, or mental condition or impairment. The subjects moved through a sequence of four high-jump barriers six times, as quickly as possible, negotiating the barriers any way they wanted. They also went through the course without the barriers as quickly as possible to establish a baseline movement time.

Results and comments
Relative to their own baseline, the fourth-graders moved through the obstacle course significantly faster than the kindergarteners, whereas the kindergarteners (matched by mental age) navigated the course significantly faster than the preschool children with intellectual disability. In addition, significant differences were found between the typically developing kindergarteners and the preschool children with intellectual disability for two sets of perceptual variables: percentage error and the slopes of two identified transitions from one mode of locomotion to another. These results and further analyses showed that at least some of the movement problems experienced by children with intellectual disability can be attributed to perceptual difficulties, and established the potential of the present methodology in examining perceptual sensitivity in a movement context in children with intellectual disability and TDC. Burton's findings suggested that differences between the two groups were explained more by perceptual difficulties than movement problems: more to do with 'knowing what' to do rather than 'knowing how' to do it.

Research that spans almost 75 years from the 1930s (Tizard and O'Connor 1950) to the present has focused on the cognitive deficits of this group and the influence that cognitive deficits have on motor performance. The central issue is the 'slowness' and inherent 'variability' of a host of performance measures that distinguish between those diagnosed as intellectual disability and their typically developing peers. These differences were documented by researchers in the 1930s (Tizard 1953, Tizard and Loos 1954), and similar conclusions from research in each decade since, from the 1950s, 1960s, and 1970s up to the present day, report these finding within a theoretical framework known as information processing.

Reaction time and movement time
On the performance of individuals diagnosed with intellectual disability on tasks that recorded reaction time and movement time, all reported that individuals with intellectual disability had difficulties in responding quickly and accurately on motor tasks that ranged in levels of difficulty and complexity. The attempt by researchers here was to both investigate the nature and scope of this response slowness and determine if some elements of this slowness were trainable or should be considered 'hard-wired', that is resistant to training. The response rate of participants with intellectual disability is slower than normal controls and becomes increasingly so as the number of response choices increases. This manifestation of both Hick's law (Hick 1952) with respect to reaction time and Fitts' law (Fitts 1954, Fitts and Peterson 1964) with respect to movement time is well documented in the research literature. Studies by Hoover et al (1981) and Wade et al (1984) report on both the reaction time and movement time of individuals diagnosed with intellectual disability for tasks requiring both speed and accuracy. Similarly, Sugden and Gray (1981) reported on movement times for males with mild intellectual disability (chronological age 13 years, cognitive age 9 years). They showed that the males had larger absolute movement times than their typically developing peers (reported by Sugden 1980) and their movement times were more related to their cognitive age than their chronological age. Yet, the basic principles of Fitts' law were found with a log linear relationship between the index of difficulty and MT, as measured by the formula $\log(2A/W)$, where A was the distance moved and W was the width of the target. However, the slope of the regression line for the males with intellectual disability was steeper than for the TDC, indicating that as the task increased in difficulty the increase in movement time was greater for them than for the TDC. A final interesting finding was that for the males with intellectual disability, just as in the TDC, the reaction times did not increase

with movement difficulty prior to the movement. One can make the same interpretation as with the TDC that this was a simple reaction time task and the males knew in advance what the movement was going to be.

Another example of this type of research (Wallace et al 1978) found that children with intellectual disability are slower than age-matched controls on both reaction- and movement-time tasks. Again, movement time increased with the level of movement difficulty, but reaction time stayed relatively constant throughout all conditions. The 'slowness' problem in individuals with intellectual disability permeates their skill performance across a wide range of ontogenetic activities. As a result, it is a serious constraint on their opportunities to be gainfully employed, their level of independent living, and their ability to participate in sport and recreation, all of which are important avenues to develop friendships and social networks. These limitations of motor skill performance become a serious impediment to overall social development.

From the perspective of employability the application of task analysis is one approach to maximize opportunities for individuals with mild to moderate intellectual disability. Task analysis of certain kinds of assembly-line work was reported by Wade and Gold (1978). Participants in this study responded positively to structured training protocols for the purpose of a bicycle brake assembly task. The research reported by Hoover et al (1981) and Wade et al (1984) demonstrated that movement time can be reduced in populations of participants with intellectual disability with training and that focused practice can positively influence the conservative speed/accuracy trade-off typical of participants with intellectual disability reported in the research literature.

Published motor skills research reports reliable differences between individuals with intellectual disability and their typically developing peers in both the performance and the learning of several motor skill variables such as the accurate tracking of a target; the timing accuracy required for precise movement control (Wade 1980); and understanding and using augmented feedback (Hoover et al 1981). The general conclusion has been that individuals with intellectual disability are 'clumsy'; display a reduced performance level across a range of skilled activities; take longer (require more trials) to reach a performance criterion level; and exhibit greater variability in the process.

Variability
Variability can take many forms, and indeed one can argue that variability is not simply a hindrance to performance but, when learning a skill, certain forms of variability may be beneficial. For example, when we perform an action, we can arrange the limbs, or constrain the degrees of

freedom, to achieve a specified skill outcome in different ways. The variability of the response may be seen as an advantage when confronted by novel situations. However, the kind of variability we are discussing here is different, and can be divided into two parts. The first is group variability, which involves a particular subgroup of the general population being more variable, that is recording a higher standard deviation, than the population at large. This is what we often find in a population of children with intellectual disability. The second is the variability within the individual (intravariance). This type of variability represents an individual being unable to consistently perform the skill. With reference to an individual child with intellectual disability, he or she cannot perform in a systematic manner in the process of acquiring a particular skill.

An example of one type of variability in motor performance on a coincidence-timing task was shown by Sugden et al (1983). They worked with a group of children with mild intellectual disability (IQs ranging from 55 to 70) whose performances were evaluated and compared with those of a group of chronologically age-matched peers and a third group of younger participants matched for cognitive age.

Overall, the mean performance of the children with intellectual disability was twice that of their chronologically matched peers and was essentially the same as the cognitive-age-matched group. Variability was expressed by calculating a coefficient of variation ([standard deviation/mean]×100). Again as a group, the children with intellectual disability were more variable; however, when the five least variable and five most variable children were removed from each of the three groups a different set of results were obtained. The five most variable children from the intellectual disability group and the cognitive-age-matched controls were much more variable than the chronologically age-matched control group. These results not only show higher performance variability for children with intellectual disability and younger cognitive-age children compared with older ones, but the results have important implications for the analysis of data with the suggestion that, rather than relying on total-group analysis, subgroup analysis might provide better insights regarding performance. These results are shown in Figure 9.6.

With respect to slowness of response and variability of performance, both the phylogenetic and the ontogenetic aspects of motor behaviour in individuals diagnosed with intellectual disability share common traits. As noted earlier, the bulk of the research reported in the literature concerning the motor behaviour of persons with intellectual disability, both children and adults, has focused on those individuals with Down syndrome, who typically record

IQ scores that range between 50 and 75. The reason being that individuals in that IQ range can reliably complete the experimental protocols used, as well as understand and follow the necessary instructions to participate in such studies.

Movement stereotypies
For those individuals diagnosed with intellectual disability and with IQs below 50, research is limited in terms of the research protocols that can be attempted. One characteristic that has received quite a lot of empirical attention is stereotypy. Stereotypic behaviour is common among the population with intellectual disabilities, especially those with IQs that place them in the moderate to profound category (IQ 50 and below). Individuals living in institutional settings have an especially high incidence of such behaviours. As with the repetitive 'pacing' of caged animals in a zoo, institutionalized individuals also exhibit repetitive behaviours such as rocking and head-banging, and waving. These behaviours form classes of activities that are both rhythmic and likely provide self-stimulation for the individual. The debate whether such activities are abnormal or normal is ongoing. Newell (1997) provides an excellent review of this issue with respect to the stereotypic behaviour that is characteristic of profound intellectual disability, but also stereotypic behaviour that is a direct result of neuroleptic medication (tardive dyskinesia). The use of drugs to treat and control people with severe intellectual disability has produced, over the long term, a class of movement disorders known as *tardive dyskinesia*, characterized by both rhythmic and jerk-like movements, especially facial, and around the eyes, lips, and tongue.

In terms of studying motor development, stereotypic behaviour is clearly different from what we might consider a motor act, which has a specified intent to achieve an outcome, for example buttoning a shirt or throwing a ball through a ring. Nevertheless, as Newell (1997) points out, 'from a behavioral standpoint, superfluous involuntary rhythmical motions exist in both drug induced tardive dyskinesia and non-drug induced repetitive behavior' (pp. 289–290).

Summary and future directions
By way of summary, the study of motor development, with respect to individuals diagnosed with intellectual disability, has produced a great deal of disparate research findings. It is clear that both motor and general cognitive behaviours are limited as a direct function of the level of disability, as measured by an IQ score. That being said, the range of abilities and the range of IQ scores are not closely correlated. Furthermore, not all individuals who are poorly coordinated and appear clumsy are diagnosed

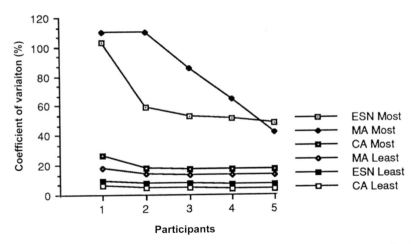

Fig. 9.6 Coefficient of variation for the five most variable and five least variable children arranged by rank order for children with moderate intellectual disability (ESN), cognitive age (CoA), and chronological age of typically developing children (CA) (Sugden et al 1983).

with intellectual disability. No single theory can account for a unified set of conclusions with respect to the motor development of this population. It is also true to say that no single theory drives practice for those who provide training and therapeutic intervention for our citizenry with intellectual disability. Much of the research on intellectual disability has been restricted to an isolated segment of the population. The research on individuals with Down syndrome may not be typical of the population with intellectual disability at large. The need to differentiate between aetiology and severity remains a challenge for both the research community and the clinicians who seek to improve both treatment and the quality of life of this group of individuals.

The research and clinical evaluation of individuals diagnosed with intellectual disability shows that from both a motor and an intellectual perspective they lag behind their typically developing peers, especially with respect to their ontogenetic skill sets, compared with their phylogenetic skill development. This places serious constraints on their ability to acquire the skills of daily living and gain independence for both living and employment. One can ask the question as to why this is the case and a number of answers are possible.

First, one can make the point that any constitutional damage during the developmental period is not always going to be so selective that it impacts only the cognitive and intellectual systems. Thus, in any population of individuals with severe to profound difficulties, it will be the rule rather than the exception that there is some form of constitutional problem, be it genetic, chromosomal, or undifferentiated brain damage. Second, this argument is more difficult to make with children showing more mild

intellectual difficulties when only a small proportion will have a known constitutional problem, and as we have seen, many of them are indistinguishable from their typically developing peers in the performance of motor skills. Third, for those that do show additional motor difficulties, one can make the argument that most motor skills contain elements of 'knowing' as well as 'doing' and by definition this group has difficulties with that. Finally, the concept of embodied cognition (one that we have supported throughout this book) argues that the separation of the motor and cognitive domains is not one that appears reasonable.

The issues discussed in this chapter describe a variety of research studies and instruments pinpointing the problems that create the barriers that prevent persons with intellectual disability from living an independent life. Having said that, it should also be noted that great progress has been made from the days, not so long ago, when individuals with IQ scores in the 60 to 70 range typically found themselves living in institutions for most of their adult lives; this was especially true for persons with Down syndrome. Modern approaches to providing community living environments and employment opportunities have improved dramatically the quality of life for many of our citizens with intellectual disability. In addition, government action has mandated an increased level of educational services that is more inclusive as to the educational experiences that children with intellectual disability can receive. From a practical point of view opportunities have increased with respect to education, independent living, and social and recreational development. This is another example of the model and philosophy that we have portrayed throughout: the person–task–environment transaction, or, to put it more bluntly, the motor skill outcomes or problems of any child, rarely, if ever, reside solely in the person, child, or adult. From a research perspective progress has been quite slow. Children with intellectual disability do have motor impairment, but they do develop and do not, as a group, remain static at the bottom end of any developmental scale. Like TDC, some develop fast at the beginning and then slow down, whereas others are slow beginners and speed up. As with other disabilities, participation is a crucial factor in their development and this involves the changing environmental and task variables.

Newell (1997) summarized the state of our knowledge with respect to the study of intellectual deficits as follows:

> We are a long way from understanding the limits of motor performance and training effects on the movement speed in people with mental retardation. The relation between hypertonia and slowness of movement has not been sufficiently explored experimentally inspite of its intuitive theoretical link. The examination of training or long term practice studies would also be useful to help unravel the source of constraint on movement speed in people with mental retardation.
>
> (p. 300)

Since Newell's (1997) review little has changed; we are writing this text in 2013 and, while motor skills research on individuals with developmental disabilities has remained somewhat dormant, there are new ideas and approaches that can influence the way forward. Throughout this text we have referred to the concept of 'embodied cognition' (the relationship between motor activity, or action, and cognitive development). We described in Chapter 4 of this book how behavioural flexibility developed in growing children primarily through them learning the limits of their motor abilities, and how this directly connected to a broader development of their cognitive abilities. The development of ecological task analysis (ETA) (Davis and Burton 1991) is influencing how we assess movement problems in people with intellectual disability. The central tenet of ETA focuses more closely on the relative rather than the absolute performance relationships in analysing motor behaviour. An excellent example of this would be the stair climbing study by Warren (1984) entitled 'Perceiving affordances: visual guidance of stair climbing'. In this study Warren (1984) reports that the absolute analysis of the participants in this study would suggest that the taller individuals switched from a bipedal to a quadrupedal pattern of climbing stairs at a significantly higher stair height than the shorter participants (see Fig. 9.7a). However, when a

relative analysis was computed by dividing the maximum stair height by the leg length of the participants the two groups of subjects did not differ with respect to their transition point of changing from bipedal to quadrupedal, as can be seen in Figure 9.7.

The 'take-home message' here is that a relative analysis reflecting this dynamic relationship yields a different conclusion. The small relative difference (88% of leg length) contrasts with the between-groups analysis that readily differentiated at an absolute level of analysis, showing the differences between the short and tall participants. Clearly, how we choose our measurement instruments greatly influences our results and conclusions. Similarly, how we choose our intervention programmes will take into consideration the same kinds of variables (see Chapter 12).

This is an important feature of employing a dynamical systems approach to understanding problems of coordination and control in all individuals irrespective of their intellectual abilities. The departure point from the more traditional approach to studying motor behaviour is to recognize that perception is directly connected to action, and not separate from it. Studies of motor behaviour of people, both typically developed and those with a range of intellectual disabilities, have usually investigated specific modalities, and have not studied performance or learning paradigms from the perspective of functional information. Traditional models of (indirect) perception required the presence of symbols and devices in the neurology to determine meaning to what is perceived. An ecologically influenced dynamical systems approach views perceptual information as coupled directly to action. Accordingly, the way we measure the variables of interest are different when contrasting these two approaches. Davis and Van Emmerik (1995a,b) noted that *extrinsic* measures are absolute measures of time, distance, or energy, whereas *intrinsic* measures are taken in reference to an actor, assuming the coupling relationship between perception and action. This is illustrated in the Warren (1984) study presented in Figure 9.7. This kind of analysis and style of inquiry has been essentially absent from research on the motor development of those children diagnosed with intellectual disability. A welcome exception to date has been the work by Ulrich and coworkers (see Box 9.1) who employed the 'stepping reflex' paradigm with young infants with Down syndrome. As was the case with the research studies featured in Box 9.1, other functional relationships might well be present in the coordination dynamics of children with intellectual disability. Understanding intellectual disability from a more contemporary theoretical perspective will not be any less challenging, but the field of candidate variables will be different.

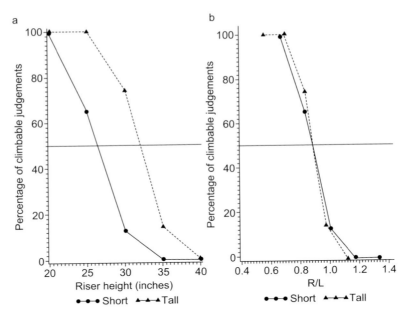

Fig. 9.7 Mean percentage of 'climbable' judgments as a function of (a) riser height and (b) a ratio of riser height (R) divided by leg length (L). Reproduced with permission of the publisher from Warren (1984).

REFERENCES

Adolph KE (2005) Learning to learn in the development of action. In: Lockman J, Reiser J, editors. *Action as an Organizer Of Learning and Development: The 32nd Minnesota Symposium of Child Development*. Hillsdale, NJ: Lawrence Erlbaum Associates, pp. 91–122.

Adolph KE, Berger SE (2006) Motor development. In: Kuhn D, Siegler RS, editors. *Handbook of Child Psychology, Volume 2: Cognition, Perception and Language*, 6th edition. New York: Wiley, pp. 161–213.

APA (2000) *Diagnostic and Statistical Manual of Mental Disorders: DSM IV*, 4th edition text revision. Arlington, VA: American Psychiatric Association.

Bayley N (1993) *Bayley Scales of Infant Development*, 2nd edition. San Antonio, TX: Therapy Skill Builders.

Burton AW (1990) Assessing the perceptual–motor interaction in developmentally disabled and non-handicapped children. *Adapted Phys Activity Q* 7: 325–337.

Butterworth G, Cicchetti D (1978) Visual calibration of posture in normal and motor retarded Down's syndrome infants. *Perception* 7: 513–525. http://dx.doi.org/10.1068/p070513

Carr J (1970) Mental and motor development in young mongol children. *J Ment Defic Res* 14: 205–220.

Charlton JL, Ibsen E, Lavelle BM (2000) Control of manual skills in children with Down's syndrome. In: Weeks D, Chua R, Elliot DG, editors. *Perceptual-Motor Behavior in Down Syndrome*. Champaign, IL: Human Kinetics, pp. 25–48.

Cowie VA (1970) *A Study of Early Development of Mongols*. Oxford: Pergamon Press.

Cunningham C (1979) Aspects of early development in Down's Syndrome infants. PhD dissertation, University of Manchester, Manchester, UK.

Davis WE, Burton AW (1991) Ecological task analysis: translating movement behavior theory into practice. *Adapted Phys Activity Q* 8: 154–177.

Davis WE, Kelso JAS (1982) Analysis of "invariant characteristics" in the motor control of Down's syndrome and normal subjects. *J Motor Behav* 14: 194–211.

Davis WE, Van Emmerik REA (1995a) An ecological task analysis approach for understanding motor development in mental retardation: philosophical and theoretical underpinnings. In: Vermeer A, Davis WE, editors. *Physical and Motor Development in Persons with Mental Retardation* (*Medicine and Sport Science*). Basel: Karger, pp. 1–32.

Davis WE, Van Emmerik REA (1995b) An ecological task analysis approach for understanding motor development in mental retardation: research questions and strategies. In: Vermeer A, Davis WE, editors. *Physical and Motor Development in Persons with Mental Retardation* (*Medicine and Sport Science*). Basel: Karger, pp. 33–67.

Emerson E, Hatton C (2007) Contribution of socioeconomic position to health inequalities of British children and adolescents with intellectual disabilities. *Am J Ment Retard* 112: 140–150. http://dx.doi.org/10.1352/0895-8017(2007)112[140:COSPTH]2.0.CO;2

Fitts PM (1954) The information capacity of the human motor system in controlling the amplitude of movement. *J Exp Psychol* 47: 381–391. http://dx.doi.org/10.1037/h0055392

Fitts PM, Peterson JR (1964) Information capacity of discrete motor responses. *J Exp Psychol* 67: 103–112. http://dx.doi.org/10.1037/h0045689

Henderson SE (1986) Some aspects of the development of motor control in Down's syndrome. In: Whiting HTA, Wade MG, editors. *Themes in Motor Development*. Dordrecht, The Netherlands: Matrinus Nijhoff, pp. 69–72.

Hick WE (1952) On the rate of gain of information. *Q J Exp Psychol* 4: 11–26. http://dx.doi.org/10.1080/17470215208416600

Hoover JH, Wade MG, Newell KM (1981) Training moderately and severely mentally retarded adults to improve reaction and movement times. *Am J Ment Deficiency* 85: 389–395.

Landesman S, Ramey C (1989) Developmental psychology and mental retardation. Integrating scientific principles with treatment practices. *Am Psychol* 44: 409–415. http://dx.doi.org/10.1037/0003-066X.44.2.409

Latash ML, Corcos DM (1991) Kinematic and electromyographic characteristics of single-joint movements in Down syndrome. *Am Retard* 96: 189–201.

Lee DN, Lishman JR (1975) Visual proprioceptive control of stance. *J Hum Movement Stud* 1: 87–95.

Lejeune J, Turpin R, Gautier M (1959) Mongolism: a chromosomal disease (trisomy). *Bulletin de l'Academie Nationale de Medecine* 143: 256–265.

Moss SC, Hogg J (1981) Development of hand function in mentally handicapped and non handicapped preschool children. In: Mittler P, editor. *Frontiers of Knowledge in Mental Retardation, Volume 1.* Baltimore, MD: University Park Press, pp. 35–44.

Newell KM (1997) Motor skills and mental retardation. In: MacLean WE, editor. *Ellis' Handbook of Mental Deficiency, Psychological Theory and Research.* Mahwah, NJ: Lawrence Erlbaum Associates, pp. 275–308.

Newell KM, Scully DM, Tenenbaum F, Hardiman S (1989) Body scale and the development of prehension. *Dev Psychobiol* 22: 1–13. http://dx.doi.org/10.1002/dev.420220102

Odem SL, Horner RH, Snell ME, Blacher, J (2007) The construct of developmental disabilities. In: Odem SL, Horner RH, Snell ME, Blacher J, editors. *Handbook of Developmental Disabilities.* New York: Guildford Press, pp. 3–14.

Savelsbergh G, van der Kamp J, Ledebt A, Planinsek T (2000) Information-movement coupling in children with Down syndrome. In: Weeks D, Chua R, Elliott D, editors. *Perceptual-Motor Behavior in Down Syndrome.* Champaign, IL: Human Kinetics, pp. 251–275.

Stott DH, Moyes FA, Henderson SE (1984) *The Test of Motor Impairment.* San Antonio, TX: The Psychological Corporation.

Sugden DA (1980) Movement speed in children. *J Mot Behav* 12: 125–132.

Sugden DA, Gray SM (1981) Capacity and strategies of educationally subnormal boyson serial and discrete tasks involving movement speed. *Br J Educ Psychol* 51: 77–82. http://dx.doi.org/10.1111/j.2044-8279.1981.tb02457.x

Sugden DA, Keogh JF (1990) *Problems in Movement and Skill Development.* Columbia, SC: University of South Carolina Press.

Sugden DA, Rose C, Weir J (1983) Variability of motor performance and learning in normal and ESN(M) children. *Phys Educ Rev* 6: 42–51.

Sugden DA, Wann C (1987) The assessment of motor impairment in children with moderate learning difficulties. *Br J Educ Psychol* 57: 225–236. http://dx.doi.org/10.1111/j.2044-8279.1987.tb03156.x

Thelen E (1986) Treadmill-elicited stepping in seven-month-old infants. *Child Dev* 57: 1498–1506. http://dx.doi.org/10.2307/1130427

Thelen E, Ulrich BD (1991) *Hidden Skills: A Dynamic Systems Analysis of Treadmill-Elicited Stepping during the First Year.* Monographs of the Society for Research in Child Development, 56, No. 223.

Tizard J (1953) The effects of different types of supervision on the behavior of mental defectives in a sheltered workshop. *Am J Ment Deficiency* 58: 143–151.

Tizard J, Loos FM (1954) The learning of a spatial relations test by adult imbeciles. *Am J Ment Deficiency* 59: 85–90.

Tizard J, O'Connor N (1950) The employability of high-grade mental defectives. *Am J Ment Deficiency* 54: 563–576.

Ulrich BD, Ulrich DA (1995) Spontaneous leg movements of infants with Down syndrome and nondisabled infants. *Child Dev* 66: 1844–1855. http://dx.doi.org/10.2307/1131914

Ulrich BD, Ulrich DA, Collier DH (1992) Alternating stepping patterns: hidden abilities of 11-month-old infants with Down syndrome. *Dev Med Child Neurol* 34: 233–239. http://dx.doi.org/10.1111/j1469-8749.1992.tb14996.x

Ulrich DA, Ulrich BD, Angulo-Kinzler RM, Yun J (2001) Treadmill training of infants with Down syndrome: evidence-based developmental outcomes. *Pediatrics* 108: 1–7. http://dx.doi.org/10.1542/peds.108.5.e84

United Nations Children's Fund (2006) *The State of the World's Children 2006: Excluded and Invisible.* New York: UNICEF.

Wade MG (1980) Coincidence anticipation of young normal and handicapped children. *J Motor Behav* 12: 103–112.

Wade MG, Gold MW (1978) Removing some of the limitation of MR workers by improving job design. *Human Factors* 20: 339–348.

Wade MG, Hoover JH, Newell KM (1984) Training RT and MT of moderately and severely retarded persons in aiming movements. *Am J Ment Deficiency* 89: 174–179.

Wade MG, Van Emmerik REA, Kernozek TP (2000) Atypical dynamics of motor behavior in Down Syndrome. In: Weeks D, Chua R, Elliot DG, editors. *Perceptual-Motor Behavior in Down Syndrome.* Champaign, IL: Human Kinetics, pp. 277–303.

Wallace SA, Newell KM, Wade MG (1978) Decision and response times as a function of movement difficulty in preschool children. *Child Dev* 49: 509–512. http://dx.doi.org/10.2307/1128718

Warren WH (1984) Perceiving affordances: visual guidance of stair climbing. *J Exp Psychol Human Perception Performance* 10: 683–703. http://dx.doi.org/10.1037/0096-1523.10.5.683

WHO (1992) *International Statistical Classification of Diseases and Related Health Problems, Volume 1,* 10th edition. Geneva: World Health Organization.

10
MOTOR DEVELOPMENT IN CHILDREN WITH OTHER DEVELOPMENTAL DISORDERS

Introduction to developmental disorders

THE FIELD OF DEVELOPMENTAL DISORDERS
The concentration within this section of the book has been on disorders that are entities in themselves and for which there are ample bodies of literature describing and analysing their motor characteristics. Children with atypical physical resources such as cerebral palsy and developmental coordination disorder (DCD), those with visual limitations, and those with learning/intellectual difficulties are obvious choices for inclusion. However, there are groups of children who do not fit neatly into these categories and for whom various labels have been given, including specific learning disability, learning disabilities, learning disorders, and developmental disorders. The terminology is constantly changing and this is made more complex by the terms used differing across countries. In addition, it is difficult to draw a boundary line around all of these children as they evidence different characteristics from each other, yet one could look outside of formal labels and note that they have fundamental difficulties in those abilities that are evident before different labels are given at school age. For example, in the years before school parents and others may notice difficulties with language, problems with social and emotional situations, problems with attention, and overactivity. When the children reach school age they become more evident when comparisons are made with other children in a more formal setting.

There is a wide range of developmental disorders in children ranging from specific difficulties to more general ones, with terminology differing across countries, especially the USA and UK. Some children experience difficulties across a wide range of skills, such as most academic areas and often those in the social domain, and score low on tests of intelligence. In the UK these children are called 'children with (general) learning difficulties',

whereas in the USA the term 'mental retardation' is often employed. In Chapter 10 we have referred to them as *children with intellectual disabilities*.

In the UK children who have difficulty with a particular skill or group of skills are referred to as 'children with specific learning difficulties', whereas in the USA the term 'learning disorders' is used. The focus in this chapter is on the latter group of children falling into the category of children with specific learning difficulties, and in most cases, although not in all, the difficulties some children experience in the developmental period are unexpected when viewed across the whole ability spectrum of the child. In this chapter these children are referred to as having developmental disorders.

At first glance it would appear to be relatively simple to separate the children with developmental disorders by stating that they have average or near average intelligence, but that they have a specific difficulty in an area of functioning. However, as Hulme and Snowling (2009) point out, it is not so easy when there is a continuum of children's profiles that run from a very specific deficit through to a total profile of difficulties. In addition, there is the vexed issue of how to conceptualize co-occurring characteristics. Most children with a specific learning difficulty, such as in attention, will also show other difficulties, such as in motor ability. The question then becomes to what degree do these co-occurring characteristics have to show before the profile emerges as one of general learning difficulties.

These and other issues are raised at various points throughout this chapter, which concentrates on four groups of children within the broad description of *developmental disorders* with a specific learning difficulty. They are better known by their formal labels of:

- dyslexia
- autistic spectrum disorder (ASD)

- attention-deficit–hyperactivity disorder (ADHD)
- specific language impairment (SLI).

There has been some mention of these disorders in other chapters, particularly in Chapter 9, in which the issues of comorbidity and co-occurring characteristics have been noted. In this chapter more detail on each condition is presented with that particular condition being the dependent variable under analysis with respect to ability in motor skills. At first glance it does appear that these are separate and disparate groups in that they address specific and separate areas of human functioning.

- *Dyslexia* is associated with the literacy skills of reading, writing, and spelling, with shortcomings in phonological processes being a common feature.
- *ASD* is of a different nature to the others as it contains some children who are severely impaired across a wide range of functioning – language, social, motor, cognitive, and others – for whom low cognitive ability is not a characteristic, but their social and personal skills still make communication, interaction, and daily functioning very difficult.
- *ADHD* as the name suggests has as its core characteristic an impaired attentional system that is accompanied or not by hyperactivity.
- *SPL* involves a difficulty with expressive and/or receptive language, often appearing to be out of line with overall functioning in other domains.

All of these developmental disorders will show co-occurring characteristics with motor performance being one of them.

These developmental disorders all share characteristics that are debatable. For example, in all there is discussion and often disagreement concerning identification, assessment, diagnosis, and intervention. These areas might include such topics as cut-off points, thereby leading to differing prevalence rates; whether the condition is best described as a continuum or a category, the question asked is: is it distinct from typically developing children or is there a continuum, in which case a cut-off point becomes almost arbitrary? What are the issues surrounding comorbidity and co-occurring characteristics, and is it possible to give a dual diagnosis? Are there underlying characteristics, either biological substrates or cognitive processes, that link the commonly co-occurring conditions? It is not possible to take every one of these issues and develop it fully, but they are seen as real dilemmas that researchers and clinicians may wish to address and are explored in parts of the chapter.

- The first part of the chapter introduces the concept of developmental disorders by presenting two analyses of the whole field:
  - First we look at possible biological and cognitive substrates and examine the phenomenon of co-occurring characteristics, which appears to pervade all developmental disorders, and includes cognitive causal modelling and some *specific theories* surrounding description and causation. It does this by offering a framework that can be used to portray each of the developmental disorders by distinguishing among biological, cognitive, and behavioural variables (Morton 2004) as well as so-called environmental influences, with an emphasis on the underlying biological and cognitive substrates. In this way it is possible to make descriptions and comparisons within and between conditions by ensuring that like-for-like issues are being addressed.
  - The second part looks at the *concept of discrepancy*, one that permeates many developmental disorders, and uses the example of dyslexia to tease out some of the subtleties of this concept. When the discrepancy concept is used, there is the assumption that the child has intelligence within the typical range and that the observed disorder is surprising in this light. On the surface this appears to be relatively straightforward but it does hide a number of nuances that make it less simple than first portrayed.
- The second part of the chapter contains sections on each individual condition, starting with the relevant definitions and core characteristics and followed by the motor characteristics of that condition.

UNDERLYING BIOLOGICAL AND COGNITIVE SUBSTRATES

This section examines some general issues related to all developmental disorders that often generate controversy and are linked in different ways to biological and cognitive substrates. Some of the issues here are elaborated in the sections addressing specific conditions.

Co-occurring difficulties

Many of the children who are diagnosed with a developmental disorder such as dyslexia or ADHD will also evidence other difficulties. Some children may have only a few difficulties of minor importance, whereas others may have numerous difficulties that are more serious in nature. There is a continuum of the number and extent of co-occurring difficulties. At some point this continuum raises the issue of whether there are comorbid conditions. A simplistic way to look at the difference between comorbid conditions and co-occurring characteristics is by defining comorbidity as two possibly related but separate diagnoses within a child, such as ADHD and dyslexia. With co-occurring conditions, the child has a primary diagnosis of a disorder such as dyslexia but with attentional and social problems as co-occurring and possibly a common aetiology, but not enough for a full diagnosis. Kaplan et al (2006) presented an alternative analysis when they addressed the three terms of 'comorbidity', 'co-occurring conditions', and 'continuum'. They defined comorbidity with its original meaning, indicating the presence of at least two diseases or disorders that are independent of each other. Kaplan et al (2006) prefer the term co-occurrence because they assert that there are common assumptions about aetiology, taking results from their work on atypical brain development as evidence.

A fundamental question to ask concerning co-occurring characteristics is why they should be present. We know that, if we take any developmental disorder and look at its characteristics that are not a part of the primary defining criteria, we will still obtain a higher prevalence of those co-occurring characteristics than in a typically developing population. In our chapter on DCD we noted the co-occurring characteristics that were present but with DCD as the focal point. In this chapter an overlapping, but slightly different, line is taken, with the four developmental disorders being the primary focus, followed by an examination of their effects on motor abilities. Note that in all four disorders, motor impairment is not a primary focus and in some cases not included in the diagnostic criteria. However, the motor characteristics are described as part of a number of other assessments when evaluating a child with a particular pattern of behaviour, whereas at other times motor abilities are specifically addressed. We have noted that there is a distinction between the terms of comorbidity and co-occurring characteristics but this varies among those who use the terms. To ease this confusion, the term co-occurring characteristics is used here simply to mean that a named disorder may have other behavioural characteristics, which may or may not have a common aetiology, and a dual diagnosis has not been given.

In Chapter 8 on DCD the concept of co-occurring conditions was described, noting that in the majority of cases this was the rule rather than the exception. This is interesting in the light of a move to identify more specific conditions such as the ones we note – DCD, SLI, ADHD, dyslexia, and ASD – even though clinically we find that comorbidity or co-occurrence is often present. There is a case for looking at so-called 'pure' cases, with recent literature looking at the value of this approach as it often presents a clearer picture of the condition itself

(Peters and Henderson 2008). In addition, as Peters and Henderson (2008) show, these 'pure' cases help in planning intervention programmes involving such actions as setting targets, objectives, and priorities, all being carried out within the motor domain. Certainly, if we are presented with a child who has 'pure' motor problems, the intervention and indeed the prognosis will be different from a child who has a co-occurring attention difficulty or has some problem with personal and social interactions. Undoubtedly there are children who have a profile that shows their motor skills to be impaired and that is the only characteristic.

The more usual situation, however, as Hill (2005) notes, is that motor problems are prevalent in the four disorders of dyslexia, ASD, ADHD, and SLI even though they are not central for their diagnosis. There are a number of reasons why co-occurrence should be present:

- An impairment, such as lack of attention, may play an important and specific role in another area such as movement.
- Neuromaturational delay may give rise to and underpin deficits across various domains; in other words there is a shared risk factor or an overlap between the risk factors.
- There is a direct neural cause for co-occurrence between motor and cognitive development, which relates to a tight relationship between the cerebellum and the frontal cortex.
- There is also the possibility that one disorder creates an increased risk for another.
- There is the possibility that co-occurrence itself is a meaningful syndrome (Caron and Rutter 1991, Hill 2006).
- Caron and Rutter (1991) note that we have an artificial subdivision of syndromes, one disorder may be the early signs of another, overlap of disorders is bound to occur if the disorders are thought of as dimensional and not categorical, and often the same behavioural characteristic appears in more than one diagnostic category.

Whenever a child shows co-occurring characteristics the implications are far reaching. From the building of a profile of strengths and weakness, through setting targets and objectives, to the establishment of priorities, which is the first of these activities to be addressed, there will be corresponding alterations to the intervention programme.

Cognitive causal modelling
One way to examine causation of overlapping conditions is to use the model shown earlier by Morton (2004).

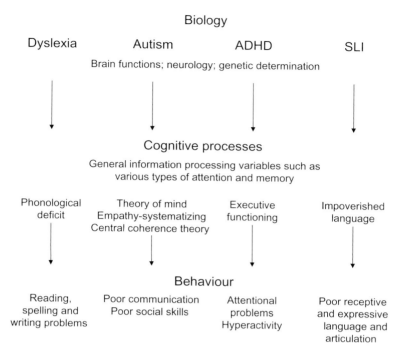

Fig. 10.1 Adaptation of the Morton (2004) model showing examples from the four disorders.

Morton has made the proposal that cognition is the link between behaviour and biology and is a crucial part of the puzzle. In various parts of the book we have used the Morton (2004) working on a model devised in conjunction with Frith (Morton and Frith 1995) as a way of looking at developmental disorders, proposing that cognitive processes are the intervening or mediating processes between the biological level and what we see at the behavioural level. This model is utilized in Figure 10.1.

Morton's model is presented here in adapted form under the main headings of biology, cognitive processes, and behaviour across the four developmental disorders of dyslexia, ASD, ADHD, and SLI.

Morton is emphasizing that cognition could be an intervening variable between biological substrates, such as the brain, and the observable behaviour. Our line agrees, noting that by proposing that the co-occurring conditions seen across developmental disorders, and the overlap of characteristics, may be a function of common underlying abnormalities in underlying biological substrates or the mediating cognitive variables.

- In *dyslexia* the intervening cognitive processes between the biology of genetic differences and possible brain differences and the behaviours of difficulty in learning to read and spelling could involve a phonological deficit or an appropriate grapho-phonemic relationship not learned.

- In *ASD* cognitive processes, such as the theory of mind (Baron-Cohen et al 1985), central coherence difficulties, empathizing and systemizing (Baron-Cohen 2008), and/or executive functioning, may be intervening and mediating variables among brain differences and the behaviours of impaired pretend play, delay in language acquisition, and socially strange behaviour that we often see in this group of individuals.

- In *ADHD* a proposed intervening variable has been executive functioning, with debate about how much influence this actually has. Some individuals have proposed that it is a core characteristic (Barkley 1997), whereas others claim it accounts for no more than one-third of cases.

- In *SLI* the core behavioural characteristics of articulation, receptive and expressive language, are again underpinned through cognitive processes and underlying biological substrates. Candidate cognitive variables include phonological working memory, declarative memory, and temporal processing.

A cognitive concept such as executive control involves higher-order strategies including planning, organization, and recruitment of memory strategies. This top-down view of context is one that could underpin all of the developmental disorders. Such a concept would become an explanatory variable as to why the characteristics of one disorder often appear in another.

Deficits in attention, motor control, and perception, atypical brain damage, and cerebellar delay

During the 1980s, the first of a series of important studies was conducted in Sweden examining children with perceptual motor and attention deficits. The children were selected at 6 years of age and followed longitudinally for nearly two decades (RH Gillberg and Rasmussen 1982, C Gillberg et al 1983, Rasmussen et al 1983). The children, who started by being described as having 'minimal brain dysfunction', moved to being called DAMP, 'deficits in attention, motor control, and perception', and, as the children were followed over the years, there were a number of studies showing the relationships among attentional problems, perceptual difficulties, and motor problems (C Gillberg 1998). In 2000, Rasmussen and C Gillberg presented the results of their longitudinal study that started in the 1980s and found, for example, 60% of children in their study to have both DCD and ADHD. Of particular importance for intervention was the finding that, by 22 years of age, those children who had both ADHD and DCD (*DAMP*) tended to have worse outcomes than either condition alone. The argument from the team is that there is a generalized disorder that underlies a number of 'labelled' conditions and that we should move away from these discrete disorders and simply look at the sum total of symptoms. A direct causal link was not made to an underlying neurological dysfunction, but there was an assumption that brain disorder was present. The selection of children was restricted to those with problems in the domains of attention, perception, and motor with conditions such as dyslexia or SLI not being associated, but *DAMP* was related to problems in the classroom.

A similar line to this was taken by Kaplan et al (1997, 1998, 2001) who proposed an underlying framework to explain some of the co-occurring characteristics that were regularly seen; however, in this case the underlying framework was specifically biological in nature. In a group of children with developmental disorders nearly 25% could fall into all three categories of dyslexia, DCD, and ADHD, whereas 22% had dyslexia and DCD, and 10% had both DCD and ADHD (Kaplan et al 1997). From these and other similar statistics they developed a conceptual framework that they called atypical brain damage, a term they used as an umbrella label to describe the developmental disorders and their relationships to each other. This was a shift back to the time when the terms minimal brain damage and minimal cerebral dysfunction were used to describe the children despite no actual cerebral damage being found. However, Kaplan et al (1998), while acknowledging that specific areas of the brain have not been conclusively found to underlie developmental disorders, propose that the damage is diffuse rather than localized and that the concept of separate developmental disorders is probably not correct but that they are all reflections of a generic underlying brain dysfunction. Visser (2007) notes that the term 'variable expressivity', one that is borrowed from genetics, is useful in describing a common underlying variable, in this case brain damage, that can go some way to explaining the high rate of comorbidity in children with developmental disorders. However, Visser (2007) also points out that, although it can explain comorbidity, it has rather less success at explaining 'pure' cases of developmental disorders and suggests that pure cases of particular conditions may differ not only in behavioural symptoms but also in some underlying pathology.

The possibility of the same biological substrates underlying more than one human ability has been explored by other writers. Diamond (2000) notes that, although motor and cognitive development have usually been studied separately, they may be interrelated and fundamentally intertwined, a point we have made with the work on embodied cognition in Chapter 1. Typically, the dorsolateral prefrontal cortex is arguably responsible for many cognitive functions, whereas the cerebellum is considered critical for motor development. However, Diamond (2000) argues that each of these structures overlaps the other in functions for motor and cognitive skills, with her evidence coming from neuroimaging studies, work with patients with brain damage, and the literature on developmental disorders, including ADHD and DCD, dyslexia and SLI, and movement disorders. From this work she suggests that motor and cognitive functions may not be as separate as previously thought, with the underlying biological substrates of the cerebellum and the prefrontal cortex being primarily responsible for their interrelatedness. She also suggests that the caudate nucleus, a C-shaped structure within the basal ganglia paralleling the lateral ventricle, may have a cognitive function, as well as its well-known motor responsibility with the neurotransmitter dopamine, of choosing appropriate movements, muscles, and force parameter.

In a similar vein, Fawcett and colleagues proposed that there may be cerebellar difficulties culminating in reading, spelling, and articulation problems and these are also associated with motor difficulties (Fawcett and Nicolson 2002). Later in the section on dyslexia, this line is elaborated and the topic has been examined by Bishop (2007), who looked at programmes specifically designed to cure cerebellar developmental delay, thought to be a cause of dyslexia, ADHD, dyspraxia, and Asperger syndrome. Although she acknowledged that the cerebellum may be involved in some difficulties, she nevertheless argued that it was premature to say that the cerebellum was the cause rather than an associated characteristic and that these difficulties may even be a result of limited experience of handwriting in those children with poor overall literacy skills. She notes quite correctly that many children with dyslexia, for example, do not have balance problems. Her research focus examines the Dore Achievement Centre, which makes various claims about training the cerebellum through motor activities and the consequent improvement in children's skills. Bishop (2007) notes 'the gaping hole…is a lack of evidence that training on motor co-ordination can have any influence on higher level skills mediated by the cerebellum' (p. 654). Work in a different but related vein using perceptual motor tasks brings up to date other papers over the last 30 years that have failed to establish a direct effect that is related to motor training (Kavale and Forness 1995).

The presence of co-occurring characteristics is a common phenomenon in the field of developmental disorders, and motor performance is one of the most prevalent and important. The explanations for this vary and should all be considered, and, at the moment, there is partial support for most theories, but no one theory can itself explain the totality of this co-occurrence. In their review paper, Green and Baird (2005) outline the detail of many studies involving motor and other abilities in children and propose different categories for overlapping conditions. Those with emotional/personal/ADHD and conduct disorders are placed in a category they label 'psychopathology'; those with reading and scholastic difficulties they label 'learning'; and those with speech and language impairment they label 'development'. They make the very valid point that how one measures motor ability and what is included in any text will influence the amount and type of co-occurring characteristics that may accompany it. This chapter is about children with these co-occurring characteristics: they are children who are identified with a particular primary disorder and who also have associated motor difficulties.

Figure 10.2 illustrates the four developmental disorders that are covered and the possible overlap with each other and with motor difficulties.

DISCREPANCY CONCEPT

In many definitions of children with developmental disorders there is a statement noting that the difficulty appears to be out of line with other areas of functioning, which leads to the complex area often known as the discrepancy

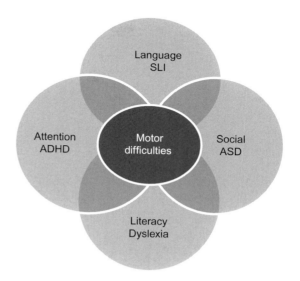

Fig. 10.2 Co-occurring characteristics of children with developmental disorders.

concept. This has been applied to many of the above disorders in varying degrees, and here the example of dyslexia is taken to illustrate some of the complexities surrounding the concept of discrepancy.

In definitions of dyslexia there is often a clause that alludes to the disorder being unexpected when viewed across the spectrum of abilities the child possesses. In other words the child is assumed to be of normal or above intelligence and the abilities of literacy associated with the condition of dyslexia are out of line when compared with this.

International Classification of Diseases 10 (ICD-10; WHO 1992) notes with respect to a specific reading disorder:

> Criterion A (1) a score on reading accuracy and/or comprehension that is at least 2 standard errors of prediction below the level expected on the basis of the child's chronological age and general intelligence, with both reading skills and IQ assessed on an individually administered test standardized for the child's culture and educational system.
>
> (WHO 1992, p. 176)

Early work on this was reported by Rutter and Yule (1975) who, in their Isle of Wight study, found it hard to establish clear cut differences at the behavioural level between children with specific reading difficulties and those who were simply generally poor readers, with both groups having similar reading patterns. In line with ICD-10 criteria (although bearing in mind that these were published almost 20 years after the Isle of Wight study), a group of children with dyslexia were identified only when intelligence was taken into account. Although multiple measures of the child's functioning are always collected, a discrepancy between reading and intelligence is, according to the same criteria, the cornerstone of assessment and diagnosis. The procedure is to obtain a measure of a child's literacy skills, which usually includes determining reading age with some assessment of writing and spelling. This is usually accompanied by a standardized test of intelligence, for example the Wechsler Intelligence Scale for Children (WISC). The scores of the two modes of assessment are compared to see if there is any discrepancy between the two. Thus, if, for example, a reading score of 70 is obtained on a reading test with a mean of 100 and a standard deviation (SD) of 15 and a score of 105 with similar mean and SD is found on an IQ test, an argument could be made that there is a discrepancy and this profile would play a major part in any diagnosis. This discrepancy is often examined through regression analysis or an analysis involving a discrepancy of two standard errors.

However, these measures also hide a number of complications and they have made the discrepancy notion a debateable one. For example, how discrepant do scores have to be before any pronouncement is made? If a child is borderline moderate learning difficulty, where one might expect some difficulty with reading, but the reading score is lower than this expectation, does this make the child dyslexic? Or what about a very high level of IQ and an average reading score, showing a clear discrepancy between the scores, with reading being of an average level but well below what one would expect from the measured IQ? In addition there may be children who have poor reading scores relative to their cognitive ability for reasons other than a specific reading difficulty, such as not speaking the language, school absences, or poor teaching, or it may simply be the case that the subculture of the child does not value reading and therefore there is little emphasis on it in the community outside of school (Morton 2004). This method also does not does not pick up those children who compensate by reading very slowly with huge effort, but accurately. Finally, with respect to reading, for a discrepancy concept to be totally accurate, there would need to be a very high correlation between reading and intelligence and, as the correlation is only around 0.6, this does raise a few concerns.

To educators and other practitioners as well as parents, the discrepancy concept has a logical feel to it: that of a particular ability being out of line with other abilities or the overall ability of the child, that is, there is some unexpectedness about it. Many practitioners are comfortable with a discrepancy definition of some sort

for a starting point for their investigation. However, it is not straight-forward and has been criticized. In this chapter it will crop up several times and it is clearly a useful concept, but caution is advised about invoking it as immutable. In the case of dyslexia, the above-named tests of IQ and reading ability are often used but are employed in conjunction with other measures, such as phonological impairment, to arrive at a more complete picture of the child. The same is true with other developmental disorders, and the concept is invoked to varying degrees of certainty.

In the following sections, each of four developmental disorders is defined and their primary characteristics described. It is not the object of this chapter to present the close detail and every argument and debate about definition in each disorder. For that references are given for the reader to take this further as he or she wishes. However, it is pertinent to outline and describe the generally agreed definitions and note some of the areas of controversy, such as the discrepancy concept described above. The definitions, characteristics, and criteria for diagnosis of each of the disorders are taken from either the *Diagnostic and Statistical Manual of Mental Disorders 4th Revision Text Revision* (DSM-IV-TR; APA 2000) or ICD-10 (WHO 1992). These manuals are the two that are the most widely consulted, and, although there are some differences between them in terms of terminology and some definitional discrepancies, they generally agree on the important issues. When describing the four conditions, we have chosen the one we believe to be most appropriate for that condition and referred to the other when there is significant discrepancy.

Individual developmental disorders

DYSLEXIA

Definitions and core characteristics

Definitions
Both ICD-10 (WHO 1992) and DSM-IV-TR (APA 2000) allude to conditions that would include dyslexia. ICD-10 (WHO 1992) uses the term *specific disorders of scholastic skills*, which includes specific reading and spelling disorders as well as specific disorders of arithmetic, and directly uses the discrepancy concept in the definition, proposing that 'a criterion that involves a child in a reading or writing test scoring two standard deviations below what would be predicted from the child's age and general intelligence' (p. 174).

All other possibilities of underachievement should be excluded such as school experiences or sensory deficit.

DSM-IV (APA 1994, p. 51) uses the term *reading disorders* and again invokes the discrepancy concept but is less specific than ICD-10, only requiring that 'the criterion of reading/writing levels to be "substantially below" that what would be expected from a child's age, intelligence and experience'.

It also notes that in oral reading there are errors involving substitutions, distortions, and omissions and that it is slow with comprehension errors. In both manuals exclusionary clauses are present such as it not being due to a visual or other sensory deficit. Very much in line with this is a definition by Reid (2007), which is one that has numerous parts and has provided the basis for his laudable intervention work in educational circles in the field of dyslexia:

> Dyslexia is one of several distinct learning disabilities. It is a specific language based disorder of constitutional origin characterised by difficulties in single word decoding usually reflecting insufficient phonological processing. The difficulties are often unexpected in relation to age and other cognitive and academic abilities; they are not the result of generalised disability or sensory impairment. It is manifest by variable difficulty with different forms of language often including in addition to problems in reading, a conspicuous problem in acquiring proficiency with writing and spelling.
>
> (p. 3)

This definition is very much concerned with language and phonology as the cognitive processes involved and also with the concept of discrepancy. However, not all definitions invoke the discrepancy concept. In 1999 the British Psychological Society set up a working party on 'Dyslexia, Literacy and Psychological Assessment' and adopted the following working definition:

> Dyslexia is evident when accurate and fluent word reading and/or spelling develops very incompletely or with great difficulty. This focuses on literacy learning at the 'word level' and implies that the problem is severe and persistent despite appropriate learning opportunities. It provides the basis for a staged process of assessment through teaching.
>
> (BPS 1999, p. 8)

Here the problem is seen as a difficulty at the word level with an assumption that it can be addressed separately from other areas such as comprehension, for example (Morton 2004). The definition above does not invoke discrepancy as a criterion but it does specify adequate and appropriate learning opportunities, which would include the formal teaching side, but excludes a cultural expectation of reading success. Snowling and Maughan (2006) summarize some of the arguments surrounding the discrepancy concept by noting that there has been concern about its usage. First, they note that the correlation between reading and intelligence is relatively modest: as we noted earlier, usually this hovers around 0.6, which leaves a fair proportion of performance unaccounted for. Second, the differences between poor readers who have low IQs and high IQs do not appear to be significant. Third, the prognoses for readers who have unexpected failures and those who do not are relatively similar.

The above debates whether or not a discrepancy concept is useful, but it does not hide the fact that it remains the usual approach to take when studying dyslexia. It is an approach that aims to exclude those with a general learning difficulty and concentrates on those for whom failure in reading is, by other measures, unexpected. It is hoped that through this approach the specific cognitive deficits that are the causes of the reading problems will be established (Hulme and Snowling 2009).

The prevalence of dyslexia using the discrepancy definition is in the range of 4% to 8% in English-speaking countries, with the prevalence being higher in inner-city areas and males outnumbering females by as many as three to one (Snowling and Maughan 2006). Prevalence varies with age and peaks at around 9% to 11%, with some children having overcome their reading problems by adolescence, and others still continuing to have problems in spelling and writing (Snowling and Maughan 2006).

Core characteristics

There is some agreement on the core features of dyslexia. There is difficulty in literacy, particularly in reading but also in spelling and writing; this difficulty is often unexpected when other measures are considered, and, although it is not a global problem across the child's abilities, there are associated difficulties. There is an assumption in the early years that language is a central difficulty leading to decoding, phonological, reading, and spelling difficulties. Children with dyslexia are often reported to have difficulties in processing, such as in tasks requiring short-term memory or perceptual tasks. There is a belief that poor phonology lies at the heart of the difficulty in many children with dyslexia, with the children showing great difficulty in mapping speech sounds to letters. This is particularly important in the early stages of reading, in which decoding and phonological processes are primary.

In the later stages of reading, meaning, fluency, and language start to become more important. Typically, in the early years, children with dyslexia show impairment in phonological skills and are poor on tasks such as 'nonwords' or in changing words by removing or adding letters at the beginning, middle, or end of words. Thus changing a word, such as 'chair' to 'hair' or 'char' by the removal of a letter, becomes difficult. Similarly, taking a word such as 'hat' and changing it to 'bat', 'pat', 'has', 'had', or 'what', 'that', and 'hate', a task that typical readers will perform quite easily, becomes difficult and a major chore for children with dyslexia (Reid 2007, Hulme and Snowling 2009).

Hulme and Snowling (2009) propose a triangular model as a metaphor for reading single words with the three parts of the model being phonological (sound), orthographic (print), and semantic (meaning).

The phonological and semantic systems are part of typical language development and are established before a child goes to school, whereas the orthographic system seems to only develop as a consequence of learning to read, with the phonological deficit theory being the one that is most supported by the research evidence. Hulme and Snowling (2009) conclude that 'The dominant theory at the present time is that the core deficit in dyslexia is a deficit in the way spoken words are represented in the brain (the phonological representation hypothesis)' (p. 69). This deficit can be the result of a number of pathways ranging from speech perception deficits, to the establishment of articulatory motor programmes, to the relationship between speech perception and speech production mechanisms.

Genetic influences have been investigated because of the high rate of occurrence in families, with DeFries and Alarcon (1996) reporting figures from the Colorado Twin Study of 68% concordance for monozygotic twins and 38% for dizygotic twins, indicating a moderate genetic influence. Owing to the known heterogeneity in children with dyslexia, it was thought unlikely that there is a single gene for the condition. More recently, however, Cope et al (2005) and Harold et al (2006) have made progress towards locating a single gene as the focal point for dyslexia. Both dyslexia and general reading difficulties are thought to have a genetic component, with molecular genetics and chromosomal research being ongoing together with some brain imaging work looking at neural substrates. Finally, as with other disorders, social influences and classroom experiences play a part (Rutter and Maughan 2002), with these influences being a crucial part of our triangular model of influences involving the child's resources, the environmental context, and the type and manner of task presentation.

It has been noted that children with dyslexia often show similar difficulties to those children who are just slow-to-learn readers, which brings up the question of how discrete a group children with dyslexia are. The concept of dyslexia then presents two possible pictures. The first is one of an unbroken continuum of reading ability and disability from those who are slow-to-learn readers to those with dyslexia. This is known as the *continuum* or *dimensional* model. The second is one of a natural break between good and poor readers or different types of poor readers and this is known as a *categorical* model. Many writers who specialize in dyslexia favour the dimensional model and yet continue to use categorical terms as they are of functional use. Hulme and Snowling (2009) point out that it is not just in cognitive disorders that this occurs, with examples in medicine such as weight and blood pressure leading to categorical labels of obesity and hypertension when clearly there is a dimensional element to both of these. In order to use a categorical label, some kind of cut-off has to be established. In many cases the cut-off, if not arbitrary, does have some fluidity in its interpretation. For example, one could simply say the lowest 5% of any curve of reading scores could be placed in a dyslexia category. This has a face-valid logic to it but little statistical validity. To do this one could take two standard deviations below the mean (identifying 2.28%) and use that figure. This does not of course allow for a discrepancy definition of dyslexia, and, to invoke this concept, one would have to examine the difference between a measure of ability (e.g. IQ score) and a reading score such that the lowest 5% or 2.28% was a function of this difference. It is pertinent to point out that using such a difference score will produce some error in the results because, as previously noted, for a difference score to be totally accurate a very high correlation between reading and IQ is required and the relationship is only moderate. Here the term dyslexia is used for descriptive purposes, tacitly acknowledging a categorical model, but recognizing that a dimensional model is preferred as it provides a more fine-grained analysis of the domain of reading difficulties.

The prognosis for reading disorders has focused on three areas (Snowling and Maughan 2006):

- The first area of persistence shows that indeed the problems do continue unless there is effective intervention even though the core difficulties may change from reading to spelling.
- The second area of concern has been the impact reading has on other academic areas and psychosocial outcomes. In terms of the impact on academic achievement, the key factor seems to be a supportive family background. In terms of psychosocial

outcome, there is some evidence of higher rates of mood swings and trait anxiety in those with reading disorders.

- The third area of concern relates to antisocial behaviour and this does not seem to be a direct result of dyslexia.

Dyslexia, despite being a controversial topic, is a condition that is widely recognized and requires specific intervention strategies. Whether these strategies are substantially and fundamentally different from those employed with children who are simply poor readers is open to debate.

Dyslexia and motor problems

Reading and motor problems

There is a strong history of children with reading and other literacy problems having a higher incidence of motor difficulties in the early work of Orton (1937) and others (Denkla 1974, Gubbay 1975, Rutter and Yule 1975). During the 1990s there was a drive in Alberta, Canada, to improve the understanding of the nature and aetiology of developmental disorders. Large groups of children were included in a cohort composed mainly of those with learning and/or attention difficulties. None of them was referred for coordination difficulties, but the children who took part in studies were examined for other difficulties co-occurring with their reading and attention problems (Kaplan et al 1998). Here only the co-occurrence of motor problems with reading difficulties is reported. The study worked with 224 children with reading/attention difficulties and 155 controls all between 8 and 16 years of age. All children were tested for cognitive ability and motor performance and given several standardized tests of reading ability.

The children were organized for types of difficulties:

- evidence of deficits in basic reading skills
- deficits in reading comprehension
- deficits in phonology.
  Complete data were available for 162 children:
- 53 children being 'pure' cases of one disorder;
- 47 met none of the criteria for a diagnosis of a disorder; and
- 62 were 'comorbid' cases.
  Of the comorbid cases
- 22 (13%) met the criteria for both reading difficulty and DCD; and
- 23 (14%) met the criteria for reading difficulty and ADHD and DCD, giving a total of 27% of the children having both reading and motor difficulties.

The reading difficulties were not specified directly as dyslexia but the study does indicate that co-occurring characteristics of reading with motor difficulties are commonly seen.

Automatization deficit hypothesis

In a series of articles, Nicolson and Fawcett (Nicolson and Fawcett 1990, Fawcett and Nicolson 1995, 1999, Nicolson et al 2001) have proposed that motor problems and abnormalities in muscle tone are common symptoms in the majority of children with dyslexia. Their research led them to propose the automatization deficit hypothesis (ADH), which emerged from their work on dual-task paradigms. This work involved the primary task of balancing on a beam and was followed by a second task, such as counting backwards, which was performed while the participant was balancing on the beam. They found that children with dyslexia were very poor when the second task was introduced, whereas the control children had no such problems. This led them to propose that the reason for this was because the children with dyslexia could not automate the first skill, thus leading to a decrement in performance. Some support was given to this by Yap and van der Leij (1994).

The ADH led Fawcett to go further by looking at the structures in the brain that may be responsible for this, and she came to the conclusion that there is a deficit in the cerebellum that in turn leads to cerebellar difficulties culminating in reading, spelling, and articulation problems (Fawcett 2002). The cerebellum has been often noted as a centre for motor control particularly for balance tasks, and the lack of automatization on the balance beam in children with dyslexia is proposed as a result of cerebellar dysfunction. If this is true, there are logical sequelae with children with ADH resulting from a cerebellum impairment being more easily distracted, lacking sustained attention to the task, and showing other comorbid difficulties. However, at this point, it should be noted that the ADH as a cause of dyslexia has led to some substantial debates in the literature surrounding the validity of this notion (Ramus 2004). Earlier in the chapter we noted the criticism of this line of thinking by Bishop (2007), arguing that currently the evidence surrounding a direct cerebellar involvement is not strong enough to warrant implementation of interventions based on this approach.

There is, however, good evidence showing the overlap between dyslexia and motor difficulties, even if the causal relationship is not proven. However, a final note of caution should be given as not all studies have reported this. In the famous Isle of Wight study by Rutter and Yule (1975) there was the interesting finding that children with general reading problems, those who had problems commensurate with their overall ability, had a higher incidence of motor problems than those with a specific reading difficulty, the dyslexic group. Indeed the former group had far more co-occurring problems in general than the dyslexic group and an explanation for this could be that the children with general reading difficulties were of general low ability and their motor ability was commensurate with this, whereas in children whose reading is poor and out of line with their overall ability one may expect motor skills to be satisfactory.

Thus, when we examine motor problems in typically developing children and children with dyslexia, we can conclude that there appears to be a higher prevalence found in children with dyslexia. However, whether this higher prevalence is evident when compared with a group of poor readers not identified as dyslexic is open to question.

AUTISTIC SPECTRUM DISORDER

Definitions and core characteristics
From the middle ages we have known about the condition we now call autism, and, in the 18th century, classic cases were described by such people as John Haslam in England and Jean Itard in France (C Gillberg 2000). However, wider attention to the condition was brought about by the pioneering work of Kanner (1943) and Asperger (1944), and since then people with ASD have presented parents, teachers, therapists, and researchers with surprises, puzzles, frustrations, and delight. The term ASD has come into common usage to describe a full range of children who have at their core a problem with socializing and would include classic or low-functioning autism, Asperger syndrome, and high-functioning autism, with the latter two being extremely difficult to separate.

Children within the ASD are clearly different from other groups of children, and, as the title suggests, there is a spectrum of characteristics and core features that are now generally agreed to fall into three groups, which have come to be known as the *triad of impairments*, with abnormal or impaired development being evident before the age of 3 years in at least one of three areas.

Both ICD-10 and DSM-IV allude to the above triad. Box 10.1 summarizes the three areas.

These three characteristics are part of the definition of autism, but only the second and third relate to people with Asperger syndrome, who generally have levels of intelligence and language within a typical range, although the idiosyncrasies of language even in children with Asperger syndrome do show and make difficult that part of communication that involves social interaction. In general, Asperger syndrome is viewed as being milder than classic autism, and children with Asperger syndrome are often difficult to differentiate from children who have come to be referred to as having 'high-functioning autism'. For reviews on autism, the following are recommended: Trevarthen et al (1996), C Gillberg and Coleman (2000), Frith (2003) and C Gillberg (2006). C Gillberg (2006) in particular notes many of the conundrums with the above definition and diagnosis, noting that in clinical practice it is hard to keep exactly to this set of guidelines and that their own set of guidelines particularly for Asperger syndrome is often used in practice.

The triad of impairments do conflate to a certain degree around social interaction, with language being viewed as a social communication process surrounding a person's own individual agenda, and the solitude of obsessive interest in single objects, etc. being also a social manifestation. The issue of joint attention with another person is seen as a marker for social interaction but also for being able to consider the world from another person's viewpoint. In children with autism joint attention development is delayed and impaired, thus inhibiting shared activities and facilitating self-obsessions.

Controversies: one continuum? Is the increase in the number of cases real?
There has been a long-standing debate as to whether full-blown autism and Asperger syndrome are on the same continuum, and, although there are pros and cons of this, the assumption here is that they are related, although with distinct differences. The research criteria from ICD-10 (WHO 1992) on Asperger syndrome notes that there should be no clinically significant general delay in spoken and/or receptive language or cognitive development. However, as we noted earlier, communication is often intrinsically related to social interaction, which is a defining problem characteristic of children with Asperger syndrome. Single words should have developed by 2 years of age and communication by 3 or earlier. It is now clearly recognized as a clinical condition and conceptualized as the highest variant of autism, but it does have a high variability in outcomes through the lifespan (C Gillberg and Coleman 2000). Differentiating Asperger syndrome from classic autism does not present many problems because the language capabilities are so different, but they are not so different from high-functioning autism, and thus differentiating between this group of children and those with Asperger syndrome is more difficult. At the time of going to press, the draft version of DSM-V has one continuum for all children with autism and Asperger syndrome.

During the last decade there has been a significant increase in the number of cases of autism identified, but

---

Box 10.1 A closer examination

Triad of impairments in autistic spectrum disorder

- The first characteristic is that there is impairment in communication with a delay in language acquisition and poor use of verbal and non-verbal means of communication (not Asperger syndrome). This can range from an almost total absence of language to echolalia or other forms of repetitive language. About one-third of individuals never speak in communicative clauses (C Gillberg 2006), and even children with high-level autism or Asperger syndrome have difficulty with understanding the concept of what is being said even though they are quite correct in the syntactical structure of their spoken language. Very often non-verbal language is also affected, being described as clumsy or awkward (C Gillberg 2006).

- The second is that there is some impairment in socializing with the children, showing a range of reciprocal interactions that range from the aloof to passive to odd, deviant, and delayed. This may involve misinterpreting signals, not understanding others' viewpoints, and odd gazing and staring. This often develops into a lack of friendships and an apparent lack of concern about this (C Gillberg 2006), although children with higher-functioning are often concerned about their inability to sustain friendships, and this could be reflected in depression levels seen in this group versus other adults.

- The third is the field of functional or symbolic play with the presence of restricted and stereotypical behaviour, with a lack of imagination, rigidity of thought and behaviour, and a reliance on routines. Stereotypies such as rocking, finger flicking, head banging, and hand flapping are commonplace. When routines are broken the incident is often accompanied by tantrums varying in content and intensity according to the ability of the child, with older children having violent episodes. Children with higher-functioning autism often have very narrow interests ranging from lengths of rivers to pop stars of the 1960s to rail and bus schedules. Occasionally some come through as savants with great skill in areas such as mathematics, art, or music (Frith 2003, C Gillberg 2006).

---

is this a real increase? Frith (2003) notes that our understanding of the condition, which has included more milder cases and those with Asperger syndrome, has altered the prevalence. Studies in the early 1960s found around 5 cases per 10 000, whereas in 2002 Wing and Potter reported between 8 and 30 classic cases per 10 000 and 60 per 10 000 on the spectrum. C Gillberg (2006) concludes that the current prevalence is between 50 and 100 per 10 000, with full-blown autism accounting for one-third of this and either Asperger syndrome or high-functioning autism constituting the remainder. Frith (2003) believes that this increase is mainly due to the newer diagnostic criteria and our increasing awareness. There is also some evidence that we may be swapping categories, with some areas reporting increases while decreases are observed in other conditions such as severe learning difficulties. There are significant sex differences in prevalence with a male:female ratio ranging from 3:1 to 6 or 9:1 depending on whether it is classic autism, in which the sexes are closer, or high-functioning autism, which affects substantially more males. C Gillberg (2006) proposes that females on the spectrum are underdiagnosed and often instead receive diagnoses for other disorders such as eating or anxiety.

Aetiology: biology, cognitive theories, and environment

When causation is examined there are mixed conclusions with some within the field of genetics backing up the prevalence statistics in families. These show that in twins there is 5 to 10 times the normal likelihood of the second twin being diagnosed after the first and a higher concordance in monozygotic than dizygotic twins. In full-blown autism there are comorbid characteristics with learning difficulties being a major one. This is not surprising with figures of 35% being the norm for those with IQs below 70 (Fombonne 1999). However, it is also known that some children with ASD have fluctuating profiles on the WISC and others, particularly those with Asperger syndrome and high-functioning autism, have good school intelligence but poor world or 'street' intelligence.

There are a number of theories as to why children with autism behave and act in the way they do. It is simple to write down the behavioural characteristics of the children, such as the triad of impairments, and it is similarly easy to examine the underlying biological substrates even if at the present time we do not have the answers. However, these do not tell us why the child is behaving in the way he or she does, and for this explanation we have to return to the Morton (2004) model and examine the intervening mediating cognitive variables. Four brief explanations are presented.

- The first explanation is one that has been with us for over 20 years and is referred to as the theory of mind (Baron-Cohen et al 1985). The theory of mind involves the ability to place oneself in someone else's shoes and take their position: it is about mentalizing and taking the view of someone else, imagining their thoughts, feelings, and motivations. Through a large number of experiments, the most famous being the 'Sally-Anne Studies', this theory proposes that children with autism and Asperger syndrome are delayed in their development of theory of mind leaving them with what Baron-Cohen (2008) now calls 'mindblindness'. Baron-Cohen gives several examples of this including pretend play in which the typical 2-year-old understands when pretending that others are also pretending. The child with autism is very much delayed in this. Another example he gives shows a typical 9-year-old being able to figure out that they might hurt others' feelings, whereas children with Asperger syndrome of normal intelligence are delayed by around 3 years on this task.

- A second theory that has been proposed is one that we have already mentioned – that of executive control or executive functioning. Executive functions are seen as higher levels of control and action and involve activities such as flexibility of response, inhibiting responses, high-level decisions, and planning and organization. Executive functioning involves taking a top-down view of the world, taking context into account: a construct of how we view the world, not necessarily how it actually is. The executive functioning deficit account of autism locates many of the behaviours seen in the disorder as being associated with poor executive functioning (the cognitive variable), with particular difficulties seen in planning, cognitive flexibility, generativity, and inhibition of prepotent response (for a review see Hill 2004a,b). These will have direct negative consequences for day-to-day behaviours and thought processes in which we have to switch between different perspectives ('I would prefer to have lunch and then meet with Jane to finish our report, but Jane has to leave in an hour so she would prefer to finish our report first') and will affect how we plan our actions ('what order am I going to do a series of tasks in order to get dressed and to work on time?')

  Situations such as these demand that the person takes a holistic view of the issues, is aware of the plan of action and of other people's needs, and is aware of what has been achieved and reformulates the plan as required. Frith (2003) proposes that these two accounts have both self-consciousness and self-awareness as central features, with individuals with ASD knowing massive amounts of detail about themselves but not about others. She notes that this lack of context to the mental states of others is what makes the ASD conditions so difficult.

- A third theoretical proposal is that children with ASD lack a central cohesion (Frith 1989), and thus they are more likely to deal with a large number of small issues rather than being able see the bigger picture and the whole scene. Their preference is for a bottom-up as opposed to a top-down approach and can be seen as linked to the executive control variable described earlier. Frith and Happe (1994) proposed that children with autism tended to focus on the small details of any situation/object rather than the whole picture, which typically developing individuals tend to do. This obsession with detail in some children with autism may be a reason why some develop extraordinary skills in one specific area and bring with them the label of 'savant'.

- Baron-Cohen has recently taken these theories and tried to unify them into what he calls the 'empathizing–systemizing theory' (Baron-Cohen et al 2003, Baron-Cohen 2008, 2010). In this he proposes that the social and communication difficulties seen in ASD can be explained by deficits in *empathy*, while referencing the strengths often seen in their skill in *systemizing*. Thus a child with autism would need to be judged according to two scales. On one they would show a lower than average ability in the area of empathy, but in the other they would score highly on systemizing. It then becomes the discrepancy of performance between these two constructs that determines whether a child is autistic or not. The first of these constructs, that of impairment of empathy, can go a long way to explaining the social communication difficulties in autism. On the other hand, the concept of systemizing can explain the strengths of children with autism in terms of their attention to detail and unusually narrow interests.

It should be noted that, for most researchers, each of the accounts outlined above does not need, necessarily, to be seen as mutually exclusive, and, indeed, there is accumulating evidence that the different features of the autism triad will be explained by different biological and therefore cognitive components.

In the early years of research into autism it was speculated that environmental factors in the form of cold aloof parenting may be a factor. It is possible that workers in the field were following work in the 1950s and 1960s on attachment theory. However, this line of thinking has all but been abandoned, except in rare cases, in favour of biological and cognitive underpinnings, even if the biology is not yet as specific and as detailed as we would like. Hulme and Snowling (2009) note that environment has received little attention of late because of advances in biology and cognition but that there are cases of severe deprivation of social interaction producing autistic-type behaviours. Rutter (1999) reported of Romanian children who were adopted into the UK, many of them from orphanages with severe deprivation, that 6% were producing autistic-type behaviours. The single case study of 'Genie' (Curtiss 1977), found in an upstairs room at 13 years of age with virtually no social and language interaction, also reports of some autistic-type behaviours. There is no suggestion in either of these studies that this deprivation produces classic cases of autism, but it merely reminds us that severe deprivation no matter how rarely seen can produce behaviours that we would only typically see in autism.

Autistic spectrum disorder and motor problems

There are particular difficulties with respect to specifically identifying motor difficulties in an ASD population due to the nature of the DSM-IV criteria, in which Criterion C states that a diagnosis of DCD is ruled out in the presence of a pervasive developmental disorder or ASD. This does not mean that motor problems cannot be identified, but it makes difficult the exact specification of them, such as a DCD comparison. Green et al (2009) note that there are diagnostic variances in clinical settings, with some children with social and communication disorders and motor problems receiving a diagnosis of ASD whereas others are referred to as DCD, with social and communication disorders listed as a secondary characteristic.

A question to be asked is why there may be links between children with ASD and motor impairment, and for that we need to look at how the characteristics of ASD could impinge and influence motor performance. It is recognized that there is a higher percentage of motor problems in children with ASD than in age-matched peers. To try to explain why, it is useful to look at the explanatory model of Morton (2004) that we have been using. It is thought that ASD has biological origins and we also know that, in general, where there is some constitutional/organic problem, it often has multiple effects. We also know that in children with lower abilities the incidence of motor impairment increases, and, as many children with ASD show this lower ability, it would be expected that

there would be a higher percentage of motor difficulties in an ASD population. If we move to the cognitive level of Morton's model (see page 283), we note the characteristics of poor executive function, a poverty of social skills, and a diminished theory of mind. All of these on certain motor tasks, such as those that involve planning and organization, taking consideration of others, and seeing a bigger picture in context, would leave the child with ASD at a disadvantage on these tasks and suffering a subsequent decrement in performance.

Green et al (2009) note that many studies have shown that, in children with ASD, motor problems are relatively common. The figure of how many are impaired differs according to which criteria are being used for the level of impairment and also the degree of involvement and severity of the children with ASD. Miyahara et al (1997) note that 22 out of 26 children with Asperger syndrome were at least two standard deviations below the mean on the Movement Assessment Battery for Children (Henderson and Sugden 1992). It is not only the high percentage of children with ASD showing additional motor problems but also the difference in the nature of their movements. Idiosyncratic actions, such as walking on the outside of the feet, and associated movements, both often viewed as indicators of soft neurological signs, have been found to be more prevalent in children with ASD than in controls (Jansiewicz et al 2006).

These findings are summarized by Green et al (2009) who report on a number of potential anomalies in some previous studies. First, they note that most studies appeared to be conducted with specific samples, occasionally rather modest in number of children with ASD, rather than a comprehensive sample across the range of the spectrum. In addition, it is well documented that children low on the intellectual scale perform poorly on motor tests and children with ASD cover the whole spectrum of intelligence. Finally, many of the samples were hospital based, often showing high levels of difficulties and comorbidity. In their study, Green et al (2009) examined a large population-derived sample of children with a wide range of IQ levels and abilities. This study is examined in Box 10.2.

The Green et al (2009) study confirms the higher incidence of motor problems across the range of ASD. This is in agreement with studies that have shown motor deficits early in infancy, as evidenced by problems in crawling and walking, in individuals with autism (Teitelbaum et al 1998), and also difficulties later in childhood such as poor coordination, clumsy gait, and slow reaction and response speed (Hallet et al 1993, Noterdaeme et al 2002, Jansiewicz et al 2006). Green et al (2009) also provide some speculation as to the underlying reasons for this

Box 10.2 A closer examination

Impairment in movement skills of children with ASDs: Green et al (2009)
The study had three aims:

- to measure how common movement impairments are in a large population-derived group of school-aged children, including those with ASD and those with both borderline and well-defined intellectual disabilities;
- to examine the association between severity of movement impairment and adaptive behaviour, independent of IQ;
- to assess the properties of the Developmental Coordination Disorder Questionnaire (DCDQ) for parents in identifying children with poor motor skills, as assessed by the Movement ABC (MABC).

Methodology
Participants: Participants were a subsample of the Special Needs and Autism Project (SNAP) drawn from a total population of around 57 000 children aged 9 to 10 in south-east England. From this all children with a clinical diagnosis of pervasive developmental disorders were included (223 males and 32 females). These children were given a comprehensive diagnostic assessment-standardized test and clinical observation, and parental assessments of autistic symptoms, language, and IQ were given. From this subsample of 255, 158 were diagnosed with ASD (autism 81; other ASD 77) and were included in the study.

Measures and procedures: All children were assessed on MABC and only those who completed all items continued in the study. This left 101 children in the study: 89 males and 12 females; 49 with autism and 52 another ASD. The parents of 97 of the 101 children who completed the MABC completed the DCDQ, which is a 17-item survey of a wide range of gross and fine motor functions, ball skills, and planning and organizational abilities. IQ was measured by the WISC-III-UK or by Raven's standard or coloured progressive matrices. If WISC full scale was not available, IQ scores were obtained through the Raven's standard. No direct testing was possible with five children, all of whom had Vineland adaptive behaviour scores less than 20 and were given an IQ score of 19, reflecting a profound intellectual disability. For analysis of the MABC scores the children were divided into two IQ groups: less than 70 with a mean of 57 (n=35); greater than 70 with a mean of 90 (n=66). Parametric (analysis of variance; t-tests) and non-parametric measures (χ^2) together with correlations were used to analyse the findings according to the layout of the data.

Results and discussion
On MABC, 80 of the 101 children were below the fifth centile indicating a definite movement problem. A further 10 were between the 5th and 15th centiles indicating borderline difficulties, and 11 had no problems. The autism group and the wider ASD group had similar percentages of movement problems, 82% and 77%, respectively, but when analyses of variance were calculated on all of the scores the autism group performed poorer than the wider ASD group. The low IQ group had a very high percentage (97%) of movement difficulties and scored poorer than the higher IQ group. Only one child in the lower IQ range did not have a movement difficulty, as defined by the MABC. The authors assert that the reason why there is a high percentage of motor problems in the autistic population is because of the underlying brain functions, and, although they acknowledge that in the low IQ group a lack of understanding of the instructions may have had an effect on the MABC, they did not believe it could account for the almost total motor impairment seen in this group. A surprising finding for the authors was the lack of association between everyday adaptive behaviours and motor impairments once IQ was accounted for. The DCDQ was moderately acceptable as a screening tool when compared with the MABC with a specificity of 75% and sensitivity of 66%. Finally the study showed that the children with ASD were more impaired on timed task, suggesting that complexity of motor task may be important in this population.

by suggesting that biological substrates may underpin a number of difficulties in autism, of which motor problems may be one of many.

Earlier in this section we suggested that the deficit in motor performance may be related to the more cognitive characteristics of the condition, such as theory of mind, lack of empathy, or other constraints related to effective communication, which is one of the core features of the ASD condition. Imitation of gesture is often part of an assessment of motor praxis, and this and difficulty with this is often seen in children with ASD (Rogers et al 1996, Mostofsky et al 2006). Imitation is an interesting action to perform in that it does require a theory of mind, empathy, and some joint attention on the part of the individual. It has been suggested by Williams et al (2005) that this deficit is related to a poor mirror neuron system, which is crucial to imitation. The question raised is whether the motor deficit observed across the board in individuals with ASD is one specifically related to imitation or a more general praxis disorder. Dziuk et al (2007) examined this problem by looking at the relationship between basic motor skill deficits and impaired imitation of gestures. Their groups of children either had high-functioning autism or Asperger syndrome and were matched to typically developing controls. Their findings showed that, after controlling for age and IQ, the ASD group showed that basic motor skill had significant effects on praxis gesture production. However, there was still a decrement in gesture performance between the ASD group and the typically developing controls after accounting for the poor motor skill performance, and that gesture performance is worse than what would be predicted from the level of motor skill. This suggests that abnormalities outside of the usual neurological substrates underpinning movements are responsible for the additional decrements in gesture performance. The authors speculate on the various brain regions responsible for this and conclude with the statement that 'dyspraxia may be a core feature of autism, or a marker of the neurologic deficits that underlie the disorder' (Dziuk et al 2007, p. 738).

Aside from the evidence for a biological influence on the development of ASD per se, there is also some evidence for a biological component to the performance on motor tasks in individuals with ASD at the level of brain structure and function. A functional magnetic resonance imaging (fMRI) study showed atypical activation in adults with ASD compared with matched controls in a visually paced tapping task (Miller et al 2001). More recently, structural brain differences in ASD have also been linked to motor performance, with increased white matter volume predicting motor impairment. The opposite correlation between brain structure and task performance was found in controls (Mostofsky et al 2007). Finally, fMRI has revealed differences in brain activation in children with ASD versus controls when performing a finger tapping task (Mostofsky et al 2009).

In summary, there is good evidence for the existence of a range of motor difficulties in ASD and, because of the range of difficulties in the autistic population from mild to very severe, there is a concomitant range of problems with motor coordination. This evidence comes from biological and cognitive investigations and suggests the presence of a pure motor deficit in some individuals with ASD, as well as motor difficulties appearing as a consequence of non-motor cognitive processes (such as executive dysfunction). Additionally, and as with any disorder, there will be a developmental component to the observed difficulties such that difficulties in early life will have an impact on the development of a whole range of skills as the child's environment and interactions with the world are moulded to some extent by their skills and difficulties.

ATTENTION-DEFICIT–HYPERACTIVITY DISORDER

Definition and core characteristics

Throughout history there have been references to children who would fit into this category from Dr Heinrich Hoffman's 'Fidgety Phil' in 1844, through George Still's lecture to the Royal Society of Medicine in 1902 describing some children as having 'serious problems with sustained attention', to William James talking of deficits in 'inhibitory volition…and sustained attention' (1899). The concept of hyperactivity is one that has been studied with interest, and particularly in the 1960s and 1970s when the 'hyperactivity syndrome' became a focus. From there the line of thought changed slightly with attention seen as the variable most under examination, leading to the terms attention deficit disorder and ADHD. This has led to the current DSM-IV criteria (APA 2000), parts of which are listed below.

- A persistent pattern of inattention or inattention and/or hyperactivity that is more frequent and severe than peers.
- It is present before 7 years of age but later observation of symptoms is often the case.
- Symptoms are present in at least two settings – home, school, and work.
- It interferes with social, academic or work functioning.
- It is not better described by either a pervasive developmental disorder or mental disorder.

DSM-IV (APA 2000) presents two lists of behaviours in order to elaborate these criteria. The first one involves those that are concerned with inattention such as 'easily distracted' and notes that six or more must be present in the last 6 months to a point that they are disruptive and inappropriate for the developmental level of the child. The second list is concerned with hyperactivity, such as is often 'on the go' or often acts as if 'driven by a motor', coupled with impulsivity, such as responding before full information has been given, and has to be present according to the same criteria as above in inattention.

Based on these and the criteria three types of children are identified:

- *combined type*: if both the criteria for the two lists are met for the last 6 months;
- *predominantly inattentive type*: if the first list is met but not the second;
- *predominantly hyperactivity impulsive type*: if the second is met but not the first.

Typical characteristics of the three types are shown in Box 10.3. It is not a complete list but an illustration of the behaviours that are commonly seen.

The ICD-10 (WHO 1992) definition is slightly different from the one by DSM-IV, but the two sets of criteria clearly relate to the same disorder in children. It is the rules for making a diagnosis that are different. For ICD-10 the condition is labelled hyperkinetic disorder and requires all three of the main behavioural problems of attention deficit, overactivity, and impulsiveness for a diagnosis. Thus the ICD-10 criteria are met only for the combined type in DSM-IV.

A range of prevalence figures has been given and these vary according to how the condition is assessed, the country in which it is assessed, which phase of education the child is in, and the criteria being used. Using the DSM-IV criteria, prevalence rates of up to 19% have been reported, but the usual range is between 3% and 5% with differences between studies usually attributed to different cut-off points rather than differences in populations (Buitelaar 2002, Taylor 2006). Ratios for male:female

---

Box 10.3 A closer examination

Typical characteristics of the three types of ADHD

Predominantly hyperactivity–impulsivity
- restless in their seats, squirming, and constantly moving, often around the classroom;
- always on the go as if 'driven by a motor';
- find keeping still difficult and uncomfortable;
- constant need to touch articles and people and engaging in activities such as noisily tapping pens and pencils;
- occasionally hit other children;
- move or answer a question before the full information is presented;
- difficulty in waiting to take turns;
- make inappropriate comments in class with little regard for consequences; and
- engage in activities that are immediate and have little payoff, as opposed to delaying actions with potentially higher payoffs.

Predominantly inattentive
- have difficulty concentrating for any length of time and are easily bored;
- are easily distracted by events or objects not connected to task;
- rush through work and make many careless mistakes by not giving appropriate attention to detail;
- move constantly from one short task to another;
- constantly misplacing items, losing pencils, not following instructions.

Combined type
- In this type the child meets the characteristics of both of the above types.

These characteristics are required to be inappropriate for developmental age and are required to be seen in at least two settings: home, school, play, work.

prevalence are in the region of 2.5:1 to 4:1, depending on whether they are clinical or population studies with the higher figure usually found when measuring hyperkinesis. There is also some suggestion that females are less likely than males to be referred (Taylor 2006).

The condition often runs in families with those who have first-degree relatives with the condition having an increased risk of three- to fivefold. There are a number of genes that have been identified as being possibly influential such as genes for dopamine receptors 4 (DRD47-repeat allele) and 5 (DRD5 148bp-allele) and the dopamine transporter gene (DAT1 10-repeat allele) (Taylor et al 2004). Each of these slightly increases the risk, emphasizing that in a complex disorder such as this a multitude of aetiological factors will contribute to the final outcome. There are the usual environmental risks with increased prevalence associated with low birthweight, prenatal exposure to toxins, and some idiosyncratic food reactions (Taylor et al 2004). In addition, through the use of structural and functional imaging techniques, various parts of the brain, such as the frontal, temporal, and parietal regions of the cortex as well as the basal ganglia, have been found to show some abnormalities (for a review see Taylor et al 2004). A dynamic gene–environment interaction seems likely, although because of the varying nature and therefore lack of certainty about symptoms this interaction is very difficult to disentangle. There appears to be an assumption that behaviour is complex and influenced by genes of a small and cumulative effect together with environmental influences.

ADHD has a history of comorbid difficulties and this is not surprising considering that attention to the task or person is an essential prerequisite to learning. Thus, if you are off task or easily distractible or doing other things, such as fiddling with objects or moving around a classroom to no apparent purpose, it would be surprising if there were no co-occurring difficulties. In a review of the condition specifying European clinical guidelines (Taylor et al 2004) note that the coexistence of other difficulties is common, noting in particular those of conduct disorder, emotional disorders, specific learning disorders, pervasive developmental disorders, tic disorders, DCD, bipolar disorder, and substance abuse. Again various prevalence rates for comorbid difficulties are available but the following give some flavour to the issue. The rates of overlap with dyslexia have shown ranges from 35% to 50% (Dykman and Ackerman 1991, Semrud-Clikeman et al 1992); in all surveys, one-third of children with ADHD have been noted to have problems in reading, spelling, and mathematics unaccounted for by low intelligence (Szatmari et al 1989). An obvious area of disability is in the social area with many showing oppositional defiant

disorder, conduct disorder, and predisposition to anxiety (Barkley et al 1990, Taylor et al 1991) and around 22% being described as socially disabled (Green et al 1997, 2001). In addition, in their study, Fitzgerald and Corvin (2001) found that 21% of children with ADHD met the full criteria for Asperger syndrome and 36% showed 'autistic traits'. Kaplan et al (2001) turn around the statistics in a different manner and report that if a child meets the criteria for ADHD they have an 80% chance of having one other disorder.

The description so far has concentrated on those traits in ADHD that are seen at the behavioural level. If these are examined within the framework of the Morton and Frith model specifying the levels of biology, cognition, and behaviour it is possible to speculate on the underlying cognitive substrates. The most prominent that appears here is that of *executive control*, which results in attentiveness because of the lack of flexibility in allocation of the attentional resource. Executive control is a term that has a wide variety of meanings but fundamentally it is a cognitive process that works '*top down*', that is, as the name suggests, the process involves taking a large view of the situation and recruiting resources to accomplish a particular task. This can involve planning and organizing and both of these processes are often used when executive control is being mentioned. Hulme and Snowling (2009) state that it contains four separate but correlated factors:

- response inhibition and execution – the ability to curb a natural reaction to respond too quickly and inappropriately;
- working memory and updating – the ability to use working memory in a pragmatic manner, particularly on a task which requires holding in store one piece of information to be used in sequence to accomplish a task;
- set shifting and task switching – the ability to move from one part of a task to another or from one task to another, again in an appropriate manner, not in any random fashion, which is actually a characteristic of the condition; and
- interference control – the ability to ignore an interference that would be detrimental to performing a task.

Thus when a response requires it to be inhibited, or an appropriate shifting response is required from one task to another, or when sustained attention is required, the child has difficulties with both of these situations (Schachar et al 1995, Barkley 1997). The response inhibition model is very much one that is favoured by researchers such as Barkley who has a model with behavioural inhibition at the core (Barkley 1997). The term executive function has a number of meanings all related to being in control of events and oneself; the ability to take control of environmental stimuli rather than be constantly driven by them. When a child is being assessed for possible ADHD, information is collected usually by checklist or interview from parents, teachers, friends, and the children themselves (e.g. Conners' Rating Scales; Conners 1996). In addition, tests involving an assessment of executive function are also used with tasks such as the stop-signal task (Solanto et al 2001), which as the name suggests assesses response inhibition, and the Tower of Hanoi, which involves planning a sequence of actions.

Attention-deficit–hyperactivity disorder and motor problems

We have noted above that the overlap between ADHD and DCD or motor problems is quite common. Kaplan in her work uses the term 'atypical brain development' and her rationale for this rests much on the overlap between DCD and ADHD. In 2006 Kaplan et al reviewed a series of investigations they had conducted consisting of three sets of analyses with school-aged children for the co-occurrence of DCD, ADHD, and reading difficulty. In the first analysis they looked at those children with DCD who also met the criteria for reading difficulty and ADHD, with the overlap ranging from 13% for those who also met the criteria for ADHD to 36% for those who met the criteria for both ADHD and reading difficulty. Put another way, 82% of children with a diagnosis of DCD met diagnostic criteria for either reading difficulty or ADHD. This basically says that the vast majority of children with a diagnosed movement difficulty will also have some co-occurring problem. Their second analysis showed that children with ADHD were more likely to have co-occurring disorders in visual and motor skills, in behaviour, and day-to-day functional tasks. From this, and other work that looks at the overlap of symptoms, Kaplan and colleagues have proposed that co-occurrence and continuum are better terms than the one currently used, comorbidity. They view the term atypical brain development described earlier as one that can shed light on the aetiology and co-occurring symptoms.

It is not surprising that children with ADHD have co-occurring difficulties that could be the result of an underlying biological substrate or a cognitive process, or simply a result of the child missing information, if the co-occurrence is with a classroom activity such as reading. Martin et al (2006), for example, showed through parent questionnaires that there is a suggestion of some overlap in the genetic aetiology of ADHD and DCD. Kedesjo and C Gillberg (2001) argue that, even in a population sample, pure cases of ADHD without co-occurring difficulties

are rare. In their study of 409 children, 15 (3.7%) were diagnosed with ADHD; 47 (10%) were diagnosed as 'subthreshold' ADHD, that is a minor form of the condition; and 352 had no ADHD. When the total group was tested for DCD using DSM-IV criteria (APA 1994), in both the full-blown ADHD group and the subthreshold group 47% had DCD (absolute numbers 7 and 20, respectively). In the rest of the group with no ADHD the prevalence rate was 9% with 30 diagnosed.

Children with ADHD have been found to have a variety of motor problems. In a number of studies, van der Meere and colleagues (Seargeant and van der Meere 1988, van der Meere et al 1989, 1992) found difficulties in children with ADHD in motor decision making, motor adjustments, and motor preparation. Some have found problems with slower reaction times (Reader et al 1994), and others have found overall motor performance measured by tests, such as the Bruininks–Oseretsky Test of Motor Proficiency (BOTMP; Bruininks 1978), to be significantly lower for children with ADHD than their age-matched peers (Whitmont and Clark 1996). The deficits that children with ADHD show cover both fine motor control, as measured by graphomotor tests (Marcotte and Stern 1997), and the gross motor skills of running, hopping, jumping, etc. (Harvey and Reid 1997).

There is overwhelming evidence to show that children with a diagnosis of ADHD have more motor difficulties than a typical sample of age-matched peers. There are some elements of motor problems in the diagnosis of ADHD, with DSM-IV having as part of the criteria some movement activities, such as constant motion, but these do not allude to quality of movement. Depending on how this is interpreted, it could mean there would be an apparent increase in the co-occurrence of ADHD and DCD as a function of this. Having motor problems in the diagnostic criteria of ADHD may reflect overlap in the conditions of ADHD and DCD, but it could also reflect the behavioural consequences of the cognitive impairments. This is particularly the case in the hyperactive child, who often moves before the full information is given. However, one should not think that all children with hyperkinesis have poor motor difficulties; indeed one has only to look at some of our most talented sports people to see overly active individuals with superb control of their motor skills.

An investigation into the relationship between characteristics of ADHD and motor proficiency was undertaken by Tseng et al (2004) and this study is shown in detail as an example in Box 10.4.

The evidence is clear that a child with ADHD is more likely to have co-occurring difficulties in the motor domain or even have a dual diagnosis of ADHD and DCD, and reports from clinical settings are giving indications

Box 10.4 A closer examination

Relationships among motor proficiency, attention, impulse, and activity control in children with ADHD: Tseng et al (2004)

Aim

The aim of this study was to investigate the relationship between motor proficiency and the core problems of ADHD by objectively measuring inattention and impulsivity in addition to parent and teacher rating scales, as used in previous studies. It was designed to investigate the influence of inattention, impulsivity, and hyperactivity on gross and fine motor skills.

Methods

The participants were 84 children between the ages of 6 and 11 years: 42 diagnosed with ADHD (36 male; mean age 8y 2mo) matched with 42 without DCD (36 male; mean age 8y 3mo). If the children were on medication, this was stopped 24 hours before the testing sessions. BOTMP (Bruininks 1978) was used to test gross and fine motor performance with the Activity Rating Scale for Parents (ARP) (Hsu et al 1982) and the Activity Rating Scale for Teachers (Hsu et al 1982) used to acquire information from significant others about the behaviour of the children. In addition, the Gordon Diagnostic System (Gordon 1991) was used to measure sustained attention and impulse control in the form of a vigilance and delay task in a computer game.

Results

On BOTMP the means for gross motor tasks were 52 (ADHD) and 59 (controls) and for the fine motor 63 (ADHD) and 69 (controls), both being significantly different. When the gross and fine motor tests were broken down into subtests, it was only balance that was the significant gross motor subtest, with no differences between the groups on running speed and agility and bilateral coordination. For the fine motor tests, only the visual motor control part was significant.

When the relationships among attention, impulse control, activity level, and motor proficiency were measured it was found that gross motor variables correlated significantly with ARP, correct responses, and commission errors, whereas fine motor skills correlated with efficiency ratios, correct responses, and commission errors. The best predictors of gross motor skills were correct responses accounting for 34% of the variance, with others accounting for 56% of the total variance. For fine motor skills the best predictor was again correct responses, accounting for 33% of the variance.

Discussion

Overall, the children with ADHD performed less well than the controls on total measures of both fine and gross motor tests but not on all of the subtests. In addition, the predictions from the tests showed that attention level, impulse control, and activity level are predictors of deficits in motor skills in children with ADHD. The authors suggest that two alternative reasons can explain the relationship between ADHD and motor skills as measured in this study. First, poor attention interferes with motor proficiency, as reflected in BOTMP scores, but does not indicate a primary motor deficit. Alternatively, problems in impulse control, inattention, and hyperactivity may be primary deficits that co-occur or even cause motor problems.

that a diagnosis will vary across different contexts. The evidence we have comes from studies looking at motor abilities from instruments such as BOTMP, described in Box 10.4, and from other work that takes prevalence data to look at percentage of overlap of two conditions or a primary condition with co-occurring characteristics (Kadesjo and Gillberg 2001).

A detailed approach was taken by Pereira et al (2000) who investigated the performance of children with a diagnosis of ADHD in tasks involving motor memory representations. They note that motor difficulties in ADHD seem to affect handwriting and that variables surrounding precision grip can be usefully examined to understand the motor control mechanisms in children with ADHD.

Their work in this study follows on from other work by the authors in which they examined neural control mechanisms for lifts with a precision grip in typically developing children and those with cerebral palsy (Eliasson et al 1991, 1992, 1995, Forssberg et al 1991, 1992; see Chapter 7). The task was to take an object with a wide base that can be altered by weight and has transducers attached to it to measure the load and grip force. The Pereira et al study comprised 25 males with ADHD (9 'pure' and 16 with additional motor coordination difficulties) and 25 age-matched peers with no history of behaviour or learning difficulties, dyslexia, or psychological and social adaptation problems. The mean age of both groups was approximately 11 years and 6 months. The basic task was to lift the object with thumb and first finger and place it inside a box; this task was varied to examine basic coordination, anticipatory control of force, and stability of force output. The ADHD group with additional motor problems (ADHD+) had more disturbed motor control than either the control group or the ADHD group without motor difficulties, with the authors indicating that the ADHD+ group exhibit a specific motor dysfunction that is not present in the other two groups. The authors suggest first that poor performance on tasks involving anticipatory control may be a function of inefficient memory processes. Second, they reject the proposition that behavioural abnormalities of motor control in children with ADHD are due to a lack of inhibition in frontal–striatal circuits influencing executive functions, and propose that in some children with ADHD (in this study the ADHD+ group) these are due to poor neural motor control functions.

It is reasonably well established that in children with ADHD there is a higher prevalence of motor disorders. The reasons for this are multiple and range from biological through cognitive to behavioural ones. The situation is made more complex by the existence of many children with a diagnosis of ADHD who are perfectly adequate in their motor skills.

SPECIFIC LANGUAGE IMPAIRMENT

Definitions and characteristics
SLI is the label given to children who have difficulties with various aspects of language. It is specific in that most of the definitions invoke the discrepancy concept, noting that their difficulty with oral language is not in accordance with their level of intelligence and ability in non-language areas. There is great variability in the condition with some having speech difficulties, others having difficulties with the social use of language, and some who have no real communication difficulties despite their speech being problematic. Usually identification of SLI involves a standardized language test, in which the child will score low, often specified statistically such as two standard deviations below the mean, alongside a non-verbal IQ test, in which the child will score within the typical range, above 80 for example. In all cases conditions such as deafness are ruled out.

Johnson and Beitchman (2006) use ICD-10 for the definition and characteristics of specific developmental disorders of speech and language impairment concentrating on the three areas of speech articulation disorder, expressive language disorder, and receptive language disorder. In typically developing children these three areas show some variability but with evidence of word comprehension (receptive language) appearing late in the first year of life and before expressive language. For children with SLI the most notable feature of their early language is that it has a delayed onset and a slow rate of development.

Johnson and Beitchman (2006) define *speech articulation disorder* as a significant delay or impairment in learning to correctly pronounce speech sounds but without expressive or receptive language problems. The ICD-10 category is similar but not identical to the DSM-IV-TR category of phonological disorders that appears under Communication disorders. It often involves the substitution of one sound for another or the total omission of a particular sound, often the final consonant. Prevalence should be below 2% to 3%, as ICD-10 uses a cut-off of two standard deviations, with between two and four times more males than females. A slow rate of speech sound development is a key characteristic starting with babbling at around 6 months of age and progressing to recognizable first words between 12 and 18 months of age. A child with a speech articulation disorder develops in a similar manner to typically developing children but slower and with some idiosyncrasies in patterns. Although a child with articulation problems can be identified early, it is more common for the child to be around 4 years of age before a diagnosis, mainly because between 2 and 4 years of age there is such variety in children's pronunciations. It is important to diagnose accurately particularly with respect to whether expressive or receptive language is also a problem, as prognosis of the comorbid variety is less optimistic than articulation on its own.

With *expressive language disorder* there is a significant delay or impairment in the use of language relative to cognitive age; receptive language is not affected to the same degree and speech articulation may or may not be affected with about a 40% overlap. Again prevalence rates are around 3% with male:female ratios ranging from 2:1 to 5:1. The main clinical features are delays in starting to talk and being slow in expanding the vocabulary as well as differences in the types of speech that are produced.

For example, there may be disorders in the content of speech and a smaller vocabulary than what is typically observed. There may be differences in form with syntax being incorrect and other grammatical errors – such as incorrect word endings, plurals, tenses, and pronouns. Problems with use of language often involve not being able to extend conversations and being limited to short sentences or phrases and words. Quite a large proportion of those with expressive language disorder also have an articulation disorder making the condition more serious and longer lasting. The factors that are speculated for the causes of expressive language disorder have been speculated to be those outlined above for articulation disorder as well as specific linguistic factors, such as poor phonological working memory, and other more general cognitive factors, including difficulties with temporal processing (Johnson and Beitchman 2006).

Receptive language disorder involves a child being delayed or impaired in understanding language when compared with the child's overall cognitive ability. There are numerous exclusions from this such as aphasia, dysphasia, and autism. There is a range of severity with some children even having problems with individual words in the most severe cases. Again with ICD-10 there is a prevalence rate of around 2% and again a male:female ratio between 2:1 and 4:1. They have difficulty learning the meaning of new words and have difficulty with questions and instructions, with the result that answers to queries or other responses are often not related to the topic at hand and in some cases appear nonsensical. Again like expressive disorders the difficulties they show may exhibit in problems with content, form, or use of the language with the result that their vocabulary becomes small with a reduced capacity for abstract ideas and concepts. These limitations often limit the amount of understanding and these translate into problems with language in daily life. The overlap with speech articulation problems is in the region of 40% to 60% (Johnson and Beitchman 2006).

Hulme and Snowling (2009) note that linguists and psychologists have rather different views on the nature and causes of the disorder. Linguists, they state, would argue that the root of the problem lies in a specific linguistic area such as grammatical knowledge. This view tacitly places language in a different place to other cognitive functions, with it operating independently. Psychologists, on the other hand, see the problems as being based on an impaired cognitive processing system with the tacit view that language is not independent but operates dynamically with other areas of cognition. Both views have their pros and cons with the independent language system failing to explain how and why the subcomponents responsible for language, and which are postulated as the cause of the

problems, fail to develop in the first instance. Processes such as speed of processing, phonological difficulties, and auditory processes rooted in cognitive explanations pose problems for the definition of SLI, being out of line with other non-verbal processes and abilities. In other words, if the problem involves general cognitive functions such as speed of processing, why isn't SLI simply a function/characteristic of general learning difficulties?

As with many other disorders the exact aetiology of SLI is not known, and we presented the Morton (2004) model earlier in the chapter to elucidate the connections between possible biological substrates and behaviour with cognitive processes as the intervening variable. Suggestions for aetiology have included genetic factors: there is good evidence that the condition is highly heritable. The usual standard of comparing monozygotic twins to dizygotic twins with and without the condition showed monozygotic twins to be more concordant for SLI (Tomblin and Buckwalter 1998). Impoverished language experience such as language in the home would also appear to be a factor often in conjunction with genetic or neurological dispositions, subtle auditory problems, and speech mechanisms or motor control problems (Johnson and Beitchman 2006). For many children the problems disappear by around 8 years of age with or without treatment, although the prognosis is better for those who have treatment. There are some minor residual difficulties but they do not impede intelligibility (Johnson and Beitchman 2006). When articulation disorders persist in conjunction with other language disorders they often serve as a marker for more serious and pervasive difficulties.

Specific language impairment and motor disorders
In the field of SLI there has been much work on the severity of the language impairment, linking it to motor ability (for a review see Hill 2001) and in particular to children's awkwardness and clumsiness, with authors such as Bishop and Edmundson (1987) finding a relationship between a peg moving task and language impairment. There have been suggestions that motor and language deficits may arise from a common underlying cause, with various possibilities being noted. For example, common brain areas may be implicated (Hill 2001). Genetic factors may also play a role (Bishop 2002); it is well known that there is a genetic influence in SLI with increased concordance rates in monozygotic twins (Bishop et al 1996) and genetic influences on behavioural performance on the Children's Nonword Repetition test (Bishop et al 1996). In addition, there are also suggestions of a common underpinning to deficits in the language and motor domains (Bishop 2002). However, genes are not uniquely involved, as there is some evidence of environmental

influences on performance on certain tests that are performed poorly by those with SLI. Cognitive variables must also be involved and some cognitive explanations may explain the co-occurring features of motor and language impairment. In an early attempt to identify putative mechanisms of co-occurrence between language and motor deficits, Powell and Bishop (1992) analysed the relationship between SLI and motor difficulties, examining three possible hypotheses as to why this relationship may exist in children with SLI. First, the left hemisphere hypothesis predicts lateralized impairments on motor tasks and normal performance on visual discrimination tasks; second, the slow rate of processing hypothesis predicts deficits only in the production of rapidly changing movements but not for those such as balance that do not involve rapid movements; third, the imperfect visual perception hypothesis predicts similar deficits in children with SLI and children with motor difficulties in visual discrimination and motor tasks, in both static and changing environments. A group of children with SLI performed poorly on tests of motor ability compared with a control group, confirming a relationship. However, there was no evidence of lateralized impairment and the motor deficits did not include only rapid movements. Only the imperfect visual perception hypothesis showed promise, but the authors queried this, as have subsequent writings. Powell and Bishop (1992) argue that the relationship in this study could have been due to poor visual perception or some other factor, such as attention, as the tasks used were of little intrinsic interest. Other common factors were speculated, but the authors conclude that no one factor associated with information processing stages could account for the whole of language and motor and indeed attentional variables.

More recently, a further cognitive theory has been proposed to explain the behavioural features of SLI, the declarative/procedural memory model. In this account, Ullman (2001) proposes sharing of the declarative memory network in the context of impairment in the procedural memory network. In language terms, they propose that this would lead to intact lexical knowledge but impaired syntactic knowledge. They suggest that this impairment arises from abnormal development of the neural structures forming the procedural memory system, specifically the frontal/basal ganglia circuits. This network is known to subserve the learning and execution of motor and cognitive skills, especially those involving sequencing, and has been implicated more recently in grammar learning and use (e.g. Ullman 2001, Ullman and Pierpont 2005). It should also be noted that it is, as yet, unclear whether there will be one unifying explanation for the language and motor deficits seen in SLI or whether, as was noted above with respect to autism, there are a number of valid explanations for different categories of behavioural symptoms, with varying underlying cognitive and biological causes (cf. Ronald et al 2006).

In two related articles (Hill 1998, Hill et al 1998), both quantitative and qualitative performance on motor skills were compared in two groups, one with SLI and the other with DCD. The study, which uses mainly quantitative data, is shown in Box 10.5.

When the data were examined from a qualitative point of view involving independent raters of the movements to establish reliability, the types of errors made by the children with SLI, children with DCD, and younger children were very similar (Hill et al 1998). For intransitive gestures to imitation only the children with DCD produced more errors than their typically developing peers (Hill et al 1998). The performance of the two groups under study – SLI and DCD groups – were very similar and three explanations were offered: first, that language has a specific role in representational tasks; second, the similarity may be because of the anatomical contiguity of the neural substrates underpinning language and motor abilities; and third, it may be that common to both conditions is some underlying immaturity of the brain. Hill et al (1998) suggest this may a reason for overlapping rather than distinct disorders and propose that in all such studies a younger typically developing group should be included.

Movement and language have certain similarities. They are both naturally developing abilities in children that under typical circumstances do not have to be taught but occur in all countries across a variety of contexts. They are generative in nature in that different movements or words can be used to achieve the same ends. They are both flexibly used and involve generalization skills and are fundamental to our activities of daily living. There is obvious overlap between the two, but, again, there are children with language difficulties whose movements are perfectly adequate and vice versa.

Summary

In a number of places in Chapters 7–12 of the book we have argued the case for any developmental disorder having co-occurring characteristics. In the case of movement skill abilities, it does not matter whether one starts with a diagnosis of motor difficulties such as DCD, or a different developmental disorder diagnosis such as the four summarized in this chapter; the end result is the same, with co-occurring difficulties usually being the rule rather than the exception.

In all of the four developmental disorders, there is a higher prevalence of movement skill difficulties than in a typically developing population. The actual prevalence

Box 10.5 A closer examination

A dyspraxic deficit in SLI and DCD? Evidence from hand movements: Hill (1998)
Children with difficulties such as SLI often show motor deficits, and two of the aims of this article were to determine whether the movement skills of children with SLI were the same or different from those with DCD and to determine whether the performance in these two groups was due to pathology or developmental delay.

Methodology
In this study, 72 children were assigned to one of four groups:

1   children with SLI
2   children with DCD
3   age-matched control children
4   younger control children.

Children with SLI were selected following comprehensive psychological and medical evaluations, including the Raven's Progressive Matrices and the CELF-R (Clinical Evaluation of Language Fundamental Fourth Edition) Repeating Sentences. The DCD group were included from referrals in a particular region followed by the MABC test. The two control groups were selected from local primary schools and had age-appropriate scores on standardized tests of non-verbal and language ability.

The children were asked to mime representational gestures, both transitive (requiring the use of an object such as using a comb) and intransitive (not requiring an object, such as a wave or a salute). All gestures were completed to verbal command or imitation. This gave four conditions: transitive verbal command; intransitive verbal command; transitive imitation; intransitive imitation. One point was awarded for a correct response and zero for an incorrect response giving a total of six for each condition (six tasks in each category).

Second, the children were required to copy a series of unfamiliar hand postures and sequences. The children copied to action from immediate memory unless unsuccessful, in which case the posture or sequence was repeated and the children were asked to imitate it concurrently. This was done a second time if unsuccessful. For single postures a score of 2 was given for a correct response and 1 if correct on the second attempt. For a fail, 0 was awarded. For multiple hand postures, 3 was given for correct from memory at the first attempt; 2 for correct from imitation on the second attempt; and 1 for a correct response to concurrent imitation on the third attempt. For a fail, 0 was awarded. The gestures are shown in Figure 10.3.

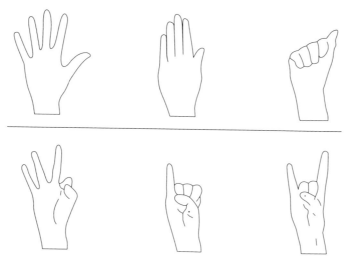

Fig. 10.3 Gestures for imitation. Reproduced with permission of the publisher from Hill EL (1998).

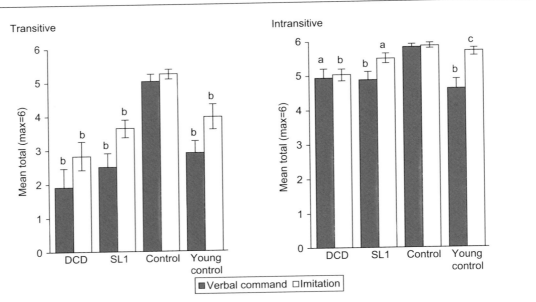

Fig. 10.4 Mean scores for representational gestures. Reproduced with permission of the publisher from Hill EL (1998).

Results

Mean scores for the representational gestures are shown in Figure 10.4.

All children performed more poorly in the transitive than in the intransitive conditions and in verbal commands to imitation. Children with DCD and SLI produced more errors than their age-matched peers and were similar in performance to the younger group.

Scores for the hand posture tasks showed no differences between the groups suggesting a ceiling effect of the tasks. Some differences in latency (speed of response) were obtained.

Discussion

Children with DCD and SLI were found to be dyspraxic only on the tests of meaningful gesture production (representational gestures) and not on copying unfamiliar hand postures. Both groups were poorer in the representational gestures than their age-matched peers and were similar to a younger group, and the author states that the poor performance of the SLI group was not due to a lack of understanding of the task. The almost equivalence of the DCD and SLI groups to the younger group led the author to suggest that the poor performances of the SLI and DCD groups were due to poor maturation of development and not neurological impairment, but, to confirm this, she suggested that longitudinal studies should be implemented. The author argued against using the term 'dyspraxic' with its roots in neurologically impaired adults as it implies 'qualitative abnormality in development which is not, as yet, justified by the empirical data' (Hill 1998, p. 394).

of motor difficulties differs across the disorders, with, for example, most children with low functioning/classic autism showing movement difficulties, whereas children with disorders such as dyslexia simply showing a higher prevalence. This can be due to the disorder or the manner in which co-occurring movement problems are assessed.

The reasons for the co-occurrence again vary. In classic autism, it could be that some underlying biological variable drives the autism and also affects the movement skill production system. There is also the possibility of some generic biological problems and there is variability in which function is affected, with other functions present but less involved. In others it could be a cognitive difficulty such as executive control or attention as seen in ADHD. In SLI the difficulty that is underpinning speech production, for example, could also affect other motor tasks such as those involving fine and gross motor skills.

The increase in prevalence of motor difficulties in these developmental disorders could be interpreted in another way that is speculative. In Chapter 1, we detailed the concept of embodied cognition, noting that motor and cognitions are not totally separate entities. To perform motor skills one has to 'know' something as well as 'do' something. In a similar vein, one could note that in order to 'know' something movement is hugely beneficial; the

influential article by Campos et al (2000), 'Travel broadens the mind', nicely encapsulates this. It is too much of a jump to propose that one causes the other, but the relationship between these seemingly disparate human abilities is difficult to ignore. The real question is where these relationships originate: are they biological, cognitive, or simply the behavioural manifestations of environmental contexts?

REFERENCES

APA (1994) *Diagnostic and Statistical Manual of Mental Disorders: DSM IV*, 4th edition. Washington, DC: American Psychiatric Association.

APA (2000) *Diagnostic and Statistical Manual of Mental Disorders: DSM IV*, 4th edition text revision. Arlington, VA: American Psychiatric Association.

Asperger H (1944) Autistic pathology in childhood. Annotated and translated in: Frith U, editor (1991) *Autism and Asperger Syndrome*. New York: Cambridge University Press, pp. 37–92.

Barkley RA (1997) Behavioral inhibition, sustained attention and executive functions: constructing a unifying theory of ADHD. *Psychol Bull* 121: 65–94. http://dx.doi.org/10.1037/0033-2909.121.1.65

Barkley RA, Du Paul GJ, McMurray B (1990) Comprehensive evaluation of attention deficit disorder with and without hyperactivity as defined by research criteria. *J Consult Clin Psychol* 58: 775–789. http://dx.doi.org/10.1037/0022-006X.58.6.775

Baron-Cohen S (2008) Theories of the autistic mind. *Psychologist* 21: 112–116.

Baron-Cohen S, Leslie A, Frith U (1985) Does the autistic child have a 'theory of mind'? *Cognition* 21: 37–46. http://dx.doi.org/10.1016/0010-0277(85)90022-8

Baron-Cohen S, Richler J, Bisarya G, Guranathan N, Wheelwright S (2003) The systemising quotient. *Phil Trans Royal Soc* 358: 361–374. http://dx.doi.org/10.1098/rstb.2002.1206

Bishop DVM (2002) The role of genes in the etiology of specific language impairment. *J Communication Disord* 35: 311–328. http://dx.doi.org/10.1016/S0021-9924(02)00087-4

Bishop DVM (2007) Curing dyslexia and attention deficit hyperactivity disorder by training motor coordination: miracle or myth? *J Paediatr Child Health* 43: 653–655. http://dx.doi.org/10.1111/j.1440-1754.2007.01225.x

Bishop DVM, Edmundson A (1987) Language-impaired 4-year-olds: distinguishing transient from persistent impairment. *J Speech Hearing Disord* 52: 156–173.

Bishop DVM, North T, Donlan C (1996) Nonword repetition as a behavioural marker for inherited language impairment: evidence from a twin study. *J Child Psychol Psychiatry* 37: 391–403. http://dx.doi.org/10.1111/j.1469-7610.1996.tb01420.x

BPS (1999) *Dyslexia Literacy and Psychological Assessment: Report by the Working Party of the Division of Educational and Child Psychology of the British Psychological Society*. Leicester: British Psychological Society.

Bruininks RH (1978) *Bruininks–Oseretsky Test of Motor Proficiency*. Circle Pines, MN: American Guidance Service.

Buitelaar JK (2002) Epidemiology: what have we learned over the last decade? In: Sandberg S, editor. *Hyperactivity and Attention-Deficit Disorders*. Cambridge: Cambridge University Press, pp. 1–39

Campos JJ, Anderson DI, Barbu-Roth MA, Hubbard EM, Hertenstein MJ, Witherington D (2000) Travelling broadens the mind. *Infancy* 1: 149–219. http://dx.doi.org/10.1207/S15327078IN0102_1

Caron C, Rutter M (1991) Comorbidity in childhood psychopathology: concepts, issues and research strategies. *J Child Psychol Psychiatry* 32: 1063–1080. http://dx.doi.org/10.1111/j.1469-7610.1991.tb00350.x

Conners C (1996) *Conners' Rating Scales – Revised*. London: Psychological Corporation.

Cope N, Harold D, Moskvina V, et al (2005) Strong evidence that KIAA0319 on chromosome 6p is a susceptibility gene for developmental dysfunction. *Am J Hum Genet* 76: 581–591. http://dx.doi.org/10.1086/429131

Curtiss S (1977) *Genie: A Psycholinguistic Study of a Modern-Day "Wild Child"*. New York: Academic Press.

DeFries JC, Alarcon M (1996) Genetics of specific reading disability. *Ment Retard Dev Disabil Res Rev* 2: 39–47. http://dx.doi.org/10.1002/(SICI)1098-2779(1996)2:1<39::AID-MRDD7>3.0.CO;2-S

Denkla MB (1974) Development of motor coordination in normal children. *Dev Med Child Neurol* 16: 729–741. http://dx.doi.org/10.1111/j.1469-8749.1974.tb03393.x

Diamond A (2000) Development and cognitive development of the cerebellum and frontal cortex. *Child Dev* 71: 44–56. http://dx.doi.org/10.1111/1467-8624.00117

Dykman RA, Ackerman PT (1991) Attention deficit disorder and specific reading disability: separate but overlapping disorders. *J Learn Disabil* 24: 96–103. http://dx.doi.org/10.1177/002221949102400206

Dziuk MA, Gidley Larson JC, Apostu A, Mahone EM, Denkla MB, Mostofsky SH (2007) Dyspraxia in autism: association with motor, social and communicative deficits. *Dev Med Child Neurol* 49: 734–739. http://dx.doi.org/10.1111/j.1469-8749.2007.00734.x

Eliasson AC, Gordon AM, Forssberg H (1991) Basic coordination of manipulative forces of children with cerebral palsy. *Dev Med Child Neurol* 33: 661–670. http://dx.doi.org/10.1111/j.1469-8749.1991.tb14943.x

Eliasson AC, Gordon AM, Forssberg H (1992) Impaired anticipatory control of isometric forces during grasping by children with cerebral palsy. *Dev Med Child Neurol* 34: 216–225. http://dx.doi.org/10.1111/j.1469-8749.1992.tb14994.x

Eliasson AC, Gordon AM, Forssberg H (1995) Tactile control of isometric fingertip forces during grasping in children with cerebral palsy. *Dev Med Child Neurol* 37: 72–84. http://dx.doi.org/10.1111/j.1469-8749.1995.tb11933.x

Fawcett AJ, Nicolson RI (1995) Persistent deficits in motor skill of children with dyslexia. *J Motor Behav* 27: 235–240. http://dx.doi.org/10.1080/00222895.1995.9941713

Fawcett AJ, Nicolson RI (1999) Performance of dyslexic children on cerebellar and cognitive tasks. *J Mot Behav* 31: 68–78. http://dx.doi.org/10.1080/00222899909601892

Fawcett AJ, Nicolson RI (2002) Children with dyslexia are slow to articulate a single speech gesture. *Dyslexia Int J Res Pract* 8: 189–203. http://dx.doi.org/10.1002/dys.222

Fitzgerald M, Corvin A (2001) Diagnosis and differential diagnosis of Asperger syndrome. *Adv Psychiatric Treatment* 7: 310–318. http://dx.doi.org/10.1192/apt.7.4.310

Fombonne E (1999) The epidemiology of autism: a review. *Psychol Med* 29: 769–786. http://dx.doi.org/10.1017/S0033291799008508

Forssberg H, Eliasson AC, Kinoshita H, Johanson RS, Wrestleing G (1991) Development of human precision grip. I: Basic coordination of force. *Exp Brain Res* 85: 451–457. http://dx.doi.org/10.1007/BF00229422

Forssberg H, Kinoshita H, Eliasson AC, Johanson RS, Wrestling G (1992) Development of human precision grip. II: Anticipatory control of isometric forces targeted for object's weight. *Exp Brain Res* 90: 393–398.

Frith U (1989) *Autism: Explaining the Enigma*. Oxford: Blackwell.

Frith U (2003) *Autism: Explaining the Enigma*, 2nd edition. Oxford: Blackwell.

Frith U, Happe F (1994) Autism: beyond theory of mind. *Cognition* 50: 115–132. http://dx.doi.org/10.1016/0010-0277(94)90024-8

Gillberg C (1998) Hyperactivity, inattention and motor control problems: prevalence, comorbidity and background factors. *Folia Phoniatrica et Logopaedica* 50: 107–117. http://dx.doi.org/10.1159/000021456

Gillberg C (2006) Autistic spectrum disorders. In: Gillberg C, Harrington R, Steinhausen HC, editors. *A Clinician's Handbook of Child and Adolescent Psychiatry*. Cambridge: Cambridge University Press, pp. 447–488. http://dx.doi.org/10.1017/CBO9780511543807.017

Gillberg C, Coleman M (2000) *The Biology of the Autistic Syndrome*. London: Mac Keith Press.

Gillberg C, Calrstrom G, Ramussen P, Waldenstrom E (1983) Perceptual motor and attentional deficits in seven-year-old children. Neurological screening aspects. *Acta Paediatrica Scand* 72: 119–124. http://dx.doi.org/10.1111/j.1651-2227.1983.tb09675.x

Gillberg RH, Rasmussen P (1982) Perceptual motor and attentional difficulties in six-year-old children: background factors. *Dev Med Child Neurol* 24: 752–770. http://dx.doi.org/10.1111/j.1469-8749.1982.tb13697.x

Gordon M (1991) *Instruction Manual for the Gordon Diagnostic System (GDS): Modell III-R*. de Witt, NY: Gordon Systems.

Green D, Baird G (2005) DCD and overlapping conditions. In: Sugden DA, Chambers ME, editors. *Children with Developmental Coordination Disorder*. London: Whurr, pp. 93–118.

Green D, Charman T, Pickles A, et al (2009) Impairment of movement skills of children with autistic spectrum disorders. *Dev Med Child Neurol* 51: 311–316. http://dx.doi.org/10.1111/j.1469-8749.2008.03242.x

Greene RW, Biederman J, Faraone SV, Sienna M, Garcia-Jetton J (1997) Adolescent outcome of boys with Attention Deficit Hyperactivity Disorder and social disability: results from a 4-year longitudinal follow-up study. *J Consult Clin Psychol* 65: 758–767. http://dx.doi.org/10.1037/0022-006X.65.5.758

Greene RW, Biederman J, Faraone SV, et al (2001) Social impairment in girls with ADHD: patterns, gender comparisons, and correlates. *J Am Acad Child Adolesc Psychiatry* 40: 704–710. http://dx.doi.org/10.1097/00004583-200106000-00016

Gubbay SS (1975) *The Clumsy Child: A Study of Developmental Apraxic and Agnostic Ataxia*. Philadelphia, PA: Saunders.

Hallet M, Lebiedowska MK, Thomas SL, Stanhope SJ, Denkla MB, Rumsey J (1993) Locomotion of autistic adults. *Arch Neurol* 50: 1304–1308. http://dx.doi.org/10.1001/archneur.1993.00540120019007

Harold D, Paracchini S, Scerri T, et al (2006) Further evidence that the KIAA0319 gene confers susceptibility to developmental dyslexia. *Mol Psychiatry* 11: 1085–1091. http://dx.doi.org/10.1038/sj.mp.4001904

Harvey WJ, Reid G (1997) Motor performance of children with attention-deficit hyperactivity disorder: a preliminary investigation. *Adapt Phys Activ Q* 14: 189–202.

Henderson SE, Sugden DA (1992) *Movement Assessment Battery for Children: Manual*. Sidcup: Psychological Corporation.

Hill EL (1998) A dyspraxic deficit in specific language impairment and developmental coordination disorder? Evidence from hand and arm movements. *Dev Med Child Neurol* 40: 388–395. http://dx.doi.org/10.1111/j.1469-8749.1998.tb08214.x

Hill EL (2001) Non-specific nature of specific language impairment: a review of the literature with regard to concomitant motor impairments. *Int J Language Communication Disord* 36: 149–171. http://dx.doi.org/10.1080/13682820010019874

Hill EL (2004a) Executive dysfunction in autism. *Trends Cogn Sci* 8: 26–32. http://dx.doi.org/10.1016/j.tics.2003.11.003

Hill EL (2004b) Evaluating the theory of executive dysfunction in autism. *Dev Rev* 24: 189–233. http://dx.doi.org/10.1016/j.dr.2004.01.001

Hill EL, Bishop DVM, Nimmo-Smith I (1998) Representational gestures in developmental coordination disorder and specific language impairment: error types and the reliability of ratings. *Hum Movement Sci* 17: 655–678. http://dx.doi.org/10.1016/S0167-9457(98)00017-7

Hsu CC, Lin JC, Kuo SL (1982) A preliminary study of the activity level of Chinese children aged three to eleven years. *Science Monthly* 10: 363–381 (in Chinese).

Hulme C, Snowling MJ (2009) *Developmental Disorders of Language Learning and Cognition*. Chichester: Wiley-Blackwell.

Jansiewicz EM, Goldberg MC, Newschaffer CJ, Denckla MB, Landa R, Mostofsky SH (2006) Motor signs distinguish children with high functioning autism and Asperger's syndrome from controls. *J Autism Dev Disord* 36: 613–621. http://dx.doi.org/10.1007/s10803-006-0109-y

Johnson CJ, Beitchman JH (2006) Specific developmental disorders of speech and language. In: Gillberg C, Harrington R, Steinhausen H, editors. A Clinician's Handbook of Child and Adolescent Psychiatry. New York, NY: Cambridge University Press, pp. 388–416.

Kadesjo B, Gillberg C (2001) The comorbidity of ADHD in the general population of Swedish school-age children. *J Child Psychol Psychiatry* 42: 487–492. http://dx.doi.org/10.1111/1469-7610.00742

Kanner L (1943) Autistic disturbances of affective contact. *Nerv Child* 2: 217–250.

Kaplan B, Crawford S, Cantell M, Kooistra L, Dewey D (2006) Comorbidity co-occurrence continuum: what's in a name? *Child Care Health Dev* 32: 723–731. http://dx.doi.org/10.1111/j.1365-2214.2006.00689.x

Kaplan BJ, Crawford SG, Wilson BN, Dewey DM (1997) Comorbidity of developmental coordination disorder and different types of reading disability. *J Int Neuropsychol Soc* 3: 54.

Kaplan BJ, Wilson BN, Dewey DM, Crawford SG (1998) DCD may not be a discrete disorder. *Hum Movement Sci* 17: 471–490. http://dx.doi.org/10.1016/S0167-9457(98)00010-4

Kaplan BJ, Dewey DM, Crawford SG, Wilson BN (2001) The term 'comorbidity' is of questionable value in reference to developmental disorders: data and theory. *J Learn Disabil* 34: 555–565. http://dx.doi.org/10.1177/002221940103400608

Kavale KA, Forness SR (1995) *The Nature of Learning Disabilities*. Hillsdale, NJ: Lawrence Erlbaum Associates.

Marcotte AC, Stern C (1997) Qualitative analysis of graphomotor output in children with attentional disorders. *Child Neuropsychol* 3: 147–153. http://dx.doi.org/10.1080/09297049708401373

Martin NC, Piel JP, Hay D (2006) DCD and ADHD: a genetic study of their shared aetiology. *Hum Movement Sci* 25: 110–124. http://dx.doi.org/10.1016/j.humov.2005.10.006

van der Meere J, van Baal M, Sergeant J (1989) The additive factor method: a differential diagnostic tool in hyperactivity and learning disability. *J Abnorm Child Psychol* 17: 409–422. http://dx.doi.org/10.1007/BF00915035

van der Meere J, Vreeling HJ, Sergeant J (1992) A motor presetting study in hyperactive, learning disabled and control children. *J Child Psychol Psychiatry* 33: 1347–1354. http://dx.doi.org/10.1111/j.1469-7610.1992.tb00954.x

Miller LT, Missiuna CA, Macnab JJ, Malloy-Miller T, Polatajko HJ (2001) Clinical description of children with developmental coordination disorder. *Can J Occup Ther* 68: 5–15.

Miyahara M, Tsukii M, Hori M, et al (1997) Brief report: motor incoordination in children with Asperger syndrome and learning disabilities. *J Autism Dev Disord* 27: 597–602. http://dx.doi.org/10.1023/A:1025834211548

Morton J (2004) *Understanding Developmental Disorders*. Oxford: Blackwell. http://dx.doi.org/10.1002/9780470773307

Morton J, Frith U (1995) Causal modelling: a structural approach to developmental psychopathology. In: Cicchetti D, Cohen DJ, editors. *Developmental Psychopathology, Volume 1: Theory and Methods*. New York: Wiley, pp. 357–390.

Mostofsky SH, Dubey P, Jerath VK, Jansiewiecz EM, Goldberg MC, Denkla MB (2006) Developmental dyspraxia is not limited to imitation in children with autistic spectrum disorders. *J Int Neuropsychol Soc* 12: 314–326. http://dx.doi.org/10.1017/S1355617706060437

Mostofsky SH, Burgess P, Gidley Larson JC (2007) Increased motor cortex white matter volume predicts motor impairment in autism. *Brain* 130: 2117–2122. http://dx.doi.org/10.1093/brain/awm129

Mostofsky SH, Powell SK, Simmonds DJ, Goldberg MC, Caffo B, Pekar JJ (2009) Decreased connectivity and cerebellar activity in autism during motor task performance. *Brain* 132: 2413–2425. http://dx.doi.org/10.1093/brain/awp088

Nicolson RI, Fawcett AJ (1990) Automaticity: a new framework for dyslexia research? *Cognition* 35: 159–182. http://dx.doi.org/10.1016/0010-0277(90)90013-A

Nicolson R, Fawcett A, Dean P (2001) Developmental dyslexia: the cerebellar hypothesis. *Trends Neurosci* 24: 508–511. http://dx.doi.org/10.1016/S0166-2236(00)01896-8

Noterdaeme M, Mildenberger K, Minow F, Amorosa H (2002) Evaluation of neuromotor deficits in children with autism and children with a specific speech and language deficit. *Eur J Adolesc Psychiatry* 11: 219–225. http://dx.doi.org/10.1007/s00787-002-0285-z

Orton ST (1937) *Reading, Writing and Speech Problems in Children*. New York: WW Norton & Co.

Pereira HS, Eliasson A-C, Forssberg H (2000) Detrimental control of precision grip lifts in children with ADHD. *Dev Med Child Neurol* 42: 545–553. http://dx.doi.org/10.1017/S0012162200001031

Peters JM, Henderson SE (2008) Understanding developmental coordination disorder and its impact on families: the contribution of single case studies. In: Sugden DA, Kirby A, Dunford C, editors. Special issue of *International Journal of Disability Development and Education: Children with Developmental Coordination Disorder* 55: 97–112.

Powell RP, Bishop DVM (1992) Clumsiness and perceptual problems in children with specific language impairment. *Dev Med Child Neurol* 34: 755–765. http://dx.doi.org/10.1111/j.1469-8749.1992.tb11514.x

Ramus F (2004) Neurobiology of dyslexia: a reinterpretation of the data. *Trends Neurosci* 27: 720–726. http://dx.doi.org/10.1016/j.tins.2004.10.004

Rasmussen P, Gillberg C (2000) Natural outcome of SDHD with developmental coordination disorder at age 22 years. *J Am Acad Child Adolesc Psychiatry* 39: 1424–1431. http://dx.doi.org/10.1097/00004583-200011000-00017

Rasmussen P, Gillberg C, Waldenstrom E, et al (1983) Perceptual motor and attentional deficits in seven-year-old children: neurological and neurodevelopmental aspects. *Dev Med Child Neurol* 25: 315–333. http://dx.doi.org/10.1111/j.1469-8749.1983.tb13765.x

Reader M, Harris EL, Scheuerholz LJ, Denckla MB (1994) Attention deficit hyperactivity disorder and executive dysfunction. *Dev Neuropsychol* 10: 493–512. http://dx.doi.org/10.1080/87565649409540598

Reid G (2007) *Dyslexia*, 2nd edition. London: Continuum.

Rogers SJ, Benetto L, McEvoy R, Pennington BF (1996) Imitation and pantomime in high functioning adolescents with autistic spectrum disorders. *Child Dev* 67: 2060–2073. http://dx.doi.org/10.2307/1131609

Ronald A, Happe F, Price TS, Baron-Cohen S, Plomin R (2006) Phenotypic and genetic overlap between autistic traits at the extremes of the general population. *J Am Acad Child Adolesc Psychiatry* 45: 1206–1214. http://dx.doi.org/10.1097/01.chi.0000230165.54117.41

Rutter M (1999) Resilience concepts and findings: implications for family therapy. *J Fam Ther* 21: 119–144. http://dx.doi.org/10.1111/1467-6427.00108

Rutter M, Maughan B (2002) School effectiveness findings 1979–2002. *J School Psychol* 40: 451–475. http://dx.doi.org/10.1016/S0022-4405(02)00124-3

Rutter M, Yule W (1975) The concept of specific reading retardation. *J Child Psychol Psychiatry* 16: 181–197. http://dx.doi.org/10.1111/j.1469-7610.1975.tb01269.x

Schachar R, Tannock R, Marriott M, Logan G (1995) Deficient inhibitory control in attention deficit hyperactivity disorder. *J Abnorm Child Psychol* 23: 411–437. http://dx.doi.org/10.1007/BF01447206

Seargeant JA, van der Meere J (1988) What happens after a hyperactive child commits an error? *Psychiatry Res* 24: 157–164. http://dx.doi.org/10.1016/0165-1781(88)90058-3

Semrud-Clikeman M, Biederman J, Sprich-Buckminister S, Lehman B, Faraone S, Norman D (1992) Comorbidity between ADHD and learning disability: a review of and report in a clinically referred sample. *J Am Acad Child Adolesc Psychiatry* 31: 439–448. http://dx.doi.org/10.1097/00004583-199205000-00009

Snowling MJ, Maughan B (2006) Reading and other disorders. In: Gillberg C, Harrington R, Steinhausen HC, editors. *A Clinician's Handbook of Child and Adolescent Psychiatry.* Cambridge: Cambridge University Press, pp. 417–445.

Solanto MV, Arnsten AFT, Castellanos EX (2001) *Stimulant Drugs and ADHD.* Oxford: Oxford University Press.

Szatmari P, Boyle M, Offard DR (1989) ADHD and conduct disorder: degree of diagnostic overlap and differences among correlates. *J Am Acad Child Adolesc Psychiatry* 28: 865–872. http://dx.doi.org/10.1097/00004583-198911000-00010

Taylor E (2006) Hyperkinetic disorders. In: Gillberg C, Harrington R, Steinhausen HC, editors. *A Clinician's Handbook of Child and Adolescent Psychiatry.* Cambridge: Cambridge University Press, pp. 489–521.

Taylor E, Sandberg S, Thorley G, Giles S (1991) *The Epidemiology of Childhood Hyperactivity: Institute of Psychiatry Maudsley Monograph.* Oxford: Oxford University Press.

Taylor E, Dopfner M, Sergeant J, et al (2004) European clinical guidelines for hyperkinetic disorder – first upgrade. *Eur Child Adolesc Psychiatry* 13: 1–30. http://dx.doi.org/10.1007/s00787-004-1002-x

Teitelbaum P, Teitelbaum O, Nye J, Fryman J, Maurer RG (1998) Movement analysis in infancy may be useful for early diagnosis of autism. *Proc Natl Acad Sci USA* 95: 13982–13987. http://dx.doi.org/10.1073/pnas.95.23.13982

Tomblin JB, Buckwalter P (1998) The heritability of poor language achievement among twins. *J Speech Hearing Res* 41: 188–199.

Trevarthen C, Aitken KJ, Papoudi D, Roberts JZ (1996) *Children with Autism: Diagnosis and Interventions to Meet their Needs.* London: Jessica Kingsley.

Tseng MH, Henderson A, Chow SMK, Yao G (2004) Relationship between motor proficiency, attention impulse and activity in children with ADHD. *Dev Med Child Neurol* 46: 381–388. http://dx.doi.org/10.1017/S0012162204000623

Ullman MT (2001) The declarative/procedural model of lexicon and grammar. *J Psycholinguist Res* 30: 37–67. http://dx.doi.org/10.1023/A:1005204207369

Ullman MT, Pierpont EI (2005) Specific language impairment is not specific to language: the procedural deficit hypothesis. *Cortex* 41: 399–433. http://dx.doi.org/10.1016/S0010-9452(08)70276-4

Visser J (2007) Subtypes and comorbidity in developmental coordination disorder. In: Geuze RH, editor. *Developmental Coordination Disorder: A Review of Current Approaches.* Marseille: Solal, pp. 9–25.

Whitmont S, Clark C (1996) Kinaesthetic acuity and fine motor skills in children with attention-deficit-hyperactivity disorder: a preliminary report. *Dev Med Child Neurol* 38: 1091–1098. http://dx.doi.org/10.1111/j.1469-8749.1996.tb15072.x

WHO (1992) *International Statistical Classification of Diseases and Related Health Problems, Volume 1,* 10th edition. Geneva: World Health Organization.

Williams J, Thomas PR, Maruff P, Butson M, Wilson PH (2005) Motor, visual and egocentric transformations in children with developmental coordination disorder. *Child Care Health Dev* 32: 633–647. http://dx.doi.org/10.1111/j.1365-2214.2006.00688.x

Wing L, Potter D (2002) The epidemiology of autistic spectrum disorders: is the prevalence rising? *Ment Retard Dev Res Rev* 8: 151–161. http://dx.doi.org/10.1002/mrdd.10029

Yap RL, van der Leij A (1994) Testing the automatization deficit hypothesis of dyslexia via a dual task paradigm. *J Learn Disabil* 27: 660–665. http://dx.doi.org/10.1177/002221949402701006

11
CHILDREN WITH VISUAL IMPAIRMENT

Role and nature of vision

VISION AND MOVEMENT

Whichever theoretical perspective one takes on the control and coordination of movement, there are two connected fundamental issues that form a central core of research endeavour. The first of these concerns what information that will aid the planning and execution of movement is available, and how it is utilized. The second concern is how the execution of movement itself is mobilized. As we have presented in Chapters 1–6 of this text, the various models of motor control view these in a different manner. The global field that invokes information processing models would have a component approach to these issues with input information from sensory–perceptual systems progressing through some central motor programming operations to the execution of the motor act. An explanation from a more dynamical systems approach would view perception and action as inseparable without a breakdown into subcomponents. Throughout this text the latter is the favoured view, but the important information that the processing approach has given us is recognized.

However, whichever viewpoint is favoured, the role of vision as part of the system is a crucial element in the control and coordination of movement. Full visual ability provides a template against which other senses can be interpreted, whereas impaired or loss of vision restricts our ways of knowing about objects and events in space. Thus, when individuals have impaired or loss of vision, it is appropriate to examine how this impairment or loss impacts upon their motor skills. In children, development involves change over time and an examination of how blind children develop and progress without vision through the various phases of their lives helps us understand how loss of vision affects motor performance and development and how it relates to development overall. This in turn provides the information upon which

stake- and fundholders can make decisions about appropriate support.

Role of vision

A starting point is to note that vision is not essential for all movements and blind and visually impaired individuals do cope with many of the motoric demands placed upon them in numerous ways. First, there is the visual guidance of movement using the visual functions that are available. Second, other ways that this is accomplished include tactile guidance of movement using the feeling through the feet, guidance with the hands and arms, indirect tactile guidance being afforded by changes in the characteristics of the surrounding air, when approaching a barrier or wall, and the indirect guidance which is afforded when using techniques such as the long-cane method. Third, there is auditory guidance of movement using passive echolocation and active echolocation. Many blind individuals are competent at echolocation and fully recognize their abilities and skills, with many children who are blind from birth or from an early age fully recruiting their visual cortex and dorsal stream functions in a way which is likely to be entirely different from those who have previously used vision to recruit visual guidance of movement. Some work has shown that the visual brain is recruited with extraordinary topographic accuracy by the specific auditory signals from both passive and active echolocation.

However, vision is a fundamental and important sense, providing information in a variety of ways. In Chapter 2 we outlined in detail the role of vision and a summary of this role is provided below.

Vision provides:

*   an *instant and simultaneous picture of the environmental context*, showing where objects and people are located in the environment whether stationary or moving;

- predictability of events involving processes such as anticipation and coincidence, allowing us to greet and meet the outstretched arms of a child or take evasive action for impending danger;
- a controlling process for the movement itself, for example by providing information to guide the hand towards a cup or when driving a car;
- feedback enabling the correction of errors about the end-product or ongoing movement;
- redundancy in terms of allowing many ways of knowing the same thing from different angles, distances or verifying information from other sources.

The importance of vision in movement is demonstrated by the term perception–action coupling, which is often used to describe the close connection between the eyes and the hands or feet in actions such as writing and drawing, driving a car, or kicking and trapping a ball, emphasizing the link between the eyes and limbs and body. This link between vision and action has been found across many contexts to involve both temporal and spatial coupling of the limbs and body and eyes.

Loss/impairment of vision
It follows from the role of vision that, if it is impaired or lost, the contributions that it makes to movement are either degraded or lost. This is not to say that compensation is not made and that individuals who are visually impaired cannot satisfactorily engage in typical daily activities with success. However, it does mean that there is some extra effort or cost to the alternative ways of achieving what an adequate visual system typically provides. It is our view that this extra effort should be aided by changes in the environmental context that support the blind individual in their activities of daily living. This is very much in line with our model of task–environment–child as the unit of analysis for movement outcomes.

Loss or impaired vision hinders the exact specification of objects or persons in the environment, whether that is near space, which can be reached by hand, or far space in travelling from one place to another. Loss of vision places larger demands on other systems to recognize not only objects and persons but also shapes, colours, and textures and limits the temporal and spatial predictions that can be made.

Without vision there is an important source of information missing, which then places an extra demand on other sensory systems to provide this information; often this information is not rich, with an additional load on the other sensory systems. This in turn can stress the other systems so much that they do not work at capacity. A good example of this is the use of sound to locate objects, with the person using this facility having to work harder to produce less accurate results. Loss of vision also makes essential the availability of environmental sources for movement control and feedback to compensate for this loss. The ongoing monitoring of an action such as reaching and grasping is no longer available through visual means and requires other sources of information that are not usually as efficient or as effective as vision.

Activities that involve communication are impaired without vision. Body language and facial expressions can be detected only by vision and such intellectual activities as reading are limited; braille is around one-quarter of the speed of sighted reading and such activities as skimming and scanning, which require fast sequential or simultaneous input and processing, are extremely limited. In addition, these limitations may have a deleterious effect on motivation. Most of these are indirect outcomes of vision that build up and often lead to some form of difficulty in personal and social development. However, an important point to remember is that there is not a linear relationship between the severity of impairment and the consequent level of performance, as there are many other variables to consider that come into play to affect the overall movement skill. Characteristics such as motivation, persistence, resilience, and personality all interact with the severity of performance to provide the level of movement competence. A final point to stress is that many of the limitations can be moderated by the amount of support society is prepared to invest in altering the environment such that the individuals can participate freely in activities of daily living.

When there is absence of sight, motivation to move is substantially reduced because the child seemingly has no place to go. They have little sense of the nature of the environment to 'lure' them into it through movement. To summarize, loss or impairment of vision

- hinders the exact specification of objects or persons;
- places an extra demand on other sensory systems and external sources for control and feedback of movements;
- impairs communication through body language or facial expression;
- impairs motivation to move as there appears to be 'nowhere to go'.

How does vision provide information?
Chapter 2 again provides detail of some of the ways in which vision provides information. The following summarizes some of this detail.

- *Central (foveal) vision*: detects environmental information in the middle 2 to 5 degrees of the visual field.
- *Peripheral vision*: detects visual information in a wider field, around 200 degrees horizontally and 160 degrees vertically.
- *Optical flow*: aids in detection of moving objects or change in the optical array.
- *Ventral stream*: specifies the layout of the environment.
- *Dorsal stream*: responsible for visual control of movement (often called the visual action system).
- *Time to contact (tau)*: aids fast actions such as ball catching by the increase in retinal size as the ball approaches.
- *Bearing angle*: the angle between a moving object, the interception point, and the individual trying to intercept it; it is considered an on-line strategy.

Vision's importance in the performance and learning of motor skills cannot be overemphasized because it provides information in so many different ways. No other sense can do this for us and when we are deprived of vision or visual input is degraded it follows that movement skills are more difficult to learn and perform and that motor development may change in children who are either blind or having some form of visual impairment. It also follows, in our view, that society in general could make increased effort to change the environmental context for blind persons, thus facilitating their overall participation in typical daily living activities.

THE NATURE OF VISUAL IMPAIRMENT/BLINDNESS

Definitions

The nature of visual impairment can vary from total absence of any light perception to various degrees of loss that affect visual acuity, field of vision, or visual functioning. Sugden and Keogh (1990) note that definitions of visual impairment can vary depending on whether they are being used for legal or functional purposes. Most developed countries now have legislation that protects and provides for those with disabilities, and legal definitions of visual impairment are often used to determine the kind of support that an individual may require in order to function effectively at school and later at work. Functional purposes often specify the extent to which individuals may participate in day-to-day activities, although the two are often conflated with many employers/community services being required by law to make reasonable adjustments to support active participation by all in typical daily activities.

Definitions vary across countries and often by examiners, and Table 11.1 shows a number of ways in which

TABLE 11.1

Classification of severity of visual impairment

Category of visual impairment	Visual acuity with best possible correction
1	20/70 to 20/200 (feet), 6/18 to 6/60 (metres)
2	20/200 to 20/400 (feet), 6/60 to 3/60 (metres)
3	20/400 to 5/300 (feet), 3/60 to 1/60 (metres)
4	5/300 (feet) or 1/60 (metres) to light perception
5	No light perception
9	Undetermined or unspecified

Adapted from ICD-10 (WHO 1992).

visual impairment has been defined. The usual way to define varying degrees of blindness is by examining visual acuity and field of vision. Visual acuity is usually measured by the examination of an object from various distances to achieve clarity. The term 20/20 (6/6m) is often used to describe typical vision with correction meaning that a person can see an object clearly at 20 feet (6m), in a similar manner to what would be expected in a normally sighted individual. A person with 20/200 (6/60) vision is legally blind and would have to stand 20 feet (6m) away to see an object with the same degree of clarity as a person with normal vision standing 200 feet (60m) away. Visual field is often used as an addition to visual acuity and usually defines as blind those individuals with less than 20 degrees field of vision with the norm being 180 degrees.

In Table 11.1, the term 'low vision' comprises Categories 1 and 2, the term 'blindness' Categories 3, 4, and 5, and the term 'unqualified visual loss' Category 9. When the extent of the visual field is also used, individuals with a field greater than 5 and less than 10 degrees around a central fixation are placed in Category 3, and those with a field less than 5 are in Category 4 even if central acuity is not impaired.

Prevalence and incidence

In previous chapters (in particular Chapter 7 'Cerebral palsy') the terms prevalence and incidence have been described in some detail. A simple explanation is that incidence of blindness is the occurrence of new cases at a particular time in a specific sample. For example, it could be the number of cases of blindness in newborn infants in the state of California during the first 3 months of 2008. Alternatively, as blindness or at least visual impairment is often correctly associated with advanced age, it could be the number of persons aged 60 and over in the UK who became visually impaired or blind during the year 2008.

Prevalence of visual impairment is the total number of persons in a population at a particular time, such as the number of blind persons in Australia in 2008. Incidence can change rapidly from year to year particularly if there has been some medical advance, whereas prevalence changes slowly because prior occurrences remain in the total count or are removed slowly by death or improved vision (Sugden and Keogh 1990).

Blindness in children is a relatively rare occurrence making prevalence data difficult to obtain because large samples are required to provide population-based statistics. It does appear to vary with socio-economic status and under-5 mortality rates. Gilbert and Foster (2001) report that, in low-income countries with high under-5 infant mortality rates, the prevalence can be 1.5 per 1000, whereas in high-income countries with low under-5 mortality rates, the prevalence is around 0.3 per 1000. Gilbert and Foster (2001) also report that the number of blind children in the world is estimated to be around 1.4 million with around three-quarters of them living in the poorest regions of Africa and Asia.

Incidence data are also difficult to obtain, as they require large longitudinal studies that have chronicled children's progress from birth with accurate registers of the blind. Gilbert and Foster (2001) suggest that in developed nations the incidence has declined, but there are no reliable figures from developing nations. However, Gilbert and Foster (2001) also note that, in developing nations, a high proportion of blind children die within a few years of becoming blind, thus potentially underestimating the number of prevalent cases.

Causes of blindness
The difficulties that are encountered in obtaining accurate statistics for prevalence and incidence are mirrored when examining causes. Gilbert and Foster (2001) report on two classifications systems, one according to site of any damage and the other on underlying aetiology. These are reproduced in Table 11.2.

Caution is recommended by Gilbert and Foster (2001) when interpreting these data, as, for example, in developing countries the data are obtained from schools for the blind and not all blind children are in school, offering a potential bias. In addition, schools for the blind usually contain children 6 to 15 years of age who could have missed recent innovations such as immunization against measles. Finally, the figures may be misleading because many children with visual impairment have damage to the brain as the underlying cause. The reason why the statistics do not appear in WHO figures is that the collection of such information has failed to include such children.

TABLE 11.2

Estimates of blindness worldwide by anatomical site and aetiological category

	Number of cases
Site of abnormality	
Retina	380 000
Cornea	260 000
Whole globe	250 000
Lens	190 000
Optic nerve	140 000
Glaucoma	90 000
Uvea	40 000
Other	50 000
Total	1 400 000
Aetiological category	
Hereditary disease	420 000
Childhood factors	280 000
Perinatal factors	100 000
Intrauterine factors	40 000
Unknown	560 000
Total	1 400 000

Reproduced with permission of the publisher from Gilbert and Foster (2001).

Within these limitations there is also evidence to show regional variation in the cause of blindness. For example, in some of the poorest developing nations, causes that predominate are corneal scarring due to vitamin A deficiency, measles, ophthalmia neonatorum, and harmful effects of traditional remedies. In contrast, in the USA 19% of 2550 children in schools for the blind were cortically blind and 12% had visual loss from optic atrophy or optic nerve hypoplasia. Throughout the world cataract, retinal diseases, and congenital abnormalities are important causes with a suggestion that genetic causes are also important (Gilbert and Foster 2001). A sad commentary on these statistics is that much of blindness could be prevented and the control of blindness is considered a high priority within the WHO's 'VISION 2020: The Right to Sight' programme (WHO 1998).

A common cause of visual impairment in children is damage to the brain, and, as noted earlier, these children are not often included in the statistics. In this context, damage to the posterior parietal area, in particular, gives rise to problems with using vision to guide movement or optic ataxia. In its milder form of dorsal stream dysfunction affected children show clumsy behaviour and problems with visual search. In its severe form there can be profound impairment of visual guidance of movement along with reduced visual acuity commonly associated with lower visual field impairment.

In the context of visual neglect, which can be due to posterior parietal damage (most often affecting the right side of the brain and the left side of the body), lack of recognition of the existence of the visual world on the contralateral side compounds the visual difficulties and can culminate, for example, in children being unable to walk in a straight line by means of visual guidance.

With retinopathy of prematurity the presumption may be made that the impairment of vision is entirely due to eye disease. However, a significant proportion of such children have profound problems with orientation that are very likely to be due to damage to the periventricular white matter in the brain, which in turn is impairing the central organization of the internal map of the surrounding world, leading to problems with navigation.

In Chapter 2 we detailed how the ventral and dorsal visual streams provide information about the environment and help control movement, respectively. There are some blind children whose cerebral visual impairment has spared the dorsal stream. Such children are rare but are remarkable in their capacity to move freely through a visual world that they have limited conscious awareness of. In addition, it is important to recognize that those who are blind recruit the visual brain to alternative perceptual functions, and it is possible that the dorsal and ventral streams continue to function for the purposes of parallel processing information and guidance of movement (dorsal) and recognition and orientation (ventral), but without a visual input.

This chapter is concerned with the movement skills of children who are blind, but, as with many categories of disability, blind individuals show a number of co-occurring characteristics and, although they are not defining characteristics, they are certainly important when individual profiles are being drawn and when interventions are being planned. Many of these are noted in the next section when movement development is described.

Movement development in blind children

A starting point when studying motor abilities in children who are blind is to examine how motor development occurs and describe the similarities and differences between them and sighted children. Often the study of development in young blind children has been carried out with the aim of examining cognitive and personal development, because of the possible carry over into inadequate emotional adjustment often seen later in life (Sugden and Keogh 1990). Thus, when motor development has been studied in blind infants, it has often been examined as an independent variable and to determine how it affects other areas of development, and not always as a dependent variable in its own right.

A logical analysis of movement skills would indicate that blind children, because of a paucity of information through vision, will have difficulties in two major areas. First, there is the problem of moving in *near space*, with objects and people who are in reach. Blind infants must rely on other senses to assist them in this area. Sugden and Keogh (1990) have called this 'entering the environment' and without the sight of an object to 'lure' the infant into action, even with non-visual cues, there is not the richness of information and motivation that vision can supply. Second, there is a difficulty with moving in *far space* in areas that are beyond touch and involve moving the whole body into the environment, an aspect of functioning often called 'orientation and mobility'. Both of these provide quite strong challenges for a child who is blind.

Degree of blindness is not the only variable to be considered when evaluating the functional ability of blind persons. Age at onset is an important factor, with loss of vision at an early age or from birth meaning fewer visual memories are available for interpreting data from other sensory sources. In addition, later onset of blindness means that an individual has developed other skills such as language that may be useful in coping with the loss of vision (Sugden and Keogh 1990).

EARLY MOVEMENT SKILLS AND NEAR SPACE AND ENTERING THE ENVIRONMENT

The early movement skills of the blind child are characterized within the first year by manipulating near space, that is, within reach of the child when stationary such as lying, sitting or standing. During this period the infant also starts to move into the environment with all of the variables associated with this move coming into play. This section describes and analyses this period, and later in the chapter a description is given of orientation and spatial mobility in later childhood and how the individual moves in far space. It is recognized that the boundary lines between these two sections are somewhat blurred and overlapping.

Developmental arrests

Classic work by Fraiberg (summarized in her book in 1977) has provided many observations into the motor development of the child who is blind. For example, some of her descriptions show that some blind infants progress quite well in the early months but then develop what Fraiberg calls *developmental arrests*. She observed blind children from birth who, after progressing well, reached 'road blocks', which often involved not moving or reaching into the environment but sometimes moving on later, showing that this was simply a delay. Others remained in that situation for a considerable period of time and often did not progress beyond that particular point. Fraiberg (1977) considers that the individual capacity to adapt is the key to how adequately blind children cope with the obstacles that appear to be present due to lack of vision. Her work is very much concerned with social, emotional, and personal development of such constructs as ego development and sees the restrictive movement development as a major variable for successful personal and social development. It is the difference in the personal set of child resources that Fraiberg examined, but her work also has serious implications for the other two transacting points of our triangle, presented throughout this text, namely the tasks presented to the child and the environmental context. Sugden and Keogh (1990) concur with this noting that the development of motor capabilities in blind children is constrained by limitations in the environmental context, their ability to adapt, and their personal and social adaptations.

One very observable early action of any child in near space is reaching and grasping; this is a motivational action with the child having a goal to achieve, something in the environment to reach, and vision is the obvious source of information for that motivation. When vision is not present, nor compensated by another source, the motivation for reaching and grasping is greatly reduced. Fraiberg was a strong believer in the visual 'lure' of the environment to encourage and motivate the child to move and explore, and stressed that non-visual sensory inputs do not provide the same or sufficient spatial, directional, or motivational information. This in turn produces delays in fundamental motor skills, such as reaching and grasping, limiting and delaying the child's entry into the environment.

A classic example of this is the case of Toni, who appeared to find a way around what Fraiberg called road blocks by possessing a great adaptive capacity that was not present in the other blind infants Fraiberg and Freedman (1964) studied. Toni rolled over at 17 weeks, could sit briefly by 22 weeks, and sat without support at 7 months, and, although she seemed ready to crawl, would only rotate on her stomach. This was described by Fraiberg and Freedman (1964) as pinwheel locomotion, with it being more of a pleasurable activity and self-stimulation rather than a means of locomoting. It appeared she had nowhere to go (Sugden and Keogh 1990). This was addressed by Fraiberg and Freedman by placing Toni in a walker, which soon led to her moving into the environment. This is another instance where the modification of the task brings out previously unseen qualities in the child's resources and functional capabilities.

Posture and manual skills

Adelson and Fraiberg (1974) studied the development of 10 children (five females and five males) who were blind from birth with no more than minimal light perception. The children on entry into the project were between 1 and 11 months of age and finished between 2 and 6 years; thus there was a great variability in the times each child was studied for, but they were visited twice a month and were recorded on video once a month. Sugden and Keogh (1990) compared the data reported by Adelson and Fraiberg (1974) with normative data from Bayley (1969) and Frankenburg and Dodds (1969) and the results are shown in Figure 11.1.

Postural norms for the blind children were slightly delayed but within a typical range, but self-initiated mobility tasks, apart from rolling over, were markedly delayed with the blind children being mainly beyond the 95th centile for typically developing children. Thus, although the children had postural control involving sitting and standing and the precursors of walking were on schedule, they were not using these to enter into the environment. Adelson and Fraiberg call this phenomenon 'road blocks'. Fraiberg (1977) reports of individuals who had all the skills needed to produce forward movement but did not use them even when tempted by toys and sounds.

A similar situation was reported by Fraiberg (1977) when she described reaching and grasping in the children, a skill that also requires the child to move into the environment. When manual skills were examined, the blind infants progressed within typical ranges for skills such as the pincer grip and exchanging from hand to hand, although Fraiberg (1977) did report that the blind infants appeared to do less with their hands. However, the real difference was observed in reaching and grasping for an object in the environment with blind infants showing marked delays, and Fraiberg concluded that the blind infants had all the necessary prerequisites for reaching and grasping but without the necessary lure or incentive to do so.

Sound is the medium that is key to providing a sensory lure for blind infants and it is known that auditory location is present at or shortly after birth (Freedman and Fisher 1968 and DA Sugden's personal observation 10 minutes after the birth of his daughter in 1980). Blind infants localize but in a different manner to sighted ones, with the latter making more head orientations than the former, and, although sound does specify location, it is not as accurate as vision, and more importantly it does not give as full a description of the object or situation with the consequent result that motivation to move is not as great (Sugden and Keogh 1990).

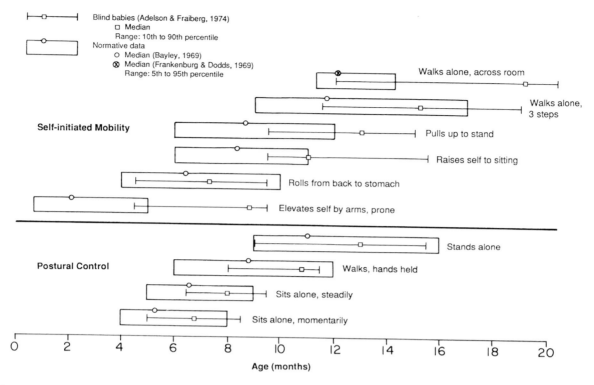

Fig. 11.1 Blind and sighted infants on achievement of selected aspects of postural control and self-initiated mobility (Sugden and Keogh 1990).

Fraiberg believes that development is fundamentally different for blind infants, with adaptation towards competence through change being achieved in different ways and adjustments having to be made to overcome road blocks. She also makes the point that these disruptions in one area of development affect other aspects of development and in particular the secondary influences on the emotional, personal, and social development of blind infants. In her text *Insights from the Blind* (1977), when describing prehension, she poses the question: 'What is "out there" to a blind infant under six months of age?' (p. 157).

She presents a picture of the blind infant being deprived of the rich input that a sighted infant obtains, being restricted to such experiences as tactile through the mother, for example, or her voice. Being devoid of pictures, objects, and persons to look at, tactile experiences appear in a random fashion seemingly without a logical progression that can be obtained from vision. There is an absence of contact-seeking behaviour and gestures of reach. She describes sounds and noises as being 'out there' but concludes that in the first 6 months of life this does not yet indicate a person or object. When the blind child drops or loses a toy it is no longer there and Fraiberg states

that this world of the blind infant is one that is 'a world of evanescent objects, a world of magic, in which persons and things are subject to capricious causality' (p. 158).

Fraiberg (1977) notes that a sighted infant can unite the experiences of sound and touch before the age of 4 months and can turn towards the sound with an expectation that is rewarded with the visual array. She has observed this turning to sound in a blind infant aged 2 months, but this is extinguished because there is nothing to keep it going, and by 6 months of age this has disappeared. Thus the blind infant at 6 months of age does not spontaneously localize through sound, and more importantly does not appear to be able to attribute substantiality to objects through sound alone. Much of the work of Fraiberg (1977) takes motor development, examines the similarities and differences between sighted and blind children, but then extends it into general development, noting that this becomes a conceptual problem with the difficult task of knowing the identity of a person or an object when only partial information is presented.

Fraiberg (1977) has presented us with fine detail of the children she worked with and in Boxes 11.1 and 11.2 there are descriptions of Robbie gleaned from nearly 30 pages in her text.

Box 11.1 A closer examination

Robbie recovering an object through sound alone in the first year of life: Fraiberg (1977)

- Robbie was first seen at 23 weeks with a diagnosis of bilateral agenesis of the optic nerves but no other congenital difficulties.
- Search for tactile object at 7 months, but, at this stage, the hand remains motionless after object is removed with no vocal protest or expression of displeasure and no attempt to 'follow' the object. However, at this age there is the start of pantomime behaviour immediately previously experienced with the object. Following this Robbie starts to make search movements (7–8mo).
- At 8 to 11 months search patterns for tactile objects become more organized but at the beginning of this period they are not coordinated with the sound.
- No search from sound cue until 11 months; before this age Robbie behaves as though there is nothing there with the hand remaining motionless. Neither bell nor rattle activates the hand in any way and there is no orientation towards the sound.
- At 8 to 11 months there is no gesture of search or reach for object but the fingers are starting to be activated in a pantomime grasping movement.
- At 11 months he begins to reach for and recover objects on sound alone and shows the beginnings of creeping behaviour in pursuit of sound-making objects.
- Fraiberg notes that the stages of Robbie's prehension can be generalized to the whole group and believes they are important for the study of ego development in the blind infant. Sound is not the same as vision and does not facilitate the development of object permanence; tactile experiences alone cannot also serve the construction of object concept, and together sound and touch do not provide the comprehensiveness of vision, leading the child to make deviations in his or her development.

Fraiberg (1977) also reported in detail on the children's development of posture and locomotion and other gross motor skills. She notes that there is a stop–start character to the normal pattern of gross motor development that is confusing to the researcher and distressing to the parent. Some posture, such as head support, is fine but others such as raising the head when placed on the stomach is very much delayed and this is not a function of lack of strength or coordination of the arms, neck, or back. The blind infants sit within the normal range of time but do not progress to the next stage of movement initiation with ease. Creeping is markedly delayed and development is slowed down. Towards the end of the first year there is supported walking by holding hands, but walking independently, which occurs as much as 3 months after hand-held walking in the sighted child, often does not occur for another 8 or 9 months. Box 11.2 is a summary of the gross motor development progression from Fraiberg (1977).

The work by Fraiberg and colleagues, although 30 to 40 years old, is still relevant today with the emphasis on meticulous recording and rich detail. Since these studies were conducted there have been others that have examined similar developmental progressions and elaborated on some of the earlier findings. For example, Prechtl et al

(2001) in Holland examined early motor development in blind infants, showing that the effect of being blind differs at various ages and across different movements. In Box 11.3 there is a closer examination of this study.

The work by Prechtl et al (2001) shows the knock-on effect of lack of vision with other senses such as proprioception and vestibular functions not having vision to aid in calibration. It also reported that all postural control was delayed after 3 months of age in blind children and not just those actions that aided moving into the environment, a finding that was not reported by other researchers.

Troster et al (1994), for example, note the Fraiberg studies that reported that, compared to sighted children, blind children were delayed in locomotor skills (crawling and walking) and fine motor skills (reaching and grasping) whereas postural development (sitting and standing) was within a typical age range. Troster et al (1994) attribute the delays to the lack of visual perception and visuomotor coordination. It would be expected that in activities such as crawling and reaching the lack of visual input would give the child no reason to move, whereas postural skills only require limited integration of distal sensory information. However, Troster et al (1994) argue that it is well known that sighted infants and children use vision for

---

Box 11.2 A closer examination

Gross motor development: Fraiberg (1977)

0 to 4 months

Unlike the sighted child, the blind infant did not move his or her head from side to side but kept it centred and sound did not make any difference. Parents reported that the blind children lay in the prone position with no sustained effort to lift the head or brace the arms on the floor, and this continued to be delayed by as much as 6 months.

4 to 8 months

The sighted child gains full mastery of the sitting position and the blind child can show good sitting position. The blind child can also roll from back to stomach, but he or she cannot use his or her own mobility to get closer to a toy, and even noise from the toy made no difference to some children. For creeping (locomoting on hands and knees) the blind infants were 6 months delayed compared with the sighted infants.

8 to 12 months

The sighted infant at this age is making fast progression from crawling to creeping to independent walking, but the blind child is delayed in this move to independent mobility. The blind child may sit and walk within a typical range and supports him or herself on hands and knees but does not initiate movement to change these positions. The problem is not lack of motor impetus, because there are many stereotypical movements in this age range; rather, it is in the transition between activities, such as from independently sitting to moving out of that position, that the delay occurs. Fraiberg (1977) interprets this as lack of motivation to move because of the absence of vision.

Further progression

Gross motor development, such as reaching and grasping, progressed differently in blind children. The neuromuscular development appeared to be within typical range, but there was considerable delay in self-initiated mobility. This in turn limits the ability to independently explore and to discover rules that govern relationships, objects, and events in the external environment.

---

postural purposes (Lee and Aaronson 1974, Butterworth and Hicks 1977). This lack of visual perception requires the blind child to have some kind of compensation, such as the postural system, in the early stages of development, with the vestibular and proprioceptive systems taking control so that there are only slight delays in posture and balance compared with sighted infants. However, it is difficult for goal-directed movements into distal and even proximal space to be compensated for by these systems. In these circumstances the outcomes are viewed as a result of blindness – specific developmental conditions.

It is worth considering this in the light of the model that has been presented throughout this text, which proposes that outcomes are the result of a transaction between the resources of the child, the task, and the environment in which the child is operating. In this case the child has depleted resources, having no vision, and, although auditory cues may help, they are not nearly as powerful as visual ones and thus the child continues to experience

delays in fundamental skills. Therefore, there has to be a search to find new ways, probably through new technology, that may provide increasingly substantial compensation. Brain damage cannot be ruled out as a cause of delay of motor milestones in blind children, as some will have a degree of cerebral palsy and other causes of motor delay, such as low birthweight. With these variables in mind, Troster et al (1994) reported on a longitudinal study of 10 congenitally blind children in the first 3 years of their lives, reporting on their motor development. The study is shown in Box 11.4.

Troster et al (1994) examined the particular case of deviations in standing up, noting that the lack of vision coupled with a restriction to the vestibular and proprioceptive systems at a particular point in development would be particularly disadvantageous when changing positions. It is also worth noting the results of the Prechtl et al (2001) studies in which there was also a poverty of calibration of the vestibular and proprioceptive systems because vision

Box 11.3 A closer examination

Role of vision in early motor development – lessons from the blind: Prechtl et al (2001)
The authors note that blindness has effects other than a lack of vision, with problems caused by a lack of calibration with other sensory systems, such as vestibular and proprioception, and particularly in how important visual information is for early motor development. They note that this has been known for some time, but in many previous studies blind children were included who had additional known brain damage. In this study they obtained video recordings of blind children who did not have any signs of brain damage.

Method
In total 14 children were selected who had severe blindness, checked by ophthalmological examination, but no evidence of brain damage, checked by careful neurological examinations and weekly ultrasound checks together with magnetic resonance imaging or computed tomography. Some had light perception and three had residual pattern vision at the lowest level. Of the 14 children, 13 were repeatedly video recorded during their first year of life and five also during the preterm period. One infant was only recorded during the preterm period. There were also recordings of four of the children from the second and third years of life. The scheduling of recordings was a function of availability not study design.

Results
During preterm and term there were no distinguishing features to indicate effects of blindness, with spontaneous movements appearing typical, and no differences in isolated leg and arm movements, stretches, yawns, trunk, and head rotations or starts and twitches (an example is Fig. 11.2).

However, differences began to emerge around the start of the third month of post-term age, with head lift in prone position being poor or absent. Pull from supine to sitting positions was delayed with head lag continuing to 6 or 7 months of age. Vestibular control was also lacking when the infant was tilted forwards or backwards with the head not being kept in the horizontal plane, as is typical. The authors suggest that this is due to a lack of visual calibration of the labyrinthine system thereby degrading the vestibular process. However, as in sighted infants, the head was centre in the midline at 8 to 10 weeks suggesting that this process is due not to vestibular systems but to sensory control by neck sensors.

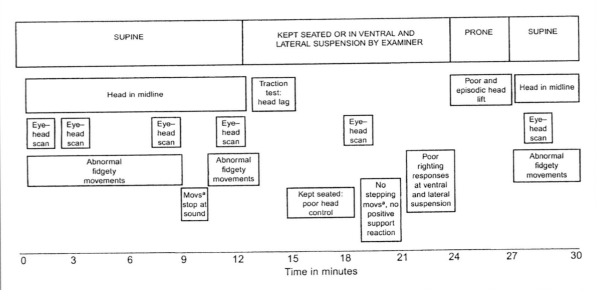

Fig. 11.2 Role of vision in early motor development: lessons from the blind. Reproduced with permission from Prechtl. General movement assessment as a method of developmental neurology: new paradigms and their consequences. *Dev Med Child Neurol* 43: 836–842, 2001. Mac Keith Press.

All blind children had disturbed fidgety movements; these are small, usually graceful movements of the arms and legs and occasionally trunk. In the blind children these movements were jerky and larger in amplitude and lasted longer, until 10 months of age in some cases, as opposed to disappearing at 15 weeks typically. The authors interpreted this as a lack of integration of visual and proprioceptive systems.

The blind infants had poor fine motor skills, as would be expected with no visual monitoring, but, in addition, when compared with sighted infants who did not look at their hands they were still more immature and clumsy. Again this could be explained by the lack of integration between vision and proprioception.

An interesting finding was the search and scanning actions by the head and eyes of the blind infants, which were identical to those of the sighted infants although the coordination disappeared. When they sat upright and an object was placed in their hand they immediately orientated their head to 'look' at the object, suggesting this facility is built in and not the result of any visual process.

All the blind children were delayed in gaining postural control with problems not only with head control and sitting but also a long-lasting ataxic instability of the trunk and head when brought to sitting, which often lasted until the children were 12 to 14 months of age. This was attributed to lack of visual input to the cerebellar vermis and cortex.

Discussion

There was no effect of blindness until the third month of life and the authors suggest that this is because at this age a major transformation of neural development takes place becoming more adaptive requiring vision to work with other sensory systems such as the vestibular mechanisms. They conclude that there are delays in motor development in blind infants and that these delays are due to the lack of vision, emphasizing that motor patterns are dependent on the normal functioning of sensory systems. This confirms the delay in motor development in blind infants from early in life. There is a recommendation that strategies to compensate for the lack of calibration of the vestibular and proprioceptive systems should be part of therapeutic programmes.

was absent. These difficulties are compounded by the motivation issues and the failure to anticipate danger, noted above, leading blind children to hesitate to stand up or walk even though they possess the necessary neuromuscular maturity.

The two studies are different in that they look at different ages, but they do overlap with some of their assessments. For example, sitting in the Prechtl et al (2001) study occurred around 12 to 14 months of age, whereas raise to sitting in the Troster et al (1994) study occurred in the term blind infants at the comparable 13 months of age; both of these are delayed by around 5 months. However, they do arrive at different conclusions with Prechtl noting that all posture is delayed, whereas Troster finds that some postural tasks were within typical limits, particularly those involving simply the accomplishment of a basic posture, with delays experienced predominantly in the tasks in which the child had to change posture from basic position to another. These differences are important as Prechtl is noting a fundamental neurological problem in all postural activities, whereas Troster et al (1994) are proposing that the real differences only occur when the child has to move elsewhere from a current position, which is in turn limited by lack of vision, but not the neural structure controlling

movement. The variety of the ages of the children, the variety of different tasks, and the known variability within the population of blind individuals may all have contributed to this difference.

Troster et al (1994) also note an interesting deviation in the motor development of blind children in that nearly all of them, full and preterm, skipped the crawling phase and only moved on all fours after they had taken their first steps, and thus missing the crawling phase seems to be a characteristic of blind children. They offer three explanations for this:

- At the normal time of crawling the blind infants do not have an object concept that allows them to link auditory perceptions with real objects, so there is no incentive to explore.
- The head is in an exposed position when crawling, and the hands cannot be used to identify and avoid objects, an explanation supported by half of the blind infants first crawling backwards.
- Vestibular information is more precise when upright than when horizontal, thus encouraging a vertical position.

Box 11.4 A closer examination

Longitudinal study of gross motor development in blind infants and preschoolers: Troster et al (1994)
This study is part of a larger longitudinal study tracking the perceptual, motor, socio-emotional, cognitive, and language development of 10 congenitally blind children from the first year of life to age 7 years, with three aims: to describe the development of blind children in these areas; to develop an early intervention and parent counselling programme; and to evaluate this intervention programme. The report in this study concentrates on the motor development of the blind children in the first 3 years of life.

Sample
The 10 children were blind from birth and at best had only light perception. Five were born at term and five pre-term with the latter having low birthweights between 650 and 1115g and a period of gestation of 26 to 29 weeks. Paediatric neurological examinations were conducted once a year and indications of brain damage were seen in one term child and four of the preterm infants. Table 11.3 compares the median age of development of postural skills of the blind infants with norms for sighted infants.

Results
The term blind infants on posture were within 95% of the age range of the sighted children. On average they could stand approximately 2 months later than sighted infants but were more delayed on the self-initiated tasks of changing posture and position. The real difference however was in the preterm blind infants, with sitting occurring 4 months later than sighted children and standing 20 months later and over 8 months for sitting up by themselves. For both term and preterm blind infants there was a longer delay between standing and maintaining balance and getting up and standing by themselves – 4 months for term infants and 17 months for preterm infants, compared with 1.6 months for sighted children (Fig. 11.3). Figure 11.4 takes the comparisons of development further by looking at locomotion. Term blind children walk around 4 months later than sighted children and crawl in a coordinated manner 9 months later. These developmental delays were much longer in the preterm blind children.

Discussion
This was a small sample of blind children, but the results show that, in the early development of posture and balance, term blind children show only slight delays. However, they show a much greater delay when they have to change posture of initial locomotion, but by the end of the second year of life all term blind infants were able to stand up and walk without support. These were very similar to Fraiberg's studies (1977). An interesting finding was that the gap between term and preterm blind children was greater than that between term blind and sighted

TABLE 11.3
Postural development in blind (preterm and term) and sighted infants

	Term blind infants	Preterm blind infants	Sighted children
Sits alone steadily	Typical at beginning of study	10	6.6
Stands holding on	Typical at beginning of study	12.5	7.6
Stands alone firmly	15.5	33.0	13.1
Raises to sitting	13.3	17.0	8.3
Stands up by furniture	12.0	18.0	8.6
Stands up	17.0	36.0	12.6
Coordinated crawling	19.0	22.5	9.7
Walks three steps alone	15.5	26.5	11.7
Walks upstairs with help	17.5	34.3	16.1

The ages of the preterm infants were corrected for preterm birth. Adapted with permission from Troster et al (1994).

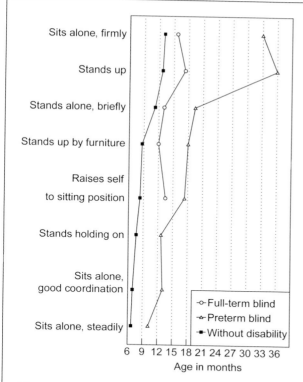
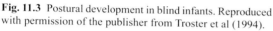

Fig. 11.3 Postural development in blind infants. Reproduced with permission of the publisher from Troster et al (1994).

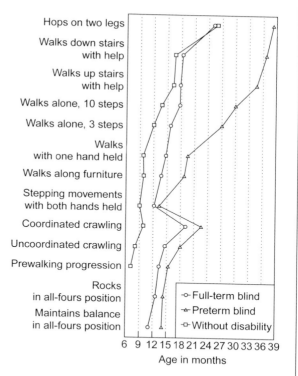

Fig. 11.4 Locomotor development in blind infants. Reproduced with permission of the publisher from Troster et al (1994).

children, with preterm birth possibly being a greater risk to delayed motor development than blindness. Thus blind children are at risk of delayed motor development because of their blindness and because of preterm birth. The preterm infants could be at risk of brain damage, an assumption partially supported by the neurological examinations but only confirmed in one infant. The authors conclude that the interaction between blindness and preterm birth poses a greater threat to early development than when the two risk factors are individually added together. Additional work involving perceptual and cognitive tasks could help throw more light on this interaction and on how global development is affected, and not just motor.

Other early signs of motor development delays or deviance have been noted in blind children, although the evidence is not clear cut. For example, there is some indication that blind children show degrees of hypotonia. Jan et al (1975) examined 180 visually impaired children, with IQs above 80 and no clinical diagnosis of neural impairment for signs of impairment, by looking at palpitating muscles and resistance during passive movements. There was a general tendency for the younger children to show hypotonia and the condition was also related to degree of blindness, with 61% of the legally blind children being hypotonic compared with 39% in the partially sighted group. Early movement skill development was also related to hypotonia with 80%

of the non-hypotonic group sitting within typical limits compared with 30% to 40% in the hypotonic group. In addition, clinical abnormalities were shown in 40% to 75% of the hypotonic group but only in 5% of the non-hypotonic group. Why hypotonia and blindness are connected is one area that has not been satisfactorily answered, but the authors argue that it is not a result of the causes of blindness but is more likely to be acquired in blind children owing to their being less mobile and more passive (Jan et al 1975). Although this is a possible answer, it is lacking in firm evidence and does not address the whole picture, such as why some blind children who are passive and not overly mobile are not hypotonic.

Variability in motor development

Other longitudinal studies have looked at preterm blind infants and the variability in their individual progression. Early studies by Parmelee et al (1958, 1959) made observations on 10 preterm blind infants from 18 to 75 months in different situations together with formal tests and interviews with parents. All infants were assessed early and diagnosed as blind, but one male made improvement such that there was useful vision in one eye. Sugden and Keogh (1990) note that this illustrates the difficulty in making an early assessment of what later vision will be, although they note that improvement of vision only occurs for a small percentage of children. The children were tested on a number of standardized developmental instruments and marked significant motor milestones such as walking and feeding with a spoon. There was great variability in when these milestones were achieved with a range of walking without support from 14 months, which is within typical limits, to 32 months, which is beyond normal variation data. Five of the infants walked before 18 months, but none walked earlier than the mean age for walking in typically developing children, which is 12 to 14 months. No relationship was found between the locomotion skills and the degree of blindness in this group of children. Feeding with a spoon ranged from 24 months to 48 months with another 3 of the 10 children not accomplishing this task.

Parmelee et al (1958, 1959) reported what we now know that individuals blind from birth are at greater risk of emotional and social difficulties and felt that delayed intellectual development was a function of this emotional disturbance. What was not examined or considered was whether the intellectual difficulties were a result of the preterm birth and possible brain damage and not just the blindness. Variability in a group such as this is expected, and the three comments below are selected from the final evaluation summaries of the children by Sugden and Keogh (1990).

Child A

No vision. Doing very well in a regular school; rides a bike, ice skates, explores toys fully and played game with a ball.

Child B

No vision. Mentally and socially advanced; should do well in an integrated school programme; play was extremely complex and conversation expansive.

Child C

No vision. Retarded, primarily on the basis of emotional disturbance; intellectual potential probably near normal; exploration of toys is very limited and seems to be withdrawn; emotional problems may contribute to poor behavioural functioning.

(p. 53)

The evidence is mixed with regard to blind children reaching for objects and crossing the midline, two major indices of manual activity. On the one hand, some work has shown that at 3 months of age a typical child will show midline interaction and at 5.5 months can transfer an object from hand to hand. However, at that age a blind infant is only showing chance engagement of midline activities (Fraiberg 1977). Warren (1994) reports a similar situation with reaching and grasping and concludes that, although the evidence about manual behaviour is mixed, there is some developmental lag, although not to the extent that is reported by Fraiberg (1977). He concludes by noting the variability within samples and proposes working with the larger samples where the variance is based upon larger numbers offering more stability.

The studies on motor development in blind children raise a number of questions; not least are the ones surrounding the role of vision in motor development and the consequences of the loss of this facility. To provide a frame of reference for this it is useful to return to the model of *child resources*, *environmental context*, and *task* with a closer look at the child resources. Typically, when the child resources are being examined, an analysis of those structures that act as constraints on movement are analysed. This would include neurological, biomechanical, and morphological variables as these are the obvious ones. However, there are more social and personal qualities that also have an effect on motor development and one of the more important ones is motivation. A typically developing child is motivated to move into the environment certainly in the first instance by what he or she sees, and with this facility being absent, blind children are less motivated than their sighted peers particularly to change posture and position, such as lifting their head when lying on their stomach or to initiate locomotion. It is as though there is nowhere to go. In addition, not only is there a lack of motivation to move but there is also a disincentive because they cannot anticipate or evaluate dangerous situations, and one bad experience can increase anxiety about moving and lead to a reluctance to engage in self-initiated locomotion. Thus when examining constraints on blind children's motor development it is important to examine the full range of intrinsic constraints involving those that are directly responsible for movement together with those that have a more indirect influence such as cognitive variables. These all, in turn, interact with the external constraints provided by the task presentation and context.

LATER MOVEMENT SKILL DEVELOPMENT

Development of spatial knowledge in blind children

This chapter has reported how blind children can be within typical limits for movement skills, such as basic posture and balance and standing, but as soon as the child has to move into the environment there are delays. Thus, the blind child is later than the sighted child in moving into the environment and has fewer and different skills once he or she is in that context. The development of spatial skills is crucial once the blind child is in the environment, with this development involving knowing location, direction, and distance of objects as well as knowing about one's own position in space. The development of spatial knowledge involves *near space*, including knowledge of body parts and body schema as well as starting to move in areas that are within normal reach of the body, and *far space*, which involves travel. Far space also involves knowledge of one's own body, with directions such as up or down, left or right, and in front or behind being first related to one's own body before locating it from an environmental perspective. Eventually, knowledge of spatial relations develops to a point in which spatial relations are made in reference to other persons or objects, with this development being the result of directions, memory for locations, and features to form internal spatial layouts or cognitive maps when an individual cannot see the travel route (Sugden and Keogh 1990). The distinction between near and far space is an obvious one to make in blind children. In near space an egocentric referencing system may be sufficient for functionality as the blind child has touch for all objects and persons within the vicinity to use as cues for information, and it may be sufficient, though not rich, for many purposes. However, the hand–arm linkage is not useful for far space unless it is being used in conjunction with some type of locomotion.

Warren (1994) describes the course of spatial development in blind children noting that in infancy it is rooted and organized with respect to the self, as opposed to sighted infants who begin to utilize some external structure that does not depend on their own location. This continued in early childhood with an emphasis on egocentric referencing of spatial information and the differences emerging between near- and far-space strategies and capabilities, with better performance when the movements could be related to body-centred proprioceptive cues, whereas their performance in far space was poorer because the blind child does not possess a reliable metric for external far space. However, Warren (1994) suggests that the ability to use external strategies does improve with age and this improvement with age is one of three factors in the near space literature that are influential in the performance of blind children. A second factor is the rather obvious one that any residual vision tends to be beneficial, and, third, those children who have had some visual experience early in life perform better than those who are blind from birth. In far space knowledge is better for those locations that are closer and local, and performance deteriorates when the distance is increased, and again those with some visual experience either from early vision or residual vision are better equipped (Warren 1994). These are just two of the variables that show performance in the area of far space to be variable across the population of blind children, with exceptional individuals occasionally producing outstanding performances by breaking free of the limitations that normally accompany blind individuals, and instead adopting their own strategies that facilitate the development of external spatial relations.

Blind children have performed equally well as sighted children in knowing spatial information from non-visual sources, but this is usually in familiar contexts in near space in a stable environment (Sugden and Keogh 1990). In far space this is rarely the case, notwithstanding some exceptional individuals and blind children who, as noted, take a more egocentric orientation and spatial perspective involving less use of external cues. Birns (1986) showed that blind children were capable of knowing perceptual constancies about spatial relationships but that they have difficulty with conceptual space, in how objects will appear from another viewpoint. She did report again the consistent finding of variability with some blind children achieving adequate representation of space. It is these individual variations that are proving to be puzzling, and it would be particularly enterprising to find out what was special about the blind children who did develop within a typical range. Earlier work by Millar (1981) showed that blind children, when compared with blindfolded sighted children, use more self-referent information when testing memory for spatial locations and proposed that external relations that are normally seen are obviously unavailable to the blind child, who thus uses spatial location strategies based upon body-related information. Millar (1981) also noted that the use of different spatial strategies was more related to visuospatial experience rather than age, again drawing attention to the multiple variables that are influencing the performance of blind children on motor tasks and why so much variability is found.

Work by Millar (1979, 1981, 1985) has explored how both sighted and blind children of an older age use spatial cues and kinaesthetic cues to locate targets and objects and has examined the relationship between kinaesthetic cues and spatial coding in the representations of object locations. An example of this is given in her work in which sighted but blindfolded children and blind children were asked to play a game involving remembering the end-point of a movement no matter where it started (Millar 1985). A common situation for a blind person is having to remember a situation or location once and then having to perform it again, such as reaching and grasping objects, receipts, or money while shopping, and Millar (1985) points out that this is not learning a skill, which is by definition 'relatively permanent', but simply a temporary memory for a location. Therefore, invoking action plans or schemas is not involved, but the studies do raise questions about how coding and monitoring of movement information are related to practice and/or change in context.

She suggests that children's coding strategies depend on their assessment of the information that is available from the task and from longer-term experience. This again is directly in line with the model persistently presented throughout this text, which states that it is not simply the child resources that affect movement outcomes but also the manner in which the task is presented.

Millar has taken her work on sensory systems, coding, and everyday activities into her text *Reading by Touch* (Millar 1997), in which she explores the world of reading by touch in blind persons, noting at the beginning that this is the most important means of written communication for blind persons. She notes a number of contradictions and raises important questions about the basis of perception by touch, stating that, while braille is relatively difficult to learn and tends to be slow, it can become fast and fluent. She stresses the importance of movement for coding shapes, contrasting active to passive movements, and the type of exploratory movement that any shape affords as well as the frames of reference that are available, such as object-centred frames based on cues external to the individual and egocentred cues that arise from information within the body framework. Both of these frames of reference are used by the blind in multiple ways in order to make sense not just of braille but of many objects and locations in near space. Readers with a particular interest in blind persons reading braille are recommended to consult Millar's (1997) book.

So far this reliance on an egocentric perspective rather than an objective external representation has been portrayed as a contributor to the impaired mobility and orientation capability of blind children. This may be true in a comparative sense with sighted persons, but these egocentric perspectives appear to be functionally useful strategies to employ in the light of their lack of vision (Sugden and Keogh 1990). They are clearly not too limiting in near space, with manual skills performed in stable and predictable environments that do not require an objective spatial perspective. However, when the blind person is travelling in far space, an objective viewpoint is useful in conjunction with a cognitive map and young blind people do have difficulties when having to rely solely on this cognitive map. This is explored further in the next section.

Orientation and mobility
The activity of moving into far space presents huge challenges for blind persons. Travelling in the environment usually means walking for blind persons, but it can mean running or even riding a bicycle. Whatever means is being employed, the blind person finds that unexpected or unfamiliar situations are particularly difficult. This is obvious in that anticipation of events is limited by the loss of vision, which leads to the blind person having to solve travel problems as they occur rather than by the usual method of anticipation through the visual mode. This in turn places a large stress on any information processing system the blind person is using, such as attentional or memory overload, and makes great demands of a person's cognitive mapping ability.

Early work by Cratty (1971) examined the subskills that are necessary for orientation and mobility and noted three that would be necessary for effective orientation:

- detection of environmental, surface, and path changes;
- accuracy of forward travelling motion – that is resistance to veering;
- directional changes at rest and in motion.

He found that these appeared to be relatively discrete and separate skills with low correlations between tests. Some of the findings were very interesting such as a downhill gradient being better detected than an uphill one, and a curve in a pathway was not generally detected unless it was part of a circle that had a circumference of less than 12.2m, which has obvious implications when a blind person reaches a kerb junction with a curved edge. Cratty (1971) compared his blind group to a blindfolded sighted group on such activities as simply trying to walk in a straight line and found the phenomenon of veering to be common. In both groups veering was as much as 35 degrees to the left or to the right with the direction of veer being constant within an individual. The further the individual walked the greater the veering, which increased as the pace of walking slowed down, and blind individuals who used a dog for travel assistance veered more than the ones who used a cane. This pioneering work by Cratty (1971) found that a large number of errors were made by the blind people, with, for example, choosing a new direction and veering contributing 35% or more to a blind person's travelling problems. He did engage the blind people in training regimes that substantially improved some of their subskills, but he did not measure the impact these made on the overall travel performance (Sugden and Keogh 1990).

As noted earlier, there is much variability in the mobility skills of blind children, and this variability can be due to multiple factors, such as the length of early visual experience or the availability of any residual vision. Warren (1994) poses the question as to what the developmental continuities between early movement skills in infancy and the major motor milestones, such as walking and running in childhood, are, and suggests that it would be logical to think of precocious infants as having better locomotor skills later in childhood. He also believes that training and intervention studies give some evidence of the importance of experience in the development of spatial behaviours crucial for orientation skills.

Sugden and Keogh (1990) take up the idea that, when studying mobility and orientation, the concept of information processing space has much to offer. They make the point that without vision blind travellers cannot locate objects and people with nearly as much efficiency and effectiveness and thus have to engage in additional processing of information, replacing vision with other sensory modalities leading to a narrowing of attention and without a full picture of events. In turn this increases the demands made upon other facilities, such as short-term memory, making it difficult for the blind person while travelling to pay attention to all of these pieces of information. Sugden and Keogh (1990) comment

> Processing load increases for blind travellers often to the point of overload. Thus, blind travellers not only lack visual input, they must use more of their processing capacity to make use of the sensory input they can obtain. More must be done to know less.

> (p. 60)

When measuring mobility, the usual criteria are efficiency and safety, both being translatable into errors during experimentation. Safety errors are usually calculated by the involuntary hitting of objects or people or straying from a designated pathway. Efficiency errors are calculated by measuring total travel time, which is made up of walking time and percentage of walking time against stopping or delaying (Sugden and Keogh 1990).

Shingledecker (1978, 1983) used travel routes to identify errors made and the load on the information processing system and incorporated a dual-task paradigm involving reaction times, with the blind person being required to press a button on a hand-held panel while performing travel tasks. The study involved 15 participants in three groups:

- one group were given verbal instructions for the route (preview group);
- one group practised a known route (same group);
- and the third group walked a new route (new group).

The preview group did better than the other two, making fewer errors, and had better efficiency scores. The results of inserting a secondary task were striking, with the group having more non-responses, more errors, and slower reaction times. The higher information load of walking a new route slowed down their reaction times. Shingledecker (1978) noted that this group did not know what was coming up next and had less time to respond, and also had to be constantly alert and processing information when no obstacle was present. The preview group made fewer errors presumably because they had some idea of what was coming and had more attentional capacity to do the secondary task. Sugden and Keogh (1990) interpreted these results as Shingledecker (1978, 1983) did: by invoking an information processing model that takes the resources of the child as really the only variable. They note that blind travellers have to rely on internal cognitive maps of a travel route, placing a great demand on short-term memory.

However, not all current researchers would agree with this assertion, and another way to analyse this is not in terms of processing space but through an analysis from a dynamical systems viewpoint in which perception and action are intrinsically linked and there is not a system of processing through various components, such as attention or short-term memory and motor programmes (see Chapter 1). In this approach, the environment affords or invites action with the child and the environment being the unit of analysis and not just the child. The environmental match between the two is the important issue, and, if one is degraded, then the whole suffers as a result. For example, normally the environment affords action according to the size of the body and its parts, with a bench inviting sitting for adults, jumping off for those in childhood, and cruising round holding on for young toddlers. Without vision this affordance is missing and the whole child–environment synergy is disturbed. Proponents of this point of view would not allude to processing space being overloaded but to the child–environmental match

Box 11.5 A closer examination

Use of auditory cues by blind persons: Emerson and Sauerburger (2008)

Emerson and Sauerburger (2008) investigated the use of auditory cues by considering to what degree the auditory detection of approaching vehicles was affected by the ambient level of sound, the sound level and speed of approaching vehicles, and the physical features of the environment such as hills, bends in roads, trees, and other obstacles.

Procedures

Sites for the study that reflected different environmental conditions and ambient sound levels were chosen. Participants were not asked to actually cross the street but to indicate by raising their hand when they first heard a vehicle approach, and the time was measured from this to when the vehicle actually passed the person. Crossing the road with normal walking was also estimated, with the difference between the above time and this measure used as a 'safety margin'. There were six environmental conditions under which the blind persons made these judgements, ranging from no obstacles and a baffle obstructing the sound, through a minor bend in the road, and increasing in difficulty to a severe bend, a hill, and a heavily tree-lined approach.

Results

The results examining the amount of safety margin varied from 6 seconds with a straight road, through 3 seconds on a minor bend or hill, to 0 seconds for a major bend. These results support having as quiet an environment as possible, and even in ideal circumstances little noise was required to affect the person's ability to detect oncoming traffic.

Discussion

Emerson and Sauerburger (2008) note that environmental features such as hills and bends affect the ability to detect oncoming traffic, but these environmental variables only account for one-third of the variance in detection times. They also note that, if a different (wider) street is used or encountered, the detection times will remain the same, but the safety margins will be smaller because of the longer crossing. In addition, sound levels will differ significantly across situations, this time affecting detection times, and, if louder, will make the safety margins worse. The final recommendation is training for blind persons to analyse each situation individually and not just rely on the features considered in this study.

being disturbed; it is not just one part of the system that has gone astray, but the whole system is now different from what it is in a sighted child.

Travelling in the community

It is logical that pedestrians who are visually impaired or blind use their hearing to detect approaching vehicles and gaps in the traffic. The strategy of 'cross when quiet' is one that is customarily used. However, this is not always a failsafe strategy, as often even when it is quiet approaching vehicles cannot be heard well enough to judge whether the gap in the traffic is long enough to cross. This has been examined in more detail with attempts to define the parameters that would enable blind persons to make decisions about crossing the street or not in the absence of traffic control. Guidelines such as 'all clear' and 'all quiet' are useful when a blind person has good walking

pace, the traffic is light, the street is narrow, traffic speeds are low, and there are no obstacles that would mask a person's ability to hear the traffic. In Box 11.5 there is an example of the effect of auditory cues and knowledge of approaching vehicles.

Since the early studies on orientation and route finding, such as the Cratty studies (1971), there has been the advent of the use of global positioning devices, which has helped individuals to store and retrieve information about specific locations. Loomis and colleagues at the University of Santa Barbara as long ago as 1985 (unpublished paper but reported in Ponchilla et al 2007) were involved in examining the usefulness of technology in this area and developed a personal guidance system for people with visual impairments (Golledge et al 1991). A global positioning system (GPS) receives information from 24 satellites that circle the earth and transmit radio signals that, when coupled with a geographic information system (GIS), can be used to locate the position of someone who is carrying a GPS receiver. A GIS stores information on physical landscapes such as rivers and mountains as well as roads and buildings. Thus GPS–GIS combinations can be used to give people access to names and locations of services such as shops, banks, etc. As soon as these became readily available the opportunities that these systems might offer to visually impaired individuals became obvious. Two recent studies examining the possibilities are described below; they are both small-scale experiments but show the possibilities these systems may offer in the future.

Marston et al (2007) examined the use of a haptic display, that is vibration, as well as audition, with the former offering potential in a noisy environment when the critical sound is masked by other sounds. Haptic displays can be vibrostimulators often worn around the waist or an electronic compass attached to a visor on the head with a vibrotactile stimulator worn on the wrist. Thus when the head faces the correct location there is corresponding stimulation on the wrist. In addition, there was also a small earbud that delivered a chime sound. All the participants (eight adults with varying degrees of blindness) followed a route with six turning points, and when they were on or off course they received a tactile or auditory cue. The time they took to walk the various routes was recorded along with the number of errors. There were a number of conditions, ranging from haptic and audition on and off alone to combinations, and there were no statistical differences between the conditions. The conclusion from this was that a simple binary signal whether tactile or auditory was sufficient for accurate route finding. Signals identifying off-course were preferred to on-course signals and were rated as more natural. Thus, a wide range of devices work well for individual impairments and different options are available to suit different needs.

Ponchilla et al (2007) worked with three individuals examining their ability to use BrailleNote GPS (BGPS). The first experiment looked at the ability of participants to regain orientation in a familiar neighbourhood after being deliberately disorientated, and the second was to measure the ability of an experienced user to locate a target house in each of three levels of electronic intervention. In the first experiment all individuals took a consistently shorter amount of time using GPS, and one was unable to re-orientate without it. In addition, there was an increased efficiency rate of finding the target house as measured by feet per second. In the second experiment, an experienced BGPS user was asked to locate five target houses with and without GPS and demonstrated that even in extremely familiar areas the GPS technology was advantageous. These were single-subject design experiments and do not necessarily generalize to a wider population, but they do demonstrate the possibilities for these systems, which can be used for simple functions with only a little training. In the first experiment, the ability of an individual to re-orientate him- or herself with 100% accuracy in less than 1 minute is not only very significant but also empowering.

Orientation, mobility, and travelling in the community are crucial aspects of any person's life whether sighted or not. They enable visits to places of interest, social interaction, and recreational and work-related opportunities, with the converse of restricted opportunities being the case when mobility is hindered. The capabilities of the person are just one part of the overall competence that blind individuals exhibit when travelling, and these are now beginning to be enhanced with various forms of additional aids, thereby changing the whole person–task–environment dynamic.

PHYSICAL ACTIVITY AND CHILDREN WITH VISUAL IMPAIRMENTS

Physical activity in children can help to increase their quality of life by enhancing physical, emotional, and mental well-being. Throughout this chapter the challenges that blind children face in developing fundamental motor skills as well as the later orientation and mobility challenges have been noted. Blind children are less likely to engage in physical activity, and very often adequate instruction and support is not forthcoming, leading to lower levels of physical activity due to lack of practice and participation (Lieberman and McHugh 2001). Unless there is some other constitutional damage caused by, for example, low birthweight or preterm birth, blind children have the same potential to develop motor skills and healthy fitness levels as their peers. Lieberman et al (2009) notes that, despite the lack of trained personnel to work in physical education with blind individuals, there are opportunities for teaching particular skills, such as jumping rope as described in Box 11.6.

Participation in sporting activities is a highly social activity and is often viewed as an important socializing environment for children and for teaching children interpersonal skills as well as physical competence, both of which contribute to the child's self-esteem. Children with disabilities often have low self-esteem and require enhanced self-concept to feel competent enough to participate in children's games and sports (Shapiro and Dummer 1998). Children with visual impairments generally have fewer opportunities for participation, which may be due to a number of factors including fewer friendships, exclusion from groups, differences in physical appearance,

---

Box 11.6 A closer examination

Teaching jump rope to children with visual impairment: Lieberman et al (2009)
This study aimed to examine jump-rope performance in children with visual impairment. Of the 71 children who took part, 18 had B-1 loss, 14 had B-2 and 39 had B-3. As defined by the United States Association for Blind Athletes, B-1 athletes have no functional vision; B-2 athletes have visual acuity less than 20/400 or a visual field of less than 5 degrees; and B-3 athletes have a visual acuity of 20/200–20/400 or a visual field of 5–20 degrees. A number of variables were examined that may influence the jumping.

First, *jumping surfaces* were examined with two mats, one grey (46 by 46cm) and the other blue with yellow sloping edges (109 by 109cm). The latter was rated as 10% more helpful in maintaining their position than the grey mat, but the children did not feel either mat interfered with their jumping and most (80% plus) said the mats helped.

Second, five different types of *jump rope* were used: plastic beaded; plastic-coated wire; flexible plastic cord; plastic beaded with a quarter of a hula hoop hung at the centre of the rope; and JumpSnap, a battery powered, talking ropeless jump rope, which measured time jumped, number of completed jumps, and calories burned. There are two plastic handles that the jumper uses, which contain small plastic balls that provide feedback to the jumper, but there is no rope. Each one of the jump ropes was rated by the children using a 5-point Likert scale. The ropeless jump rope was rated as the safest by 80% of the children, and the best for their own skill level, followed by the adapted hula hoop rope and then the flexible plastic cord. The ropeless jump rope also had the most comfortable grip and was rated best overall by the group.

Third, *instructional modifications* were suggested as helpful to the children in achieving their optimum skill level. These included *whole–part–whole* instructions involving a demonstration of the whole skill through residual vision or by touch, followed by breaking it down into parts and finally building it back up to the whole again. *Physical guidance* was also used, which involved a simple tap on the knee to remind the child to jump or moving the child's arm in the whole swinging motion. Tactile modelling involves the child feeling the instructor's movements in order to obtain the necessary information for their participation.

Fourth, *modifications of the environment* were made. One method was *to cut the rope in half* to eliminate timing or height of the jump; occasionally, for a child who was having difficulty holding the rope, it *was tied to the hand*; *mat*s were employed to ensure the child stayed in a designated area; in order to encourage a rhythmic jump, *sound sources* from music and metronomes were used; in cases in which the child had an additional physical disability such as cerebral palsy, *only one hand was used* with the other end of the rope tied to a door handle or another child held it and jumped at the same time. *Group* or *Double-Dutch jumping* was occasionally employed with the child being a turner.

Comment
This is a study that classically illustrates the model we have shown throughout the text. The child comes with a certain set of *resources*, such as having no vision or some residual vision. The *environment* is modified in numerous ways by making different demands on the child and by employing different types of adaptive equipment of ropes and mats. Finally, *task* or *instructional modifications* are made that best match the needs and capabilities of the child.

---

and poorer performance on fitness activities and motor skills. However, these are all connected to the resources of the child and some researchers have found that these are not the only variables and may not be the most important ones. Lieberman et al (2002) found that physical education teachers lacked the professional preparation for teaching children with visual impairments and were generally uninformed about equipment, assessment, and modifications in teaching such as through differentiation.

Many of these general findings were queried by Shapiro et al (2008) who examined perceived competence, ratings of importance of physical appearance, athletic competence, and social acceptance and global self-worth in a group of 43 children of mixed ages from 8 to 18 years. The somewhat surprising results showed that none of social acceptance, athletic competence, and physical appearance domains appeared to be perceived as important, and the authors note that this is the first study they

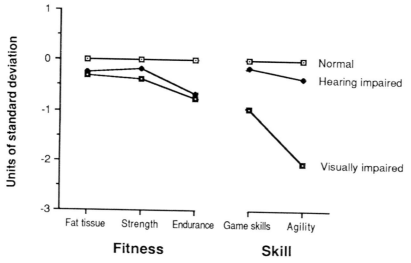

Fig. 11.5 Mean performance of typically developing, hearing-impaired, and visually impaired youths aged 10 to 17 years. Redrawn from data reported by Winnick and Short (1982) and Sugden and Keogh (1990).

have seen that used Harter's multidimensional scales with a disability population to have found this. The low rating for athletic competence was of concern to the authors because it may suggest that children with visual impairment may choose not to participate in such activities, thereby posing a potential health risk. They discounted the importance of these variables while maintaining a high overall self-worth score. Lieberman et al (2002) suggest that the global self-worth may have come from specialized schools and camps where they are given individual attention and are encouraged and supported to participate and develop positive self-esteem. Such concepts as self-worth and quality of life in general are often an outcome of a variety of sources, and, with respect to physical activity, a question to ask is whether physical activity and related variables are indeed related to quality of life. Holbrook et al (2009) quantified physical activity, body composition, and quality of life in middle-aged visually impaired men and women and examined the relationship between these variables. They found that it was not possible to predict quality of life from physical activity level, severity of visual impairment, or the combined influence of these variables. Thus, currently, the evidence is mixed with respect to participation, physical competence, and self-worth in blind individuals. However, this mixed evidence should not undermine our aims and goals that involve creating contexts and environments that facilitate inclusion and participation in all aspects of life, including recreation and physical activity.

Most of the work on fitness and sport skills has been limited to maximum performance measures such as how far the children can throw or how fast they can

run (Sugden and Keogh 1990). Work by Winnick and Short (1982) examined some of these variables in blind, deaf, and typically developing children and young adults, providing assistance for those unable to see lines or directions of throw or the place to jump from and placement of obstacles. Fitness levels were lower for the visually and hearing impaired groups than for the typically developing children, and this is probably related to these two groups being less active, as there is really no reason to suppose that a sensory deficit leads to greater amounts of fatty tissue and less of lean tissue. In games and agilities, as shown in Figure 11.5, the children who were visually impaired performed significantly worse. This is supported by endurance runs being reduced substantially by practice and motivation (Sugden and Keogh 1990). Performances in general movement skills by the visually impaired group were substantially poorer than those of the hearing impaired group, who were only marginally less competent than the typically developing group.

These studies (Winnick and Short 1982, Lieberman et al 2002, Holbrook et al 2009) raise questions about the relationships among visual impairment, physical activity, both real and judged, and quality of life as well as such personal variables as self-esteem. The picture we are seeing over and over again is the one that is commensurate with the *child resources–task–environment* model. The outcomes do not reside solely in the resources of the child, as we have seen how modifiable these are with the assistance of the clever use of environmental and task variables.

There is strong evidence that blind children are at risk of poor physical fitness, but it appears that this is not a direct consequence of their visual impairment and is instead due to a lack of participation. There is great variability in the opportunities that blind children have to participate in physical exercise, and it appears that the more opportunities there are, the more the blind individual reaches levels of fitness that would be considered typical. In addition, another variable seems to be encouragement, with the rather obvious but necessary statement that the more an individual is encouraged, the more participation is evident.

Summary

The literature on blind individuals is diverse with the good reason that from birth through adulthood and into old age the demands of the environment that involve vision change substantially. Thus, when the model of child resources–environment–task is employed each one of these plays a differential role at different stages of the person's life. For example, when a term blind infant is observed for posture in the early months, there is some delay but many milestones are within the typically developing range. However, if the blind infant is preterm with evidence of neural abnormalities there is substantial delay, presumably the preterm birth being the prime cause but interacting with the lack of vision. As soon as the young infant has to move into the environment, not only is there substantial delay but there also appears to be a strong personal and emotional connection, with motivation being affected and the child having 'nowhere to go'.

The development into early and later childhood brings with it a whole new set of challenges. The fundamental skills of walking, running, and many manual skills are within the capability of the blind child, but without vision providing the lure, the invitation, and the motivation, the developing child's actions become limited. In dynamical systems terms, the environment is not spontaneously affording actions from the child, and, in order for this to occur, the environment and the task have to be modified to provide that affordance. The information on the ability to use spatial cues and to orientate and be mobile is not only severely hindered by the lack of vision, but also more attention from other senses is required and produces poorer results. This then hinders the mobility of the individual and also affects other personal qualities such as motivation and self-esteem.

Sugden and Keogh (1990) suggested the presence of movement stereotypies that are so often present in blind children and which, by their inappropriate social connotations, serve to limit the movement experiences of blind children. Rhythmical movement stereotypies are relatively common in blind children with Eichel (1979) reporting that only 4 out of 28 children studied did not engage in them, and Sugden and Keogh (1990) suggested that these behaviours are important in limiting experience in the same sense that echolalia can limit experience in speech and language development.

The term 'blindisms' is an interesting one in that in its very name it implicates blind persons when in fact the movements that are referred to are no different in blind people from those observed in sighted individuals. These behaviours are stereotypical and repetitive and can include eye rubbing, head turning, hand gestures, and larger body movement such as rocking and swaying. They could also involve more complex sequences of movements (Warren 1994). Children who are blind or with visual impairment do engage in these movements, which can have not only an inhibiting effect on normal social interactions but also cause the children to miss some part of any presentation in the physical world that may be interesting or informative, and could be dangerous to the child. The reasons for the mannerisms could be that they are self-stimulatory to the various sensory systems, such as rocking to the vestibular system, and it is often observed that under conditions of stress these mannerisms increase. Warren (1994) cautions against automatically trying to reduce the incidence of these as the children themselves are usually quite effective in regulating their amount of self-stimulatory behaviour and in avoiding overstimulation, and he urges sensitivity on the part of both parents and professionals in this area.

The obvious way to support the blind individual when personal resources are limited is to provide support in the environment or through task modifications such that they can more readily participate in the activities of daily living. Thus, research shows that natural environments differ in how they provide auditory information, with trees, hills, and bends all masking to some extent traffic noise, thus hindering the blind individual. An awareness of this and training to recognize these are all part of any support system. The advent of global positioning devices is starting to make a big impact on the mobility and orientation activities of blind individuals, and this type of technology will only increase, thus making the environment a safer and easier place for the person to navigate. In recreational activities both the task and the environment can be changed substantially in order to facilitate participation, with the jump-rope study being a good example of this. The motor development of blind individuals is driven by the child resources in the first instance, but from a very early age the amount of support that is provided by modifications of the task and the environment can make substantial differences to the daily lives of blind individuals, and variations in this support are often a cause of the known high individual variability in blind persons' motor development.

REFERENCES

Adelson E, Fraiberg S (1974) Gross motor development in infants blind from birth. *Child Dev* 45: 114–126. http://dx.doi.org/10.2307/1127757

Bayley N (1969) *The Bayley Scales of Infant Development.* New York: Psychological Development.

Birns SL (1986) Age at onset of blindness and development of space concepts: from topological to projective space. *J Vis Impairment Blindness* 80: 577–582.

Butterworth G, Hicks L (1977) Visual proprioception and postural stability in infancy: a developmental study. *Perception* 6: 255–262.

Cratty BJ (1971) *Movement and Spatial Awareness in Blind Children and Youth.* Springfield, IL: Charles C Thomas.

Eichel VJ (1979) A taxonomy of mannerisms in blind children. *J Vis Impairment Blindness* 73: 167–178.

Emerson RW, Sauerburger D (2008) Detecting approaching vehicles at streets with no traffic control. *J Vis Impairment Blindness* 102: 747–760.

Ferrell KA, Trief E, Dietz SJ, et al (1990) Visually impaired infants research commission consortium (VIIRC): first year results. *J Vis Impairment Blindness* 84: 404–410.

Fraiberg S (1977) *Insights from the Blind.* New York: Basic Books.

Fraiberg S, Freedman D (1964) Studies in the ego development of the congenitally blind child. *Psychoanalytic Study of the Child* 19: 113–169.

Frankenburg WK, Dodds JB (1969) The Denver developmental test. *J Pediatr* 71: 181–191. http://dx.doi.org/10.1016/S0022-3476(67)80070-2

Freedman SJ, Fisher HG (1968) The role of the pinna in auditory localisation. In: Freedman SJ, editor. *The Neuropsychology of Spatially Oriented Behaviour.* Homewood, IL: Dorsey Press, pp. 135–152.

Gilbert C, Foster A (2001) Childhood blindness in the context of VISION 2020 –the right to sight. *Bull World Health Organization* 79: 3.

Golledge RG, Loomis JM, Klatzsky RL, Flury A, Yang X (1991) Designing a personal guidance system to aid navigation without sight: progress on the GIS component. *Int J Geographic Information Systems* 5: 373–395. http://dx.doi.org/10.1080/02693799108927864

Holbrook EA, Caputo JL, Perry TL, Fuller DF, Morgan DW (2009) Phycial activity body composition and perceived quality of life of adults with visual impairments. *J Vis Impairment Blindness* 1: 17–29.

Jan JE, Robinson GC, Scott E, Kinnis EP (1975) *Visual Impairment in Children and Adolescents.* New York: Grune & Stratton.

Lee DN, Aaronson E (1974) Visual proprioceptive control of standing in human infants. *Percept Psychophys* 15: 529–532. http://dx.doi.org/10.3758/BF03199297

Lieberman LJ, McHugh E (2001) Health-related fitness of children who are visually impaired. *J Vis Impairment Blindness* 95: 272–287.

Lieberman LJ, Housten-Wilson C, Kozub FM (2002) Perceived barriers to including students with visual impairments in general physical education lessons. *Adapted Phys Activity Q* 19: 364–377.

Lieberman LJ, Schedlin H, Pierce T (2009) Teaching jump rope to children with visual impairments. *J Vis Impairment Blindness* 103: 173–178.

Marston JR, Loomis JM, Klatzsky RL, Golledge RG (2007) Nonvisual route following with guidance from a simple haptic or auditory display. *J Vis Impairment Blindness* 101: 203–211.

Millar S (1979) The utilization of external and movement cues in simple spatial tasks by blind and sighted children. *Perception* 8: 11–20. http://dx.doi.org/10.1068/p080011

Millar S (1981) Self-referent and movement cues in coding spatial location by blind and sighted children. *Perception* 10: 255–264. http://dx.doi.org/10.1068/p100255

Millar S (1985) Movement cues and body orientation in recall of locations of blind and sighted children. *Q J Exp Psychol* 37A: 257–279.

Millar S (1997) *Reading by Touch.* London: Routledge. http://dx.doi.org/10.4324/9780203359440

Norris M, Spaulding PJ, Brodie FH (1957) *Blindness in Children.* Chicago: University of Chicago Press.

Parmelee AH, Cutsforth MG, Jackson CL (1958) Mental development of children with blindness due to rentrolental fibroplasia. *Am J Dis Child* 96: 641–654.

Parmelee AH, Fiske CE, Wright RH (1959) The development of ten children with blindness as a result of retrolental fibroplasia. *Am J Dis Child* 98: 198–220.

Ponchilla PE, Rak EC, Freeland AL, LaGrow SJ (2007) Accessible GPS: reorientation and target location among users with visual impairments. *J Vis Impairment Blindness* 101: 389–401.

Prechtl FR, Cioni G, Eispieler C, Bos AR, Ferrari F (2001) Role of vision in early motor development: lessons from the blind. *Dev Med Child Neurol* 43: 198–201.

Shapiro DR, Dummer G (1998) Perceived and actual basketball competence of adolescent males with mild mental retardation. *Adapt Phys Activ Q* 15: 179–190.

Shapiro DR, Moffett A, Lieberman LJ, Dummer G (2008) Domain-specific ratings of self-importance and global self-worth of children with visual impairments. *J Vis Impairment Blindness* 102: 232–244.

Shingledecker CA (1978) The effects of anticipation on performance and processing load in blind mobility. *Ergonomics* 21: 355–371. http://dx.doi.org/10.1080/00140137808931733

Shingledecker CA (1983) Handicap and human skill. In: Holding D, editor. *Human Skills.* New York: Wiley, pp. 227–256.

Sugden DA, Keogh JF (1990) *Problems in Movement Skill Development.* Columbia, SC: University of South Carolina Press.

Troster H, Hecker W, Brambring M (1994) Longitudinal study of gross-motor development in blind infants and pre-schoolers. *Early Child Dev Care* 104: 61–78. http://dx.doi.org/10.1080/0300443941040105

Warren DH (1994) *Blindness and Children: An Individual Differences Approach.* Cambridge: Cambridge University Press. http://dx.doi.org/10.1017/CBO9780511582288

WHO (1992) *International Statistical Classification of Diseases and Related Health Problems, Volume 1,* 10th edition. Geneva: World Health Organization.

WHO (1998) *Global Initiative for the Elimination of Blindness.* Geneva: World Health Organization.

Winnick JP, Short FX (1982) The physical fitness of sensory and orthopedically impaired youth. Project UNIQUE final report. Brockport, NY: Department of Physical Education and Sport, State University New York.

12
ASSESSMENT AND INTERVENTION FOR CHILDREN WITH MOVEMENT DIFFICULTIES

Assessment and intervention

Throughout the text there has been an emphasis on the development of children, whether typical or atypical, being a function of the interaction between the child's resources, the context in which any activity takes place, and the type and manner of the presentation of any tasks. In this chapter there are descriptions and analyses of the twin and interrelated processes of assessment and intervention, and in both of these the same interactive effects of child resources, environment, and task hold true. Even though the object of any exercise is the child with movement difficulties, it is not sufficient just to take into consideration the resources of the child. For example, when assessing a child with movement difficulties, it is obvious that collecting information on the child's resources is a crucial area and, as described later in the chapter, this can be done in multiple ways and indeed information from different sources would appear to be the most logical way of building up a total picture of the child. However, in addition, a description of the environmental context of the child's world is also a necessity for all appropriate and relevant information to be considered: first for

assessing the child and second for planning intervention. Similarly, the types of tasks the child has been exposed to, is good at, and is having difficulty with, and how they have been presented, are also relevant variables when deciding how intervention should proceed. These guide how goals, objectives, and priorities are decided for future presentation of tasks. It is indeed a dynamic system with all parts contributing to the whole; many of the parts are within the child but also many reside outside of the child and are in the control of other significant persons. The model that has been portrayed throughout the text is shown below in Figure 12.1.

The two processes of *assessment* and *intervention* are specific processes with different methodologies, but they are linked. There is a firm belief that, without detailed and accurate assessment of the child and his or her ecology, the chances of successful intervention are slim. The children who are being assessed are having difficulties on a wide range of tasks, and, thus, collecting information or accurate assessment of the child and the context in which he or she operates are crucial steps towards successful intervention. In this way the two processes are

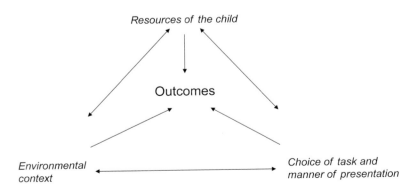

Fig. 12.1 Triad of transactions on movement outcomes.

intrinsically linked. In another way they are linked in that, during and following intervention, there is a need to see how much, if any, improvement has taken place, and, for that, some form of assessment is necessary.

The format of the chapter is such that *assessment* and *intervention* are taken separately but with the knowledge that they are interrelated. We have used the terms *assessment* and *intervention* as these are the ones in common usage, but we also use the terms *collecting information to plan a programme* and *implementing a programme* (Sugden and Henderson 2007) at various points in the chapter. In each section, general descriptions and principles of both assessment and intervention are taken and followed by examples of clinical and educational practice.

For the obvious reasons of space, there is no attempt to be comprehensive in presenting all modes of assessment and intervention for children with movement difficulties. For example, in children with cerebral palsy, there is no coverage of techniques, such as botulinum toxin, or of any surgical procedures, two prominent intervention methods for these children. What are covered are the general principles and variables associated with assessment and intervention, with specific examples given to show how they operate in a clinical or educational setting. Boxes throughout the chapter show practices in both assessment and intervention.

Purposes of assessment

Assessment is the systematic collection of information about the child and his or her environment, and the integration of the various parts such that a total picture can be used for a number of purposes. These purposes involve the following (Burton and Miller 1998):

- diagnosis and categorization of the child leading to services and support;
- planning intervention for the child;
- examining the child over time to determine what changes have taken place;
- enabling feedback to be given to significant others;
- assessment used to evaluate a particular type of intervention; and
- assessment that provides an overview of the type of environment the child is situated in.

DIAGNOSIS AND CATEGORIZATION OF THE CHILD LEADING TO SERVICES AND SUPPORT

Very often services for a child with movement difficulties are dependent upon a diagnosis being given. Thus, a child with cerebral palsy or developmental coordination disorder (DCD) is assessed often in order for a recommendation to be given from health or education to obtain

the extra resources or support necessary for the child. It is important not only for supporting the child but also to ensure that there is efficient use of resources in a field where heavy demands are made with respect to finance. Accurate assessment can help to ensure this. This process does lead to the child having a label and the advantages and disadvantages of labelling a child are well known. The major advantages include an understanding of the condition and a pathway to ensure that the child receives some form of help that otherwise would not be available. The cons include those associated with exclusion and being different, self-fulfilling prophecies, and the limiting of ambition.

PLANNING INTERVENTION FOR THE CHILD

A complete assessment of the child and his or her ecology is directly beneficial to the planning for the type of intervention that is deemed necessary. This is a crucial part of the support system with detailed and comprehensive coverage of the child's capabilities provided by a number of different sources: the child, parents and family, school, and health services. The use of a number of different methodologies provides a total picture of the child, and enables a complete profile of the child to be developed. For any intervention, it is recommended that both strengths and weaknesses are noted with strengths being used to help the child participate and be an asset to improve areas where there are weaknesses. All of this information is used, together with the environmental circumstances in which the child is living, involving home, school, community, and the health service, showing the possibilities from the close environments such that objectives can be set and priorities developed.

EXAMINING THE CHILD OVER TIME

Children are dynamically changing individuals and continued assessment of some type is helpful to see what is happening to the child over time. Examples observed in the developing child and how objectives, priorities, strengths, and weaknesses change as he or she progresses from early childhood through to emerging adulthood strengthen the need for continuous monitoring. When this is twinned with the type of environment the child is situated in, it provides more useful information to the therapist or teacher about whether to change any intervention procedure and/or when to stop it.

ENABLING FEEDBACK TO BE GIVEN TO SIGNIFICANT OTHERS

Involving significant individuals, especially the child and parents, is crucial to the overall success of any intervention programme. Without feedback being cascaded, there is a void in the help that can be given. In addition, feedback is a two-way process: the results of assessment can be given to the parents and teachers who in turn can provide information that can be obtained only in their particular environmental niche. It is particularly important that feedback is given to the child in a form that can be readily understood. The child is the central person throughout the process, and it is beneficial for him or her to be involved in goal setting and other choices that need to be made.

ASSESSMENT USED TO EVALUATE A PARTICULAR TYPE OF INTERVENTION

Very often a programme is enacted involving a particular type of intervention, and assessment is necessary to examine the efficacy of the programme. Does it work? Is it suitable for all children or a specific subset? Does the success of the programme justify the cost? This can be done at various levels from the assessment of an individual programme for the child to a much larger school district level, moving through various sized groupings en route. There are examples in the field of developmental disorders where large-scale programmes have been implemented, such as the TEACCH Autism Program (Mesibov et al 2004).

ASSESSMENT OF THE TYPE OF ENVIRONMENT

A description of the child's environmental circumstances, such as home routines, community, and school support systems, is a key action for the planning of appropriate intervention. In this case, it is collecting information rather than simple assessment. We maintain that without a knowledge of and partnership between the home life and those planning intervention, any attempt at intervention is likely to be limited (Bernheimer and Keogh 1995). Information regarding the ecology of the child is desirable, as outcomes from similar conditions will differ according to the environmental context.

The term assessment is one that is in common use, but we do recognize that it leads one to think in particular ways. In many instances, particularly when looking to provide a programme of intervention, the phrase 'collecting information' might be one that is more suitable, as this is a more appropriate term when describing the child and analysing the environmental context (Sugden and Henderson 2007).

The field of intervention

The term intervention has been chosen from a range of possibilities – remediation, therapy, management, teaching, and others that are used in the literature – yet we believe that these alternatives do not quite capture the

breadth of the approaches that come under the heading of intervention. We are firm advocates of an 'ecological approach' to intervention (Sugden and Henderson 2007), which covers many of the specific approaches to intervention. This approach describes how intervention is not always delivered by an experienced and skilled professional, and does not always occur in a recognized and designated therapy session, but includes other methods as well. Thus, intervention can be a tight experimental design with strong controllable methodological procedures. Other interventions have at their roots clinical practice and schools in real-life situations with some interventions being a combination of both. It is difficult to dichotomize the two approaches as the dividing line is quite blurred. However, there is a range of approaches to intervention that vary in their origins – medical, educational, social – and employ methodologies that also vary. The following sections briefly overview two such approaches.

QUASI EXPERIMENTAL DESIGNS

In many fields, such as medicine and psychology, a tight experimental design is often undertaken in which the variables that are free to vary are kept to a minimum. Thus, in a classic randomized controlled study, groups will have been randomly selected to receive a particular form of treatment and compared with other groups who received a different type or none at all. This is a popular and strong method for testing such variables as medication and doses of the same. When working with young children, it often is difficult for the controls to be so tight, but this method does attempt to provide good control over extraneous variables. The intervention is usually delivered by skilled professionals, for example occupational therapists or physiotherapists, and is often used to test a particular method. Much of our empirical evidence is obtained from these types of intervention studies, and the results of many of these studies are often pulled together in a meta-analysis to group several studies together and give stronger indications of effectiveness of particular interventions. An example of this would be the meta-analysis performed by Pless and Carlsson (2000) that looked at children with DCD. The studies in this group still vary according to the kinds of comparisons that are made with control groups, yet they provide valuable information on the overall type of approach.

The description of intervention above is one in which there has been as much internal control as possible, with an attempt to eliminate any variables that may make the results appear ambiguous or due to some extraneous factor. However, by keeping this tight control, there is a risk of the intervention being more divorced from the reality of

---

Box 12.1 A closer examination

Kinaesthetic approach to intervention: Simms et al (1996a,b)
The primary aim of these two studies was to investigate the effect of kinaesthetic training on children with DCD (labelled 'clumsy' in the studies).

Subjects

In the *first study* (Simms et al 1996a) there were two groups of children, 10 in each group. The groups were matched by IQ, motor impairment scores, and kinaesthetic sensitivity. Both groups were identified as having movement difficulties.

In the *second study* there were three groups of children, 12 in each group, and again all were matched on chronological age, verbal IQ, scores on kinaesthesis, and motor competence.

Procedure

In the *first study* both groups had kinaesthetic training, as proposed by Laszlo and Bairstow (1985), and also a period of no training, one group having the training while the other one had no training with a switch over after 10 days. This involved 10 days of training for 20 to 25 minutes each day, working on both kinaesthetic acuity and kinaesthetic perception and memory. There was an immediate post-training test and one 3 months later.

In the *second study* two of the three groups were given intervention, one of the groups receiving kinaesthetic training and the second receiving cognitive affective training, while the third group did not receive any intervention.

Results

For the immediate post-training test in the *first study* after the first period of intervention, both groups improved on both kinaesthetic measures and overall motor competence. This pattern repeated after the second period of intervention. This was unexpected as the ones who were given kinaesthetic training could not be distinguished from those who were not.

In the *second study* both groups that received intervention improved in performance and did not differ from each other, whereas the group that did not receive intervention did not alter in performance.

Discussion

At the end of the *first study*, because the control group improved as much as the intervention group, a decision was taken to undertake a second study. The improvement in both groups in the first study was attributed to an effect of the assessment procedure.

The results of the second study showed that both types of intervention improved the performance of the children, and the authors recommend that in future studies the exact content of the intervention should be specifically examined to determine what causes the effect.

---

a real-life situation. For this reason, in some intervention studies, the situation is made more lifelike with children working in schools in their daily lessons and activities or at home with their parents. In these studies the situation is more 'real', but then of course additional variables play a part. For example, in the tightly controlled studies the length of intervention is often noted: how many times and exactly what is done in each session is carefully described. An example of this type of study is Simms et al (1996a,b) in Box 12.1.

CLINICAL, SCHOOL, AND EXPERIENTIAL APPROACHES
As the methods move closer to real-life situations, such as in clinics or classrooms, it is often the case that the individuals who are working with the children may be parents or teachers, and the measures noted above are not as formally enforced. There are still measures taken, but, because of the nature of the environmental context, the controls are not as tight as the ones described in quasi-experimental designs, and many of these parameters become more variable and more difficult to influence. However, the great advantage of clinical and experiential

studies is that they are set in real-life situations and are not constrained by tight rigid influences, which may make the situation seem artificial.

Thus there becomes a continuum from a study with tight internal controls, with the possibility of a lessened real-life situation, to one in which some of the controls are lifted and the study becomes more externally valid but variables become freer, thus making it more difficult to be confident that the results are for the reasons the study set out to investigate. These include other types of interventions in which there is no formal assessment of the outcomes and children are simply engaging in everyday activities. Assessment then becomes the *collection of information* as opposed to testing. This is part of an *ecological approach* with children being involved in community sport (simple participation); family activities involving recreation and leisure such as hiking, cycling, and swimming or even the day-to-day running of the house where they are involved in cooking, setting the table, washing up, or even gardening; and, finally, hobbies such as construction kits, computer games or other indoor activities that include motor components (Sugden and Henderson 2007).

There is an acceptance of these activities as participation in normal daily living, but it is also known that, if the condition under question is a lifelong condition, it follows that any intervention should be multifaceted with parts of it being conducive to everyday living and the routines and culture of the family. Thus there may be specialist help in the form of occupational therapy but with the knowledge that this therapy is only infrequently available. The recommendation from an ecological perspective is that intervention should involve specialist and non-specialist help plus the self-regulation and goal setting of the child. The specialist help, such as from a therapist, can provide formal support, giving practices for the child to engage in. The therapist cannot oversee the child in these, and thus they have to be either supervised by someone else, such as a parent or teacher, or the child internalizes them and self-regulates them into their daily routines. In addition, the child also participates in the daily activities involving motor tasks around the house and in social and recreational settings. An example of this is shown in Box 12.2.

The two Sugden and Chambers studies are examples of field studies that have definite aims with some control over variables. However, total control is not possible because, although diaries were kept by the parents and teachers, there was no exact control of what they did in the sessions, how many sessions they did, and for how long. Yet the studies were conducted in a natural environment in a typical daily setting, making them ecologically strong.

A summary of the two approaches is presented in Figure 12.2, noting that they are not dichotomous but represent a continuum of external and internal controls and validity.

Principles underlying types of assessment and intervention

The number of assessment instruments and intervention procedures and packages is almost endless and it would be a fruitless exercise to try to describe all of them. Thus the approach in this part of the chapter is to place a structure on the various modes of both assessment and intervention that will encapsulate the various systems and methodologies. In order to do this there is reference to the Morton (2004) model that has featured prominently in this and other chapters, and in doing so we are taking a liberty with the model as we will use it in a manner different from what was intended. The original model of Morton (2004) had a three-level approach to describing and explaining developmental disorders: the biological level was shown with cognition as a second level moving through to the behavioural level. The major feature of this three-level approach was Morton (2004) proposing that cognitive variables were appropriate as explanations or intervening mechanisms linking the biological and behavioural signs (Fig. 12.3).

The approach modifies the assumptions and characteristics of the Morton model and takes each one of the three levels and describes how the various approaches to assessment and intervention may fit into one of these. We recognize that many will not have an exact fit and may involve more than one level, but it will provide some structure and logic to the various methods and will aid when evidence for their effectiveness is analysed. This approach is not totally novel: some evaluations of the effectiveness of both assessment and intervention have been carried out using dichotomies such as process versus product methods or process versus task approaches (Henderson and Sugden 1992, Polatajko et al 1995a, Sugden and Wright 1998, Pless and Carlsson 2000, Wilson 2005, Polatajko and Cantin 2006, Sugden 2007). These are presented later in the chapter, but here there is a breakdown of assessment and intervention into the three camps of biology, cognition, and behaviour.

Assessment and Intervention Using Biological Foundations

The basic tenet of these approaches to both assessment and intervention is that biology or brain functions are the core of the problem, and, if these can be accurately assessed and intervention directly aimed at them, the problem is more likely to be solved. The essence here is

---

Box 12.2 A closer examination

Intervention: the role of parents and teachers in children with DCD: Sugden and Chambers (2003, 2007)

Questions

These studies asked three questions. First, can teachers and parents with help carry out an intervention programme for children with DCD? Second, can children with DCD be helped in this way? Third, are there some children for whom extra and possibly different intervention is necessary?

Children

Over a period of nearly 4 years 31 children took part in the study; five children dropped out leaving 26 who were followed through. All children were assessed for DCD according to *Diagnostic and Statistical Manual of Mental Disorders 4th Revision* criteria (APA 2000). Teachers originally chose children who had movement problems and these children were tested on the Movement ABC test and checklist to satisfy Criteria A and B with the exclusionary Criteria C and D also being satisfied (see p. 225).

Procedure

After the children were first tested there was a period of 8 weeks with no intervention followed by a second test to ensure that no improvement had taken place with no intervention. Then half of the children had intervention from parents and half from teachers for sessions of 20 to 30 minutes duration, a minimum of 3 to 4 times a week for a period of 8 weeks. At the end of this first intervention period they were tested again and the groups swapped over with the parents taking the teachers' group and vice versa for 8 weeks as before. Following this they were tested again followed by five separate testing sessions over the next 2 years. After the first assessment the following individual profiles developed:

- strengths, weaknesses, and priorities
- abilities to work on activities and ways to present (later)
- principles from ecological intervention (Sugden and Henderson 2007)

From these, guidelines were given to the parents each week.

Results

The 26 participants who followed through with the study formed three groups:

- 14 stayed out of lowest 5% – 10 out of lowest 15%
- eight of the children were variable in their responses, with five staying out of the diagnostic category as long as intervention continued. Thus a total of 19 out of 26 improved as long as intervention was present
- two had only minor changes and two children stayed in lowest 5% – no improvement

Conclusion

- Teachers and parents with help can enact a programme of intervention for children with DCD.
- A majority of children with DCD can be helped in this way.
- Some children will need more specific intervention.
- As yet it is not possible to predict, pre-intervention, which children will benefit from the intervention process and stay out of the DCD category post intervention.

---

not in the observed behaviour or the cognitions, although they are seen as a direct consequence of the primary target of assessing and moderating underlying biological substrates. The advantages of such approaches are obvious: if specific biological structures can be identified and assessed accurately, it follows that intervention should address these structures. An underlying assumption, and one that is inherently attractive, is that, by targeting the fundamental biological/neurological structures, many if not all of the behavioural and cognitive functions are possibly addressed.

Using this logic, assessment procedures and programmes of intervention have been directed at specific areas of the brain, from brainstem through the cerebellum

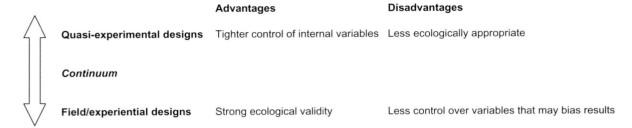

Fig. 12.2 Research designs for intervention. Drawn from data reported by Winnick and Short (1982).

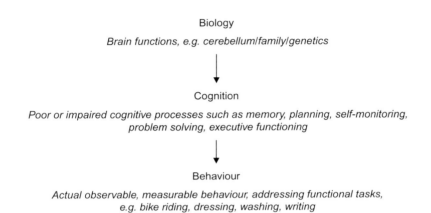

Fig. 12.3 Morton's (2004) causal model of developmental disorders (adapted for assessment and intervention).

to the higher cortical levels. In the intervention process, activities and exercises are given that are purported to directly address these structures. It is as though the assessment and intervention procedures have a 'built-in' generalization propensity with a few specific and direct procedures that can be generalized to many behaviours. Most of these approaches have this assumption either explicitly or implicitly included (e.g. Fawcett and Nicolson 1995).

Obvious examples in the assessment of this type of approach would be imaging and a neurological examination. In recent years various forms of imaging have been employed as a more direct measure of brain activity. These advancements have led to a greatly increased understanding of brain functions. They still do not provide us with total answers, as we have good examples of children with 'normal' scans who present us with motoric difficulties and the converse of children with 'abnormal' scans who appear to be functioning appropriately. However this field is moving forward very quickly with examples over the last 20 years from work in the area of cerebral palsy and more recently in DCD (Bax et al 2006, Zwicker et al 2009). The neurological examination is an interesting one in that most of the time we are looking at biological markers that could lead to behavioural actions; for example,

damage to parts of the cerebral cortex can lead to the various forms of cerebral palsy with movements that show spasticity, dystonia, or ataxia. When a neurological examination/assessment is being made, there is almost a paradox in that the converse is being employed with behavioural symptoms examined as signs of biological damage.

Some intervention systems within this biological framework often go further than simply saying that they modify the behaviour through stimulating brain functions, by proposing that they actually change the brain structure, that is re-educate the brain by utilizing its well-known plasticity. These will then have a concomitant effect on both cognitions and behaviour. These proposals are both logical and laudable, but they are not universally accepted and have been questioned. First, many conditions have unknown biological origins and therefore the targeting of specific areas becomes rather a hit-and-miss affair. Second, we know that some areas of the brain have more than one cognitive and behavioural outcome. Third, some conditions are known to have more than one constitutional possibility for their origin. In a later section there will be an examination of the theoretical and empirical evidence for this approach together with an elaboration of many of these points.

ASSESSMENT AND INTERVENTION USING COGNITIVE PROCESSES

Cognitive processes as proposed by Morton (2004) can be mediating variables between biology and behaviour and are a logical proposal as they make an attempt to model how the same or different biological factors can lead to atypical or indeed typical behaviour. In one important way, the use of cognitive processes as a basis for both assessment and intervention of motor disorders has much in common with the one describing biological substrates. At the core is a belief that, by identifying and targeting these processes, the results will generalize to a number of behavioural signs and symptoms. Again this is a laudable aim as we know that, in children with motor and indeed other difficulties, the lack of spontaneous generalization appears to be a core characteristic. Thus procedures assessing and intervening with cognitive functions have arisen, addressing sensory processes, attention and memory functions, and such processes as executive function and numerous areas of self-regulation and goal setting (Hoare and Larkin 1991, Henderson and Sugden 1992, Polatajko et al 1995a, Wilson and McKenzie 1998). In this section we also include the important area of sensory functions, as these have played a major role in the assessment and intervention programmes of a number of children with different types of movement difficulties (Hulme et al 1982, Laszlo and Bairstow 1985, Lord and Hulme 1987, Sigmundsson et al 1997, Hill 2005).

The advantage of the cognitive programmes, such as the ones addressing biology, is that, if the processes are accurate, generalization to a number of related behaviours would appear to be the logical outcome. The drawback to these proposals is the debate surrounding whether indeed the processes are related to the behaviours and, if so, how? Again the theoretical and empirical evidence is analysed in a later section.

ASSESSMENT AND INTERVENTION USING BEHAVIOURAL FUNCTIONAL TASKS

This approach, on the surface, is the easiest to explain in that the assessment and intervention methods are aimed directly at the behaviours that are proving to be difficult for an individual child. It has strong face validity to it: if the child has difficulty with a task, the difficulty is first assessed in detail and then an intervention programme aimed at that behaviour or group of behaviours is created. It appears to have a face-valid logic, but of course there are drawbacks, the biggest of which surrounds the notion of time and generalization. A child during his or her lifetime acquires a huge number of skills that are evident in the behaviours they show. It is evident that there is not enough time to formally learn all of these skills or all of

the variants of one particular type of skill; it is known that children pick up skills incidentally through their day-to-day experiences without formally being taught. To formally be assessed on or learn each skill is impossible, and thus teaching every individual behaviour is clearly not an option. The result of this is that teaching for transfer becomes the major issue, and this is a difficult and complex task. Methods of assessment usually try to identify 'classes of events' so that one or two activities are utilized to represent a much larger group that is being assessed. This notion of classes of events is also utilized alongside task analysis in intervention to try to overcome the difficulty with generalization (Polatajko et al 2001a, Larkin and Parker 2002, Schoemaker et al 2003, Sugden and Henderson 2007).

The three types of approaches, biological, cognitive, and functional, have different purposes and thus show different advantages and disadvantages. However, it can be argued that they are all linked by the concept of transfer or generalizability. In the first two, generalizability is an implicit outcome because the methods are dealing with underlying functions or processes, and the assumption is that these underlying structures or processes will underpin many behavioural activities. However, there is the disadvantage of not precisely knowing whether the underlying functions and the structures and processes are directly connected to the observable behaviour and in what way. With functional behaviours, the corollary is the case. There is the obvious advantage of dealing with the exact difficulty in the form of a functional task, but with the drawback that the vexed problem of generalizability has to be faced.

A summary of the three types of approaches is shown in Table 12.1.

Although it is possible to find pure approaches, as shown in the categories above, many assessment and intervention approaches will include a mixture. For example, some intervention approaches will concentrate on functional activities and will also include in their methodology the use of cognitive strategies such as self-regulation, memory activities, self goal setting, and generalization skills (Henderson and Sugden 1992, Polatajko et al 2001a,b, Sugden and Henderson 2007).

Validity and reliability

The twin concepts of validity and reliability are fundamental to how we can judge the quality of any data, whether from assessment protocols or from the results of intervention studies. Together they provide measures of how confident we can be with the data that have been collected and the uses that can be made of it. They are usually applied to assessment instruments, but, as assessment is

TABLE 12.1
Biological, cognitive, and behavioural approaches to assessment and intervention

Approach	Emphasis	Advantages	Disadvantages
Biological	Brain/neural system genetics	Strong on generalization	Lack of direct evidence for specific effect
Cognitive	Processes such as perception memory, attention, problem solving, self-monitoring	Strong on generalization	Insufficient direct evidence for specific effect
Behavioural	Functional tasks such as cycling, writing	Strong on ecological validity and functional tasks	Evidence required for generalization effect

used to examine the results of intervention, they are also an integral part of the intervention process.

VALIDITY

The validity of a test, instrument, or measure used in intervention is the degree to which it measures what it is supposed to measure. It refers to the soundness of the interpretation of the scores. Validity is a single entity but can be broken down into four main types.

Face validity

The first is known as face validity or logical validity (Thomas et al 2005) and is claimed when the measure under question is obviously the performance being measured. Thus maximum speed of running could be measured by a 30m sprint and this would have logical validity to it as 30m is an appropriate distance to run for typically developing individuals and an approximation of maximum speed can be made for a time. However, as soon as the sprint becomes say 100m, the logic of a maximum speed test could be questioned because for many children 100m would involve endurance as well as maximum speed. Face or logical validity does have a common-sense feel to it; it is used quite often, but in many cases researchers require something a little more substantial and based on more concrete evidence.

Construct validity

A second type of validity is known as construct validity and involves 'the degree to which scores from a test measure a hypothetical construct and is usually established by relating the test results to some construct' (Thomas et al 2005, p. 197).

Any construct should be placed in a conceptual framework outlining the construct and showing how it is different from others. Factor analysis is a statistical measure that is often used to examine construct validity and can be used to show how many factors are within the construct and what these factors are; how much each factor

will contribute to the overall construct; and which tasks can best represent the factors (Burton and Miller 1998). Despite the fact that there is a breakdown of abilities, such as motor ability, into factors, we often use generic terms to give a global description of a particular type of ability. One such term is 'general motor ability', which refers to whether there is an overall construct that could be named as such. Barnett (2008) debates whether this construct exists, as many tests (BOT, Bruininks 1978, Bruininks and Bruininks 2007; MABC 1, Henderson and Sugden 1992; MABC 2, Henderson et al 2007) purport to assess overall motor ability. There is some evidence that this may exist in abilities such as timing, but others are more specific and their total is required in order to provide an overall picture of the child's competence.

Content validity

A third type of validity is known as content validity and involves determining whether the test content or other measurements adequately cover the variable under question and do not contain any extraneous variables. Does it involve the entire said variable, are some parts overrepresented, or are any parts missing? For example, if a test of general motor ability did not contain a measure of balance or ball skills or some assessment of manual dexterity, we could claim that the content validity of the test could be brought into question. Judgements about content validity are usually made by persons thought to be experts in that particular field. Thus, if one was to try to develop content validity for classroom skills, one could start by asking a group of class teachers to produce activities that were ongoing in their classroom. Although the term content validity is widespread, it is not always regarded as a true test of validity and the term content-related evidence is used as an alternative as it is a less 'firm' label than validity (Burton and Miller 1998). An example of content validity is provided by Chambers and Sugden (2006) in the development of the early movement skills checklist.

Criterion validity

The final measure of validity, that of criterion validity, comes in two forms, concurrent and predictive. The first, concurrent validity, involves comparing the measurement or test with some established measure used at the same time. Thus, a new test of motor impairment used in situ with a group of children with cerebral palsy could be compared to an established measure or test. In this way the new measure could be evaluated alongside one that has been used with confidence. This does not mean that the measures have to totally agree; there will and should be some degree of similarity between the instruments, but the new instrument may be measuring something that is peculiar to that particular situation and picks up detail or another way of looking at the problem that the old one did not.

The second type is predictive validity and as the name implies, this involves examining a test or measure against some later behaviour. Thus, if we are using a new test of motor impairment or ability and we claim that this is a measure of how competent the child is in everyday motor activities, we may use as a predictive check the views of the teacher over the next few weeks to see if the test results equate to daily living in the school. Predictive validity is often used alongside the terms *sensitivity* and *specificity*, which are employed to determine whether the placement of an individual as the result of a test is the correct decision. *Sensitivity* is a true positive, the likelihood that a positive test places the person in a given category; *specificity* is a true negative, the likelihood that a negative test places the person outside of a given category. These measurements are particularly important when decisions are being made about placement of children into various programmes. The more sensitive and specific the test for placement in a particular programme the less wastage there is of finances and other resources. Using sensitivity and specificity measures can help to ensure that all children who are true positives (sensitivity) are being catered for and none are being missed, but also that those who are true negatives (specificity) are not being included.

RELIABILITY

The other half of our twin concepts is that of reliability, which is usually defined in terms of how consistent the measure is. There is an interesting interaction between reliability and validity: a test cannot be valid if it is not reliable, but a measure can be reliable but not valid. If a test is not consistent (that is, unreliable) then it cannot be testing what it purports to test (validity). However, it can be invalid (say the content validity is not good) and still be reliable in that the test can consistently measure with confidence, but it is not measuring what it claims. The reliability of a measure often surrounds whether it can be consistently administered.

Interobserver reliability

One form of reliability, known as interobserver reliability, assesses to what degree behaviours observed and scored on the instrument by two different people are done so in the same manner with the same results. It would be expected that both assessors have had adequate training and experience with the assessment instrument such as a checklist or a standardized test.

Test–retest reliability

Another form of reliability is test–retest reliability over time, and it assesses the degree to which the same person can administer the instrument at different times with the same children and collect the same results. This form of reliability is tricky as there should not be too long a gap between the tests, as the children may naturally be changing through development, and it should not be too short a period, as the children may remember parts of the test. Correlation is the usual statistic used to determine the reliability of the measure in both interobserver and test–retest situations.

Internal consistency

Finally there is an *internal consistency* measure that uses the scores to determine the consistency *within* the test. A simple one is the split-half technique, which simply splits the test in half in some way – first half and second half or odd and even – and then calculates the correlation between the two. Other more complex and complete methods include the Spearman–Brown prophecy formula, the Kuder Richardson method, and Cronbach's alpha coefficient, the last one being the most popular method of estimating reliability in standardized tests.

A summary of validity and reliability measures is shown in Table 12.2.

Intervention is about participation and learning

In order for a child with movement difficulties to improve their skills, the two activities of *participation* and *learning* need to be addressed. They are very much interrelated in that participation is a necessary activity for learning to take place, but they are also different and different variables may affect the child's success in each one. The need for participation as a necessity for learning is linked to the fundamental principle of learning as a function of the amount of appropriate practice, which in itself is participation. The corollary is also true in that, as the child learns more skills, this new found competence places him or her in a better position to be able to participate. In

TABLE 12.2
Reliability and validity

Validity	Description and meaning
Face/logical	The performance is the measure under question from a common-sense view
Construct	The relationship of the test to a conceptual framework
Content	The content covers the variable under question with no extra ones or ones missing
Criterion	Concurrent – compare to established measure
	Predictive – examine against later outcome
Reliability	
Inter-rater	Agreement between two or more assessors
Test–retest	Agreement of same person at two different times
Internal consistency	Measures to what extent the test is internally consistent throughout

addition, participation is also an end in itself without any effect on learning. It brings independence to the child; it encourages confidence and social awareness and mixing, and, most importantly, it is a human right.

PARTICIPATION

Participation is a crucial variable in the life of a child with movement difficulties and it is one we very often take for granted when development is typical. However, when development is atypical, participation is often diminished. There is a large amount of evidence to show that children with motor difficulties do not participate as much as their non-disabled peers in movement situations – whether they are organized and structured or simply recreational. Morris et al (2006) propose two main reasons for this. First, there may be an actual or perceived lack of skill on the part of the child that prevents or hinders participation. In a world that adheres to the concept of inclusion this should not happen and the context should be flexible enough to allow all children to participate. Second, if the environment or context is not structured appropriately, this may prevent children with difficulties from participating.

Thus, in any society that considers the well-being of all of its citizens, increased participation for all should be a major objective and involves two major opportunities and advantages for children with movement difficulties. First, participation as a dependent variable in its own right provides the child with an increased sense of well-being and self-accomplishment, and from society's point of view it is a right that should be available to all. It offers the chance to interact with peers and friends and facilitates family activities such that children can increase their social skills and self-esteem as well as the important issue of being a more integral part of a group whether that

is family or friends. Second, increased participation is absolutely necessary for increased learning. If the objectives of any portfolio include skill learning or enhanced competence in motor activities, then participation is a fundamental necessity. A great tenet of skill learning is that it is dependent on the 'amount of appropriate practice' and this can only come about through increased participation.

In Chapters 7 and 8, on cerebral palsy and DCD, participation was described using the International Classification of Functioning, Disability and Health (ICF) model as a base and a move away from success being dependent upon the child's resources. Real-life situations that are personally and socially meaningful for the individual concerned are to be encouraged and this should be assessed by taking the view of the child through self-report, as well as the view of parents and significant others (McConachie et al 2008). Thus, when evaluating participation in children with movement difficulties, one not only looks at how encouraging and easily accessible contexts are but also how positive an influence they have on the child's life as viewed by all interested parties. Chen and Cohn (2003) report on how participation involves a range of activities in different contexts such as household work in the home, community-based leisure activities, and full participation in school activities. The extent to which this participation is achieved is dependent upon intrinsic factors, such as the self-worth and -esteem of the child, and the extrinsic factors of attitudes, culture, and gender issues. Chen and Cohn present a model of participation for children with DCD that can be used with any child with a movement difficulty, and a modified version is presented in Figure 12.4.

Within an ecological framework for intervention, participation is viewed as a major objective. It follows on from the levels of the ICF model (Chapter 7), and

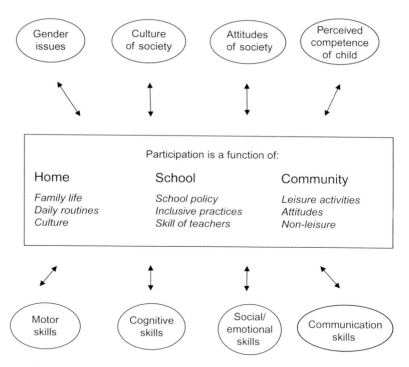

Fig. 12.4 Participation of children with movement difficulties. Adapted from Chen and Cohn (2003).

therapists are now engaging in the overall participation of children with motor difficulties in the home, school, and community settings, with this being emphasized by Sugden and Henderson (2007) with their ecological intervention and Law et al (1998) and their family-function-centred approach.

LEARNING

Fundamentally, the various methods of intervention are different approaches to aid and support children in their learning. When terms such as therapy and teaching are employed, these are the actions of the person doing the helping and supporting and indeed are the fundamentals of what is described as intervention. However, the dependent variable is learning, and, in order to obtain a more complete picture of the process of intervention and the advantages and disadvantages of the different approaches, it is first appropriate to examine what we mean by learning, based on the rather obvious logic that it is necessary to understand what the aims are before examining the methods by which these are approached.

DEFINITION AND CHARACTERISTICS OF LEARNING

What is learning?

Schmidt and Lee (2005) define learning as 'a set of internal processes associated with practice or experience leading to a relatively permanent change in the capability for skilled behaviour' (p. 320).

There are a number of important features in this definition, all of which impinge on any intervention approach:

- First, learning is associated with *internal processes*; the assumption here is that one cannot view learning, but one can infer that learning has taken place by an examination of performance at two or more points in time. Performances are one shot occurrences that are observable, whereas learning is a continuing process that can only be inferred through changes in performance. An implication of this is not to assume the child has not learned just because performance has not changed; learning may have taken place in the form of internal processes, but this has not yet translated to any change in performance. Thus a tip is to 'wait' but not for too long; this is where the skill of the teacher and therapist is shown, knowing how long to wait and taking a different course of action if performance has not changed.

- Second, learning is associated with *practice* or *experience*; it is not maturation or development, although children will learn differently at various stages of development. Learning is brought about by practice and this means a deliberate attempt to acquire skills through a formal or quasi-formal setting. It is brought about by experience and this means a more informal setting in which the child is not being 'taught' directly, but through their everyday experiences of life they are learning new skills. For the therapist and teacher this is important because many of the children they work with are not as proficient as typically developing children at this experiential learning and may require more direct teaching/therapy.

- Third, learning is a *relatively permanent change*. This does not mean the behaviour that is learned will stay there permanently. What it does imply is that the change in the capability for skilled action is relatively permanent. Again this has implications, and for the therapist and teacher means that the behaviour may have faded, but the internal processes that originally changed are relatively permanent and, with short exposure to the same situation again, the behaviour should return.

- Finally, the change is in the *capability for skilled behaviour* and not necessarily in the behaviour itself. For a variety of reasons a child may have learned the capability but chosen not to employ this facility.

Learning is a change in a set of internal processes that can only be measured through assessing performance at more than one moment in time and this gives an observable and operational measure of learning. Therefore, what are the changes in performance that indicate learning has taken place? The following list from Magill (2007) provides an indication of the range of dependent variables that clinicians and educators could use to assess whether intervention has had any effect. It is more comprehensive than measures usually taken and thus provides a more complete coverage of any changes that have occurred.

How is learning recognized?
- First, there is the measurable improvement in performance in that *skills can now be performed* that previously could not. This could quite simply be that the child with cerebral palsy can now pick up an object when beforehand this was not accomplished. This performance becomes relatively permanent.
- The child *improves* his or her score on a given task such as catching 7 balls out of 10 as opposed to 3.
- The child becomes more *consistent* in the performance of a skill. If the child was rather hit or miss in picking up an object (could do it maybe only 50% of the time) and then progresses to doing it every time, this is a measure of learning.
- The child becomes more *stable in the performance*, in the action of picking up an object, such

as overcoming any perturbation that may be present. Thus the child can reach over the top of a bowl at the breakfast table, changing the trajectory of the reach to grasp a cup.

- With learning there is an *increase in the persistence* of the child. Very often a child will stay with the task until it is accomplished if it has been accomplished previously.

- With learning the child becomes more *adaptable in the performance of a skill*. Thus reaching and grasping can be accomplished in different locations with unfamiliar objects. This occurs with 'closed skills', those that are predictable in terms of time and space, such as reaching for stationary objects, and in the performance of more complex 'open skills' in which the environment is moving and more unpredictable, such as reaching and grasping a rolling ball.

- With learning, *parts become wholes*. We very often see reaching and grasping as two separate components in children with cerebral palsy. The child manages to reach with the arm–hand linkage, but the shaping of the hand to the object is a separate and distinct skill. With learning these two actions become one. A similar example can be seen in driving. When individuals are starting to learn to drive there are a myriad of separate skills to do with looking, hand control, and foot control, with a conscious effort on each one. When they can drive, the whole task is driving, not the individual parts.

- Linked to the last bullet point is the notion of *automaticity* and doing two tasks at once. In the early stages of learning, it is usual to concentrate on one task, such as reaching for a spoon. However, as learning becomes firm and accomplished a child with cerebral palsy can reach for the spoon and talk to her brother at the same time, something that would not have been possible in the early stages of learning. The task of reaching and grasping an object has become automatic, freeing up 'space' to accomplish other tasks at the same time.

- Finally, there is the movement during the learning process from the *freezing* to the *freeing* of the degrees of freedom. In the early part of the skill learning process, the individual 'freezes' some of the potential joints and muscles such that they can be controlled. As learning progresses these are 'freed', facilitating greater flexibility and adaptability of movement. This is discussed further in the next section on Stages of learning.

These variables can be summarized as follows:

- relatively permanent achievement of a skill previously not performed;
- improvement in product scores;
- consistency in performance;
- stability in performance;
- adaptability in the performance;
- parts become wholes;
- persistency of child;
- task becomes more automatic enabling dual-task performance; and
- freezing to freeing degrees of freedom.

The variables above can be used by therapists or other professionals together with parents and friends and may be noted in formal settings or simple observations. The range of variables to use is vast because, first, they are probably necessary to cover the full range of learning that the child has encompassed and, second, because along with our view that intervention is done by multiple persons taking different roles, these variables will vary with the individual concerned.

STAGES OF LEARNING

Anyone who has been involved in supporting and enhancing children's learning will recognize that there are different parts to the learning process with big differences between the early and later stages.

This has been examined on a number of occasions and researchers have found that the typical learning curve a child exhibits is one that we describe as negatively accelerated (Fig. 12.5a). Learning as shown here is characterized by early fast learning with smaller gains later on. This type of curve has been shown to be typical across many tasks with gains going on for a number of years – although slowly.

- Much of the work has been done with adults, and thus we may see different curves for younger children, particularly those who have difficulties, such as the one in Figure 12.5b; this is a positively accelerated curve with slow learning in the first instance followed by an acceleration when the child has got the 'hang' of the task.
- A further learning process may be similar to the one shown in Figure 12.5c, in which there are two parts to the task with a plateau in the middle. All of these curves have implications for teaching and therapy with the type of instruction, demonstrations, practices, and feedback being geared to the manner in which the child is progressing on a particular task.

It is appropriate to remember that these 'learning' curves are really 'performance' curves made up of

(a)

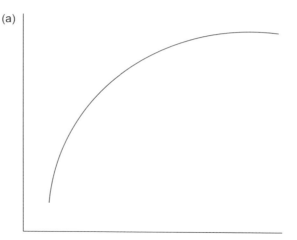

(b)

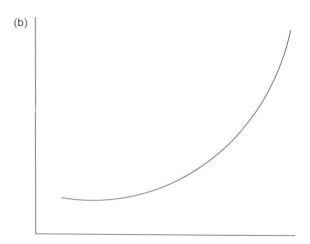

(c)

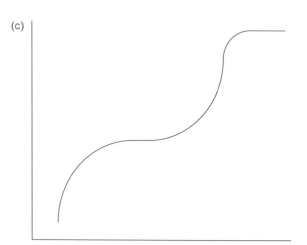

Fig. 12.5 Different types of learning curves.

measurements of performance at various times during the learning process. Also, in Figure 12.5b, in which there appears to be little learning happening during the early stage of the process, it could be that learning is happening but is not yet translated into a measurable performance.

Researchers have translated these progressions of learning into stages, with various characteristics being assigned to the various stages. There are numerous models of these and below are three: the *first* is one that is well known and frequently used in the motor learning literature; the *second* is less well known but from highly respected researchers who provide a different yet complementary model; the *third* is one that has recently become more popular and uses a totally different framework.

Model 1: Fitts and Posner (1967)

One model that has proved to be of great utility over a long period of time is the three-stage model first proposed by Fitts and Posner (1967).

- They labelled the first stage the *cognitive stage*, as this is the period when the individual is starting to understand the demands of the task and making the first attempts at practice. What is the task requiring of me? Practice here is characterized by large errors and inconsistency in performance.
- The second stage is known as the *associative stage*. Here the child understands the task and has learned to associate the demands of the task with the environmental cues. It is a period of physical practice with the errors becoming smaller as the learning progresses. Effective and efficient feedback from the therapist or teacher is essential in this stage to help the learner progress to self-monitoring of performance and the detection of their own errors.
- The final stage is known as the *autonomous stage*. In this stage the skill is now almost automatic and the child can do it with little attention and can engage in other tasks at the same time as well as keeping a consistent and high level of performance. It is a period in which learners can accurately detect their own errors, but learning is still continuing and so practice is still a crucial variable. Fitts and Posner (1967) point out that these three stages are not discrete and that there is a gradual, almost seamless movement from one to the other rather than any abrupt, sharp shift.

Model 2: Gentile (2000)

Gentile (2000) proposes a two-stage rather than three-stage model:

- In the *initial stage* the individual has to acquire two goals:
  - The *first* is the acquisition of the movement coordination pattern, which means developing the

movement characteristics to match the environmental context in which the skill is performed, such as matching the hand to the size of the glass being grasped.
  - The *second goal* is to be able to discriminate between those conditions in the environment that are essential to the task and those that are not. This first stage of the learning process involves large amounts of cognitive problem solving and could be a combination of the first and parts of the second stage of Fitts and Posner's model. At the end of this stage the learner is starting to achieve the skills but not with efficiency and consistency.
- Gentile labels her *second stage* the *later stages*, and here the learner aims for three achievements: adaptability, consistency of effort, and consistency, all of which are qualities we noted earlier in our description of what happens when we learn. In this second stage, gentile distinguishes between two types of skills to be learned:
  - For *closed skills* she advocates *fixating* basic movement coordination patterns such that they are refined and can be consistently achieved with as little effort as possible. Self-care skills such as dressing would come into this.
  - For *open skills*, however, she advocates *diversifying* movement patterns such that the learner is continuously adapting to the changing environmental conditions. Thus the learner here is constantly monitoring the contextual array.

Model 3: dynamic systems

A totally different way to look at the stages of learning is to examine the movement dynamics of the task and examine aspects of coordination. This is very much in line with the dynamical view of motor behaviour and the classic work of Bernstein (1967) and the many who have elaborated on his work (e.g. Whiting, Turvey, Kelso, Thelen). In order to move effectively and to accommodate the potentially overwhelming memory demands, it is proposed by many that the unit of movement consists of groups of muscles and/or joints that are constrained together to act as a single entity. These have been called 'coordinative structures' or synergies. This is an explanation for how we overcome the degrees of freedom problem and control the many potential degrees of freedom, the muscles, joints, motor units, that are potentially available in any movement. By constraining these into larger units, such as coordinative structures, the mover can make a generic response to a given movement problem and then attune it to the specific environmental demands. The term that is used for the recruitment of coordinative structures is

TABLE 12.3
Models of learning

Model	Stages
Fitts and Posner (1967)	*Cognitive* – understanding the demands of the task and what is required
	Associative – trial and error utilizing different forms of feedback
	Autonomous – task is performed automatically and facilitates dual-task success
Gentile (2000)	*Initial* – acquiring the movement pattern and reading the environment
	Later – fixating patterns for closed skills and diversifying for open skills
Dynamical systems	Freezing and freeing the degrees of freedom
	Flexible recruitment of appropriate coordinative structures
	Enhancing perception–action linkage

'softly assembled', indicating that they are stored ready in some global sense and then finely grained and moderated to the situation at hand.

In the early stages of learning there is strong evidence that individuals use as few degrees of freedom as possible to accomplish the task. This enables them to perform the task in some basic manner commensurate with their abilities. As learning progresses and the individual improves, he or she is able to release or free the degrees of freedom thus allowing a potentially more effective movement; he or she is more able to react to complex environmental demands and produce a better performance. One has only to look at beginning throwers, and how they fixate their trunk and stance and compare them to later, more accomplished throwers, who rotate their trunk and step forward, to notice the difference. Similarly therapists use this in their daily work by asking clients to fix parts of their body to enable a task to be completed and then show them ways to release their body parts, in order to obtain more functional responses to everyday demands. This has become known as the progression from the *freezing to the freeing of degrees of freedom* and eventually *exploiting them* (Bernstein 1967, Savelsbergh et al 2003). Recent work has shown this process to be more complex with some degrees of freedom being kept constant, whereas others are released during the learning process (Konczak et al 2009).

Intervention can be enhanced by analysing the *learning process*, as this is one of the two fundamental aims of the intervention process. Learning, as has been described, is not a unitary process as it involves not only multiple outcomes but also a number of different yet overlapping stages. These are used to illustrate that it is our belief that the empirical studies of children with movement difficulties, while carried out in a proper manner, have yet to encompass many of the variables we have outlined. Usually dependent variables are few in number and there

is little research concerning the stages of learning and how therapy may change with the progression. This is not a criticism of the studies but merely a note to say that there are many opportunities for new and different types of studies waiting to be undertaken. Indeed it is noted often in therapists' individual reports that they have observed some of the variables that have been presented. The next step is to undertake more formal evaluations of these in reports of both assessment and intervention. A summary of the models of stages of learning is shown in Table 12.3.

PRACTICE VARIABLES: HOW DOES PRACTICE INFLUENCE LEARNING?

It seems an obvious statement to make that, as we practice in order to learn, the manner in which we practice appears to be a crucial factor in the intervention process. When an intervention programme is delivered, how is practice organized? Or more logically, what are the practice variables that may impinge and influence the learning process? A number of these have been studied in great detail by researchers investigating the field of sport and in industrial settings, and these are described below.

Amount of practice

There is a substantial amount of evidence to propose that the amount of appropriate practice is a key variable in the learning of any skill, with the word 'appropriate' being of crucial importance. Throughout this text we have referred to 'experience' as being vital to outcomes of motor capability. Practice is a more formal activity than experience, which is almost incidental learning, but both would include time-on-task as a relevant variable.

The distribution of practice

What is the effect of having practice sessions that are close together and massed, versus ones that are spaced apart and distributed? It clearly depends upon the task at hand because for some tasks massing may be 5 days in a row as in bike riding practice, whereas for other tasks massing may all be in 1 day. The general conclusion is that more frequent and shorter sessions lead to better learning than longer and less frequent ones. Classic work by Baddeley and Longman (1978) investigated the best way to train postal workers on a mail sorting machine when there were 60 hours and 5 days a week available for training. Four groups were involved in the following regimes:

- Two groups practised for 1 hour each session: one with one session a day and one with two sessions a day, giving a total duration of 12 and 6 weeks, respectively.
- Two other groups practised for 2 hours each session: one with one session a day and one with two sessions a day, giving a total duration of 6 and 3 weeks, respectively.

The task goal was to be able to achieve a typing speed of 80 words per minute. Only the two groups who trained for 1 hour per session each day achieved this in the allotted 60 hours thereby suggesting that the distributed practice of only 1 hour was best when other variables were controlled. After retention tests were taken at 1, 3, and 9 months it was found that the group that massed the most training, two sessions a day of 2 hours, was worse than the other groups. This kind of choice has implications not only for the effect of the type of practice on learning but also the efficient use of therapists in a health authority. It should be pointed out, however, that all of the groups had at least one practice session a day, making at least five a week, which is very different to most intervention schedules in a clinical setting where once a week is the norm. There is little firm evidence on that kind of scheduling, but it would be logical to assume that once a week is not enough to evoke change. One could argue that practice once a week is akin to going on a diet every Thursday afternoon!

Whole versus part learning

There are various ways of presenting tasks, such as in their entirety or broken down into their components parts. This variable is well known to both teachers and therapists, and it is explained in more detail later in the chapter.

Instructions, explanation, demonstrations, and feedback

All of these involve providing information to the child in some way, either before the task has started or after an attempt has been made. These are crucial variables, and we know that the manner in which information is provided interacts with the ability of the child and the stage of learning they have reached. For example, for children with quite severe difficulties or at the earliest stage of learning, it is more useful to give them single or, at most, two points to concentrate on that are big points and easily understood. As learning progresses, so does the complexity and detail of the information provided.

Specificity and variability of practice

When one of our objectives is to teach manual skills to children with cerebral palsy, is it better to teach a wide range of skills, giving variability of practice, or is it more effective to hone in on one specific skill and get it right? The answer will vary according to the skill level of the child and the types of skills to be learned. Does the child require a specific skill or does he or she require flexibility across situations? These are the variables that dictate the answer.

Mental practice

Can mental rehearsal aid physical performance? In most studies of mental rehearsal or mental practice the literature suggests that it is better than no practice, and can be a substantial aid to performance when combined with physical practice.

More detail on practice variables can be found in Schmidt and Lee (2005) and Magill (2007).

Summary of practice variables

- *Amount of practice* – in general the more *appropriate* practice the better, but it depends on scheduling and a trade-off between small gains later on and the amount of resources required.
- *Scheduling of practice* – several sessions of shorter duration appear to be more effective than longer and fewer sessions, but this will depend upon the task involved. Logic and experience suggest that once a week is not enough.
- *Whole versus part learning* – the more a task can be learned in its entirety the better, but task analysis is used when this is not effective.
- *Instructions, demonstrations, practices, feedback* – at different stages of the learning process these are modified.
- *Variability of practice* – for skills that require flexibility of response, variability of practice is recommended.
- *Mental practice* – mental practice combined with physical practice is the best option.

SUMMARY OF PARTICIPATION AND LEARNING

At the start of this section it was emphasized that participation and learning were two overall objectives for children with movement difficulties. It does not matter who is providing the support; whether parents, teachers, therapists, and/or friends, the objective usually involves these two activities. From these two activities, other aims and goals can be achieved such as increased skill competence, social inclusion, self-esteem enhancement, or simply general well-being. The variables that influence participation are usually aligned to modification of context, such as the provision that is available for the child and the amount of support that is given. For learning, these variables are important together with the added ones of practice variables and the outcomes that are desired.

Ecological approaches to assessment and intervention

Throughout the text and at the beginning of this chapter, there has been an emphasis on the child's development – his or her strengths and difficulties – as a function of the triad of influences comprising the resources the child brings to the movement situation, the environmental context in which the movement is based, and the type of task and the manner of presentation (Fig. 12.1).

Nowhere is this triad of transactional influences more important than in the area of assessment and intervention, which has origins in numerous and disparate sources. The use of this as a basis for assessment and intervention is founded upon two fundamental assumptions. The first is that a child's difficulties rarely, if ever solely, reside in the child. Second, there is an optimism about the approach by intervening at various places in the model.

One could argue that the genesis of this approach lies in the work of Uri Bronfenbrenner who, in a series of books and articles, has shown how the ecological settings are the major drivers of overall child development (Bronfenbrenner, 1979). He stressed that development takes place through the influence of a number of 'systems' in a model for examining developing children in their natural ecology, and analysed the contexts in varying degrees of specificity from microsystems, through mesosystems and exosystems, to macrosystems that detail the influence of the environment from the specific face-to-face interaction at home and school, through to the larger, more general influence of government policy and spending. His interests lay in the dynamics of each of these and the transitions from one to another, as they are all embedded in one another.

The influence of ecological systems has been taken up by a number of authors in the motor control and development area and has developed into approaches to such activities as assessment, task analysis, and intervention, with whole texts being devoted to the same topic as *Ecological Task Analysis and Movement* by Davis and

Broadhead (2007). Other outlets are from Keogh and Sugden (1985), Newell (1986), Davis and Burton (1991), Davis and Broadhead (2007), Newell and Jordan (2007), and Sugden and Henderson (2007).

Newell and Jordan (2007) provide a recent analysis of Newell's 1986 model, which has been taken as the cornerstone of this approach. They use the term 'constraints' to mean boundaries limiting the system, which in turn can be the organism, the task, or the context. The organismic constraints include neural, biochemical, and morphological ones. Newell and Jordan (2007) make the prediction that these may also include some future manipulation of the individual's genomic make up. They describe the environmental constraints as those physical boundary conditions external to the organism, but still keep a rather 'tight' definition of environment that is not nearly as wide as Bronfenbrenner's (1979) definition. Their logic probably surrounds the notion that any action occurs at a moment in time within a particular context, whereas Bronfenbrenner would certainly look to the conditions leading up to the circumstances in which the child finds him or herself. Newell and Jordan (2007) at first place task constraints in two categories: the goal of the task and the rules specifying the constraints to realize the goal. However, they also recognize that task constraints can be what they call a 'change agent', such as a teacher or a coach who affects the learning process. This we believe would be an essential component of the triad, as they directly affect the dynamics of the movement situation as a whole.

Hultzer (2007) takes the triangular model we have repeatedly shown and fills in some of the subcomponents of each section. Thus he presents a model, such as that shown in Figure 8.4, to which we have added the barriers or facilitators in italics for the task constraints. These will be elaborated further in the section on ecological intervention on page 355.

Hultzer (2007) describes a model he calls the systematic ecological modification approach, in which he elaborates the variables associated with his ecological approach. In the text by Davis and Broadhead (2007) other examples are given of an ecological approach, such as applied to physiotherapy (Mullally and Mullally 2007); persons with neurological disorders (Vermeer 2007); empowerment in coaching (Kidman and Davis 2007); enhancing student decision making (Carson et al 2007, Taylor et al 2007); and linking with knowledge-based approaches (Wall et al 2007). For details of these, the text by Davis and Broadhead (2007) is recommended.

A comprehensive guide to ecological approaches has been developed by Sugden and Henderson (2007) as part of the overall assessment and management package Movement Assessment Battery for Children (Henderson et al 2007). This guide, entitled *Ecological Intervention for Children with Movement Difficulties*, has as its basis the triad of constraints or variables (child resources, task, and environmental context) that has been constant throughout this text. The essence of this approach is encapsulated in the quote from Sugden and Henderson (2007):

> Ecological Intervention is a way of thinking, an approach rather than a rigidly prescriptive package, which must be delivered by a highly skilled professional in a specified way. Our starting point is that intervention cannot be viewed as an add-on to normal daily life. Instead, the basic idea is that intervention should be an integral part of daily living with different individuals playing different, but equally important roles.
>
> (p. 3)

This approach is covered in detail in the section on *intervention* on pages 355–357.

Approaches to assessment and collection of information

Earlier in the chapter it was stressed that assessment covered many purposes such as planning for intervention, diagnosis and categorization, and examining the child over time. With these and other purposes, it is not surprising that this diversity in purpose leads to corresponding diversity in methodologies of collecting the information, what is customarily called assessment. In this section a range of assessment methods are presented with examples and further reading offered for those who wish to engage in some of the specific methods in more detail.

In their recently published book, *Ecological Intervention for Children with Movement Difficulties*, Sugden and Henderson (2007) present a detailed summary of the kinds of information on the child that can be collected. The phases of ecological intervention comprise two parts with the first part, *collecting information to plan the programme*, presented here and the second, *implementing the programme*, later in the chapter when describing intervention. They use the term collecting information to indicate that this includes regular assessment of the child but also takes in a detailed description of the context in which the child is situated.

COLLECTING INFORMATION AND PLANNING THE PROGRAMME

Child resources

A fundamental assumption is that accurate assessment of the child and the context in which he or she functions is an essential component of the information collecting process. Starting with the child, the child's wishes are key variables in the intervention process, and this will usually include identifying functional tasks, choosing priorities, establishing targets for success, and engaging in monitoring their own progress. A full information-gathering exercise may involve the following parts:

- *Standardized tests* – these provide information on a given child in comparison with other children. They are used by professionals with appropriate training who understand the principles behind standardized testing. They compare a child against age-matched peers by providing a centile ranking of the child's performance and can help to confirm, or otherwise, the presence of a motor difficulty.

- *Dynamic assessment* – this is now quite commonplace in educational and clinical circles with the examiner taking a look at the child in context and exploring the child's upper and lower limits of competence. Very often this involves the examiner using a normative-referenced test but modifying the instructions if necessary to see exactly what the child is capable of. For example, testing a child with autism might involve providing a degree of assistance to obtain the best performance of the child, which cannot be obtained by following the instructions in the manual. The norms cannot be used under these circumstances, but through this dynamic assessment the capabilities of the child are shown if the context is modified.

- *Criterion-referenced tests* – this method examines what the child can achieve on everyday functional tasks without necessarily referring to normative data. They look at the skills or competencies the child has in their normal daily settings of school and home. They have the advantage of being easily understood by clinicians, educators, and parents, who can relate them to daily life experiences, and it can be seen how they lead directly to a programme of intervention. However, it is important to realize that daily life activities will differ according to who is identifying them.

- *Interviews* – and other input from parents, child, teacher, and significant others are a crucial part of any information-collecting exercise as they help to build up a total picture of the child in a variety of contexts. School reports on how the child functions in school are important feedback on such things as how poor coordination interferes with life in school, in the classroom with writing and drawing, in the gymnasium and physical education, and at social times out on the playground.

- *Exclusionary criteria* – if a diagnostic assessment is being followed, are there exclusionary criteria that are present? For example, if a diagnosis of DCD is being sought and the child tests below 70 on an IQ test or equivalent, the DCD diagnosis should not be given. The same applies to other conditions, such as autistic spectrum disorder, while remembering that a dual diagnosis can be given.
- *Non-motor factors* – we know that many motor difficulties are accompanied by non-motor factors, such as attention difficulties and cognitive, social, emotional, and behavioural problems, for example, and these are crucial pieces of information for setting up intervention.

From this information a *profile* of the child's strengths and weaknesses is constructed, which in turn leads to setting *objectives* for any intervention programme. It is usual for there to be several objectives that need to be placed in order of *priority*. Decisions about priorities can be made according to various strategies. One may involve the difficulty that is most distressing for a number of individuals – the child and various adults and peers. Another may involve addressing those objectives that have a knock-on effect, ones that, if accomplished, may lead to the accomplishment of others. A third may involve a 'quick win'. We know that many children with movement difficulties have a downwards spiral of failure, and, if a quick win can be arranged, this has carry-over effects to many other aspects of the child's functioning. Another strategy for choosing priorities is to look at the motivation of the child, as we know that continual failure does lead to a lack of motivation. If success can be coupled with a demonstration of effort from the child and this is acknowledged, there is a good chance this will increase the motivation of the child. Finally there is the enjoyment factor and the choice here may lay entirely with the child; choosing an activity he or she wants to engage in may help to foster some of the ones noted above.

Environmental context
The environmental context is a crucial part of the ecological model as it is well known that contextual variables have a profound effect on how well the child copes with difficulties. Ecological intervention divides the environmental context into four parts:

- *Family and home* – there is good evidence that if an intervention does not take into account the routines, dynamics, and cultural values of the home and family, the chances of success are slim (Bernheimer and Keogh 1995). This context changes over time and, by

collecting this type of information, the family can be engaged in informed decisions and the intervention process can be much better planned.
- *School setting* – schools differ across countries but most will have resources for children with difficulties. Thus information can be collected on areas such as the school's policy on special educational needs or inclusion, which may include whether there are formal procedures; what resources are available in school; what are the general practices in school; what support practices are available; and what outside help is present in the form of educational psychologists or health professionals.
- *Health services* – for many children with movement difficulties, the health services are often the first port of call and always a major factor in the intervention process. Questions that may need to be asked when collecting information include the mode of delivery of any service; whether the professionals work at a centre in school or travel to the child; whether there are any waiting lists and if so how long; and how often do the professionals get to see the child, and if it is infrequently, do they provide ongoing work that parents and teachers can engage in?
- *Community support* – this is the final part of information collection from the environmental context, and involves an assessment of potential support from the community in the form of sports clubs, sports centres, community groups, and any other help that may be available. We have seen communities organize specific training on individual skills, such as bike riding, and these have proved to be extremely successful.

This information on the environmental context of the child combines with an assessment of the child's resources to provide a total ecological picture. It details all aspects of the child and the support that is potentially available in the environment, both of which are fed into the intervention process itself (Table 12.4).

Ecological approaches recognize that, just as the child's difficulties do not solely reside within the child and are a function of tasks and environmental contexts, it follows that information about the child's ecology should be taken in order for a comprehensive picture to be obtained.

Process deficit and functional task-orientated approaches to intervention
Different terms have been used to describe the multitude of approaches that have been used in intervention studies and in clinical practice, and in order to place some form or order and structure on these they have been placed in a range of categories by different authors. Our way of

TABLE 12.4
Collecting information to plan the programme

Child resources

Standardized tests for a formal assessment of motor capabilities

Dynamic assessment to flexibly examine capabilities

Criterion-referenced tests for functional assessment of skills

Interviews with child, parent/carers, teachers, and significant others

Non-motor difficulties such as co-occurring characteristics

Environmental context

Family and home – taking account of cultural values and providing information for informed decisions by the family

School setting – school policies and practices and support systems for children with disabilities

Health services – services offered from speech therapists, occupational therapists, physiotherapists, and others

Community support – potential support from community groups, parent groups, sports clubs

Sugden and Henderson (2007).

organizing this is to divide them into the two categories of process and functional task approaches, recognizing that these are reductionist, but they do serve to place a big picture on the area. While accepting that there are more fine-grained analyses that can be conducted, we believe the simplest way to examine these is to divide the approaches into two: one approach examines the underlying factors or processes that are thought to influence skill acquisition; the second takes a more direct approach by addressing the functional skills themselves. Various reviews in the last 10 years have included, among others, these two large approaches in their analyses of interventions (Pless and Carlsson 2000, Wilson 2005, Polatajko and Cantin 2006, Sugden 2007).

PROCESS AND DEFICIT APPROACHES

These approaches have been well established in practice for a number of years and have given rise to specialist intervention programmes such as sensory integration therapy (Ayres 1979, 1989). Although many of these methods differ in certain respects, they have major fundamental principles in common, including a deficit being addressed through the remediation of some underlying process or structure. This can be a sensory process, such as vision or kinaesthesis, or can involve biological structures such as the cerebellum. However, whichever it is, the logic or principles behind the method are similar. A motor action is taken and broken down into the potential component parts. Thus an information processing model is used with a sensory input followed by some central decision making culminating with a motor component. These processes are addressed and the ones chosen are often sensory processes, which are seen to drive motor processes. The assumption is that there is some deficit in the underlying sensory processes that underpin planning functions and therefore motor performance is disrupted. Sensory integration therapy is the main approach that has emerged from this and is designed to remedy faulty sensory systems in a *bottom-up* fashion; that is, it works on the underlying processes of a skill and not the skill itself, and aims to better integrate sensory functions for any forthcoming motor action. Other approaches take a more fundamental leaning and attempt to address what the proponents believe to be the biological structures underpinning movement. Here, it is not just the sensory processes that are being addressed but the exact biological structure, such as the cerebellum or some other neural mechanism, that is being targeted. However, it is still a *bottom-up* approach, as it is working from underlying structures rather than the skill itself.

The logic behind these approaches is relatively simple and has attractiveness to it. If the underlying processes or deficits are addressed then the influence will carry over to a number of skills that are based upon these underlying processes. The proponents are working on a generalization model whereby the remediation of certain processes will transfer to many skills that have this process as part of their make-up. Thus, if sensory processes are improved, this will carry over to a number of motor skills. Similarly, if a neural structure is targeted, many improvements will be seen across a number of skills that involve this structure. Whether processes or structures are being addressed, the fundamental assumption is that they underpin a number of skills and by remediating the deficit these skills will improve. Two examples of this are the two Simms et al (1996) studies described on page 335.

Sensory integration therapy

This is a popular approach with occupational therapists and is typical of a process intervention approach. It is usually attributed to the work of Jean Ayres, who was both an occupational therapist and educational psychologist (Ayres 1979, 1989). She developed a theory of sensory integration to explain the link between the nervous system and behaviour through five basic assumptions (Roley and Jacobs 2009):

• The phenomenon of neuroplasticity, meaning the potential for change in the developing brain throughout the lifespan.

- For adequate sensory integration to occur there has to be interactions between higher cortical and subcortical areas of the brain.
- There is a natural sequence of the development of sensory integrative functions.
- There is an adaptive response to environmental demands as a consequence of the environmental context and this promotes a higher level of integration.
- To facilitate the development of sensory integration, there is an inner drive.

These five principles direct both assessment and intervention. Ayres believed that intervention should be delivered in a playful style utilizing the child's inner drive to learn and develop. The environmental context was used to facilitate vestibular, proprioceptive, and tactile sensations as well as adaptive motor responses. She utilized swings, ropes, hula hoops, rocker boards, ceiling hooks, thick mats, ramps, ladders, overstuffed pillows, vibrating toys, and objects with different textures, all designed to stimulate and integrate the sensory systems. The approach is child centred with an encouragement for intrinsic motivation and active participation. As the system has evolved over time, a number of additional goals have been identified as being consistent with a sensory integration approach, including enhanced self-concept, some cognitive, language, and academic skills, gross and fine motor skills, and enhanced family life and social participation. These are natural progressions in any intervention approach, but they do make evaluations difficult as one does not quite know whether the original aims, goals, and methods are being addressed or whether it is a combination of these together with some evolving ones that have been developed as our knowledge has increased.

In their review, at the end of a chapter on sensory integration, Roley and Jacobs (2009) first note that, although sensory integration is probably the most widely researched area of occupational therapy, the evidence for its effectiveness remains inconclusive. A major reason for this is the lack of studies that fulfil stringent research protocols. These include the lack of a homogenous sample; the lack of replicable methods that adhere to sensory integration principles; inadequate outcome measures; and finally methodological limitations such as lack of power or control groups. Roley and Jacobs (2009) conclude by suggesting that future research in this area could address which children might best respond to sensory integration therapy. For example autistic children, many of whom have a known difficulty with sensory processes, may evidence long-term benefits that are of benefit to families. In the defence of sensory integration, one could add that few, if any, intervention approaches could fulfil the research

protocols noted above, although sensory integration has had a much longer time span in which to do so.

Another way to look at this is to take a theoretical viewpoint on whether the principles upon which an approach is based are strong. Process-orientated approaches, and particularly sensory integration, are very much based on relatively old information processing models with an emphasis on the input and in particular the sensory side of the motor control process. This is made clear in the name or sensory integration, but, by comparison, it gives little attention to the cognitive decision making and the motor output side of the motor control process. This is made more complex by the activities that are used; much of sensory integration is centred upon developing and improving the manner in which incoming sensory systems integrate to eventually produce an outcome. However, the outcome does vary: sometimes it is a functional movement, but often it is not and the outcome stays with something that is not functional and indeed is often not motor, being simply a sensory process. Thus it is difficult to examine the holistic nature of the approach or approaches. Wilson (2005) makes the point that these approaches are not consistent with modern theories of motor control. When the empirical evidence is examined, the results are again inconclusive. The diagnostic and remediation programmes have been questioned on psychometric grounds and others have conducted review articles that have called into question the effectiveness of sensory programmes (Pless and Carlsson 2000, Wilson 2005, Polatajko and Cantin 2006, Sugden 2007). There were some earlier studies showing effectiveness and the methods are still popular within the physiotherapy and occupational therapy professions, but, overall, more recent theoretical, empirical, and/or experiential evidence is required to justify the level of practical engagement.

The other approaches that are included in this group are the ones that attempt to directly address neural structures. The assessment in this area is usually an eclectic mixture of neurological tests, a physical examination, and often intellectual assessment. From these, terms such as 'soft signs' or minimal brain dysfunction emerged and the programmes are similarly eclectic with structures such as the cerebellum directly addressed or more general neurological signs such as reflexes, with paradoxically both the suppression and the facilitation of reflexes being part of differing programmes.

FUNCTIONAL SKILL APPROACHES

As the name suggests, functional skill approaches involve the teaching of those skills that are required for everyday functioning in a child's life. There are a number of programmes available that take this approach.

The ones that have been shown to be most successful are those that have involved cognitive methods to teach these functional skills (Henderson and Sugden 1992, Revie and Larkin 1993, Polatajko et al 2001a, Schoemaker et al 2003, Sugden and Henderson 2007). Early approaches by Henderson and Sugden (1992) in their cognitive motor approach and Revie and Larkin (1993) in their task-specific approach employed methods that had long been popular in the motor learning domain, drawing upon research literature in the sporting arenas and in the workplace. These were followed by a popular Canadian approach that further developed the idea of working with cognitive processes allied to functional tasks (Cognitive Orientation to Daily Occupational Performance Programme, CO-OP).

Cognitive Orientation to Daily Occupational Performance Programme

In the mid-1990s a series of articles described and evaluated the CO-OP approach (Polatajko et al 2001a,b, Polatajko and Mandich 2004) in which the therapist places an emphasis on involving the child in the choice of which skills they will aim to acquire through a problem-solving exercise. It is based on functional tasks, with a first objective being motor skill acquisition, and may include activities such as handwriting, dressing, or riding a bike. A second objective is the use of cognitive strategies to solve motor problems with an examination of the strategies that are involved to support the motor skill acquisition goal. The third and fourth objectives can be combined as the former involves generalization, which Polatajko et al (2001a,b) define as using the skill under different stimuli conditions to those in which it was learned, that is in different places such as the home and school or at a different time with different people. The latter one of transfer involves using the skill as the basis for learning other similar skills. The aim of intervention is 'for the child to leave therapy with the ability to generalize and transfer the problem solving strategies and skills that have been learned in therapy into everyday life' (Mandich and Polatajko 2005, p. 231).

The essential key component of the CO-OP approach is that the child is actively engaged in the seven key features of

- *Client-chosen goals* – the child's perspective is of central importance starting with goal setting and involving self-evaluation.
- *Dynamic performance analysis* – it is highly individualistic and is based on the understanding that performance is a product of the child–task–environment interaction. The focus is on the observable skills and the environmental variables that affect performance and are aided by the appropriate cognitive strategies.
- *Cognitive strategy use* – these are the strategies that enable the child to engage in problem-solving and metacognitive activities and for generalization and transfer. These strategies are both global and domain specific. The global strategy is the use of GOAL–PLAN–DO–CHECK, which is taught in the first session and is often taught through the use of a puppet. It is first presented by the therapist and then the child takes over and initiates it. The domain-specific strategies are those that are required for a specific task and include feeling the movement, attention to the task, producing verbal motor mnemonics, and other verbal cues, as CO-OP involves a highly verbal approach.
- *Guided discovery* – this is closely related to strategy use and is used when the child gets stuck in the GOAL–PLAN–DO–CHECK sequence, with the aim that the child will attribute any success to him or herself thus increasing motivation.
- *Enabling principles* – these are used throughout the intervention programme and include 'making it fun', 'promoting learning', 'working towards independence', and 'promoting generalization and transfer'.
- *Parent/significant other involvement* – throughout the session the therapist shares the information with parents and/or significant others.
- *Intervention structure* – this involves the format of the intervention, which includes 10 sessions starting with the child identifying three goals and the therapist assessing the child on these goals. The child is then taught the GOAL–PLAN–DO–CHECK strategy and applies it to the three goals, followed by domain-specific strategies, and finally the therapist re-evaluating the child's performance.

The principles upon which the approach is based rest upon the emphasis of cognition and motor learning with cognitions bridging the gap between ability and skill level. Cognition is a mediator of skill performance and rejects such explanations as failure in crossing the midline or bilateral coordination as justifiable reasons as to why children fail motor skill tasks. As Mandich and Polatajko state 'research has shown limited effectiveness of that type of approach *(process oriented)* and often the child outgrows several bikes while waiting for the therapist to fix the underlying deficits' (2005, p. 240).

The CO-OP approach is different, with the therapist concentrating on the specific skill acquisition and leading the child through the appropriate cognitive strategies to achieve the goal they have chosen, concentrating on where the task has broken down and not being concerned

---

Box 12.3 A closer examination

Evidence for CO-OP: Mandich and Polatajko (2005)

Philosophy
The authors start with the theoretical argument that CO-OP is nested in ICF (WHO 2001), focusing on activity and participation and not disability and impairment, with the aim of improving motor skills performance and eliminating barriers in the environment to achieve this. For this it draws upon evidence from human movement science, psychology, health, and occupational therapy to achieve these objectives.

Objectives for CO-OP
Four objectives are presented:
- skill acquisition
- cognitive strategy use
- generalization
- transfer of learning.

Evidence for success
- Single-case studies with children aged 7 to 12 (Wilcox and Polatajko 1993, 1994, Martini and Polatajko 1998).
- Use of cognitive strategies for global problem solving and domain-specific strategies that were tailor made to the child's difficulties (Mandich et al 2001).
- A randomized controlled trial by Miller et al (2001) with 10 children randomly assigned to a CO-OP group or one receiving typical therapy with the results favouring CO-OP for both acquisition of skill and skill transfer.
- Studies to show that CO-OP has a positive effect on everyday life including families (Segal et al 2002, Mandich et al 2001).

---

with the underlying processes that may or may not have relevance to the skill at hand.

The evidence to support the CO-OP approach so far has been positive. The original approach was worked out with graduate students under supervision of Helen Polatajko and with various colleagues (Polatajko et al 2001a,b, Polatajko and Mandich 2004). One could argue that this process of consultation helped to provide a form of construct validity. A number of studies have provided evidence of the effectiveness of the approach. The most impressive randomized controlled trials were those of Miller et al (2001) in which children were assigned either to a CO-OP group or one that involved traditional therapy where the therapist could use any other method he or she deemed to be appropriate for the child. The findings showed, even with this small number of children, that the CO-OP group outperformed the traditional therapy group.

In 2004 Polatajko and Mandich stated that the CO-OP approach was successful in that it met the demands of parents by helping their children to succeed; therapists in that it was child centred and performance based; and administrators as it was efficient and cost effective. A summary of this evidence is presented in Box 12.3.

Ecological intervention
The approach itself (Sugden and Henderson 2007) consists of two major parts:

- collecting information and planning the programme – this has been covered in pages 350–351 of this chapter; and
- implementing an ecological intervention programme.

These two headings encompass the objectives of this chapter, namely assessment and intervention.

Implementing an ecological intervention programme
Ecological intervention involves the child's resources, the environmental context, and the task itself. Information has been collected from the first two arms of the triad, namely child resources and the environmental context, and fed into this third part, which is the actual intervention itself. This third arm of ecological intervention surrounds the task variables, choice of task, and how it is presented. There are two important and overlapping prerequisites for the whole approach:

- participation through engineering the environment; and
- successful learning through good teaching.

So far there is information on the child and the targets that have been set by him or her or others; there are data on the environment in which the child lives and the possibilities it has to offer; and there are data on the individuals involved and the role they may play. To implement ecological intervention there is involvement of the following:

- The movement coach – there is a need for a central person to argue case and take responsibility for such things as a plan of action. The movement coach is also responsible for the organization, delivery, and monitoring of ecological intervention and must negotiate with significant persons and coordinate with families. It could be someone from health, such as an occupational therapist, or from education, such as the person responsible for inclusion policies in the school.
- Organizing the context and setting the scene – this involves working with the child on the targets he or she has set and the targets others see as important; an examination of support systems and possibilities and of the individuals involved and their roles, including the organization of meetings and obtaining firm commitments; and the scheduling of practices and the communication and timetabling for action.
- Working in a meaningful context – this involves working with functional tasks that are realistic and relevant to the everyday functioning of the child and include both formal and informal activities, with an emphasis on active movements in context and passive movements being used only as a final alternative.
- Learning specific skills through task analysis, task adaptation, and expert scaffolding – task analysis and task adaptation are two of the cornerstones of intervention work. Meaningful task analysis is a great skill to have and selected parts of an example of bike riding are shown in Table 12.5 (C Dunford, personal communication, 2006). Task analysis involves breaking down the task into meaningful parts that can be achieved and seamlessly reassembled to make up the full picture. It also involves an analysis of what the child needs to know to accomplish the task and what the child needs to do. Task adaptation involves adapting the task to make it more accessible, such as using larger buttons or even Velcro for fastening.
- Instructions, practice, and feedback – this involves an examination of the factors that need to be considered

TABLE 12.5
Lead-up activities to bike riding

Standing on left, holding bike, and pushing the bike while steering

Braking to verbal command and visual target

Steering in and out of cones and around corners

With brakes, getting on and off bike

'Scooting' – sitting on bike with pedals removed on lowered seat, walking the bike followed by raising of legs

'Scooting' and steering and braking

With a handling belt, pedal with support repeating all of the above stages

Prepare pedal for push off with belt

Push off and prepare second foot to move to pedal, still with belt

Once this can be accomplished remove belt but 'shadow' support

Once confident with this, start to make context unpredictable with cones and moving others

to make the learning process as seamless as possible, and includes an examination of the phases of learning and how we present instructions, practices, and feedback during the various phases of understanding the skill, acquiring and refining the skill, and automating the skill.
- Skill generalisation – learning specific skills is not enough. Learning should be broadened through generalization – although learning functional and specific skills is one of the major aims, we are also aware that in order to gain a full repertoire of skills generalization or transfer is a necessary activity. Strategies for generalization are shown from those that affect the *learner*, such as teaching self-monitoring, to those that are *context* driven and the social support, and those that involve the *task*, such as presenting variable practice to classes of activity. These are shown in Table 12.6.
- Monitoring and evaluation – this involves two processes with the first being ongoing monitoring, which includes checking with the child whether the activities are enjoyable, progress is being made, and others feel the same. From this, targets and priorities may be realigned. The second process is the evaluation of the whole programme, incorporating the child's view, the view of the team, the test, and other data.

We have described the implementation of an ecological intervention programme in some detail as it provides a holistic approach to both assessment and intervention. It is not geared to a rigid methodology but incorporates evidence from the motor learning and development literature

TABLE 12.6
Strategies for generalization

Learner (child)	Setting of own objectives
	Self-monitoring and evaluation
	Use of a variety of cognitive strategies for memory, attention, planning, organization, self-talk
Context	Assistive questions by more competent other (scaffolding)
	Organization of the context
Task	Variability of practice
	Teach to class of activities

and clinical practice. A summary of ecological intervention principles is shown in Table 12.7.

Neuromotor task training
Another current functional approach to intervention for children with DCD is neuromotor task training (NTT) developed by Marina Schoemaker and Bouwien Smits-Englesman (Shoemaker et al 2003), and taking as its basis the work of Henderson and Sugden (1992), with their cognitive motor approach, Revie and Larkin (1993), with their task-specific intervention programme, and CO-OP (Polatajko et al 1995a), together with principles from neuromotor control theories and motor learning principles in general. The approach is based on functional tasks supported by the neuronal group selection theory (Sporns and Edelman 1993), which use both of what they call primary and secondary neuronal repertoires. During development, selection occurs and behaviour becomes less variable, but variability returns in order for the child to meet the demands of an increasingly diverse environmental context. Schoemaker and Smits-Englesman propose that this secondary or adaptive variability is less well developed in children with DCD and that practice of the appropriate

skills will enhance the correct selection of the appropriate neuronal groups through the increase of adaptive variability. The authors also use variability in the manner that Schmidt (1975) explains in his schema theory of motor learning.

NTT uses the evidence we have on how to instruct, how to practice, and how to provide feedback and base this on the stages of learning as proposed by Fitts and Posner (1967) described on page 346 in this chapter. Schoemaker and Smits-Englesman state that, in the early part of skill learning, demonstrations following the work of Bandura (1986) and observational learning are better than verbal instructions, which are more helpful in later stages, such as when the child moves into what Fitts and Posner (1967) called their associative phase. The same progression is seen in how feedback is given with a movement from a motivational guide in the early stages to one that is more informational as the skill learning progresses. Throughout these phases, NTT describes how at the motor learning process the teaching principles will differ and take into account the process of transfer.

NTT is the third approach that we have examined that shares some commonalities. It rests upon motor learning principles that were earlier espoused by Henderson and Sugden (1992), Revie and Larkin (1993) and Polatajko et al (1995). The authors have developed this using work from neuronal research (Sporns and Edelman 1993) and produced a system that shares many points with the other two approaches in this section. It has been evaluated by Schoemaker et al (2003) who with a small group of children found positive effects on both fine and gross motor skills, with the important observation that only skills that were practised improved, thus validating the task-orientated approach of NTT.

The three approaches that we have described in the functional or specific task approaches have a number of principles and other factors in common:

TABLE 12.7
Ecological intervention

The movement coach	Named person to take responsibility
Organizing the context	Organizing targets, commitments, support systems
Working in a meaningful context	Functional active tasks that are realistic and relevant
Learning specific skills	Task analysis and task adaptation
Instructions, practice and feedback	How they change as learning progresses
Learning through generalization	Teaching of cognitive strategies
Monitoring and evaluation	Looking at targets and priorities from all view points

Sugden and Henderson (2007).

361

- First, as the name implies, they address functional skills and do not subscribe to remedying underlying process deficits such as in sensory integration theory.
- Second, they all to a greater or lesser extent address the issue of transfer and/or generalization, as this is the obvious target of criticism of any method that takes functional skills. They are different in the manner in which they address this issue, but strategies, such as cognitions and variability of task and context presentation, are present in all three.
- Third, child choice and engagement, whether through goal setting, self-regulation, or monitoring, are present in all three approaches.
- Fourth, all use guidelines, in greater or lesser measures, that have been gleaned through research in other areas such as mainstream psychology and the motor learning literature.

The most recent one, ecological intervention (Sugden and Henderson 2007), is a complete system, drawing upon many of the approaches that have preceded it, including cognitive approaches (Henderson and Sugden 1992), and takes the child from first identification through to evaluation of the approach. This intervention approach transfers the information processing literature (see Schmidt and Lee 2005) to the developing child and dynamical systems approaches (see Turvey 1977, Kelso 1995), but it has not had a full evaluation of its effectiveness, only drawing upon work leading up to its publication. Partial evaluations have been made of both CO-OP and NTT, all of which have been supportive, and what is needed now is more independent evaluations of all three approaches.

One could argue that all of the approaches have evidence supporting them in the form of the theoretical underpinnings, in that all have the strong motor learning literature support both for the performance and learning of motor skills. In addition, the literature supporting specific skill or task-specific approaches is very much stronger than that supporting process-orientated methods. This does not mean to say that process-orientated approaches do not work; they may, but, at the moment, with the current approaches in that domain, they do not provide the supportive evidence.

Interventions for cerebral palsy

The interventions we have described so far could be applicable to all children showing difficulties in movement. The move towards teaching functional skills would appear to be one that goes across the ability range, whether the children have learning difficulties and associated movement problems or whether the primary condition is movement based such as in DCD. The group of children with cerebral palsy, described in Chapter 7, present a slightly different case. They are our largest category of children who have known constitutional impairment and present us with movement problems as the core of their difficulties. As such, it is not surprising that specific interventions have been tailored for this group of children. These interventions have ranged from ones that are specific to particular classes of movements such as hand functions (e.g. constraint-induced therapy) to those that are much more wide ranging and take on board the total lifestyle of the child (conductive education). It is not our intention to cover every intervention method in detail but to illustrate through examples certain principles that indicate the type of underlying theoretical foundations upon which the interventions are based.

NEURODEVELOPMENTAL APPROACHES

These approaches have been used for a long period of time and many of their variants are still in widespread practice and are possibly still the most widely used methods. In this approach, therapists focus on remedying the motor impairment that the child shows through facilitating typical development and inhibiting primitive movements such as reflexes. The classic work through the Bobath approach are examples of this (Bobath 1980). However, over the last decade, these methods have begun to be questioned. Law et al (1998) found little evidence to suggest that the inhibition of primitive reflexes promoted typical motor development. They use as an example the stepping reflex noting that its disappearance is not the result of the higher neural centre taking control but is, as described by Thelen in numerous articles (see Chapter 2), the result of a number of subcomponents such as skeletal group, weight, and fat content as well as neural maturation.

FAMILY-CENTRED FUNCTIONAL APPROACH

This type of approach is very similar to parts of the ecological approach outlined earlier in the chapter and described by Law et al (1998) who list four principles defining the approach:

- Promote functional performance – the approach is directed to functional tasks not underlying processes or trying to 'normalize' development.
- Identify periods of change – parents are the best persons to identify when a child is trying to do a new task and this is the optimal time to intervene.
- Identify and change task, environment, or child resources – very much in line with our theme throughout the book.
- Encourage practice – as much as possible in a variety of environments.

Using this approach, Law et al (1998) facilitated change in a group of children with cerebral palsy who made observable and meaningful progress during the course of intervention. They accepted that this type of approach does present challenges and there were some difficulties in identifying the focus of the initial intervention, as the families wished to change the child resources, whereas the researchers were looking towards changing the task and the environment. As with many types of intervention, there was some overlap with traditional methods – this is always the case but it is the focus and main principles and the rationale for engagement that is important. Here the focus was on family-based functional tasks, not on hierarchical neurodevelopmental sequences; it starts and ends with the family and parents and is totally in synchrony with our view following the work of Bernheimer and Keogh (1995), who state that any intervention with children evidencing difficulties is doomed to failure if it does not consider the routines and cultures of the family and enable them to make informed decisions. An example of functional and ecological approaches is described and supported by Ekstrom Ahl et al (2005) drawing upon the ecological work of Bronfenbrenner (1986), together with children's perceptual exploration of their environment and problem solving (Lesensky and Kaplan 2000). This is shown in Box 12.4.

SPECIFIC APPROACHES FOR CHILDREN WITH HEMIPLEGIC CEREBRAL PALSY

Children with hemiplegic cerebral palsy are a unique group to work with both clinically and in a research capacity. This is because one side of their body has some impairment and the other side is either not affected or, more usually, less affected. In research, this enables both capabilities and intervention to be controlled within the one individual and there are no problems with having to match children. They are in effect their own controls. In Chapter 7 we showed that, during the performance of manual skills, when children with hemiplegic cerebral palsy used both hands together, that is bimanual movements, there was some carry over from the less affected to the more affected limb (Sugden and Utley 1995, Utley and Sugden 1998, Steenbergen et al 2003). This type of research activity has clear intervention guidelines, but other research has used intervention methods that are almost diametrically opposite to the bimanual coupling research and has come to be known as constraint-induced therapy (CIT).

Constraint-induced therapy

The basic principle of CIT, which has also been used for stroke patients, is that the unimpaired limb is prevented

or constrained from moving, thus ensuring that manual activities are carried out by the impaired limb. It is based on the premise that 'learned non-use' of the affected hand occurs when individuals fail to use it. Thus by preventing the use of the unimpaired limb, the individual is forced to use, and thereby practise with, the impaired limb. Support for the method comes from Crocker et al (1997), Charles et al (2001), Willis et al (2007), and Taub et al (1999). A modified version of CIT was examined by Eliasson et al (2005) who analysed how much improvement could be expected, which children would benefit from the treatment, what age was most appropriate for treatment, and whether the results varied with the type and severity of the hemiplegia. The group of children receiving CIT wore a glove on their unimpaired hand, and the results showed that they had improved their ability to use the hemiplegic hand more than the children in the control group, but there was high within-group variability indicating that the effects were multifactorial. Age and measures at onset showed significant differences. The measure of initial hand functions before intervention at onset showed that children who were initially low improved the most, and this onset measure accounted for 31% of the variance of the results. Surprisingly, older children did better than younger ones, and again age after correction for measure at onset accounted for 31% of the variance of the results. The duration of practice did not show differences.

CIT has used different methods to constrain the unimpaired limb – glove and casts – and the general conclusion is that positive results are seen, although there is not a plethora of studies examining this method. The theoretical reasons behind this appear to be strongly related to practice effects; it is a way of encouraging the individual to use the affected limb, as the consequences of non-use are well known – eventually the limb simply becomes inert. However, there are several limitations to the method, as noted by Gordon et al (2006). First, there are few studies using randomized control trials and the type of constraint, the amount and intensity of treatment, and the evaluation measures all vary across studies. Gordon et al (2006) continue their criticism by saying that CIT was developed for adults and children have to overcome what they call developmental non-use, as they may never have effectively used their impaired limb. Second, the constraint is potentially invasive and would certainly go against any therapy that had natural contexts in daily life as a major underlying principle. Finally, they point out that many unimanual actions such as brushing teeth can easily be carried out with the unimpaired limb, and, in addition, CIT does not address bimanual activities.

Box 12.4 A closer examination

Training in daily life settings: Ekstrom Ahl et al (2005)
The aim of the study was to evaluate training in daily-life settings for preschool children with cerebral palsy with respect to:

- goal attainment
- gross motor function
- performance of daily activities
- amount of caregiver assistance required
- perceptions of parents and assistants affected by the methodology.

Method
This study comprised 14 preschool (aged 1y 6mo–6y) children with cerebral palsy and no severe learning difficulty. The children had either spastic diplegia or tetraplegia and were classified between levels II and V on the Gross Motor Function Classification System. The children were divided into two groups for ease of training and there was no control group.

Seven measurable goals were set by the parents, the child's preschool assistant, and the therapists, and graded as complete (100%), partial (50%), or no improvement (0%). Various assessment instruments were used such as the Gross Motor Function Measure-66 (GMFM) (Russell et al 2002) and a Swedish version of the functional skills and caregiver assistance scales of the Pediatric Evaluation of Disability Inventory (PEDI) (Nordmark et al 1999). Parents' and assistants' perceptions were obtained through questionnaires and diaries.

Intervention
The intervention started with a 4-day live-in period for all concerned – families and assistants – in which both theoretical and practical instructions were given. This was followed by 5 months of goal-directed functional therapy carried out in the child's normal setting at home and in preschool. Continuous dialogue was held throughout this period with help and support given, and all of the children met once a week. Group guidance sessions were given to parents and assistants in functional therapy with special attention given to enabling children to become active participants. Participants were encouraged to perform different activities in a variety of ways and different problem-solving solutions were attempted.

Results
The diaries showed that frequency of training varied considerably, which mostly reflected the goal chosen. Originally 98 goals were chosen; after 3 months of training 45 were fully met and 25 partially completed; after 5 months 76 were fully completed and 19 partially completed; and after 8 months of follow-up the goal attainment was sustained. The scores on the PEDI from the parents also improved as did the perceptions of the parents and the assistants concerning the services they had received.

Discussion
The authors stressed that functional goal-directed therapy was successful, with the goals being reached in 77% of cases and parents and assistants being positive and indicating the children had learned skills. The importance of goals was stressed, noting the importance of clarity for the children and workers and that the goals are understandable and achievable in a given time frame. The role of the parents as an important component of an ecological approach was emphasized, and the children benefited from this functional goal-directed approach.

HABIT
To address these concerns, Gordon et al (2006) have developed HABIT, hand–arm bimanual intensive training. The method uses the principle of intensive practice; targets known deficits in bimanual coordination (Steenbergen and Gordon 2006); draws upon the motor learning literature such as practice variables; and utilizes the principles of neuroplasticity, which show brain changes as a result

of types of movements. HABIT emphasizes functional skills with increasingly complex practice together with extended practice (6h a day on bimanual activities).

HABIT uses a wide range of tasks that require the use of both hands, including manipulative games, card games, video-games, some larger-limb tasks, such as carrying activities involving shoulder and arm movements, and arts and crafts. Repetitions of whole tasks are given together with graded constraints such as changing the spatial and temporal requirements (Gordon et al 2006). Whole practice of the task is used for about 15 to 20 minutes followed by, if necessary, some part practice, and the task difficulty is graded by requiring greater speed or accuracy as the situation and child's ability demand. Gordon et al (2006) argue that the approach differs from conventional therapy in two ways. First, it is more intensive with more practice, a principle gained from CIT, and long established in the motor learning literature. Second, it differs from both conventional therapy and CIT by asking children to use the involved hand as a typically developing child would. It involves active learning and problem solving for the children as they discover their bimanual capabilities. The authors recognize that implementation is not a simple matter, but the approach overall looks to incorporate the best of a number of approaches, while utilizing what we know about coordination and control, bimanual coupling, and practice variables.

The work on children with cerebral palsy typifies the work on intervention in general, with the fundamental question of whether the intervention is aimed at remediating impairment and disability or teaching functional skills. This continuum of focus, and it is a continuum rather than being dichotomous, appears in several guises. In the cerebral palsy literature it is seen when one compares a Bobath-type approach to one involving teaching everyday functional skills in families, with the emphasis on learning new skills rather than a concentration on underlying processes to remedy impairment. This is also seen in the literature on children with DCD, with the approaches of sensory integration therapy and its derivatives and the more functional task approaches of CO-OP, ecological intervention, and NTT. When one does move into the functional skills approach, the debate becomes how one best teaches it, with this being nicely shown by looking at the two different yet complementary approaches of CIT and HABIT.

Summary

Assessment and intervention are two processes inextricably linked, with each informing the other in a continuous cycle. Without accurate assessment the process of intervention is at best a chance endeavour and the emphasis in this text is on a total assessment that encompasses examining the daily context of the child as well as his or her personal resources. We have called this *collecting information to plan the programme* to emphasize the holistic nature of the process. This leads into the intervention process in which the environment and the presentation of the task are crucial variables. Together they influence the amount of participation the child engages in and subsequent learning and skill acquisition. The World Health Organization (2001) ICF framework is an important influence on our emphasis on functional skill learning as exemplified by intervention programmes such as CO-OP, NTT, and ecological intervention.

The view taken here is that assessment and intervention constantly feed into each other, and this dynamic process involves a consideration of the fact that the context the child is operating in, the influence of the environment, and how the task is presented make extraordinary differences to the child's functioning. One has only to imagine a health authority with strong occupational therapy and physical therapy services in a developmental centre working with a child with hemiplegic cerebral palsy, providing individual specialist assessment, help, and support plus advice and practical tips to schools and parents, and compare it to one that does not evidence the same support. If the former also is in a community with understanding, resources, and personnel and a school that makes diversity and inclusive practices a priority and a benefit to all children, the differences are heightened. The whole process is dynamic with the child's resources being an important, but only a single, part of the equation, determining how functional a child becomes in everyday life.

It has not been the intention to cover the wide range of assessment and intervention practices there are available but to give a flavour of ones that are utilized based upon a set of criteria. For both of the processes, clinicians and researchers are advised to look at the evidence that supports a particular assessment procedure or intervention approach, and the evidence is available from three different sources. First, there is theoretical evidence that goes to the very core of the method or procedure; second, there is empirical evidence that shows what research has said about an approach; and, third, there is experiential evidence that outlines the experiences of practitioners in the field (Sugden and Dunford 2007). Often these pieces of evidence do not seamlessly fit together but only by examining what evidence is available can we be confident about our decision-making processes.

REFERENCES

APA (2000) *Diagnostic and Statistical Manual of Mental Disorders: DSM IV*, 4th edition text revision. Arlington, VA: American Psychiatric Association.Ayres AJ (1979) *Sensory Integration and the Child*. Los Angeles, CA: Western Psychological Services.

Ayres JR (1979) *Sensory Integration and the Child*. Los Angeles: Western Psychological Services.

Ayres AJ (1989) *Sensory Integration and Praxis Test Manual*. Los Angeles, CA: Western Psychological Services.

Baddeley AD, Longman DJA (1978) The influence of length and frequency of training sessions on the rate of learning to type. *Ergonomics* 21: 627–635. http://dx.doi.org/10.1080/00140137808931764

Bandura A (1986) *Social Foundations of Thought and Action: A Social Cognitive Theory*. Englewoods Cliffs, NJ: Prentice Hall.

Barnett A (2008) Motor assessment in developmental coordination disorder: from identification to assessment. In: Sugden DA, Kirby A, Dunford C, editors. Special issue of *International Journal of Disability Development and Education: Children with Developmental Coordination Disorder* 55: 113–129.

Bax MDM, Tydeman C, Flodmark O (2006) Clinical and MRI correlates of cerebral palsy. *JAMA* 296: 1602–1608. http://dx.doi.org/10.1001/jama.296.13.1602

Bernheimer LP, Keogh BK (1995) Weaving interventions into the fabric of everyday life: an approach to family assessment. *Topics in Early Childhood Special Education* 15: 415–433. http://dx.doi.org/10.1177/027112149501500402

Bernstein N (1967) *The Coordination and Regulation of Movements*. New York: Pergamon Press.

Bobath K (1980) *A Neurophysiological Basis for the Treatment of Cerebral Palsy*. London: William Heinemen Medical.

Bronfenbrenner U (1979) *The Ecology of Human Development: Experiments by Nature and Design*. Cambridge, MA: Harvard University Press.

Bronfenbrenner U (1986) *The Ecology of Human Development*. Cambridge, MA: Harvard University Press.

Bruininks RH (1978) *The Bruininks–Oseretsky Test of Motor Proficiency*. Circle Pines, MN: American Guidance Service.

Bruininks RH, Bruininks BD (2007) *Bruininks–Oseretsky Test of Motor Perfromance*, 2nd edition. Minneapolis, MN: American Guidance Service.

Burton AW, Miller AE (1998) *Movement Skill Assessment*. Champaign, IL: Human Kinetics.

Carson LM, Bulger SM, Townsend JS (2007) Enhancing responsible student decision-making in physical activity. In: Davis WE, Broadhead GD, editors. *Ecological Task Analysis and Movement*. Champaign, IL: Human Kinetics, pp. 141–159.

Chambers ME, Sugden DA (2006) *Coordination Disorders in the Early Years*. London: Whurr.

Charles J, Lavinder G, Gordon AM (2001) The effects of constraint-induced therapy on hand function in children with hemiplegic cerebral palsy. *Pediatr Phys Ther* 13: 68–76. http://dx.doi.org/10.1097/00001577-200107000-00003

Chen HF, Cohn ES (2003) Social participation for children with developmental coordination disorder: conceptual, evaluation and intervention considerations. *Phys Occup Ther Pediatr* 23: 61–78.

Crocker MD, Mackay-Lyons M, McDonnell E (1997) Forced use of the upper extremity in cerebral palsy: a single case design. *Am J Occup Ther* 51: 824–833.

Davis WE, Broadhead GD, editors (2007) *Ecological Task Analysis and Movement*. Champaign, IL: Human Kinetics.

Davis WE, Burton AW (1991) Ecological task analysis: translating movement theory into practice. *Adapted Phys Activity Q* 8: 154–177.

Ekstrom Ahl LE, Johansson E, Granat T, Carlberg EB (2005) Functional therapy for children with cerebral palsy: an ecological approach. *Dev Med Child Neurol* 47: 613–619.

Eliasson AC, Sundholm LK, Shaw L, Wang C (2005) Effects of constraint-induced movement therapy in young children with hemiplegic cerebral palsy: an adapted model. *Dev Med Child Neurol* 47: 266–275. http://dx.doi.org/10.1017/S0012162205000502

Fawcett AJ, Nicolson RI (1995) Persistent deficits in motor skill in children with dyslexia. *J Motor Behav* 27: 235–241. http://dx.doi.org/10.1080/00222895199599441713

Fitts PM, Posner MI (1967) *Human Performance*. Belmont, CA: Brooks/Cole.

Gentile AM (2000) Skill acquisition: action movement and neuromotor processes. In: Carr J, Shepherd RB, editors. *Movement Science: Foundations for Physical Therapy in Rehabilitation*, 2nd edition. Gaithersburg, MD: Aspen.

Gordon AM, Charles J, Wolf SL (2006) Efficacy of constraint-induced therapy on involved upper-extremity use in children with hemiplegic cerebral palsy is not age-dependent. *Pediatrics* 117: e363–e373. http://dx.doi.org/101542/peds.2005-1009

Henderson SE, Sugden DA (1992) *Movement Assessment Battery for Children: Manual*. Sidcup: Psychological Corporation.

Henderson SE, Sugden DA, Barnett A (2007) *Movement Assessment Battery for Children 2: Kit and Manual*. London: Harcourt Asseement/Pearson.

Hill E (2005) Cognitive explanations of the planning and execution of movement. In: Sugden DA, Chambers ME, editors. *Children with Developmental Coordination Disorder*. London: Whurr, pp. 47–71.

Hoare D, Larkin D (1991) Kinaesthetic abilities of clumsy children. *Dev Med Child Neurol* 33: 671–678. http://dx.doi.org/10.1111/j.1469-8749.1991.tb14944.x

Hulme C, Smart A, Moran G (1982) Visual perceptual deficits in clumsy children. *Neuropsychology* 30: 475–481.

Hultzer Y (2007) Systematic ecological modification approach to skill acquisition in adapted physical activity. In: Davis WE, Broadhead GD, editors. *Ecological Task Analysis and Movement*. Champaign, IL: Human Kinetics, pp. 161–178.

Kelso JAS (1995) *Dynamic Patterns: The Self-Organization of Brain and Behavior*. Cambridge, MA: MIT Press.

Keogh JF, Sugden DA (1985) *Movement Skill Development*. New York: Macmillan.

Kidman L, Davis WE (2007) Empowerment in coaching. In: Davis WE, Broadhead GD, editors. *Ecological Task Analysis and Movement*. Champaign, IL: Human Kinetics, pp. 121–139.

Konczak J, Vander Velden J, Jaeger H (2009) Learning to play the violin: motor control by freezing not freeing degrees of freedom. *J Motor Behav* 41: 243–252. http://dx.doi.org/10.3200/JMBR.41.3.243-252

Larkin D, Parker H (2002) Task-specific interventions for children with developmental coordination disorder: a systems view. In: Cermak S, Larkin D, editors. *Developmental Coodination Disorder*. Albany, NY: Delmar, pp. 234–247.

Laszlo JI, Bairstow P (1985) *Test of Kinaesthetic Sensitivity.* London: Senkit PTY in association with Holt Rinehart & Winston.

Law M, Darrah J, Pollock N, et al (1998) Family-centred functional therapy for children with cerebral palsy: an emerging practice model. *Phys Occup Ther Pediatr* 18: 83–102.

Lesensky S, Kaplan L (2000) Motor learning – putting theory into practice. *Occup Ther Pract* 25: 13–16.

Lord R, Hulme C (1987) Perceptual judgements of normal and clumsy children. *Dev Med Child Neurol* 29: 250–257. http://dx.doi.org/10.1111/j.1469-8749.1987.tb02143.x

McConachie H, Colver AF, Forsyth RJ, Jarvis SN, et al (2006) Participation of disabled children: how should it be characterised and measured? *Disabil Rehabil* 28: 1157–1164. http://dx.doi.org/10.1080/09638280500534507

Magill RA (2007) *Motor Learning and Control: Concepts and Applications*, 8th edition. New York: McGraw-Hill.

Mandich AD, Polatajko HJ (2005) A cognitive perspective on intervention for children with developmental coordination disorder. In: Sugden DA, Chambers ME, editors. *Children with Developmental Coordination Disorder.* London: Whurr, pp. 228–241.

Mandich A, Polatajko H, Macnab J, Miller L (2001) Treatment of children with developmental coordination disorder: what is the evidence? *Phys Occup Ther Pediatr* 20: 51–68.

Martini R, Polatajko HJ (1998) Verbal self guidance for children with developmental coordination disorder: a systematic replication study. *Occup Ther J Res* 18: 157–181.

Mesibov GB, Shea V, Schopler E (2004) *The TEACCH Approach to Autistic Spectrum Disorders.* New York: Springer Verlag. http://dx.doi.org/10.1007/978-0-306-48647-0

Miller LT, Polatajko HJ, Missiuna C, et al (2001) A pilot trial of a cognitive treatment for children with developmental coordination disorder. *Hum Movement Sci* 20: 183–210. http://dx.doi.org/10.1016/S0167-9457(01)00034-3

Morris C, Kurinczuk JJ, Fitzpatrick R, Rosenbaum P (2006) Do children's abilities explain their participation? *Dev Med Child Neurol* 48: 954–961. http://dx.doi.org/10.1017/S0012162206002106

Morton J (2004) *Understanding Developmental Disorders.* Oxford: Blackwell. http://dx.doi.org/10.1002/9780470773307

Mullally G, Mullally M (2007) Using ecological task analysis in physiotherapy. In: Davis WE, Broadhead GD, editors. *Ecological Task Analysis and Movement.* Champaign, IL: Human Kinetics, pp. 219–246.

Newell KM (1986) Constraints on the development of coordination. In: Wade MG, Whiting HTA, editors. *Motor Development in Children: Aspects of Coordination and Control.* Amsterdam: Martinus Nijhoff, pp. 341–361. http://dx.doi.org/10.1007/978-94-009-4460-2_19

Newell KM, Jordan K (2007) Task constraints and movement organisation: a common language. In: Davis WE, Broadhead GD, editors. *Ecological Task Analysis and Movement.* Champaign, IL: Human Kinetics, pp. 5–23.

Nordmark E, Jarnlo GB, Hagglund G (1999) The American Pediatric Evaluation of Disability Inventory (PEDI). *Scand J Rehabil Med* 31: 95–106. http://dx.doi.org/10.1080/003655099444605

Pless M, Carlsson M (2000) Effects of motor skill intervention on developmental coordination disorder: a meta analysis. *Adapted Phys Activity Q* 17: 381–401.

Polatajko HJ, Cantin N (2006) Developmental coordination disorder (dyspraxia): an overview of the state of the art. *Semin Pediatr Neurol* 12: 250–258. http://dx.doi.org/10.1016/j.spen.2005.12.007

Polatajko HJ, Mandich AD (2004) *Enabling Occupation in Children: The Cognitive Orientation to Daily Occupational Performance (CO-OP) Approach.* Ottawa, ON: Canadian Association of Occupational Therapists.

Polatajko HJ, Macnab JJ, Anstett B, Lalloy-Miller T, Murphy K, Noh S (1995a) A clinical trial of the process-oriented treatment approach for children with developmental coordination disorder. *Dev Med Child Neurol* 37: 310–319. http://dx.doi.org/10.1111/j.1469-8749.1995.tb12009.x

Polatajko HJ, Fox M, Missiuna C (1995b) An international consensus on children with developmental coordination disorder. *Can J Occup Ther* 62: 3–6.

Polatajko HJ, Mandich AD, Miller L, MacNab JJ (2001a) Cognitive orientation to daily occupational performance (COOP): part II – the evidence. *Phys Occup Ther Paediatr* 20: 83–106.

Polatajko HJ, Mandich AD, Miller L, Macnab J (2001b) Cognitive orientation to daily occupational performance (COOP): part III – the protocol in brief. *Phys Occup Ther Paediatr* 20: 107–124. http://dx.doi.org/10.1080/J006v20n02_07

Revie G, Larkin D (1993) Task-specific intervention with children reduces movement problems. *Adapted Phys Activity Q* 10: 29–41.

Roley SA, Jacobs R (2009) Sensory integration. In: Crepeau EB, Cohen ES, Schell BAB, editors. *Willard and Spackman's Occupational Therapy*, 11th edition. Philadelphia, PA: Lippincott, Williams and Wilkins, pp. 792–817.

Russell DJ, Rosenbaum PL, Avery LM, Lane M. (2002) *Gross Motor Function Measure (GMFM-66 and GMFM-88) User's Manual.* London: Mac Keith Press.

Savelsbergh G, Rosengren K, Van der Kamp J, Verheul M (2003) Catching action development. In: Savelsbergh G, Davids K, Van der Kamp J, Bennett S, editors. *Development of Movement Coordination in Children.* London: Routledge, pp. 191–212.

Schmidt RA (1975) A scema theory of discrete motor skill learning. *Psychol Rev* 82: 225–260. http://dx.doi.org/10.1037/h0076770

Schmidt RA, Lee TD (2005) *Motor Control and Learning: A Behavioral Analysis.* Champaign, IL: Human Kinetics.

Schoemaker MM, Niemeijer AS, Reynders K, Smits-Engelsman BC (2003) Effectiveness of neuromotor task training for children with developmental coordination disorder: a pilot study. *Neural Plast* 10: 155–163. http://dx.doi.org/10.1155/NP.2003.155

Segal R, Mandich A, Polatajko H, Cook JV (2002) Stigma and its management: a pilot study of parental perceptions of the experiences of children with developmental coordination disorder. *Am J Occup Ther* 56: 422–428. http://dx.doi.org/10.5014/ajot.56.4.422

Sigmundsson H, Ingvaldsen RP, Whiting HTA (1997) Inter- and intra-sensory modality matching in children with hand-eye coordination problems. *Exp Brain Res* 114: 492–499. http://dx.doi.org/101007/PL00005658

Simms K, Henderson SH, Hulme C, Morton J (1996a) The remediation of clumsiness I: an evaluation of Laszlo's kinaesthetic approach. *Dev Med Child Neurol* 38: 976–987.

Simms K, Henderson SH, Morton J, Hulme C (1996b) The remediation of clumsiness II: is kinaesthesis the answer? *Dev Med Child Neurol* 38: 988–997. http://dx.doi.org/10.1111/j.1469-8749.1996.tb15059.x

Sporns O, Edelman GM (1993) Solving Bernstein's Problem: a proposal for the development of coordinated movement by selection. *Child Dev* 64: 960–981. http://dx.doi.org/10.2307/1131321

Steenbergen B, Gordon AM (2006) Activity limitation in hemiplegic cerebral palsy: evidence for disorder in motor planning. *Dev Med Child Neurol* 48: 780–783. http://dx.doi.org/10.1017/S0012162206001666

Steenbergen B, Utley A, Sugden DA, Thieman PS (2003) Discrete bimanual movement co-ordination in children with hemiparetic cerebral palsy. In: Savelsbergh G, Davids K, Van der Kamp J, Bennett S, editors. *Development of Movement Coordination in Children*. London: Routledge, pp. 156–176.

Sugden DA (2007) Intervention approaches in children with developmental coordination disorder. *Dev Med Child Neurol* 49: 467–471. http://dx.doi.org/101111/j.1469-8749.2007.00467.x

Sugden DA, Chambers ME (2003) Intervention in children with DCD: the role of parents and teachers. *Br J Educ Psychol* 73: 545–561. http://dx.doi.org/10.1348/000709903322591235

Sugden DA, Chambers ME, editors (2004) *Children with Developmental Coordination Disorder*. London: Whurr.

Sugden DA, Chambers ME (2007) Stability and change in children with Developmental Coordination Disorder. *Child Care Health Dev* 33: 520–528. http://dx.doi.org/10.1111/j.1365-2214.2006.00707.x

Sugden DA, Dunford CD (2007) The role of theory empiricism and experience in intervention for children with movement difficulties. *Disabil Rehabil* 29: 3–11. http://dx.doi.org/10.1080/09638280600947542

Sugden DA, Henderson SE (2007) *Ecological Intervention for Children with Movement Difficulties*. London: Harcourt Assessment.

Sugden DA, Utley A (1995) Interlimb coupling in children with hemiplegic cerebral palsy. *Dev Med Child Neurol* 37: 293–310. http://dx.doi.org/10.1111/j.1469-8749.1995.tb12008.x

Sugden DA, Wright H (1998) *Motor Coordination Disorders in Children*. Thousand Oaks, CA: Sage Publishers.

Taub E, Uswatte G, Pidikiti R (1999) Constraint-induced movement therapy: a new family of techniques with broad application to physical rehabilitation – a clinical review. *J Rehabil Res Dev* 36: 237–251.

Taylor J, Goodwin D, Groeneveld H (2007) Providing decision-making opportunities for learners with disabilities. In: Davis WE, Broadhead GD, editors. *Ecological Task Analysis and Movement*. Champaign, IL: Human Kinetics, pp. 197–217.

Thomas JR, Nelson JK, Silverman SJ (2005) *Research Methods in Physical Activity*, 5th edition. Champaign, IL: Human Kinetics.

Turvey MT (1977) Preliminaries to a theory of action with reference to vision. In: Shaw R, Bransford J, editors. *Perceiving, Acting and Knowing*. Hillsdale, NJ: Erlbaum, pp. 211–265.

Utley A, Sugden DA (1998) Interlimb coupling in children with hemiplegic cerebral palsy during reaching and grasping at speed. *Dev Med Child Neurol* 40: 396–404.

Vermeer A (2007) Ecological approach to the care of persons with neurological disabilities. In: Davis WE, Broadhead GD, editors. *Ecological Task Analysis and Movement*. Champaign, IL: Human Kinetics, pp. 247–257.

Wall AE, Reid G, Harvery WJ (2007) Interface of the KB and ETA approaches. In: Davis WE, Broadhead GD, editors. *Ecological Task Analysis and Movement*. Champaign, IL: Human Kinetics, pp. 259–277.

WHO (2001) *International Statistical Classification of Diseases and Related Health Problems, Volume 1*, 10th edition. Geneva: World Health Organization.

Wilcox A, Polatajko H (1993) Verbal self guidance as a treatment technique for children with developmental coordination disorder. *Can J Occup Ther* 60 (Conference Supplement, 30).

Wilcox A, Polatajko H (1994) The impact of verbal self guidance on children with developmental coordination disorder. *11th International Congress of the World Federation of Occupational Therapists. Congress Summaries 3*, pp. 1518–1519.

Willis AE, Reid G, Harvery WJ (2007) Interface of the KB and ETA approaches. In: Davis WE, Broadhead GD, editors. *Ecological Task Analysis and Movement*. Champaign, IL: Human Kinetics, pp. 259–277.

Wilson PH (2005) Practitioner review: approaches to assessment and treatment of children with DCD: an evaluative review. *J Child Psychol Psychiatry* 46: 806–823. http://dx.doi.org/10.1111/j.1469-7610.2005.01409.x

Wilson PH, McKenzie BE (1998) Information processing deficits associated with developmental coordination disorder: a meta analysis of research findings. *J Child Psychol Psychiatry* 39: 829–840. http://dx.doi.org/10.1017/S0021963098002765

Zwicker JG, Missiuna C, Boyd LA (2009) Neural correlates of developmental coordination disorder. *J Child Neurol* 24: 1273–1281. http://dx.doi.org/10.1177/0883073809333537

13
PERSPECTIVES ON TYPICAL AND ATYPICAL DEVELOPMENT

The 'what' and the 'how' of motor development

In this book we have presented descriptions and explanations of the developmental trajectories of children, both those with typical development and those whose developmental progress is constrained by atypical conditions. In our judgement, research on both groups of children contributes insights and ideas as to how best to formulate and deliver paedagogical and therapeutic interventions appropriate to the conditions and resources of the developing child. Chapters 1–6 of the book presented material on typically developing children. Some of the material has remained unchanged since educators and scientists first began to study motor development. The essential natural, biological, and physical growth of the individual child assumes appropriate sustenance and social and emotional support. The evolutionary and genetic history almost guarantees an acceptable growth rate that reflects what the early motor development scholars and the medical professionals termed *motor milestones*. These were the expected developmental changes common to all children from birth to adolescence. Growth charts and intellectual evaluations in both paediatrics and education are used worldwide to monitor normal growth and development. If the physical development and intellectual growth meet these expected changes across the lifespan, what in fact has changed?

The first six chapters of this book described and sought to explain the nature of change in a typical child's motor development from birth to maturity. Changes are particularly noticeable and dramatic earlier in life, as well as reasonably similar in progression, if not in rate, among individuals. Early movement development follows a general order or sequence that is similar for all infants worldwide, although the rate of development for the age of specific achievements may vary considerably for individual children. Thus, the expectation is that the developing infant will walk and handle objects in a similar progression of improvement, but some will do so

sooner, and others later. For example, the onset of walking occurs between 10 and 14 months; later movement development is sometimes less orderly, and considerable variation is observed in what individuals do and how they move to perform similar movement tasks. Throughout the developmental period, the dynamic interactions among the *child resources*, the *task* and the *environment* act both to constrain and, eventually, produce the desired movement outcome.

Chapters 7–12 of the book examined a number of circumstances that illustrate how development can change as the resources of a particular child vary. Thus, when children exhibit atypical characteristics or resources with respect to motor, sensory, cognitive, social, and behavioural ways, the nature of the dynamic interactions among the child, the task, and the environment show concomitant differences. These are not just different but transactional in that the child's available resources dynamically change the nature of the task, and the context in which it is likely to occur. The follow-on is that this is an optimistic model, with the modification of the task and the environment being able to change the resources of the child and thus modify development. It is models such as this in which health, educational, and rehabilitation professionals are starting to engage.

The change in the way we think about motor development is a consequence of the emerging theoretical accounts of *how* children acquire their changing and growing repertoires of skilled activities from the first moments of expressing their independence from their mother, such as early crawling, to the point at which they acquire a substantial degree of physical (but not social or financial!) independence. In other words, what theories best account for and can predict the growth in the child's skilful behaviour, and what are the key factors that make such growth possible? Comparing typical and atypical progress provides an important contrast that benefits a better understanding of both groups of children.

We have highlighted three important growth factors that play a crucial role in motor development:

- The *physical changes* that occur as a function of appropriate food and nutrition: bones grow longer and stronger; muscles grow in size and strength. The child experiences these changes as opportunities to move around his or her environment – crawling, cruising, and finally walking independently.
- Along with the physical growth, *brain development* produces an ever-increasing number of synaptic connections, which is made possible by the ever-increasing activities of the growing child. Typically these activities will include sensory, perceptual, and cognitive development.

These first two points illustrate the *child resources* and have been extensively described and analysed throughout the book.

- Finally, with the opportunities to move and explore their world with ever-increasing ease and efficiency, the growth of *experiential inputs* increases at an exponential and somewhat alarming rate, especially once independent locomotion is achieved. Thus, growth occurs as a function of improved biomechanics and brain development and these two growth features are enriched by an ever-widening set of experiences, which the growing child exploits to his or her advantage.

These are the two points of our transactional model, representing the *task* and the *environment*. Examples of this come not only from how the task is presented, as described in Chapter 12, but also from cross-cultural studies that show the effect of the larger social setting, including the handling of infants, the value of certain activities, such as sitting upright or smiling, crawling, and walking, and how sex characteristics are viewed.

Consistency and constancy

Keogh and Sugden (1985) proposed an alternative way to think about the general nature of change with respect to movement development: the solution of two major movement problems for the growing child, what they termed *consistency* and *constancy*.

- An initial movement problem to be resolved is the development of *movement consistency*, which will achieve a *reliable set of movements* for coping with an everyday, recurring set of movement activities. Movements become more consistent and refined with

development and in time are modified to produce more elegant solutions to a specific movement activity. *Consistency* in a basic and comprehensive movement repertoire provides the building blocks that can be used to develop more complex movements. An important difference between younger and older movers is that older movers exhibit greater movement consistency in their control of more limited and complex movements.

- A second movement problem is the development of *movement constancy*, which is the *flexible use of movement consistencies* in a variety of movement situations. *Constancy* is recognizing and using similar situations and responses and requires flexibility in both perceptual and response organization. Older movers will have more ways to move, and they will know more about mixing and matching movement solutions and problems. One could analyse this from a dynamical systems perspective, noting that constancy is about the effective flexible and adaptable recruitment of softly assembled flexible and adaptable coordinative structures for the action of catching.
- *Consistency* and *constancy* are twin concepts conceived as transactional, as each alters the state of the other. It also seems likely that developing movement constancy can help improve movement consistency. Children's play activities exemplify the difference between consistency and constancy and the existence of both in the same general situation. Children at play often repeat a movement many times, as well as 'play' with it by making it in different and unusual ways. Repetition should lead to a more consistent movement performance and a better knowledge of the movement. Playing with a movement is the flexible use of it and an achievement of movement constancy. The point is that children establish an extensive repertoire of reliable movements that can be used flexibly and adaptively, and this is best achieved with large amounts of *appropriate experience/practice*.

Environmental influence

At various times throughout the book we have stressed the importance of experience or practice, in other words time on the task. This appears to be a crucial factor in all motor development no matter what the children bring to the situation in terms of personal resources. We have evidence from a number of sources to substantiate this assertion. From the motor learning literature with adults, the amount of appropriate practice is often stated as one of the fundamental variables that influences the final movement product. Evidence from this comes from sport, dance, and work environments. We have also high-lighted the developmental work reported by researchers such as Adolph and colleagues (2003, 2008) and the broad set of converging studies reported by Campos et al (2000), which attest to the enormous change and acceleration in both motor and cognitive development as a function of achieving independent locomotion. Once achieved, self-generated exploration (which independent locomotion makes possible), the 'time-on-task' factor, expands rapidly producing large increases in the practice of the many skilled activities the child chooses to engage in. From an entirely different field, that of reading, one has only to look at the statistics of good readers compared with poor ones to recognize that 'time on task' is a crucial variable.

Thus, in order to encourage practice and experience the child requires participation; there is little, if any, learning without physical participation. We are in control of the environmental aspect of the child–task–environment transaction, and it follows that we can have a major impact upon participation and practice. There are a number of variables to consider when planning for participation:

- First, *participation choice* refers to what a child chooses to do: what types of activities or experiences are selected, including the level of skill required and how often a child seeks participation. This is the type and amount of involvement in movement experiences.
- Second, *participation effort* is what a child does when involved in an activity. Participation effort is a complex mixture of the effort that a child invests and the social conditions during the actual participation. If a child chooses frequent participation and makes a strong effort, which is supported by others, the child's movement skill should improve. A child participating without positive support has a less favourable outcome for improvement, and a child who does not participate is much less likely to show improvement.
- Third, *participation satisfaction* is what the child gets out of it. It is not much good unless the child actually feels better about him or herself following participation. Lack of participation or unfavourable participation will limit skill development, making the structuring of the environmental context an important variable in the upwards growth trajectory of the child's motor development.
- Finally, it is incumbent upon us all to make these participation experiences and opportunities a regular and easily accessible part of everyday life, not some 'add-on' activity that is discretionary in its availability.

How does development progress?

One of the distinct features of change has been to call into question the shape of the traditional motor development growth curves, which reflected a relatively smooth, upwards trajectory. This has now been shown to be less than reliable: when the sampling rates of these growth observations are recorded more frequently across time there is a noticeable increase in the variability of many motor skill changes prior to a specific developmental change (a 'new milestone'). The work of Karen Adolph and her co-workers (Adolph et al 2003, 2008) demonstrated that there was a distinct increase in variability. This is supportive of the contemporary dynamical systems view of accounting for improvement in overall coordination and control. Rather than viewing change as systematic and essentially linear, motor development reflects a large increase in variability prior to the transition to a new, more stable skill set. This is akin to the characteristics of non-linear systems discussed in chaos theory, in which a rapid increase in variability is observed prior to the transition to a new, more permanent stable state. It may be noted that, when water undergoes an increase or decrease in ambient temperature, just before boiling point is reached the surface of the water bubbles and becomes agitated, then the water suddenly changes (at 100°C), and steam is the result. In the other direction the water surface forms an almost syrup-like consistency prior to the formation of ice on the surface when freezing commences. The point here is that motor development is not especially orderly or smooth, reflecting the more contemporary dynamic systems theory of development. In this sense motor development is not a 'waiting game', waiting for the brain to trigger a developmental change; rather, it is the opportunities to explore and discover the environment in which the child finds himself or herself that push both the motor and the cognitive capacity to new heights.

Embodied cognition

This brings us to the other important message we have sought to convey in this book: namely that motor development is not an autonomous process, isolated from cognitive development; the two go hand in hand and are in fact complementary. This view, referred to as 'embodied cognition', no longer views cognition as the separate domain of abstract thinking, and no longer sees physical and motor development as a function of independent biological processes. Much of the research we have drawn your attention to in this book emphasizes the powerful connections between movement experience and cognitive development. With respect to atypical development, one of the markers of children with intellectual disability is a concomitant record of poor or delayed motor development.

Motor and cognition were once thought to be separate systems, but we now know that progress in the motor domain drives progress in general growth of cognition – defined generally as 'knowing'. The relationship between delayed motor development and the possibility of related intellectual disability has existed for some time but is rarely considered or expressed in the context of cause and effect. With the growing acceptance of embodied cognition this will change in the future, as research seeks new ways of understanding the interrelationship between motor development and the wider domain of cognitive development.

Contemporary research in motor development is only just beginning to focus on the skill acquisition of children, with special emphasis on viewing perception not as containing, individual and separate modalities such as vision, hearing and kinaesthesis but as a global capacity, albeit dominated by vision. Dynamic touch or haptics (the old term was kinaesthesis) seeks to better account for the inherent accuracy we have in making judgements of wielded objects that we cannot directly observe but only 'feel'. In essence this 'feel' reflects the perceptual sensitivity to the 'information' present in the act of wielding (the invariant properties detected in what Turvey 1996 has termed the 'inertial tensor'). This new science, in which motor development can play a part, will lead to a new method of defining what will be called 'physical intelligence', that is knowledge derived from action, a very different view than the traditional definition of intelligence that predicted success only in western styles of educational achievement (IQ scores).

The typical–atypical continuum

The title of this book, *Typical and Atypical Motor Development*, suggests that the two halves of the book are categorical and separate from each other. This is not the case; we have selected populations in Chapters 7–12 of the book as illustrations of what happens to the observable aspects of motor development when differences are present in the personal resources of the child. We like to think of these resources as a continuum rather than categorical because the same variables are important in the motor development of all children, no matter what their

resources; it is simply that the balance of these variables will change according to the needs of the individual child. In order to promote the motor development of any child, first, the *environmental context* can be modified to suit the needs of the individual child, particularly to ensure appropriate participation. Second, the choice and presentation of the *task* can be modified or varied, according to the personal resources of the child to encourage appropriate learning. Thus we began with an emphasis on the relationship between the task, the performer, and the environment and the constraints and possibilities this 'trinity' can make possible for the motor development of the growing child, and we conclude with this very same mantra!

Finally, by the very title and content of this book, we obviously believe that motor development is a crucial part of overall development. We can reinforce this by adding that studying all of motor development, whether typical or atypical, will bring us to a closer understanding of overall human development. To take a behavioural example of this one has only to try and think of anything one does during the day that does not involve motor actions. Second, movement is our *only* facility that allows us to interact with both other living beings and the environmental context. We conclude with a thought about lines from Campos and colleagues (2000) in their article '*Travel broadens the mind*':

> … in infancy, the onset of locomotor experiences brings about widespread consequences, and after infancy can be responsible for an enduring role in development by maintaining and updating existing skills [p. 150] … it is no accident that we have idioms such as 'making great strides', 'step-function improvement', and 'moving ahead' to refer to accomplishments … Locomotion connotes progress and advance, in the person's relation to the environment and in the person's mind … [and] … we tried to make a case for invigorating the investigation of the role of motoric attainments for psychological development.

(p. 212)

REFERENCES

Adolph KE, Vereijken B, Shrout PE (2003) What changes in infant walking and why. *Child Dev* 74: 475–497. http://dx.doi.org/10.1111/1467-8624.7402011

Adolph KE, Robinson SR, Young JW, Gill-Alvarez F (2008) What is the shape of developmental change? *Psychol Rev* 115: 527–543. http://dx.doi.org/10.1037/0033-295x.115.3.527

Campos JJ, Anderson DI, Barbu-Roth MA, Hubbard EM, Hertenstein MJ, Witherington D (2000) Travel broadens the mind. *Infancy* 1: 149–219. http://dx.doi.org/10.1207/S15327078IN0102_1

Keogh JF, Sugden DA (1985) *Movement Skill Development*. New York: Macmillan.

Turvey MT (1996) Dynamic touch. *Am Psychol* 51: 1134–1152. http://dx.doi.org/10.1037/0003-066X.51.11.1134

INDEX

Other titles from Mac Keith Press www.mackeith.co.uk

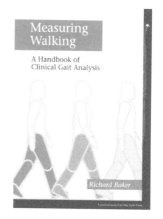

Measuring Walking: A Handbook of Clinical Gait Analysis
Richard Baker

A practical guide from Mac Keith Press
June 2013 ▪ 248pp ▪ softback ▪ 978-1-908316-66-0
£49.95 / €60.00 / $199.95

This book is a practical guide to instrumented clinical gait analysis covering all aspects of routine service provision. It reinforces what is coming to be regarded as the conventional approach to clinical gait analysis. Data capture, processing and biomechanical interpretation are all described with an emphasis on ensuring high quality results. There are also chapters on how to set up and maintain clinical gait analysis services and laboratories.

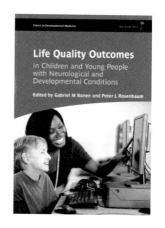

Life Quality Outcomes in Children and Young People with Neurological and Developmental Conditions
Gabriel M. Ronen and Peter L. Rosenbaum (Eds)

Clinics in Developmental Medicine
April 2013 ▪ 394pp ▪ hardback ▪ 978-1-908316-58-5
£95.00 / €120.70 / $149.95

Healthcare professionals need to understand their patients' views of their condition and its affects on their health and well-being. This book builds on the World Health Organization's concepts of 'health', 'functioning' and 'quality of life' for young people with neurodisabilities: it emphasises the importance of engaging with patients in the identification of both treatment goals and their evaluation. Uniquely, it enables healthcare professionals to find critically reviewed outcomes-related information.

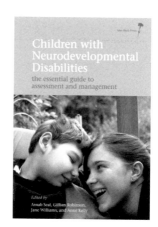

Children with Neurodevelopmental Disabilities: the essential guide to assessment and management
Arnab Seal, Gillian Robinson, Anne M. Kelly and Jane Williams (Eds)

March 2013 ▪ 744pp ▪ softback ▪ 978-1-908316-62-2
£65.00 / € tbc / $ tbc

A comprehensive textbook on the practice of paediatric neurodisability, written by practitioners and experts in the field. Using a problem-oriented approach, the authors give best-practice guidance, and centre on the needs of the child and family, working in partnership with multi-disciplinary, multi-agency teams. It provides a ready reference for managing problems encountered in the paediatric clinic.

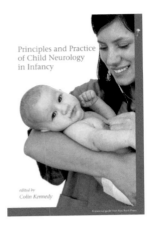

Principles and Practice of Child Neurology in Infancy
Colin Kennedy (Ed)

A practical guide from Mac Keith Press
2012 ▪ 384pp ▪ softback ▪ 978-1-908316-35-6
£29.95 / €38.10 / $49.50

This handbook of neurological practice in infants is designed to be of practical use to all clinicians, but particularly those in under-resourced locations. Seventy per cent of children with disabilities live in resource-poor countries and most of these children have neurological impairments. This book presents recommendations for investigations and treatments based on internationally accepted good practice that can be implemented in most settings.

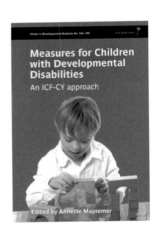

Measures for Children with Developmental Disabilities
An ICF-CY approach
Annette Majnemer (Ed)

Clinics in Developmental Medicine No 194-195
2012 ▪ 552pp ▪ hardback ▪ 978-1-908316-45-5
£150.00 / €186.00 / $235.00

This title presents and reviews outcome measures across a wide range of attributes that are applicable to children and adolescents with developmental disabilities. It uses the children and youth version of the International Classification of Functioning, Disability and Health (ICF-CY) as a framework for organizing the various measures into sections and chapters. Each chapter coincides with domains within the WHO framework of Body Functions, Activities and Participation, and Personal and Environmental Factors.

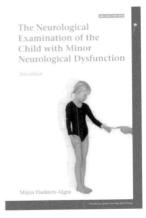

The Neurological Examination of the Child with Minor Neurological Dysfunction, 3rd edition
Mijna Hadders-Algra

A practical guide from Mac Keith Press
2010 ▪ 160pp ▪ softback ▪ 978-1-898683-98-8
£49.95 / €60.00 / $76.00

Bert Touwen's classic handbook has been updated to reflect contemporary clinical practice. This refined, sensitive and age-appropriate technique is designed to take into account the developmental aspects of the child's rapidly changing nervous system. The accompanying DVD contains videos illustrating typical and atypical performance and also provides an electronic assessment form.